AF829473

Phytomedicine and Alzheimer's Disease

Phytomedicine and Alzheimer's Disease

Edited by
Atanu Bhattacharjee
Akula Ramakrishna
Magisetty Obulesu

CRC Press
Taylor & Francis Group
Boca Raton London New York

CRC Press is an imprint of the
Taylor & Francis Group, an **informa** business

First edition published 2021
by CRC Press
6000 Broken Sound Parkway NW, Suite 300, Boca Raton, FL 33487-2742

and by CRC Press
2 Park Square, Milton Park, Abingdon, Oxon, OX14 4RN

© 2021 Taylor & Francis Group, LLC

CRC Press is an imprint of Taylor & Francis Group, LLC

Reasonable efforts have been made to publish reliable data and information, but the author and publisher cannot assume responsibility for the validity of all materials or the consequences of their use. The authors and publishers have attempted to trace the copyright holders of all material reproduced in this publication and apologize to copyright holders if permission to publish in this form has not been obtained. If any copyright material has not been acknowledged, please write and let us know so we may rectify in any future reprint.

Except as permitted under U.S. Copyright Law, no part of this book may be reprinted, reproduced, transmitted, or utilized in any form by any electronic, mechanical, or other means, now known or hereafter invented, including photocopying, microfilming, and recording, or in any information storage or retrieval system, without written permission from the publishers.

For permission to photocopy or use material electronically from this work, access www.copyright.com or contact the Copyright Clearance Center, Inc. (CCC), 222 Rosewood Drive, Danvers, MA 01923, 978-750-8400. For works that are not available on CCC please contact mpkbookspermissions@tandf.co.uk

Trademark notice: Product or corporate names may be trademarks or registered trademarks and are used only for identification and explanation without intent to infringe.

ISBN: 978-0-367-33202-0 (hbk)
ISBN: 978-0-429-31842-9 (ebk)

Typeset in Times
by Deanta Global Publishing Services, Chennai, India

Contents

Preface

Alzheimer's disease is the most common form of dementia and is a generic term for memory defect and other cognitive impairments that seriously affect daily life. Alzheimer's disease is a progressive disease, where brain regions like the hippocampus deteriorate over time, exacerbating the symptoms of dementia steadily. In its initial stages, the memory defect is mild, but, over a number of years in late-stage Alzheimer's disease, patients lose the ability to convey a message and to respond to their surroundings. Alzheimer's disease is still incurable, but current treatment strategies can temporarily reduce the symptoms and ameliorate the quality of life for the patient. Today, a universal effort, from the entire health care fraternity to personal caregivers, has come together to find better ways of slowing the progress of the disease. Rigorous emphasis has been placed on medicinal plants worldwide, which can be used to delay the progress of Alzheimer's disease, as the World Health Organization (WHO) describes them as safer and more economical than conventional allopathic medicines. Asian countries are home to a plethora of flowering plant species, which are used in codified systems of medicine, such as Ayurveda, Unani, Siddha, and Amchi, and non-codified folk medicine, which offer the most fascinating reservoir of potential new drugs. It has now become essential to explore the ethnopharmacological properties of native flora to develop extracts or lead molecule(s) as drugs for the treatment of Alzheimer's disease. In this context, this book has been developed specifically with reference to the medicinal plants and their derivatives used in the treatment of dementia and Alzheimer's disease.

Phytomedicine and Alzheimer's Disease is an up-to-date compilation of in-depth information on traditional medicinal plants and phytopharmaceuticals used in both modern and traditional medicine for the management of the difficult-to-treat and challenging neurodegenerative disease known as Alzheimer's disease written by eminent academics and researchers. Readers will find cutting-edge knowledge on the role of codified alternative systems of medicine, neurotransmitters, pre-clinical approaches, new strategies, and biochemical aspects reported to diagnose and treat Alzheimer's disease. The book highlights the mechanistic aspects of neurodegeneration in Alzheimer's disease and the role of phytochemicals as restorative agents. It also describes the chemistry, bioactivity, and the functional aspects of biologically active phytomolecules with the potential to be future drugs to treat Alzheimer's disease. The use of plant extracts and their derivatives, scientifically tested and clinically trialed, along with updates on their most recently revealed ethnopharmacological aspects, are also presented. Epigenetic modifiers associated with Alzheimer's disease, along with therapeutic and dietary interventions, are also highlighted. In addition, the pharmacognosy of species of the Annonaceae family, for developing phytomedicines for Alzheimer's disease, is described in detail.

This volume was written to attract scientists, academics, and professionals from all over the world who are engaged in plant and animal sciences, biochemistry, and life sciences, from modern clinicians to alternative medicine practitioners.

Atanu Bhattacharjee
Akula Ramakrishna
Magisetty Obulesu

Acknowledgment

The editors are grateful to the Almighty for all and showing the path to publish this book.

The editors would like to thank all the contributors to this volume, which has become a comprehensive treatise on the topic. We appreciate that the contributors are active scientists and have volunteered to share their findings and perspectives with the readers, who will benefit from learning about the implications and applications of the various topics in this book.

We are grateful to Renu Upadhyay, Assistant Commissioning Editor; Jyotsna Jangra, Editorial Assistant; and the team from CRC Press/Taylor & Francis Group, including Todd Perry, Production Editor, and Andrew Corrigan at Deanta Global, Project Manager, for their help in bringing this volume to completion in such a beautiful and appealing presentation.

The editors are thankful to our families, who have encouraged us to take up this task, and allowed us to take time off from our families. We are also grateful to our friends and academic colleagues for their support in helping in the successful completion of the book.

Dr. Atanu Bhattacharjee expresses his sincere gratitude to Assam Down Town University, Assam, India, for their support.

Dr. Akula Ramakrishna is thankful to Bayer Crop Science, Bengaluru, India, for their support.

Mr. Magisetty Obulesu is thankful to ATG Laboratories, Pune, India, for their support.

Atanu Bhattacharjee
Akula Ramakrishna
Magisetty Obulesu

Editors

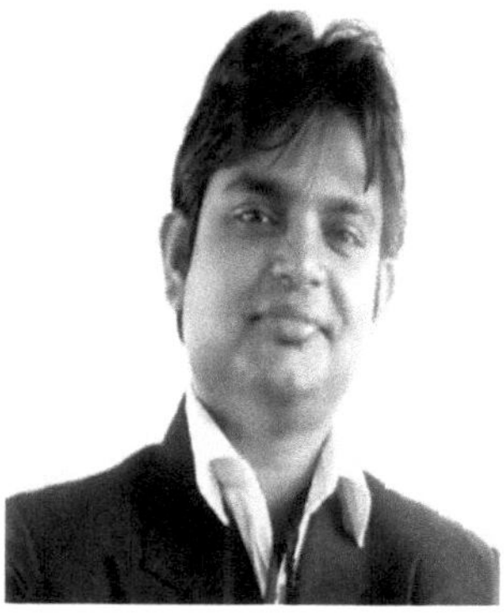

Atanu Bhattacharjee is currently working as Associate Professor in the Faculty of Pharmaceutical Science, Assam Down Town University, Assam, India. His areas of specialization include pharmacognosy and phytochemistry. Dr. Bhattacharjee holds a master's degree in pharmacognosy from J.S.S. College of Pharmacy, Ooty, India. He was the recipient of a Senior Research Fellowship from CCRAS, New Delhi. He subsequently obtained his PhD in pharmaceutical sciences from Nitte University, Mangalore (a NAAC 'A' graded University) in 2015 in the area of phytochemistry and neuropharmacology of traditional Indian medicinal plants. Dr. Bhattacharjee has worked extensively on the evaluation of the nootropic potential of Ayurvedic plants, emphasizing their effects on cholinergic neurotransmission. His research contributions include assessments of several *in-vivo* neuro-pharmacological assays and *in-vitro* cholinesterase enzyme assays, and the antioxidant potential of drugs obtained from natural sources. He is the Honorable Academic Editor of the Asian Journal of Medicine and Health, *SCIENCEDOMAIN International*, India. He is also the Associate Editor of *MedCrave Online Journal of Tumor Research*. Recently, he was elected an Editorial Board member of the journal *Integrative Trauma and Emergency Medicine*. He is a registered PhD supervisor of Assam Down Town University, India. Dr. Bhattacharjee has published more than 20 peer-reviewed research and review articles in reputed national/international journals, and has authored many chapters in books by international publishers, such as Taylor & Francis and Springer. Dr. Bhattacharjee has presented several scientific papers, attended a number of national and international conferences and delivered invited lectures in different scientific fora. He is a life-time member of the Indian Pharmaceutical Association, Mumbai, India. At present, he is an editorial team member of seven journals and reviewer for more than ten highly regarded international journals. Dr. Bhattacharjee is enthusiastically involved in scientific research on traditional medharasayana drugs in Assam Down Town University, where he is developing an active research culture.

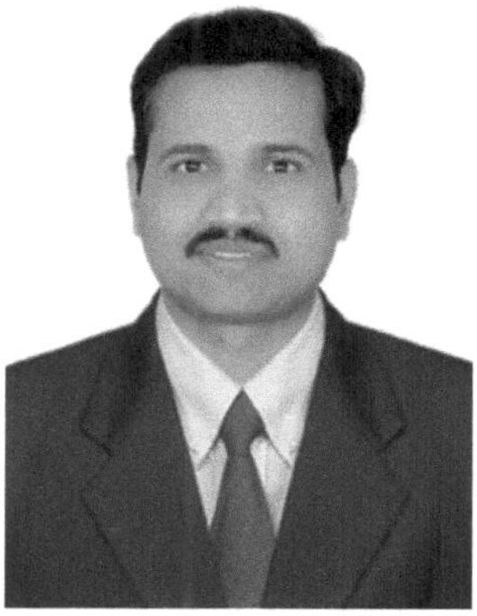

Akula Ramakrishna is currently a scientist at Bayer Crop Science, Bangalore, India. Dr. Ramakrishna holds a master's degree from Sri Krishna Devaraya University, Anantapur, Andhra Pradesh, India. He obtained his PhD in biochemistry from the University of Mysore, CSIR-CFTRI, Mysuru, India. He is a Senior Research Fellow of CSIR, New Delhi. Dr. Ramakrishna is involved in various research fields, such as plant biotechnology, biochemistry, plant secondary metabolites, food science and technology, and vegetable quality analysis. He has published a number of research papers in leading international journals and published three books, reviews, and book chapters. Dr. Ramakrishna also serves as an editorial board member and reviewer for several reputed international journals. He has presented more than 20 research papers in symposia in India and abroad, as well as several invited lectures in India. Dr. Ramakrishna attended the Fifth International Symposium on Plant Neurobiology held in 2009 in Florence, Italy, and also attended the Technical Community of Monsanto (TCM) held in 2016 in St. Louis, Missouri. He is a member of the Indian Science Congress Association and of the Society for Biotechnologists (India). He is a fellow of the Society for Applied Biotechnology, India (since 2012), and recipient of the Global Vegetable Research Excellence Award (2017), the Global Technology Recognition Award, the Rapid Recognition Award, and the Special Recognition Award from Monsanto Company Limited.

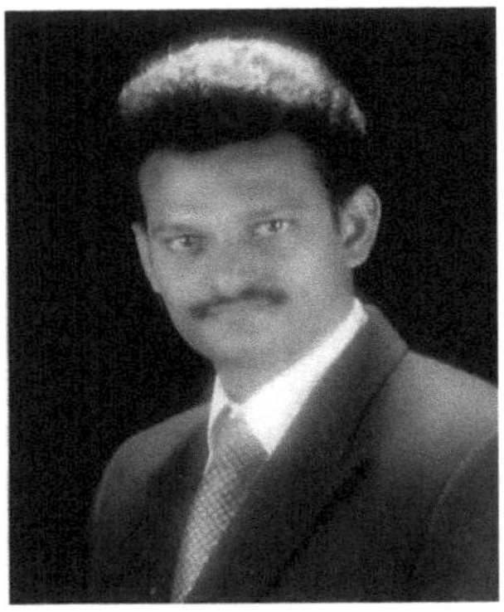

Magisetty Obulesu is currently a scientist at ATG Laboratories, Pune, India. He has 18 years of research and teaching experience. His research areas are many, including food science; pathology of neurodegenerative diseases, such as Alzheimer's disease; design of polymer-based biomaterials; and the development of metal chelators to overcome metal-induced toxicity. Mr. Obulesu's present research focuses on the development of redox-active injectable hydrogels of polyion complexes. Mr. Obulesu has carried out research into Alzheimer's disease and developed an aluminum-induced neurotoxicity rabbit model. Two books by Mr. Obulesu, a monograph entitled *Alzheimer's Disease Theranostics* (Elsevier) and an editorial collection *Alternative Medicine for Alzheimer's Disease* (Taylor & Francis) are currently in preparation. Mr Obulesu is the first and corresponding author for the majority of his articles. Mr. Obulesu is on the editorial board of several pathology journals, such as the *Journal of Medical Laboratory and Diagnosis*, the *Journal of Medical and Surgical Pathology, Annals of Retrovirals and Antiretrovirals, Kenkyu Journal of Medical Science and Clinical Research, SciFed Oncology and Cancer Research Journal*, and the *Journal of Cancer and Cure*. Mr. Obulesu is also on the editorial board of nanotechnology journals such as *SciFed Nanotech Research Letters, SciFed Drug Delivery Research, Current Updates in Nanotechnology*, and the *Journal of Nanotechnology and Materials Science*.

List of Contributors

Naheed Akhter
College of Allied Health Professionals
Government College University
Faisalabad, Pakistan

Muhammad Akram
Department of Eastern Medicines
Government College University
Faisalabad, Pakistan

Fozia Anjum
Department of Chemistry
Government College University
Faisalabad, Pakistan

Rumaisa Ansari
Department of Eastern Medicines
Government College University
Faisalabad, Pakistan

P. M. Aswathy
Human Molecular Genetics Laboratory
Rajiv Gandhi Centre for Biotechnology
Trivandrum, India

Moinak Banerjee
Human Molecular Genetics Laboratory
Rajiv Gandhi Centre for Biotechnology
Trivandrum, India

Veruska Cavalcanti Barros
Parasitology Department
Federal University of Piaui
Teresina-Piaui, Brazil

Chandana C. Barua
Department of Pharmacology and Toxicology
College of Veterinary Science
Khanapara, India

Iswar Chandra Barua
Department of Agronomy
Assam Agricultural University
Jorhat, India

Rajashri Bezbaruah
Pratiksha Institute of Pharmaceutical Sciences
Panikhaiti, India

Pobitra Borah
Pratiksha Institute of Pharmaceutical Sciences
Panikhaiti, India

Lipika Buragohain
Department of Pharmacology and Toxicology
College of Veterinary Science
Khanapara, India

Raja Chakraborty
National Education Foundation
College of Pharmacy
Lokhra, India

S. R. Chandra
National Institute of Mental Health and
Neurosciences (NIMHANS)
Bangalore, India

Bishnu Choudhury
Department of Kayachikitsa
North Eastern Institute of Ayurveda and
Homeopathy
Mawdiangdiang, India

Muhammad Daniyal
School of Pharmacy
Hunan University of Chinese Medicine
Changsha, People's Republic of China

V. S. Dendi
CHRISTUS Trinity Mother Frances Hospital
Tyler, Texas

Shilpa A. Deshpande
Department of Pharmacology
Priyadarshini J. L. College of Pharmacy
Nagpur, India

Biplab Kumar Dey
Department of Pharmacy
Assam Down Town University
Guwahati, India

Chistiane Mendes Feitosa
Chemistry and Pharmacy Department
Federal University of Piaui
Teresina-Piaui, Brazil

Fahad Said Khan
Department of Eastern Medicines
Government College University
Faisalabad, Pakistan

Samreen Gul Khan
Department of Chemistry
Government College University
Faisalabad, Pakistan

Rinki Kumari
Department of Biotechnology
Microtek College of Management and Technology
Murtazabad, India

Anindita Kundu
Department of Pharmaceutical Technology
Jadavpur University
Kolkata, India

Umme Laila
Department of Eastern Medicines
Government College University
Faisalabad, Pakistan

B. Mahendran
ATG Laboratories
Pune, India

Pooja Mailankody
National Institute of Mental Health and Neurosciences (NIMHANS)
Bangalore, India

Vinayak Majhi
Department of Biomedical Engineering
North-Eastern Hill University
Umshing Mawkynroh, India

Rupshikha Malakar
Royal College of Pharmacy and Health Sciences
Berhampur, India

Subhash C. Mandal
Department of Pharmaceutical Technology
Jadavpur University
Kolkata, India

Vivekananda Mandal
Institute of Pharmacy
Guru Ghasidas Central University
Bilaspur, India

Bhargawi Mishra
Banaras Hindu University
Varanasi, India

Naveed Munir
Department of Biochemistry
Government College University
Faisalabad, Pakistan

Alyandra de Sousa Nascimento
Chemistry and Pharmacy Department
Federal University of Piaui
Teresina-Piaui, Brazil

Ghanshyam Panigrahi
Royal College of Pharmacy and Health Sciences
Berhampur, India

Abida Parveen
Department of Botany
Government College University
Faisalabad, Pakistan

Khaleel Pasha
Department of Gastroenterology
Osmania Hospital
Hyderabad, India

Sudip Paul
Department of Biomedical Engineering
North-Eastern Hill University
Umshing Mawkynroh, India

G. K. Pratap
Department of Studies and Research in Biochemistry
Mangalore University
ChikkaAluvara, India

Mahendra Rai
Department of Biotechnology
Sant Gadge Baba Amravati University
Amravati, India

Muhammad Riaz
Sargodha Medical College
University of Sargodha
Sargodha, Pakistan

Antônia Laires da Silva Santos
Chemistry and Pharmacy Department
Federal University of Piaui
Teresina-Piaui, Brazil

Bapi Ray Sarkar
Department of Pharmaceutical Technology
University of North Bengal
West Bengal, India

Saikat Sen
Faculty of Pharmaceutical Science
Assam Down Town University
Guwahati, India

C. M. Shafeeque
Human Molecular Genetics Laboratory
Rajiv Gandhi Centre for Biotechnology
Trivandrum, India

Manjula Shantaram
Department of Studies and Research in Biochemistry
Mangalore University
ChikkaAluvara, India

Abaid Nath Singh
Udai Pratap Autonomous College
Varanasi, India

Jasmit Singh
Banaras Hindu University
Varanasi, India

Anamika Tiwari
Banaras Hindu University
Varanasi, India

Valeria Lima Silva Veras
Center of Agrarian Sciences
Federal University of Piaui
Teresina-Piaui, Brazil

Niraj S. Vyawahare
Dr. D. Y. Patil College of Pharmacy
D.Y. Patil Educational Complex
Pradhikaran, India

Sujata Wangkheirakpam
Chemistry Department
National Institute of Technology
Manipur, India

1 Annonaceae Species
A Perspective For Developing Phytomedicines for Alzheimer's Disease

Chistiane Mendes Feitosa, Antônia Laires da Silva Santos, Alyandra de Sousa Nascimento, Veruska Cavalcanti Barros, Valeria Lima Silva Veras, and Mahendra Rai

CONTENTS

ABBREVIATIONS

AChE	Acetylcholinesterase
AD	Alzheimer's Disease
ANVISA	National Health Surveillance Agency
DPPH	2,2-diphenyl-1-picrylhydrazyl
IC_{50}	Inhibitory Concentration
TBARS	Thiobarbituric Acid-Reactive Substances
WHO	World Health Organization

1.1 INTRODUCTION

The healing power of plants has been known since the human species has been on earth. Early civilizations realized that some plants contained, in their essences, active principles which, when tested in the fight against disease, empirically revealed their healing power (Badke et al., 2011; Carneiro et al., 2014).

In Brazil, the use of medicinal plants in the treatment of diseases contains influences of the indigenous, African, and European cultures, the individual contributions of which were integrated into a set of principles that aimed at treating diseases and restoring health and vitality to man (Silva et al., 2008; Badke et al., 2016). According to the National Health Surveillance Agency (ANVISA), a medicinal plant is any plant, or part of it, that contains substances or classes of substances responsible for therapeutic action. According to the World Health Organization (WHO), 80% of the world population makes use of medicinal plants. Mostly, these plants are utilized by adults and the elderly, who seek to use them for the treatment of chronic disease (Brasil, 2010; WHO, 2018).

Alzheimer's disease (AD) affects millions of people around the world. Estimates indicate that 24 million people are affected, and in the next thirty years, this number will reach 81 million (ABRAz, 2012). The treatment for AD is symptomatic and consists of attempts to restore cholinergic function, because elevation of the levels of the neurotransmitter acetylcholine has been shown to be useful in improving learning disability, one of the signs of AD. Therefore, acetylcholinesterase (AChE) inhibitory substances are widely used in the treatment of this disease (Sereniki and Vital, 2008; Feitosa et al., 2015).

There are some members of the custard apple family, the Annonaceae, whose activity against AD has been identified, although the reported effects of others are still empirical; extracts of parts of the plant and isolated substances therein are used. *Guatteria friesiana* can also be mentioned here for its wide-ranging biological activities, such as antimicrobial (Costa et al., 2008), larvicidal (Aciole et al., 2011), antitumor (Britto et al., 2012), and cytotoxic effects (Costa et al., 2013) (Table 1.1).

The Annonaceae family comprises approximately 122 genera and about 1100 species. In Brazil, about 30 genera and 260 species are used to relieve or even cure some illnesses. The family consists of trees, shrubs, and rarely, scandic shrubs (Pontes et al., 2004). In the Cerrado, it is represented by several genera and species, many of which are cultivated for their delicious fruits, such as *Annona coriacea* Mart., *Annona crassiflora* Mart. and *Rollinia emarginata* Schl. (Silva et al., 2001), and others as ornamental plants, such as *Xylopia aromatica* (Lam.) Mart. (Silva-Junior et al., 2005).

Chemically, members of the Annonaceae are known for their rich alkaloid content, but also have non-alkaloidal constituents, such as carbohydrates, lipids, amino acids, proteins, vitamins, polyphenols, essential oils, terpenes, aromatic compounds, steroids, and saponins (Leboeuf et al., 1980). Some of the alkaloids have proven biological activities. Bisbenzylisoquinolinones, for example, have antiparasitic activity, especially against *Leishmania* sp. (Munshi et al., 1972; Fournet et al., 1993), *Trypanosoma cruzi*, and *Plasmodium* sp. (Rojas de Arias et al., 1994).

Considering the beneficial effects that plants have presented in relation to the treatment of cognitive disorders, this chapter aims to present a pharmacological investigation of the natural products from plants of the family Annonaceae, that have shown activity on the central nervous

TABLE 1.1
Biological Activities of Tissue Extracts and Compounds From *G. friesiana*

Preparation	Biological Activity	Reference
Essential oils of leaves	Antimicrobial, larvicidal, antitumor, and cytotoxic	Costa et al., 2008 Aciole et al., 2011 Britto et al., 2012
Alkaloidal fraction in chloroform extract of the stem. Liriodenine	Antimicrobial	Costa et al., 2009
Guatteriopsiscine Alkaloidal fraction of leaves Neutral fraction of dichloromethane extract of leaves Methanol extract of leaves 13-Hydroxy-discretinine 13-Hydroxy-2,3,9,10-tetramethoxyprotoberberine 6,6a-Desidroguatteriopsiscine 9-Desidroxy-1-methoxy-diidroguatteriouregidine 7,8-Dihydro-8-hydroxypalmatine Palmatine	Cytotoxic	Costa et al., 2013
α-, β-, ε-, and γ-Eudesmol	Cytotoxicity	Bomfim et al., 2013

system, to help in understanding the neurochemical bases of many neurodegenerative diseases, particularly AD.

1.2 THE ANNONACEAE FAMILY

The Annonaceae family was first cataloged by Jussieu in 1789 (Hutchinson, 2004), and represents the largest family of the order Magnoliales (Sauquet et al., 2003), comprising 2500 cataloged species distributed over 135 genera, and found predominantly in tropical and subtropical regions of South America, Central America, Africa, Asia, and Australia (Chatrou et al., 2004). In South America, the members of the Annonaceae are represented by 39 genera (Hocquemiller et al., 1981). In Brazil, there are 29 genera, comprising 392 species (Maas et al., 2015) distributed in the Amazon, Mata Atlântica, and Cerrado (Maas et al., 2007).

Members of the Annonaceae are classified into four sub-families, the Anaxagoreoideae, Annonoideae, Ambavioideae, and Malmeoideae (Chatrou et al., 2012). Members of the Annonaceae family are characterized by the presence of some extremely primitive morphological features, such as flowers with numerous free parts, spiral stamens, free carpels, etc., that is why Darwin called them "living fossils" because, through some favorable circumstances, they escaped extinction and survived to the present day (Takhtajan, 1969).

These plants have several economic roles, especially in the food, wood, cosmetic, and pharmaceutical industries. The ripened fruits of several species of the Annonaceae are very much appreciated and consumed fresh or processed into products such as juices, ice cream, jellies, jams, liqueurs, and sweets (Pimenta et al., 2014). The most important and well-known genera include *Annona* and *Rollinia*, namely *A. cherimola* (cherimolia), *A. crassiflora* (marolo), *A. squamosa* (ata, fruit of the count), *A. montana* (mountain graviola), *A. muricata* (guanabana, graviola), *Annona reticulata* (countess), *R. mucosa* (biribá), *R. sylvatica* (araticum), and *R. deliciosa* (biribá) (Kessler, 1993). Figure 1.1 shows the fruits of some of these species.

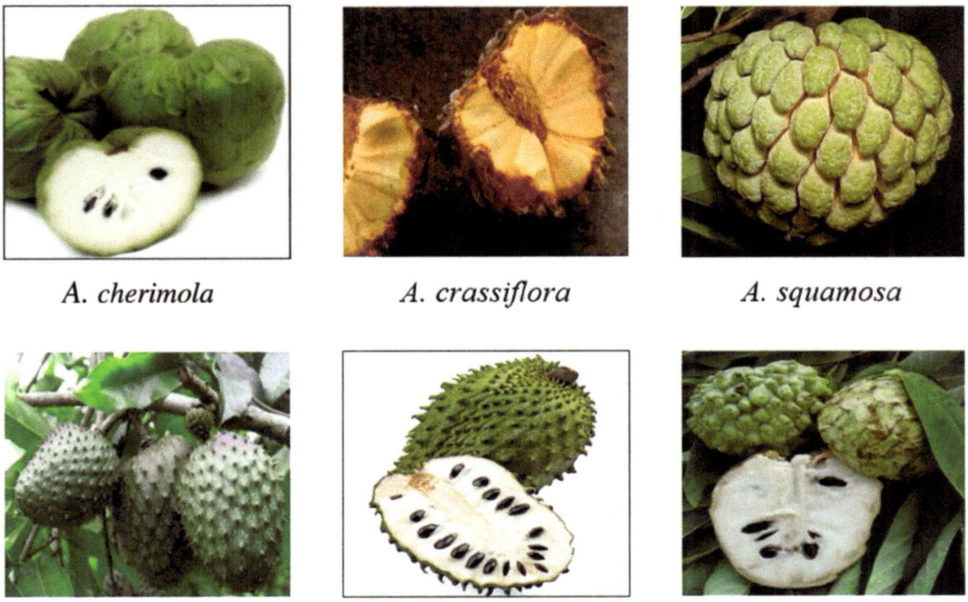

A. cherimola *A. crassiflora* *A. squamosa*

A. montana *A. muricata* *A. reticulata*

FIGURE 1.1 Fruits of some species of the Annonaceae family.

Bocageopsis spp., *Fusae longifolia*, *Guatteria megalophylla*, *G. stipitata*, *Oxandra polyanthia*, *O. lanceolata*, *Xylopia aethiopica* and *X. villosa* are economically important in terms of logging (Kessler, 1993; Sáenz, 1997; Murilo and Restrepo, 2000). In other species, the wood of their stems is used in the production of alcohol and paper (Leboeuf et al., 1980).

In Asia and Africa, the flowers of *Cananga odorata* and *Artabotrys odoratissima* are used in the manufacture of perfumes (e.g. ylang-ylang oil) (Kessler, 1993) and a large number of species of Annonaceae are used in traditional medicine, exhibiting antimicrobial activities (Alawa et al., 2003), as well as antihelminthic (Alawa et al., 2003) and antitumor activity (Alali et al., 1999), along with inhibition of platelet aggregation (Chang et al., 1998) and treatment of senile dementia (Schultes, 1993). Inhibition of the enzyme, acetylcholinesterase (AChE), is known to increase the concentration of the neurotransmitter acetylcholine in the synapses, a region of communication between neurons in the brain, which could decrease or delay the progression of symptoms in patients with Alzheimer's disease. Some plants that inhibit AChE enzyme activity belong to the family Annonaceae and will be described in Section 1.3.

1.3 PLANTS OF THE FAMILY ANNONACEAE OF POTENTIAL USE IN AD TREATMENT

Alkaloids are a class of substances that exhibit potential for anti-AChE activity. It may be noted that galanthamine, an alkaloid isolated from species of the family Amaryllidaceae, such as snowdrop (*Galanthus* spp.), is currently being evaluated as a drug in the treatment of AD (De Melo and Costa, 2005, Feitosa et al., 2015).

Annona glabra, a fruit tree native to the Americas, is widely distributed in Brazil (Padmaja et al., 1995; Galvão et al., 2016), and has demonstrated different biological activities, such as anticancer (Cochrane et al., 2008), anti-inflammatory (Siebra et al., 2009), antimicrobial and cytotoxic activities (Galvão, 2015). In addition, studies on *A. glabra* have shown the presence of active alkaloids that have been identified as AChE inhibitors. In this study, 20 compounds were isolated, of which four, from the ethanolic extract of the stem of this species, were previously unknown, namely (7S,14S)-(-)-N-methyl-10-*O*-demethylxilopinine, pseudocolumbamine, palmatine, and pseudopalmatine, and which exhibited anticholinesterase activities with half-maximal inhibitory concentrations (IC_{50}) of 8.4, 5.0, 0.4, and 1.8 μM, respectively (Tsai and Lee, 2010).

Lee et al. (2015) isolated the alkaloids (-)-anolobine and (-)-roemeroline from the ethanolic extract of the leaves of *A. glabra*, which exhibited IC_{50} values of 22.4 and 26.3 μM, respectively. Figure 1.2 shows the alkaloid structure of (-)- anolobine isolated from the leaves of *A. glabra*.

A. crassiflora is a native tree of the Brazilian Cerrado, and is popularly known as araticum, marolo, and pinha-do-cerrado (Corrêa et al., 2013, Pimenta et al., 2014). It exhibits antileishmanicidal and trypanocidal activities (Mesquita et al., 2005), as well as antioxidant (Roesler et al., 2007), cytotoxic, pesticidal, and antitumor activities (Pimenta et al., 2003).

Hidalgo (2017) evaluated alkaloids in leaf extract of *A. crassiflora* for activity against AChE. It was possible to isolate and identify the aporphine alkaloids stephalagine and xylopine (Figure 1.3). At a concentration of 100 µg/mL, xylopine (**1**) inhibited AChE activity by about 20%, whereas the same concentration of stephalagine (**2**) exhibited 75% inhibition. Structurally, the compounds are similar, xilopine has a free hydrogen and stephalagine a linked methyl.

In a study on *A. crassiflora* carried out by Melo (2017), a methanolic leaf extract exhibited a higher percentage AChE inhibition than did the individual isolated compounds described by Hidalgo (2017).

Formagio et al. (2015) carried out trials with methanolic extracts of the leaves and seeds of *A. crassiflora*; the extracts were tested at concentrations of 1.0–2.0 mg/mL and the samples were considered active when the percentage of inhibition was more than 50%. The obtained results of percentage of inhibition were 22 and 45%, respectively. The methanolic extract of seeds of *A. coriacea* was more active, with inhibition of 52%, compared with 33% for the leaf extract, whereas the related

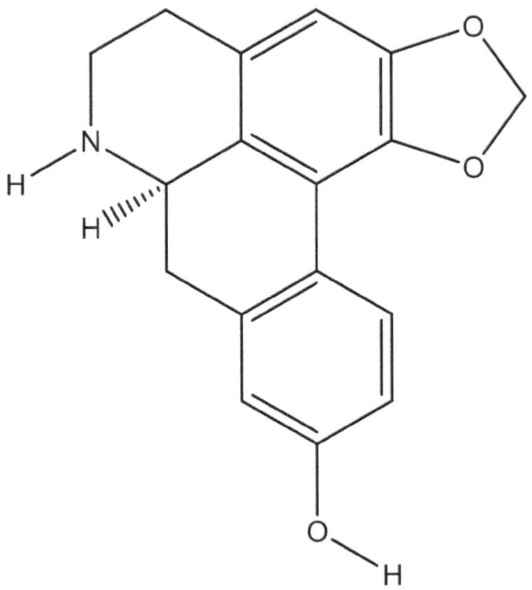

FIGURE 1.2 Alkaloid structure of (-)-anolobine isolated from the leaves of *Annona glabra*.

estefalagine (2).

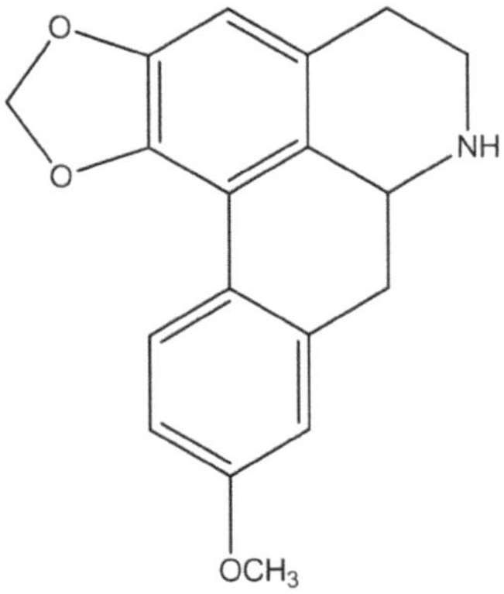

1

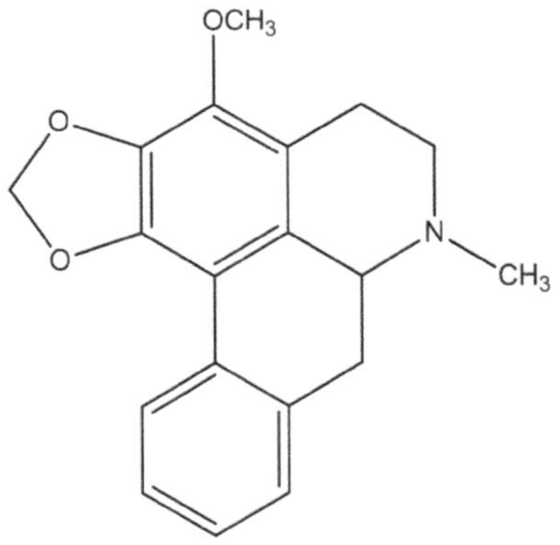

2

FIGURE 1.3 Aporphinal alkaloids isolated from *Annona crassiflora*, namely xylopine (**1**) and stephalagine (**2**).

medicinal species *Duguetia furfuracea*, also from the Annonaceae, exhibited an inhibitory value of 46% for the seed extract and 25% for the leaf extract. In High Perfomance Liquid Chromatography of *A. crassiflora* methanolic extract, the phenolics caffeic acid, *p*-coumaric acid, sinapic acid, and rutin were all present. Rutin is a flavonoid that has been recognized for its antioxidant activity and is capable of repairing damage to the central nervous system (Oliveira, 2015; Soares et al., 2005). There are reports in the literature about the acetylcholinesterase enzyme activity of rutin in *in-vitro* and *ex-vivo* studies (Fiorenza, 2011).

When the leaf extract of *Annona sylvatica* was tested, the AChE inhibition was not impressive, with only 12% inhibition, whereas, for the seeds, there was no inhibition (Formagio et al., 2015). Figure 1.4 shows the percentage AChE inhibition achieved by extracts of different parts of the plant.

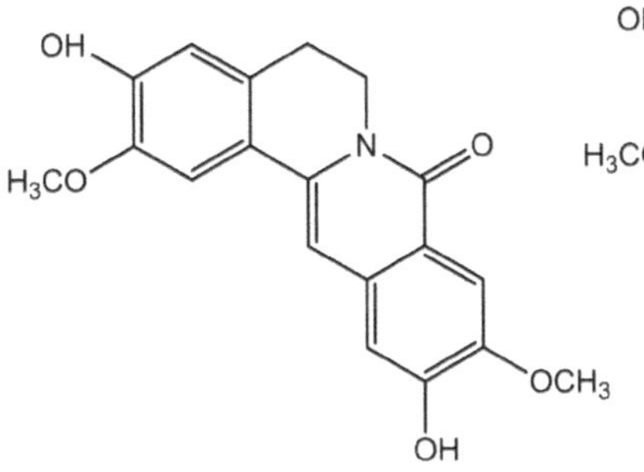

1

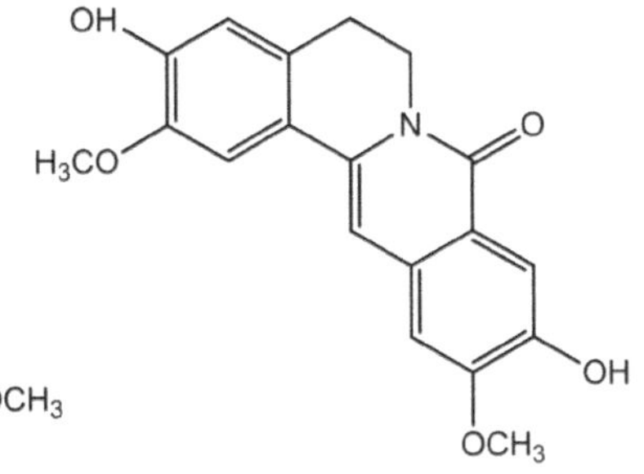

2

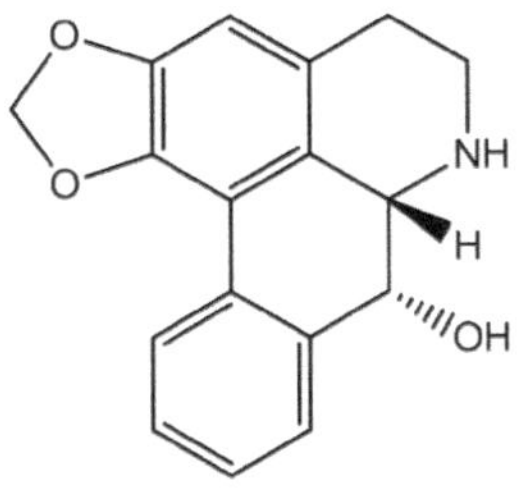

3

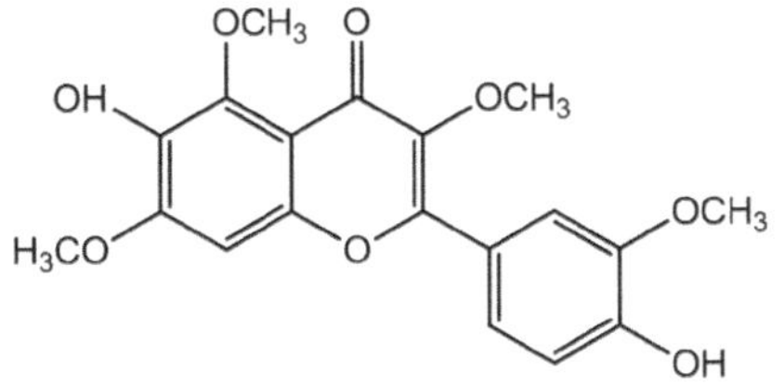

4

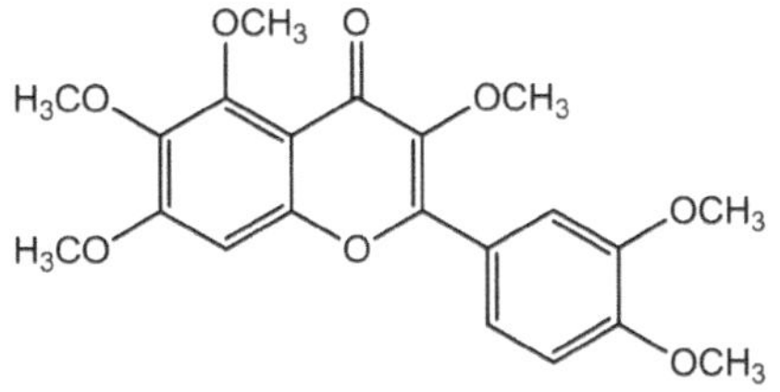

5

FIGURE 1.4 Percentage inhibition of the acetylcholinesterase enzyme of methanolic extracts of species of the Annonaceae family.

The seed oil of *Annona hypoglauca* was tested for anti-AChE activity, where 79.55% inhibition was observed. The major constituents were the fatty acids palmitic (C16:0; 16.35% inhibition), oleic (C18:1 n-9; 42.65%), and linoleic (C18:2 n-6; 29.63%). This inhibitory effect must be related to the ability of fatty acids to act against inflammatory processes, and especially, neuroinflammation, which can lead to brain disorders such as AD and Parkinson's disease (Santos et al., 2015).

Annona squamosa is a widely cultivated plant grown for its edible fruits, popularly known as ata and fruit of the count (Brito et al., 2008; Roopan et al., 2012). It is reported as having several biological activities, such as antidiabetic (Shirwaikar et al., 2004), acaricidal, insecticidal and larvicidal (Roopan et al., 2012), leishmanicidal (Vila-Nova et al., 2011), and cytotoxic activities (Vivek et al., 2012). Some authors have reported testing *A. squamosa* extracts for inhibitory effect against AChE. Bangou et al. (2011) conducted an experiment with a methanol extract of leaves, and showed 28.80% inhibition, while another study demonstrated only 0.5% inhibitory activity in an ethanol extract of seeds (Sultana, 2008).

In addition, Bangou et al. (2011) also evaluated the inhibitory activity of extracts of another species of the same genus, *Annona senegalensis*. It was confirmed that the acetylcholinesterase enzyme activity of a methanolic extract of the leaves of this plant was not impressive, with an inhibition of 2.94%.

Meliusa is another genus of the Annonaceae family, with 60 known species, and is distributed in a restricted area of Thailand (Rajkumar et al., 2016). *Meliusa thorelii* is a species with few reports in the literature and is used in folk medicine as an analgesic and aphrodisiac by Thai tribes. Despite there being no accounts of activity in extracts of this plant, Promchai et al. (2018) isolated compounds from a combined acetone extract of root and leaf tissue and tested them for their activity. Figure 1.5 shows some compounds isolated from *M. thorelii* with AChE inhibitory activity.

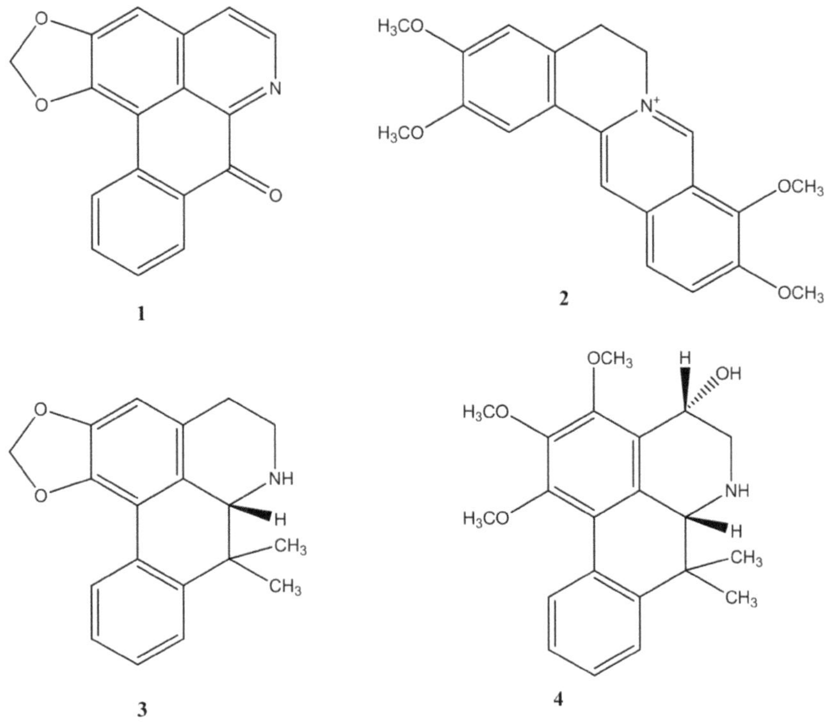

FIGURE 1.5 Some compounds with antiacetylcholinesterase activity isolated from *Meliusa thorelii.*

This work represented the first isolation and structural elucidation of compounds from *M. thorelii*, where 25 compounds were isolated with three new compounds and 22 compounds have already been reported in the literature. These three compounds were tested at a concentration of 100 mM. The aporphine alkaloids (**3**) gave greater inhibition, with values up to 50.17%, whereas the 8-oxo protoberberine alkaloids exhibited inhibition of 40.70% (**1**) and 27.93% (**2**). It has been suggested that this difference between the protoberberine alkaloids could be attributed to the positions of the methoxy and hydroxy groups in these compounds. The flavones (**4**) and (**5**) exhibited 35.60% and 38.68% inhibition, respectively. The other compounds showed a percentage inhibition of less than 30% and were therefore considered to be inactive (Promchai et al., 2018).

Guatteria blepharophylla (synonym: *Guatteriopsis blepharophylla*) is a tree, 3–6 m tall, known as "envireira" or "envira". It is found in regions of the Amazon forest of Brazil, Venezuela, Guyana, Peru, and Ecuador (Ribeiro et al., 1999). The phytochemical profile of this species is characterized mainly by the presence of alkaloids and terpenes. Among the alkaloids are *O*-methylmoschatoline, lysicamine, nornuciferine, liriodenine, isocoreximine, subsessiline, and isomoschatoline, and the terpenes include caryophyllene oxide and spathulenol. In addition, *G. blepharophylla* also contains xanthone (liquexanthone) and steroids (β-sitosterol and stigmasterol) (Costa et al., 2011).

In-vitro studies with the alkaloid isomoschatoline, isolated from the stem bark of *G. blepharophylla*, showed antifungal activity (Costa et al., 2011) and anticholinesterase activity (Feitosa et al., 2015). Its anticholinesterase activity may be relevant for the treatment of AD, justifying the selection of *G. blepharophylla* for its possible therapeutic application.

Guatteria friesiana (WA Rodrigues) Erkens & Maas (synonym: *Guatteriopsis friesiana* WA Rodrigues) is a tree native to Brazil, where it is popularly known as "envireira" and is found, in particular, in the Amazon region (Maas et al., 2015). *G. friesiana* can be identified by its cordate leaf bases (Rodrigues, 1981; Maas and Westra, 2011), dark secondary veins, and the dense covering

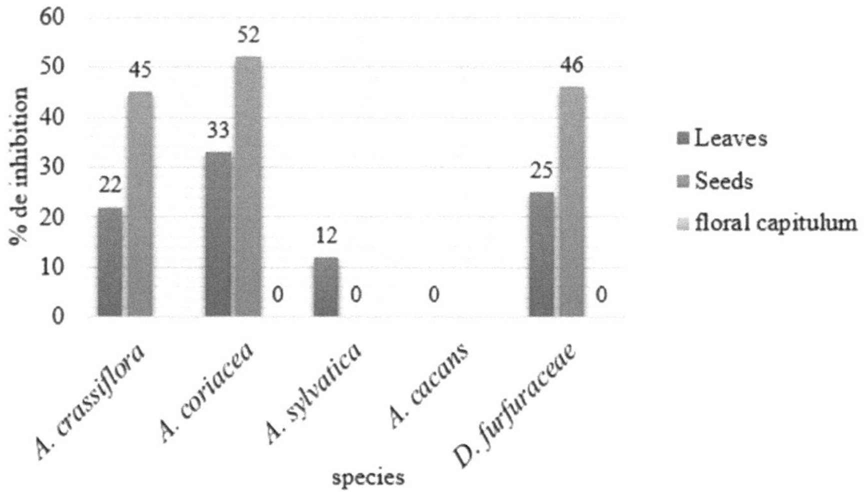

FIGURE 1.6 Alkaloid inhibitors of acetylcholinesterase isolated from species of *Guatteria, Xylopia*, and *Annona.*

of short, upright, silky hairs on young branches and flowers. Flowering occurs between the months of February and May, with fruiting from March to June (Maas and Westra, 2011).

Figure 1.6 lists alkaloids isolated from *Guatteria*, *Xylopia* and *Annona* species which have proved to be inhibitors of AChE. The compounds shown in Figure 1.6 were isolated from the alkaloid fraction of the methanolic extract of the leaves and stem of the following species: *G. friesiana, G. blepharophylla* and *Xylopia laevigata* and *Annona vepretorum*. Tests for inhibition of AChE were performed following the Ellman et al. (1961), modified by Rhee et al. (2001), on the compounds, namely liriodenine **(1)** (IC_{50} 38 µg/mL), palmatine **(2)** (IC_{50} 2.20 µM), 6,6a-dihydrodemethoxyguadiscine **(3)** (IC_{50} 339 µg/mL) and guatteriopsicine **(4)** (IC_{50} 0.3 µg/mL) (Feitosa et al., 2015). The *in-vitro* quantitative AChE enzyme assay allowed calculation of the half-maximal inhibitory concentration values for these alkaloids. These values were obtained from the initial velocity of the samples at each of five different concentrations, which was compared with the velocity of the blank, in this case, the buffer solution. Guatteriopsiscine **(4)** (IC_{50} 0.3 µg/mL) showed greater inhibition than rivastigmine (IC_{50} 1.87 µg/mL), a cholinesterase inhibitor used for the treatment of mild to moderate AD (Feitosa et al., 2015).

Guatteriopsicine, an alkaloid that, up to that point, had been found only in the leaves and stem of *G. friesiana*, has anticholinesterase and antioxidant activities (sequestering of free radicals of nitrogen and elimination of the 2,2-diphenyl-1-picrylhydrazyl radical in the DPPH antioxidant assay). This finding suggests that teas and infusions of these parts of the plant could be used in the treatment of AD, since oxidative stress plays an important role in the pathophysiology of AD (Feitosa et al., 2015). The effect of enzymatic activity on the production of free radicals and the damage to lipid membranes in the brain is a consequence of cellular damage and apoptosis. This leads to an increase in inactivation of the nuclear transcription factor kappa-B (NF-κB), a phenomenon which is associated with the neuronal degeneration that occurs in AD (Lee et al., 2005). In addition, the end result, following neuronal death, is a deficit in cholinergic, serotonergic, dopaminergic, and noradrenergic neurotransmission, with the predominance of cholinergic dysfunction (Karran et al., 2011).

The genus *Xylopia* consists of about 150 species, some of which are known for their ethnomedicinal uses and pharmacological activities. *X. aromatica* is reported to be a diuretic and is used for the treatment of skin edema. A large number of chemical compounds have been isolated from medicinal plants of the genus *Xylopia*, among them diterpenes, sesquiterpenes, alkaloids, and flavonoids (Silva et al., 2009). The species *X. laevigata* (Mart.) is popularly known as "meiú" and "pindaíba", and is a medicinal plant used widely for the treatment of pain and inflammation. Its leaves and flowers are used as an antinociceptive (Quintans et al., 2012), for its antitumor properties (Quintans et al., 2013), and as anti-inflammatory and antimicrobial (Woguem et al., 2014).

Queiroz et al. (2014) investigated the antinociception, antioxidant, and anti-inflammatory effects of essential oils from *X. laevigata* leaves in animal models. The authors found potent antioxidant (from both the DPPH and TBARS assays), anti-inflammatory and antinociceptive activities, corroborating the popular use of this plant to treat pain and inflammation. In a phytochemical screening, Feitosa et al. (2015) verified that some diterpenes isolated from *X. laevigata* exhibited anticholinesterase activity *in vitro*. All these biological activities (anti-inflammatory, antioxidant, and anticholinesterase) exhibited by extracts of this species justify its possible use for the prevention of symptoms due to AD. Anti-inflammatory substances may be used as adjuvants in the therapy of AD, as one of the characteristics observed in brain tissues of persons with AD is inflammation (Sereniki and Vital, 2008).

There are records in the literature of Annonaceae species with activities toward the central nervous system. The pyrimidine-β-carboline alkaloid annomontina, isolated from *Annona purpurea*, presented anxiolytic potential in mouse studies (Rejon-Orantes et al., 2011). The fruits and leaves of *A. muricata* (known as graviola) are used in traditional medicine as an anesthetic and natural sedative. The isoquinolinic alkaloids of the fruit of this species exhibit an antidepressant effect (Hasrat et al., 1997). *A. chemirola* is used in folk medicine as an antidepressant agent. Martinez-Vazques et al. (2012) found that alkaloids extracted from the aboveground parts of this species may promote an antidepressant effect, and suggested that it was involved in an increase in the concentration of monoamines, serotonin, and dopamine, a result that confirms the popular use of this plant for treating depression, one of the symptoms in the majority of patients with AD.

1.4 CONCLUDING REMARKS

Scientific research has shown that extracts and individual bioactive compounds isolated from plants of the Annonaceae family have anti-inflammatory, antioxidant, and anticholinesterase activity, and these properties are very important for the prevention and treatment of neurodegenerative diseases, corroborating the traditional therapeutic use of annonaceous plants.

1.5 SUMMARY

AD is one of the neurodegenerative diseases that most affect the geriatric population worldwide. Treatment consists of improvement of symptoms since no cure exists for this disease. The drugs used are inhibitors of the enzyme AChE, and studies show that preparations with antioxidant and anti-inflammatory activities have also been effective in treatment of AD patients. Many pure substances and plant extracts from species of the Annonaceae family have these biological activities and are therefore promising in the treatment of AD and other neurodegenerative diseases.

ACKNOWLEDGMENTS

The authors thank CNPq, for the scholarship awarded to Mahendra Rai (grant number 403888/2018-2), and the Federal University of Piaui, Brazil.

REFERENCES

ABRAz. *Alzheimer's Disease*. 2012. <Disponível em: http://abraz.org.br/abraz-na-midia/release-institucional-doenca-de-alzheimer>. Acesso em: July 20, 2015.

Aciole SDG, Piccoli CF, Duque JEL, Costa EV, Navarro-Silva MA, Marques FA, Sales Maia BHLN, Pinheiro MLB, Rebelo MT. Insecticidal activity of three species of *Guatteria* (Annonaceae) against *Aedes aegypti* (Diptera: Culicidae). *Rev Colomb Entomol*. 2011;37:262–268.

Alali FQ, Liu XX, Mclaughlin JL. Annonaceous acetogenins: recent progress. *J Nat Prod.* 1999;62:504–540.

Alawa CBI, Adamu AM, Gefu JO, Ajanusi OJ, Abdu PA, Chiezey NP, Alawa JN, Bowman DD. *In vitro* screening of two Nigerian medicinal plants (*Vernonia amygdalina* and *Annona senegalensis*) for anthelmintic activity. *Vet Parasitol.* 2003;113:73–81.

Badke MR, Budó MLD, Silva FM, Ressel LB. Medicinal plants: the knowledge sustained by daily life practice. *Esc Anna Nery.* 2011;15:132–139.

Badke MR, Somavilla CA, Heisler EV, Andrade A, Budó MLD, Garlet TMB. Popular knowledge: the use of medicinal plants as therapeutic form in health care. *Rev Enferm UFSM.* 2016;6:225–234.

Bangou MJ, Kiendrebeogo M, Meda NT, Coulibaly AY, Compaoré M, Zeba B, Milogo-Rasolodimby J, Nacoulma OG. Evaluation of enzymes inhibition activities of medicinal plant from Burkina Faso. *Pak J Biol Sci.* 2011;14:99–105.

Bomfim DS, Ferraz RPC, Carvalho NC, Soares MBP, Pinheiro MLB, Costa EV, Bezerra DP. Eudesmol isomers induce caspase-mediated apoptosis in human hepatocellular carcinoma HepG2 cells. *Basic Clin Pharmacol Toxicol.* 2013;113:300–306.

Brasil. *Resolução – RDC nº 10, de 09 de março, Brasília,* 2010. Ministério da Saúde: Agencia Nacional de Vigilância Sanitária.

Brito HO, Noronha EP, França LM, Brito LMO, Prado MAS. Análise da composição fitoquímica do extrato etanólico das folhas da *Annona squamosa* (ata). *Braz J Pharm Sci.* 2008;89:180–184.

Britto ACS, Oliveira ACA, Henriques RM, Cardoso GMB, Bomfim DS, Carvalho AA, Moraes MO, Pessoa C, Pinheiro MLB, Costa EV, Bezerra DP. *In vitro* and *in vivo* antitumor effects of the essential oil from the leaves of *Guatteria friesiana. Planta Med.* 2012;78:409–414.

Carneiro FM, Da Silva MJP, Borges LL, Costa JDP. Trends of studies for medicinal plants in Brazil. *Rev Sap Soc Sab Prát Educ UEG/Câmp Iporá* 2014;3:44–75.

Chang FR, Wei JL, Teng CM, Wu YC. Two new 7-dehydroaporphine alkaloids and antiplatelet action aporphines from the leaves of *Annona purpurea. Phytochemistry.* 1998;49:2015–2018.

Chatrou LW, Pirie MD, Erkens RHJ, Couvreur TLP, Neubig KM, Abbott JR, Mols JB, Maas JW, Saunders RMK, Chase MW. A new subfamilial and tribal classification of the pantropical flowering plant family Annonaceae informed by molecular phylogenetics. *Bot J Linn Soc.* 2012;169:5–40.

Chatrou LW, Rainer H, Maas PJM. Annonaceae (Soursop Family). In: Smith N, et al. (eds.). *Flowering Plants of the Neotropics.* New York, NY: New York Botanical Garden, 2004, 18–20.

Cochrane CB, Nair PR, Melnick SJ, Resek AP, Ramachandran C. Anticancer effects of *Annona glabra* plant extracts in human leukemia cell lines. *Anticancer Res.* 2008;28:965–971.

Corrêa SC, Rezende ML, Ferreira EB, Azevedo L. Marolo (*Annona crassiflora* Mart.): a study of value chain and processing. *Food Sci Technol.* 2013;33:362–368.

Costa EV, Cruz PEOD, Pinheiro MLB, Marques FA, Ruiz ALT, Marchetti GM, Maia BHL. Aporphine and tetrahydroprotoberberine alkaloids from the leaves of *Guatteria friesiana* (Annonaceae) and their cytotoxic activities. *J Braz Chem Soc.* 2013;24:788–796.

Costa EV, Marques FDA, Pinheiro MLB, Braga RM, Delarmelina C, Duarte MCT, Maia BH. Chemical constituents isolated from the bark of *Guatteria blepharophylla* (Annonaceae) and their antiproliferative and antimicrobial activities. *J Braz Chem Soc.* 2011;22:1111–1117.

Costa EV, Pinheiro MLB, Marques FA, Braga RM, Sales Maia BHLN. First report of alkaloids in the genus Guatteriopsis (Annonaceae). *Biochem Syst Ecol.* 2009;37:43–45.

Costa EV, Teixeira SD, Marques FA, Duarte MC, Delarmelina C, Pinheiro MLB, Maia BHLS. Chemical composition and antimicrobial activity of the essential oils of the Amazon *Guatteriopsis* species. *Phytochemistry.* 2008;69:1895–1899.

De Melo GO, Costa SS. Herbal natural products for the treatment of Alzheimer's disease: promise and challenge. *Rev Fito.* 2005;1:41–47.

Ellman GL, Courtney KD, Andres Jr V, Featherstone RM. A new and rapid colorimetric determination of acetylcholinesterase activity. *Biochem Pharmacol.* 1961;7:88–95.

Feitosa CM, Costa Júnior JS, Costa EV, Cavalcante NA, Silva VL. Antioxidant compounds in fruits and Alzheimer's disease. In: Chistiane Mendes Feitosa (ed.). *Medicinal Plants and Alzheimer's Disease.* Campinas: Editora Átomo, 2015, 103–122.

Fiorenza AM. Effects of rutin on the activity ofthe acetylcholinesterase and on the behavior of rats exposed to cadmium. Dissertation *of Master's Degree,* Post-Graduating Program in Biological Sciences (Toxicological Biochemistry), Federal University of Santa Maria, RS, Brazil, 2011.

Formagio ASN, Vieira MC, Volobuff CRF, Silva MS, Matos AI, Cardoso CAL, Carvalho JE. *In vitro* biological screening of the anticholinesterase and antiproliferative activities of medicinal plants belonging to Annonaceae. *Braz J Med Biol Res.* 2015;48:308–315.

Fournet A, Angelo BA, Muñoz V, Hocquemiller R, Cavé A. Effect of some bisbenzylisoquinoline alkaloids on American *Leishmania* sp. *Phytother Res.* 1993;7:281–284.

Galvão SDSL. *Avaliação da atividade antimicrobiana e citotóxica de Annona Glabra L. (Araticum).* Universidade CEUMA, 2015.

Galvão SSL, Monteiro AS, Siqueira EP, Bomfim MRQ, Dias-Souza MV, Ferreira GF, Denadai AML, Santos ARC, Santos VL, Souza-Fagundes EM, Fernandes ES, Monteiro-Neto V. *Annona glabra* flavonoids act as antimicrobials by binding to *Pseudomonas aeruginosa* cell walls. *Front Microbiol.* 2016;7:1–9.

Hasrat JA, De Bruyne T, De Backer JP, Vauquelin G, Vlietinck AJ. Isoquinoline derivatives isolated from the fruit of *Annona muricata* as 5-HTergic 5-HT1A receptor agonists in rats: unexploited antidepressive (lead) products. *J Pharm Pharmacol.* 1997;49:1145–1149.

Hidalgo EMP. Biological activities of alkaloids isolated from *Annona crassiflora* Mart. Dissertation *of Master's Degree*, Instituto de Biociências, Universidade de São Paulo, São Paulo, 2017. Recovered in October 25, 2019, de www.teses.usp.br. doi:10.11606/D.41.2018.tde-22032018-135520.

Hocquemiller R, Rasamizafy S, Moretti C, Jacquemin H, Cavé A. Anaxagoreine, a new aporphine alkaloide, isolated from two species of the genus *Anaxagorea. Planta Med.* 1981;41:48–50.

Hutchinson J. The genera of flowering plants. In: Chatrou LW, Rainer H, Maas PJM (eds.). *Annonaceae (Soursop Family)*; Smith N, et al. (eds.). *Flowering Plants of Neotropics.* New York Botanical Garden, 2004.

Karran E, Mercken M, De Strooper, B. The amyloid cascade hypothesis for Alzheimer's disease: an appraisal for the development of therapeutics. *Nat Rev Drug Discov.* 2011;10:698–712.

Kessler PJA. Annonaceae. In: Kubitzki K, Rohwer JG, Bittrich V (eds.). *The Families and Genera of Vascular Plants. II. Flowering Plants, Dicotyledons, Magnoliid, Hamamelid and Caryophyllid Families.* Berlin: Springer Verlag, 1993, 93–129.

Leboeuf M, Cavé A, Bhaumik PK, Mukherjee B, Mukherjee R. The phytochemistry of the Annonaceae. *Phytochemistry.* 1980;21:2783–2813.

Lee SS, Wu DY, Tsai SF, Chen CK. Anti-acetylcholinesterase alkaloids from *Annona glabra* leaf. *Nat Prod Commun.* 2015;10:891–893.

Lee SY, Ha TY, Son DJ, Kim SR, Hong JT. Effect of sesaminol glucosides on β-amyloid-induced PC12 cell death through antioxidant mechanisms. *Neurosci Res.* 2005;52:330–341.

Maas PJM, Maas H, Miralha JMS, Junikka L. Flora da reserva Ducke. In: Maas P, Lobão A, Rainer H (eds.). *Annonaceae Lista de Espécies da Flora do Brasil.* Jardim Botânico Rio de Janeiro, 2007. Available in:<http://floradobrasil.jbrj.gov.br/jabot/floradobrasil/FB110399>. Access in: March 03, 2015. Última edição por Lobão, A. em 13/09/2014 – 12:57:51.

Maas PJM, Rainer H, Lobão AQ. Annonaceae. In: *Lista de Espécies da Flora do Brasil.* Rio de Janeiro: Jardim Botânico do Rio de Janeiro, 2015. Available in: <http://floradobrasil. jbrj.gov.br/jabot/floradobrasil/FB1 10572>. Access in July 26, 2015.

Maas PJM, Westra LYT. A taxonomic survey of *Guatteria* section Mecocarpus including the genera *Guatteriopsis* and *Guatteriella* p.p. (Annonaceae). *Blumea.* 2011;56:113–145.

Martínez-Vázquez M, Estrada-Reyes R, Escalona AGA, Velázquez IL, Martínez-Mota L, Moreno J, Heinze G. Antidepressant-like effects of an alkaloid extract of the aerial parts of *Annona cherimolia* in mice. *J Ethnopharmacol.* 2012;139:164–170.

Melo CHS. Análises fitoquímica e farmacológica das espécies *Eugenia dysenterica* DC. (Cagaiteira) e *Annona crassiflora* Mart. (Araticunzeiro) direcionadas para doenças neurodegenerativas. Dissertation *of Master's Degree*, Federal University of Piaui, 2017.

Mesquita ML, Desrivot J, Bories C, Fournet A, Paula, JE, Grellier P, Espindola LS. Antileishmanial and trypanocidal activity of Brazilian Cerrado plants. *Mem Inst Oswaldo Cruz.* 2005;100:783–787.

Munshi CP, Vaidya PM, Buranpuri JJ, Gulati OD. Kala-azar in Gujarat. *J Indian Med Assoc.* 1972;59:287–293.

Murilo J, Restrepo D. *Las anonáceas de la región de Araracuara: estudios en La Amazonía Colombiana XX.* Bogotá: Soporte Editorial, 2000.

Oliveira GLS. Capacidade antioxidante celular da rutina frente ao dano oxidativo induzido em linhagens mutantes de *Saccharomyces cerevisiae. Rev Ciênc Farm Básica Apl.* 2015;36:461–466.

Padmaja V, Thankamany V, Hara N, Fujimoto Y, Hisham A. Biological activities of *Annona glabra. J Ethnopharmacol.* 1995;48:21–24.

Pimenta AC, Silva P, Zuffellato-Ribas KC, Koehler HS. Characterization of plants and fruit of araticum plant (*Annona crassiflora* Mart.) native to the Cerrado of Mato Grosso. *Rev Bras Frutic.* 2014;36:892–899.

Pimenta LPS, Pinto GB, Takahashi JA, Silva LGF, Boaventura MAD. Biological screening of annonaceous Brazilian medicinal plants using *Artemia salina* (Brine shrimp test). *Phytomedicine.* 2003;10:209–212.

Pontes AF, Barbosa MRV, Maas PJM. Flora Paraibana: Annonaceae Juss. *Acta Bot Bras.* 2004;18:281–293.
Promchai T, Saesong T, Ingkaninan K, Laphookhieo S, Pyne SG, Limtharakul T. Acetylcholinesterase inhibitory activity of chemical constituents isolated from *Miliusa thorelii. Phytochem Lett.* 2018;23:33–37.
Queiroz JCC, Antoniolli AR, Quintans-Júnior LJ, Brito RG, Barreto RS, Costa EV, Lima, JT. Evaluation of the anti-inflammatory and antinociceptive effects of the essential oil from leaves of *Xylopia laevigata* in experimental models. *Sci World J.* 2014;2014:1–11.
Quintans JDSS, Soares BM, Ferraz RPC, Oliveira ACAD, Silva TBD, Menezes LRA, Antoniolli AR. Chemical constituents and anticancer effects of the essential oil from leaves of *Xylopia laevigata. Planta Med.* 2013;79:123–130.
Quintans JSS, Antoniolli AR, Cardoso RSD, Prado DS, Costa EV, Prata APN, Bonjardim LR, Quintans Junior LJ. Antinociceptive effect of *Xylopia laevigata* leaf essential oil in mice – evidence of involvement of periaqueductal gray area. In: 43rd International Symposium *on* Essential Oils (*43rd ISEO*), Lisboa, 2012.
Rajkumar G, Alister M, Nazarudeen A, Pandurangan AG. *Miliusa sahyadrica*, a new species of Annonaceae from the Western Ghats, India. *Phytotaxa.* 2016;284:211–217.
Rejón-Orantes JC, González-Esquinca AR, Mora MP, Roldan GR, Cortes D. Annomontine, an alkaloid isolated from *Annona purpurea*, has anxiolytic-like effects in the elevated plus-maze. *Planta Med.* 2011;77:322–327.
Rhee IK, Van de Meent M, Ingkaninan K, Verpoorte R. Screening for acetylcholinesterase inhibitors from Amaryllidaceae using silica gel thin-layer chromatography in combination with bioactivity staining. *J Chromatogr A.* 2001;915:217–223.
Ribeiro JELS, Hopkins MJG, Vicentini A, Sothers CA, Costa MAS, Brito JM, Pereira EC. *Flora da Reserva Ducke: Guia de Identificação das Plantas Vasculares de uma Floresta de Terra Firme na Amazônica Central.* DFID, INPA, Manaus, Brazil, 1999, 816p.
Rodrigues WA. *Guatteriopsis friesiana* W. Rodrigues, nova espécie de Annonaceae para a Amazônia. *Acta Amaz.* 1981;11:49–51.
Roesler R, Catharino RR, Malta LG, Eberlin MN, Pastore G. Antioxidant activity of *Annona crassiflora*: characterization of major components by electrospray ionization mass spectrometry. *Food Chem.* 2007;104:1048–1054.
Rojas De Arias A, Inchausti A, Ascurrat M, Fleitas N, Rodriguez E, Fournet A. *In vitro* activity and mutagenicity of bisbenzylisoquinolines and quinones against *Trypanosoma cruzi* trypomastigotes. *Phytother Res.* 1994;8:141–144.
Roopan SM, Bharathi A, Kumar R, Khanna VG, Prabhakarn A. Acaricidal, insecticidal, and larvicidal efficacy of aqueous extract of *Annona squamosa* L peel as biomaterial for the reduction of palladium salts into nanoparticles. *Colloids Surf B Biointerfaces.* 2012;92:209–212.
Sáenz MS. *Catálogo preliminar comentado de la flora del Medio Caquetá.* Colombia: Tropenbos, 1997.
Santos RC, Melo Filho AV, Chagas EA. Fatty acid profile and bioactivity from *Annona hypoglauca* seeds oil. *Afr J Biotechnol.* 2015;14:2377–2382.
Sauquet H, Doyle JA, Scharaschkin T, Borsch T, Hilu KW, Chatrou LW, Thomas A. Phylogenetic analysis of Magnoliales and Myristicaceae based on multiple data sets: implications for character evolution. *Bot J Linn Soc.* 2003;142:125–186.
Schultes RE. Plants in treating senile dementia in the Northwest Amazon. *J Ethnopharmacol.* 1993;38:121–128.
Sereniki A, Vital MABF. Alzheimer's disease: pathophysiological and pharmacological features. *Rev Psiquiatr Rio Gd Sul.* 2008;30:1–17.
Shirwaikar A, Rajendran K, Dinesh Kumar C, Bodla R. Antidiabetic activity of aqueous leaf extract of *Annona squamosa* in streptozotocin–nicotinamide type 2 diabetic rats. *J Ethnopharmacol.* 2004;91:171–175.
Siebra CA, Nardin JM, Florão A, Rocha FH, Bastos DZ, Oliveira BH, Weffort-Santos AM. Potencial antiinflamatório de *Annona glabra*, Annonaceae. *Rev Bras Farmacogn.* 2009;19:82–88.
Silva DB, Silva JA, Junqueira NTV, Andrade LRM. *Fruits of the Cerrado.* Planaltina, DF: EMBRAPA/Cerrados, 2001.
Silva FLA, Oliveira RAG, Araújo EC. Use of medicinal plants by the elders at a family health estrategy. *Rev Enferm UFPE on line.* 2008;2(1):9–16.
Silva MSD, Tavares JF, Queiroga KF, Agra MDF, Barbosa Filho JM, Almeida JRGDS, Silva SASD. Alkaloids and other constituents from *Xylopia langsdorffiana* (Annonaceae). *Quim Nova.* 2009;32:1566–1570.
Silva-Júnior MC, Santos GC, Nogueira PE, Munhoz CBR, Ramos AE. *100 Cerrado Trees – Field Guide.* Brasilia, DF: Cerrado Seed Network, 2005.
Soares DG, Andreazza AC, Salvador, M. Cellular antioxidant capacity of rutin against the oxidative damage induced in mutant strains of *Saccharomyces cerevisiae. J Appl Pharm.* 2005;41:95–100.

Sultana N. Lipoxygenase inhibition by novel fatty acid ester from *Annona squamosa* seeds. *J Enzyme Inhib Med Chem.* 2008;23:877–881.

Takhtajan A. *Flowering Plants: Origin and Dispersal. Oliver & Boyd: Edinburgh. English tranl. by CJ Jeffrey*, 1961.

Tsai SF, Lee SS. Characterization of acetylcholinesterase inhibitory constituents from *Annona glabra* assisted by HPLC microfractionation. *J Nat Prod.* 2010;73:1632–1635.

Vila-Nova NS, Morais SM, Falcão MJ, Machado LK, Beviláqua CM, Costa IR, Brasil NV, Andrade Júnior HF. Leishmanicidal activity and cytotoxicity of compounds from two Annonaceae species cultivated in Northeastern Brazil. *Rev Soc Bras Med Trop.* 2011;44:567–571.

Vivek R, Thangam R, Muthuchelian K, Gunasekaran P, Kaveri K, Kannan S. Green biosynthesis of silver nanoparticles from *Annona squamosa* leaf extract and its *in vitro* cytotoxic effect on MCF-7 cells. *Process Biochem.* 2012;47:2405–2410.

Woguem V, Fogang HP, Maggi F, Tapondjou LA, Womeni HM, Quassinti L, Papa F. Volatile oil from striped African pepper (*Xylopia parviflora*, Annonaceae) possesses notable chemopreventive, anti-inflammatory and antimicrobial potential. *Food Chem.* 2014;149:183–189.

World Health Organization. *Primary Health Care*. Available in: http://sinus.org.br/2014/wp-content/uploads/2013/11/OMS-Guia-Online.pdf. Access in August 26, 2018.

2 An Alternative Approach for Anti-Alzheimer's Compounds from Plant Extracts

G. K. Pratap and Manjula Shantaram

CONTENTS

ABBREVIATIONS

Aβ42	Amyloid-beta 42
AChE	AcetylcholInesterase
AD	Alzheimer's Disease
ApoE	Apolipoprotein E
BACE-1	Beta-secretase Enzyme
BChE	Butyrylcholinesterase
β-APP	β-amyloid Precursor Protein
CNS	Central Nervous System
CSF	Cerebrospinal Fluid

FDA Food and Drug Administration
MAP Microtubule-Associated Proteins
NFT Neurofibrillary Tangles
WHO World Health Organization

2.1 INTRODUCTION

Alzheimer's disease (AD) is a progressive neurodegenerative disease, resulting in the gradual decline of a person's memory, accompanied by increasing difficulty to communicate and carry out daily activities (Pratap et al., 2017). The incidence of AD ranges from 2–4 percent of the population per year, in ages particularly from 65 to 70 years; rates may approach 5 percent for those over the age of 80 years. AD is the most common cause of dementia in the elderly and accounts for 70–80% of cases, because of poor diet and stressful lifestyle (Rodgers, 2008; Singh et al., 2011; Anand et al., 2014).

AD was the fourth-leading cause of death in 2016. It was discovered in 1906 by Alois Alzheimer, a German neurologist and psychiatrist. However, there is no cure and no effective treatment for AD (Seiguer, 2005). Nowadays, more than 42 million people suffer from AD globally and that number will be doubled by 2030. AD is characterized by the loss of neurons and by disrupted signaling between neuronal cells in the brain. The major component of the amyloid plaques in brains of AD patients is a small, 40- or 42-amino acid amyloid-beta (Aβ) peptide (Soheili et al., 2012; Ansari and Khodagholi, 2013). Aβ, the causative agent of AD, was first suggested as part of the amyloid hypothesis about 15 years ago and this is now widely accepted amongst the scientific community. AD is the most common type of presenile and senile dementia. The human β-amyloid precursor protein (β-APP) cleavage enzyme (BACE-1) is a key enzyme responsible for amyloid plaque production, which is implicated in the progress and symptoms of AD (Iriti et al., 2010; Bais et al., 2018).

AD occurs in two forms: familial and sporadic. In familial AD, mutations in genes encoding β-APP, presenilin 1, and presenilin 2 are the currently known causal factors (Selkoe, 2001). Familial AD constitutes only a small proportion (2–3%) of all AD patients (Table 2.1) (Bossy-Wetzel et al., 2004) and it has an early age of onset (younger than 60 years of age). On the other hand, sporadic AD constitutes the vast majority of AD cases and is associated with a later age of onset (70 years and older; Bertram and Tanzi, 2008). Although the specific causes of sporadic AD are still unknown, many common factors seem to be involved in sporadic AD, including aging, mitochondrial defects, environmental conditions, and insulin-dependent diabetes. In familial AD, genetic mutations accelerate the disease process (Monte and Wands, 2005; Reddy and Beal, 2005; Qiu and

TABLE 2.1
Forms of Dementia (Abbott, 2011)

Sl. No.	Dementia Form	Neuropathology	Symptoms	Dementia Cases (%)
1	AD-related dementia	Aβ plaques and NFT tangles	Memory impairment, depression, problems with judgment, and confusion.	50–80
2	Vascular dementia	Decreased blood flow to the brain and hypoperfusion	Vascular dementia is like AD, but with less effect on memory.	20–30
3	Lewy bodies	Lewy bodies are accumulations in glial and neuron cells	Similar to AD but less so to Parkinson's disease (PD) hallucinations, tremors, etc. (Houghton and Howes, 2005)	<5
4	Frontotemporal dementia	The aggregation of MAP-tau, affects the frontal and temporal lobes.	Loss of social behavior, difficulties in verbal communication.	5–10

Folstein, 2006; Tanzi and Bertram, 2008), whereas, in sporadic AD, due to the absence of genetic mutations, cellular changes that control AD progression take more time to develop (Lazarov et al., 2005). The effect of cholesterol in the development of AD is established, apart from mutations in the proteins associated with ß-APP and the presenilins, and the strongest known risk factor influencing the incidence of sporadic Alzheimer's disease is the genotype for apolipoprotein E (ApoE), the major carrier of cholesterol in the CNS (Singh et al., 2010). Persons carrying one or two copies of the *APOEε4* allele have a higher risk of developing sporadic AD. The APP can be proteolyzed directly by α-secretase and then by γ-secretase, a process that does not generate Aβ. But actions of the proteases BACE1 (β-secretase) and γ-secretase result in the production of Aβ (Corder and Saunder, 1993; Richard and Amouyel, 2001; Peters et al., 2008; Chen and Lin, 2009).

As a microtubule-associated protein tau contributes to microtubule dynamics and its main role is in the stabilization of neuronal microtubules which, in turn, provide the track for intracellular transport (Mandel and Andelkow, 1994). The molecular mechanism involves tau aggregation and is mainly represented by several post-translational modifications that modify its structure and conformational state in the neuron. Hence, the abnormal hyperphosphorylation and truncation of tau proteins have gained credence as crucial mechanisms that cause tau proteins to be a pathological unit (Kolarova et al., 2012). After neuronal damage, tau is released into the extracellular space and concentrations may be increased in the cerebrospinal fluid (CSF). Elevated CSF levels of tau occur in parenchyma diseases, including neurodegenerative as well as inflammatory diseases (Sigurd et al., 2001).

2.2 PATHOLOGICAL PATHWAYS OF AD

AD is one of the most multifactorial, complex and leading neurodegenerative disorders. Although widespread research has been conducted in the field, the exact mechanisms of its pathogenesis are still not known. Some mechanisms, like obesity, dyslipidemia, diabetes mellitus, cholinergic pathways, interleukin receptor-associated kinase 4 signaling pathway, and *Wnt* signaling pathways, are linked to AD; certain pathways are gradually gaining more importance because of their prospective role in promoting or developing AD. The pathology of AD and its symptoms, the understanding of related alterations in a number of metabolic, hormonal, and molecular pathways in AD, and targeted interventions may help those with age-related cognitive decline (Nday et al., 2018).

2.3 ROLE OF PHYTOMEDICINE IN AD

AD is an older-age, irreversible and progressive neurodegenerative disease that results in a significant loss of memory, some behavioral change, and a decline in cognitive abilities. There is no cure for AD. Presently available drugs do not cure AD, but they can control the AD symptoms (Panossian, 2016). Medicinal plants are the most effective sources of novel drugs, and the majority of the plant products that have been derived from herbal medicinal plants are already at the clinical stage of development. Currently, many scientists and researchers promote the initiative of deriving or isolating medicines from extracts of Ayurvedic medicinal plants or using individual plant constituents to treat AD (Rao et al., 2012).

An herbal drug preparation can be defined as a drug derived from a whole plant or parts of the plant (bark, leaf, root, fruit, rhizome), following development as a crude plant drug. It is useful for pharmaceutical formulation. From the Industrial Revolution and the advances in organic chemistry, there was a corresponding increase in synthetic drug production.

Ayurveda is a traditional old Indian practice medicinal practice, that involves a broad use of medicinal herbs and medicinal herbal drug preparations, and is known to treat different neurological disorders like AD, Parkinson's disease, etc. Using traditional herbal medicine to treat various neurological disorders was being practiced many years ago. Since it was recognized scientifically that the chronic inflammatory responses of the neuroglia are closely related with the AD pathology in the CNS, it has been known that medicinal herbal drugs and their constituents control anti-inflammatory activity and exhibit a potent neuroprotective activity to treat the various neurological disorders (Khan and Ahmad, 2019). Medicinal herbs are recognized as one of the most valuable resources for discovering novel beneficial bioactive compounds that can act against known targets, making use of diverse proteomics and genomics techniques followed by high-throughput screening (Kumar and Khanum, 2012). In the modern pharmacological search for effective measures against brain disorders, the center of attention is now on the herbal medicinal drugs.

According to a WHO report, traditional medicine is used by 80% of the total global population for primary health-care measures. These herbal medicines are reportedly safer and better tolerated by subjects than are synthetic chemical drugs in treating chronic illnesses, and herbal medicines have fewer side effects. In its crude drug form, the traditional herbal medicine is obtained as a standardized herbal extract, formulations derived from it, and in the form of its composite preparations (Vyawahare et al., 2008).

Current synthetic drugs, which are used as AD therapeutic options, are not completely successful in restoring the normal neural functions, due to their inability to repair the neurons that have already been damaged, or to regenerate them. Due to this feature of conventional therapy in terms of recovery from neural damage and the harmful side effects associated with administration of synthetic drugs, it is vital to look for alternative treatments in the form of herbal drugs, plant-derived drugs or medicinal plant products to treat such dangerous disorders (Mohamed et al., 2012). Plant bioactive compounds, such as flavonoids, polyphenols, etc. which are naturally antioxidative in nature, as well as possessing anxiolytic properties, are the primary choice to be employed as neuroprotective and antiamnesic agents (Ferdousy et al., 2016). Moreover, some of the neurotransmitters become autoxidized, thereby leading to reactive oxygen species (ROS) generation. Oxidative stress is one of the key features of neurodegenerative diseases, such as AD, a well-known fact that contributes majorly towards AD pathogenicity (Esposito et al., 2012). Many flavonoids, phenols, and polyphenols exert a neuroprotective efficacy, in that they can easily cross the blood–brain barrier (BBB) and scavenge the free radicals of oxygen and nitrogen present at pathological concentrations, as well as acting as transition metal ion chelators (Aquilano et al., 2008). Thus, herbal drugs and phytomedicines are potential alternative medicines for controling neurological disorders and thereby allowing damaged tissue to recover (Esposito et al., 2012). Fruits that contain flavonoids, phenolics, and polyphenolics are being chosen as a means to improve learning, memory, and cognitive abilities (Chen et al., 2013). This makes them an attractive choice as a treatment against the prevention of brain damage associated with disease conditions like AD and other such neurodegenerative diseases, which lead to a decline in neuronal apoptosis, and thereby improving learning, memory, and cognitive functions (Subash et al., 2014). Herbal extracts, plant products, and individual phytoconstituents have strengthened their position as potent free-radical scavengers that also inhibit ROS and lipid peroxidation activity. The synthetic drugs with antioxidant characteristics tend to be toxic, so that natural antioxidants are in great demand as alternative strategies. Since the chemical composition of traditional herbal medicines and herbal products reflects the physiological functions of a living organism, they are evidently more compatible with human system than are synthetic chemicals (Sen et al., 2010; Srivastava et al., 2019).

Therefore, the aim of this chapter is to understand the relationship between AD and phytomedicines, the side effects of synthetic drugs, and how to use medicinal plants as a future mainstream source of anti-AD drugs.

2.4 CURRENT TRENDS IN PHYTOMEDICINE AND HERBAL DRUGS IN AD THERAPY

In the 21st century, with the greater efficacy of the pharmacological impacts of medicinal plants, herbal medicine has been considered the future of alternative medicine for the management of human health care (Leslie, 2000). Medicinal plants play a crucial role in the development of new drugs. According to the WHO, nearly 25% of the current medicines have been isolated from traditional medicinal plants and the WHO has recognized plant medicines as vital components of human primary healthcare. Plant-based medicinal drugs have contributed revolutionarily to present-day therapeutics (Srivastava et al., 2019).

The rich traditions of herbal medicine were followed by Siddha and Ayurveda medicines in India, traditional Chinese medicine (TCM), Unani medicine in the Middle East, and Kampo medicine in Japan (Mosihuzzaman and Choudhary, 2008). Nowadays, the high demand for plant-based products, cosmetics, and food supplements is building in both developed and developing countries. The reason behind this popularity is that the natural products are less toxic, have fewer side effects, and are easily accessible at reasonable prices (Evans, 1994). Medicinal plants are considered to be rich sources of phytochemical ingredients, which play a vital role in the development of new drugs. People have been using medicinal plants to treat diseases without any scientific information or appropriate guidance for thousands of years. It has been scientifically established that every part of plants can have medicinal properties, including roots, stems, leaves, flowers, fruits, and seeds. However, it has also been witnessed that some medicinal plants are not safe for consumption because they are toxic and show side effects in the patient (Wink, 2010). In recent times, there has been a change in the universal trend, from synthetic to herbal medicine, which is claimed as "Return to Nature." Medicinal plants have been exploited since ancient times and are highly regarded all over the world as a rich source of therapeutic agents for the prevention and treatment of human ailments (Srivastava et al., 2019).

2.5 PHYTOCHEMICALS AND PHARMACOLOGICAL RESEARCH IN MEDICINAL PLANTS

There are more than 400,000 plant species on earth, representing an enormous wealth of medicinal remedies from Mother Nature. Natural products and their derivatives represent more than 40% of the content of all the drugs in current conventional therapeutics. Because of the low success rate and inadequate investment, today's conventional drugs are very expensive. Medicinal plants from a number of Indian, orthodox, western, and Chinese traditional medicinal systems have been used for treatment of different diseases, like fever, cancer, neurodegeneration, etc. One of the most extensive traditional systems to treat neurodegenerative diseases is the Indian traditional *Ayurveda* system called *Rasayana*. It is an ancient Indian medicinal system, practiced since 2000 BC, in which medicinal plants used for anti-diabetic and CNS-protective effects were well documented in classical texts of *Ayurveda* (Perry et al., 1999; Abascal and Yarnell, 2004).

Some parts of the medicinal plants, such as leaves, roots, stems, barks, flowers, and fruits are commonly rich in phenolic compounds and other secondary plant metabolites (Agarwal et al., 2015). The pharmacological properties of each plant extracts differ with respect to their different active principles, and many Indian medicinal plant composites are represented as containing neuroprotective and pharmacologically neuroactive compounds (Canevari and Clark, 2007). Recently, medicinal plants have gained wide acceptance, because of the relative absence of side effects, compared with synthetic drugs, and also to address the need to meet the requirement for medicines by the rapidly growing human population. The WHO has paid greater attention to developing herbal medicines with improved and safer therapeutic profiles (Perry et al., 1999).The therapeutic value of a medicinal plant is thus considered in terms of the interaction between one or more of its chemical constituents with the relevant disease-related system (Howes and Perry, 2003). For plant products to be incorporated into conventional medicine, both clinical efficiency and relevant biological activity need to be established (Kennedy and Wightman, 2011). AD is a potential therapeutic target, in terms of identified biological mechanisms for amelioration, which include enhancing cholinergic transmission, restricting oxidative stress, and preventing Aβ formation or toxicity (Kumar, 2006; Manyam, 1999). Some investigators have reported that a number of medicinal plants are utilized in AD treatment, including *Centella asiatica, Ginkgo biloba, Withania somnifera, Bacopa monnieri,*

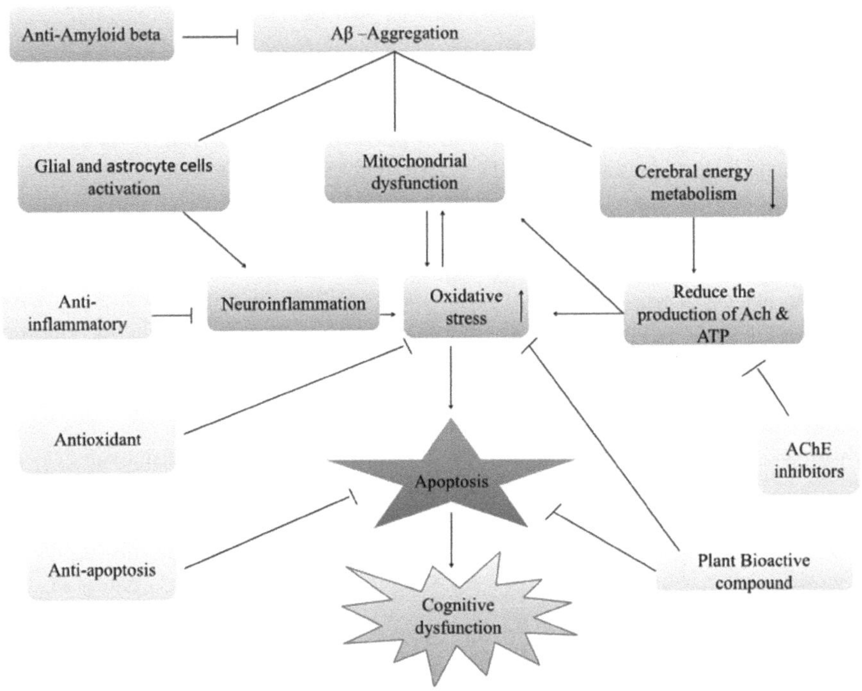

FIGURE 2.1 Various mechanisms of action and therapeutic targets of herbal drugs (Kumar et al., 2017).

Salvia officinalis, Melissa officinalis, Tinospora cordifolia, and *Glycyrrhiza glabra*, among others., and various medicinal plant-derived compounds are already being used for the treatment of AD. The most prominent examples are physostigmine, galantamine and huperzine A, where the plant-derived compounds are being used for anticholinesterase activity. More than 150 different medicinal plant species (Figure 2.1 and Table 2.2), in various preparations and mixtures, have been used in the context of age-related CNS disorders (Rao et al., 2012; Lin et al., 2016).

2.6 PHARMACOLOGICAL PROPERTIES OF PLANT COMPOUNDS

2.6.1 Phenols and Phenolic Compounds

Phenolic compounds constitute one of the most common and widespread groups of secondary metabolites in plants. The term "phenolic" or "polyphenol" can be precisely defined chemically as a substance which possesses an aromatic ring bearing one or more hydroxyl substituents, including functional derivatives such as esters, glycosides, methyl ethers, and others. Phenol itself is a naturally occurring product but most phenols have two or more hydroxyl groups (Crozier et al., 2006; Oksana et al., 2012), and health effects and activities of polyphenolic compounds. Flavonoids have been used in various medicines and food products due to their potential health benefits since ancient times and are still relevant and widely used nowadays. Many phenolic compounds present in natural foods may reduce the risk of serious health problems because of their antioxidant actions (Tewari et al., 2018).

The plant secondary metabolites are synthesized *via* biochemical pathways that are not crucial for plant development but which have biological and pharmacological significance. Naturally occurring antioxidant compounds, such as phenolics, have numerous biological activities, being potent antioxidants and free radical scavengers. Generally, plant phenolic compounds are used in treatment of certain chronic diseases, for instance, diabetes, cancers, and cardiovascular diseases, for the management of oxidative stress (Selamoglu, 2017; Lin et al., 2018).

TABLE 2.2
Selected Prominent Medicinal Plant Compounds and Plant Genera Used For the Treatment of Dementia

Sl. No	Plant Name	Active Compounds	Mechanism
1.	*Allium sativum*	S-Allylcysteine	It prevents aging, increases longevity, improves mental function and it is also used to treat CNS disorders (Anekonda and Reddy, 2005).
2.	*Areca catechu* L.	Arecoline	In a clinical study, arecoline demonstrated memory-enhancing effects in AD patients Despite initial success with *in vitro* studies, the compound failed to improve the cognitive functions in mild to moderate ADpatients (Soncrant et al., 1993; Houghton et al., 2005).
3.	*Amanita muscaria*	Muscarine	Muscarinic agonists (Alagha et al., 2014)
4.	*Angelica sinensis*	Z-ligustilide	Z-ligustilide showed protective effect against Aβ peptide-induced neurotoxicity in rats (Chao and Lin, 2011).
5.	*Astragalus membranaceus*	Cycloastragenol	A neuroprotective function against apoptosis induced by DNA damage, ischemia, glutamate, and amyloid peptide (Fanny et al., 2014)
6.	*Bacopa monnieri*	Reseperpine	It provides protection against working memory decline and against AD in the mouse model. It protects neurons from Aβ-induced cell death (Pravina et al., 2007).
7.	*Buxus hyrcana, Buxus papillosa*	Buxamine B	Inhibited AChE *in vitro* (Deka et al., 2017).
8.	*Coptis chinensis*	Berberine	Berberine inhibited both Aβ and β-secretase under *in vitro* conditions (Kim et al., 2014).
9.	*Chondrodendron tomentosum*	Tubocurarine	Nicotinic antagonists (Steinbach et al., 1995).
10.	*Cynanchum atratum*	Cynatroside-B	Significantly inhibited AChE activity (Lee et al., 2005).
11.	*Celastrus paniculatus*	Celastrine	It also shows cholinesterase inhibitory activity (Shashank et al., 2017)action.
12.	*Centella asiatica*	*Hydrocotyle sibthorpioides*	PC-12 neuron protection (Veerendra et al., 2003)
13.	*Corydalis speciosa*	Protopine	Significantly inhibited AChE activity (Kim et al., 1998)
14.	*Curcuma longa*	Curcumin, curcuminoids	Inhibition of Aβ deposition, Aβ oligomerization, and tau hyperphosphorylation in the brain of AD animal model, achieving behavioral improvement (Wang et al., 2014).
15.	*Catharanthus roseus*	Vinpocetine	Vinpocetine is protective, indicated by the significant decrease in AChE, tau, β-secretase (Ali et al., 2017).
16.	*Crocus sativus*	Crocin	Crocin possesses *in vitro* antioxidant and antiamyloidogenic properties (Papandreou et al., 2006).
17.	*Camellia sinensis*	Epigallocatechin-3-gallate	Tea consumption reduces the risk of AD, and induces an antiamyloid effect(Liu et al., 2016).
18.	*Cytisus scoparius*	Sparteine	Nicotinic antagonist (Daly, 2005)
19.	*Evodiarutae carpae*	Dehydroevodiamine hydrochloride	Cholinergic therapy in AD (Singhal et al., 2012)
20.	*Elsholtzia rugulosa*	Luteolin	Luteolin has a potentially protective effect on learning defects and hippocampal structures in AD (Wang et al., 2016).

(Continued)

TABLE 2.2 (CONTINUED)
Selected Prominent Medicinal Plant Compounds and Plant Genera Used For the Treatment of Dementia

Sl. No	Plant Name	Active Compounds	Mechanism
21.	*Elsholtzia rutaecarpa*	Dehydroevodiamine	Strongly inhibited AChE *in vitro* and reversed scopolamine-induced memory impairment in rats (Heo et al., 2002; Jae et al., 2014)
22.	*Fatoua villosa*	Zeatin	AChE inhibitory effect *in vitro* (Heo et al., 2002)
23.	*Gastrodia elata*	*p*-Hydroxybenzyl alcohol (HBA) and gastrodin (GAS)	HBA reduced inflammation and neurotoxicity. Lipopolysaccharide (LPS) treatment of macrophages induced expression of proinflammatory cytokines (TNF-α, IL-1β, and IL-6) (Wang et al., 2016).
24.	*Galanthus nivalis*	Galantamine	Cholinesterase inhibitor used in treatment of AD (Asa et al., 2011).
25.	*Ginkgo biloba*	Kaempferol, Quercetin	Significant inhibition of the Aβ42 levels in the human H4 cell line (Hawes, 2013; Bui and Nguyen, 2017).
26.	*Huperzia serrata*	Huperzine A	Memory-enhancement property (Yang et al., 2013)
27.	*Hyoscamus niger*	Hyoscamine	Muscarinic antagonists (Nana et al., 2017)
28.	*Heteromeles arbutifolia.*	Marlinic acid	Avoids Aβ-induced cytotoxicity *in vitro* studies (Zurita et al., 2016).
29.	Lamiaceae species	Rosmarinic acid	Rosmarinic acid may significantly prevent Aβ-induced memory loss. Rosmarinic acid has also been shown to protect neuronal PC12 cells to avoid Aβ-induced cytotoxicity (Ansari et al., 2013).
30.	*Lobelia inflata*	Lobeline	Nicotinic agonist (Decker et al., 1993)
31.	*Magnolia officinalis*	Biphenolic, magnolol	Inhibit AChE activity *in vitro* and have also shown to release hippocampal AChE *in vivo* (Lee et al., 2009).
32.	*Origanum majorana*	Ursolic acid	Findings suggest that ursolic acid prevents memory impairment through amelioration of oxidative stress and inflammatory response, and may offer a novel therapeutic strategy for the treatment of AD.
33.	*Panax notoginseng*	Ginsenoside Rg1	It is used to treat CNS dysfunctions and it is involved in improving cognitive abilities such as learning and memory. The activity of β-secretase was inhibited in a concentration-dependent manner and a dose-dependent reversal of Aβ-induced decreased cell viability was observed following treatment with GRg1 in PC12 cell lines *in vitro* studies (Choi et al., 2016).
34.	*Paeonia suffruticosa*	Paeoniflorin	Paeoniflorin improved radial maze performance in rats impaired by an anti-cholinergic drug (Ohta et al., 1993).
35.	*Panax ginseng*	Ginsenosides	Ginsenosides have significant inhibitory potential against AChE and BACE1 (Coelho and Birks, 2001).
36.	*Physostigma venenosa*	Physostigmine	Physostigmine has shown cholinesterase inhibition and memory enhancement properties (Lily et al., 2013).
37.	*Pilocarpus* sp.	Pilocarpine	AChE inhibitor (Robert, 2014).
38.	*Papaver somniferum*	Codeine	Alterations in the antigenic profiles of cerebral proteins activate the microglia. It shows antiAβ activity (Ahmad et al., 2018).
39.	*Polygonum minus*	Polygonumins A	AChE inhibitor (Bais and Kumari, 2018).

(Continued)

TABLE 2.2 (CONTINUED)
Selected Prominent Medicinal Plant Compounds and Plant Genera Used For the Treatment of Dementia

Sl. No	Plant Name	Active Compounds	Mechanism
40.	*Polygala tenuifolia*	Sinapic acid	Increased the activity of choline acetyl transferase in the frontal cortex of brain-lesioned rats (Balez et al., 2016).
41.	*Petroselinum crispum*	Apigenin	Neuroprotective action of apigenin against AD pathogenesis in a human disease model and *in vivo* mouse model (Li et al., 2010).
42.	*Pueraria lobata*	*Puerarin*	Puerarin has a protective effect against Aβ-induced neurotoxicity in rat hippocampus neurons *via* various mechanisms. Pre-treatment with puerarin decreased Aβ-induced cell death in cultured rat hippocampal neurons by inhibiting GSK-3β (Misiti et al., 2004).
43.	*Rheum x hybridum*	Rhaponticin	It demonstrated *in vitro* neuroprotective action against Aβ-induced toxicity. It inhibited Aβ-fibril formation and promoted Aβ clearance *in vitro* studies. The compound improved cognitive dysfunction, which is proposed to be related to its *in vivo* AChE inhibitory activities. (Du and Zhang, 1995).
44.	*Salvia miltiorrhiza*	Salvianolic acid A	Salvianolic acid A shows protection against cerebral ischemia-induced memory impairment in mice (Zhoua et al., 2011).
45.	*S. miltiorrhiza*	Tanshinone	AChE inhibitory activity in *in vitro* studies. Tanshinone improved changes induced by Aβ (1-42) in rats, including a decrease in AChE-positive fibres. Tanshinones demonstrated a wide range of pharmacological activities of relevance to AD therapy (Yina et al., 2011).
46.	*Silybum marianum*	Silibinin	Silibinin is protective against Aβ-induced oxidative stress in SH-SY5Y human neuroblastoma cells. The aggregation of Aβ was markedly inhibited following treatment with silibinin (Jayakumar and Murugan, 2016).
47.	*Solanum tuberosum*	α-Solanine	Neuroprotective activity of solanine was evaluated against ischemia in rats (Bhattacharjee, 2018).
48.	*Tabernaemontana australis*	Rupicoline	Rupicoline activity reported in the treatment of AD occurred *via* the utilization of acetylcholinesterase (AChE) and butyrylcholinesterase (BChE) inhibitors (Mishra et al., 2000).
49.	*Withania somnifera*	Sitoindosides IX	It has been suggested that the mechanism for this effect may involve modulation of cholinergic neurotransmission. It shows an anti-AChE activity (Ali, 2018).
50.	*Zingiber officinale*	Gingerols	Gingerols had a protective effect on Aβ1–42-induced damage and apoptotic death in rat pheochromocytoma cells (PC12 cells) and were investigated in the underlying mechanisms of neuroprotective effects. Gingerol significantly increased cell viability and reduced cell apoptosis in Aβ1–42-treated cells (Paula et al., 2013).

2.6.2 Flavonoid Compounds

Flavonoids consist of a large group of polyphenolic compounds having a benzo-γ-pyrone structure and are ubiquitously present in plants. Flavonoids are synthesized by the phenylpropanoid pathway (Kumar and Pandey, 2013). In nature, flavonoid compounds are found in several parts of the plant.

Flavonoids are used by plants for their growth and defense against Aβ plaques (Panche et al., 2016). Many flavonoids are easily recognised as flower pigments in most angiosperm families. Flavonoids are also present in large quantities in foods and beverages of plant origin, such as fruits, tea, vegetables, cocoa, and wine; hence they are termed "dietary flavonoids". Altogether, 6000 flavonoids have been identified, which include chalcones, flavones, flavanols, and isoflavones. These subgroups have unique major plant sources. For example, tea and onions are major dietary sources of flavanols and flavones, respectively (Wang et al., 2018).

Vegetables and fruits are the main dietary sources of flavonoids for humans, along with wine and tea. Most recent research has focused on the health aspects of flavonoids for humans. Many flavonoids have been shown to have health benefits, like free radical scavenging capacity, antioxidative activity, coronary heart disease prevention, anti-inflammatory, hepatoprotective, and anticancer activities, and some flavonoids exhibit possible antiviral activities. The flavonoids have beneficial roles in human health as well as being of significance for plants (Sharma, 2006; Agarwal, 2011; Kumar and Pandey, 2013; Tungmunnithum et al., 2018).

2.6.3 Triterpenes and Terpenoids

Triterpenoids are the most important group of terpenoids as they exhibit a wide diversity of biological activities and they are the major constituents in many medicinal plant decoctions and extracts. Some new plant bioactive compounds have been identified from traditional medicines, leading to the isolation of numerous triterpenoids with important pharmacological properties and activities (Jainendra et al., 2018). Triterpenoids are widespread in nature and can be found in vegetables, fruits, cereals, ferns, fungi, monocotyledonous and dicotyledonous plants, animals, and marine organisms. The higher plants are the major source of biologically active triterpenoids, with numerous reports showing that the Rhamnaceae, Cucurbitaceae and Apocynaceae plant families and the fungal Ganodermataceae family produce a wide variety of tetracyclic triterpenoids (Bishayee et al., 2011).The acidic function and -OH (hydroxyl) groups of the triterpenoids cannot interact with the stationary phase, as the two groups are located on the opposite sides of the compound (Parmar et al., 2013). The triterpenoid compounds found in the oleane family are erythrodiol, oleanolic acid, and β-amyrinandin, whereas those in the ursane family include uvaol and ursolic acid, with the lupane family including lupeol, betulinic acid, and botulin (Dzubak et al., 2005; Han and Bakovic, 2015; Battineni et al., 2018).

Many such triterpenoid compounds can either be used directly as bioactive compounds or modified to increase their selectivity and effectiveness. The wide range of biological activities associated with tetracyclic triterpenes and pentacyclic triterpenoids include antidepressant, immunomodulatory, anticancer, antianxiety, anti-inflammatory, memory enhancing, neuroprotective, antinociceptive, and other CNS-related actions (Chudzik et al., 2015; Peterson et al., 2011).

2.6.4 Alkaloids

Alkaloids constitute an important class of structurally diverse plant compounds that have a nitrogen atom in the heterocyclic ring, and are derived from amino acids. The term 'alkaloids' was coined by the German chemist Carl F. W. Meissner in 1819 and the word is derived from the Arabic name al-qali that is related to the plant from which soda was first isolated (Howes et al., 2003; Rinaldia et al., 2017). The alkaloid compounds are low-molecular-weight structures and make up about 20% of plant-based secondary metabolites and they have influenced human history profoundly, due to their wide range of physiological effects on animals and pharmacological properties on humans, such as anticancer and antibiotic properties, along with their potential exploitation as narcotics, stimulants, and poisons (Kaur and Arora, 2018). About 12,000 alkaloids have been isolated from the plant kingdom. Depending upon their biosynthetic precursor and heterocyclic

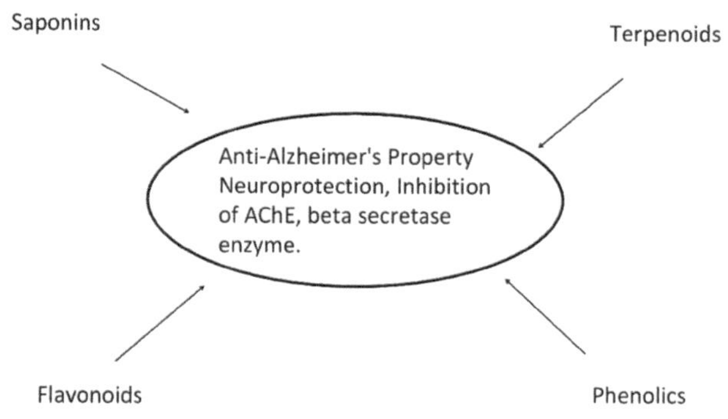

FIGURE 2.2 Flavonoids, terpenoids, saponins, and phenolics active against AD.

ring system, alkaloids have been classified into different categories, including indole, piperidine, tropane, purine, imidazole, pyrrolidine, pyrrolizidine, quinolizidine, and isoquinoline alkaloids (Ramakrishna et al., 2012; Aniszewski, 2007; Bribi, 2018). They are classified using various signatures, such as natural source or chemical nature. The biological activity of alkaloids, like cytotoxic and CNS activity, and toxicity against herbivores, include anticarcinogenic, antibacterial, antifungal, and antiviral properties in vertebrates (Wirasathien et al., 2006; Padma Kumar et al., 2009; Ramakrishna et al., 2011).

2.6.5 Lignans and Lignin Glycosides

The lignans are bioactive plant compounds, non-nutritional, non-caloric phenolic plant compounds that are found at the highest concentration in sesame and flax seeds and in lower concentrations in grains, other seeds, vegetables, and fruits (Abef and Yamauchi, 1990; Gokare and Akula, 2010). The chemistry and biosynthesis of lignans in plants present in major food sources and their metabolism in humans have been studied (Zhao et al., 2003). The plant lignans most commonly distributed in foods are lariciresinol, matairesinol, pinoresinol, and secoisolariciresinol (Houghton and Howes, 2005). Some lignans are present in foods, including medioresinol (sesame seeds, rye, and lemons), sesamin, syringaresinol (grains), and their precursor sesamolin (Rao et al., 2011). Lignans are recognized as a class of natural products with a particularly wide spectrum of important biological activities, with the main biological properties of lignans being antitumor and antiviral activities (Zhao et al., 2003; Kim et al., 2015) (Figure 2.2 and Table 2.2).

2.7 CURRENT PHYTOMEDICINE USED IN TREATMENT OF AD

2.7.1 Phenolic Compounds

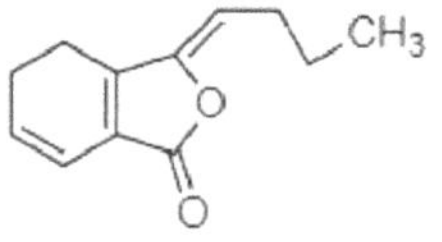

i. Z-Ligustilide

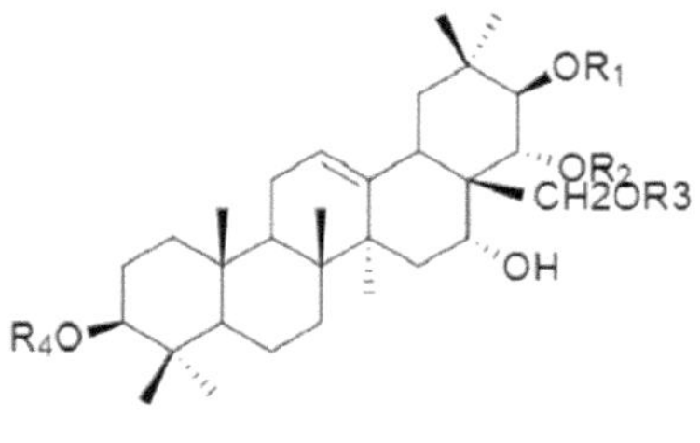

ii. Hydrrocotylesibthorpioides

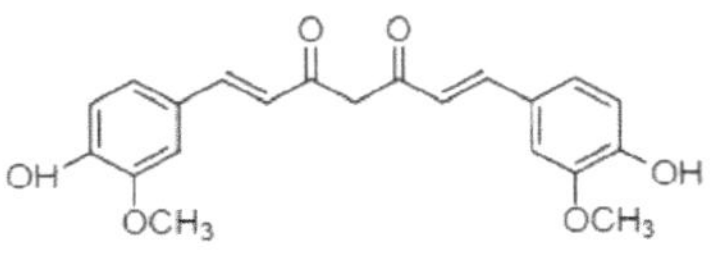

iii. Curcumin

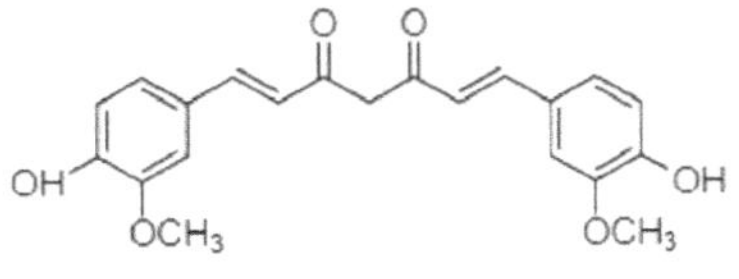

iv. Curcuminoid

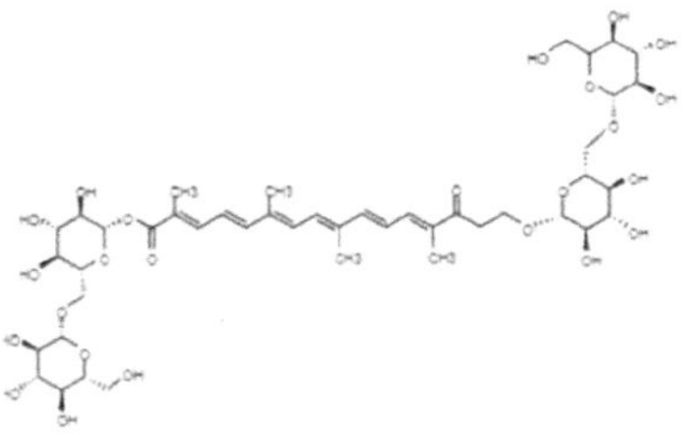

v. Crocin

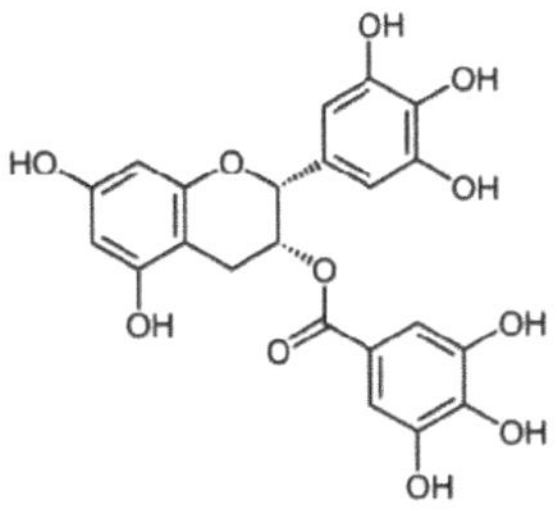

vi.Epigallo catechin-3-gallate

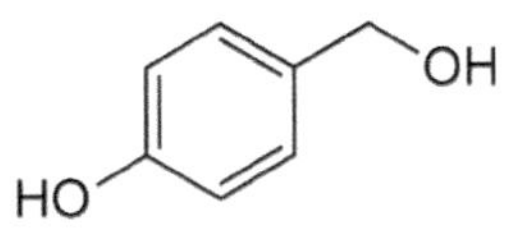

vii. p-Hydroxybenzyl

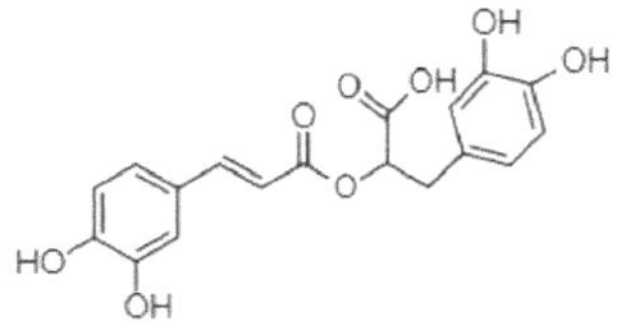

viii. Rosmarinic acid

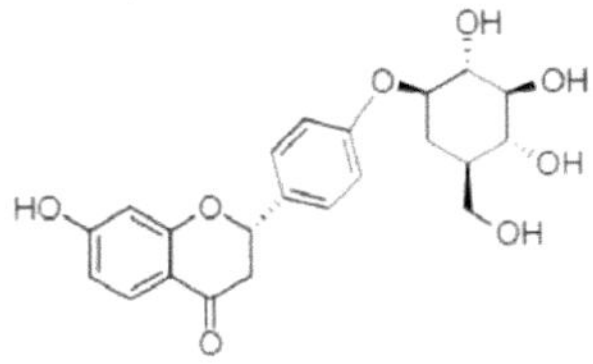

ix. Paeoniflorin

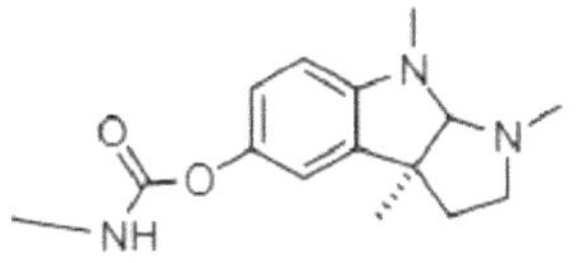

x. Physostigmine

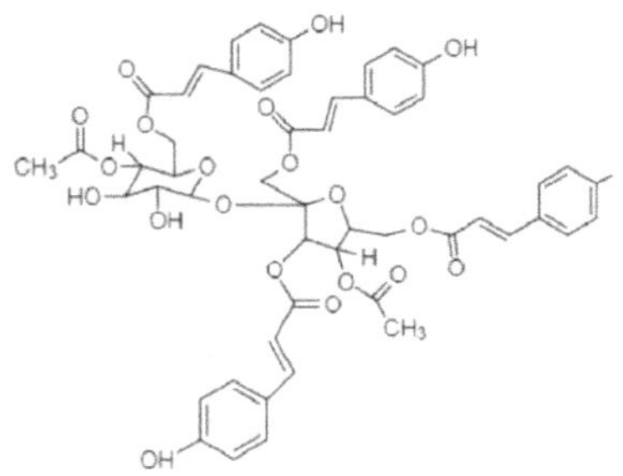

xi. Polygonumins A

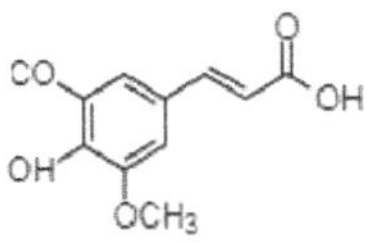

xii. Sinapic acid

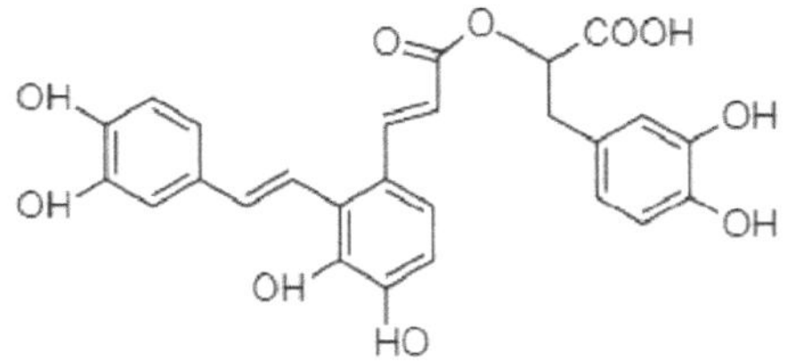

xiii.Salvianolic acidA

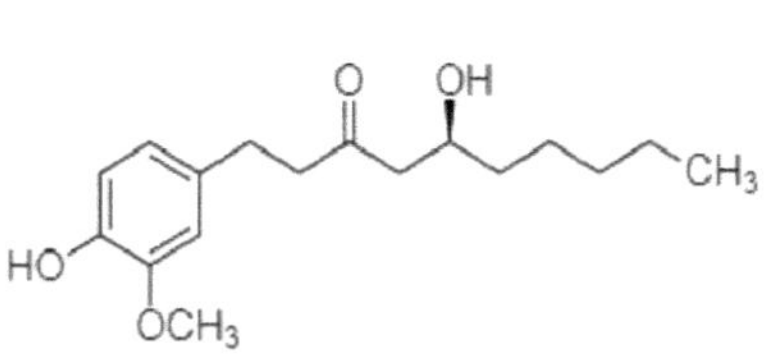

xiv. Gingerols

2.7.2 Flavonoid Compounds

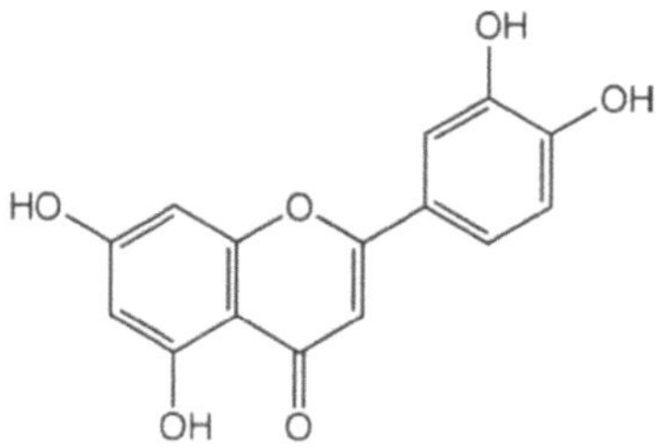

i.Luteolin

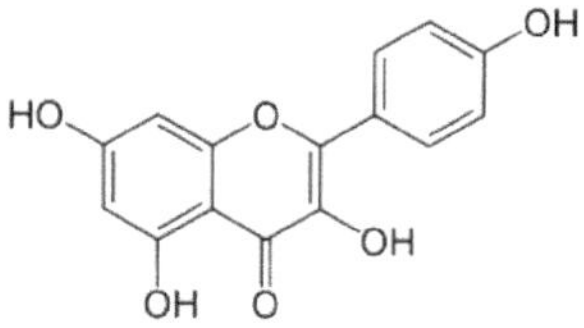

ii. Kaempferol

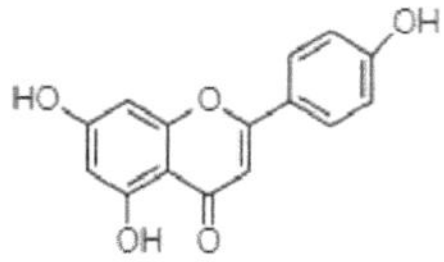

iii. Apigine

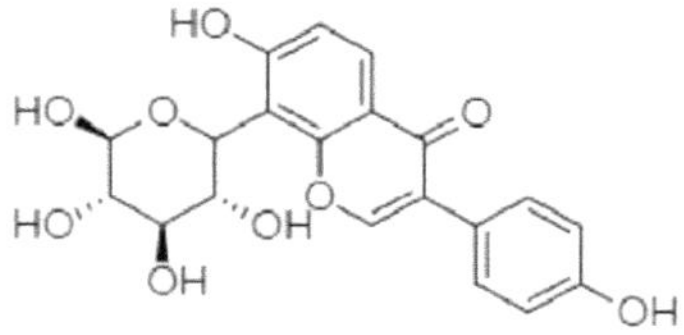

iv. Puerarin

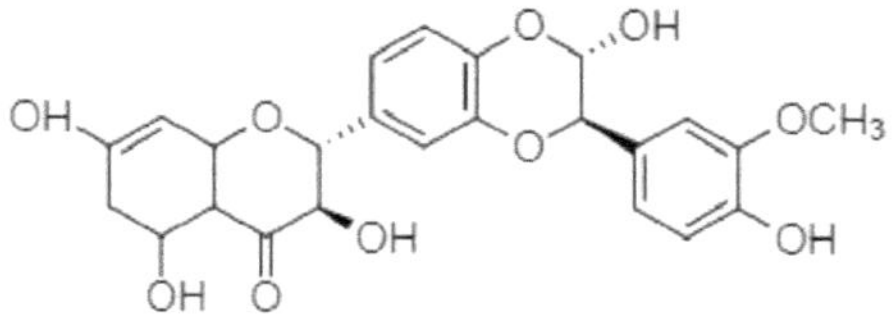

v. Silibinin

2.7.3 Triterpenes and Triterpenoids

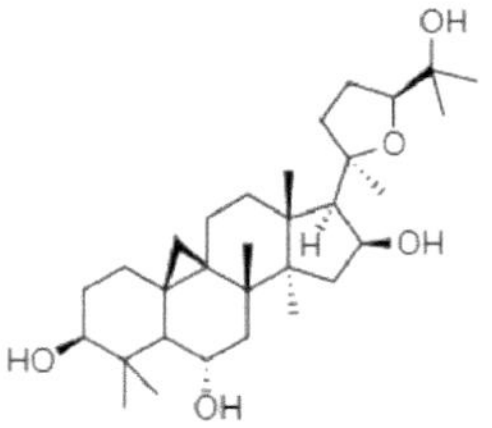

i.Cycloastragenol

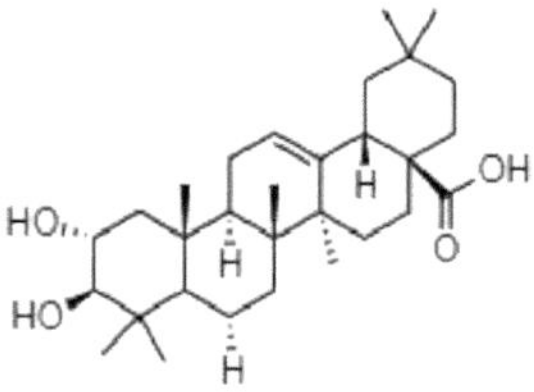

ii.Malinic acid

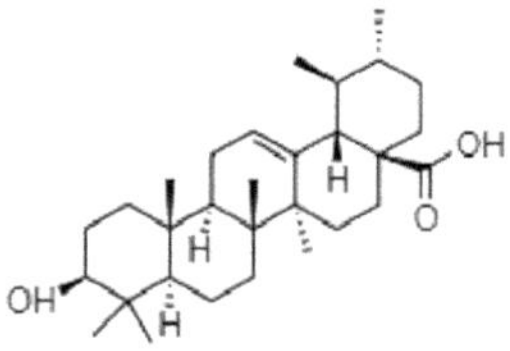

iii. Ursolic acid

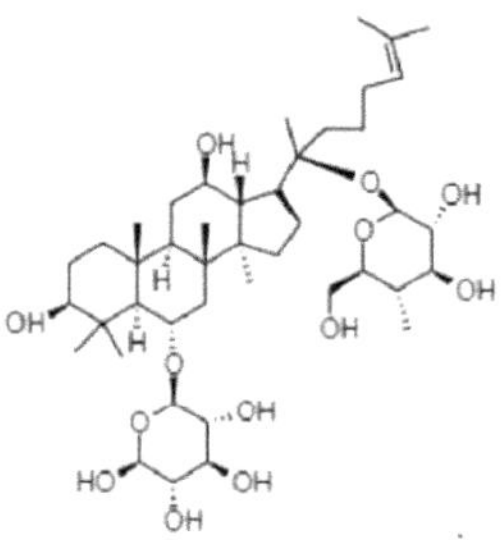

iv. Ginsenoside Rg1

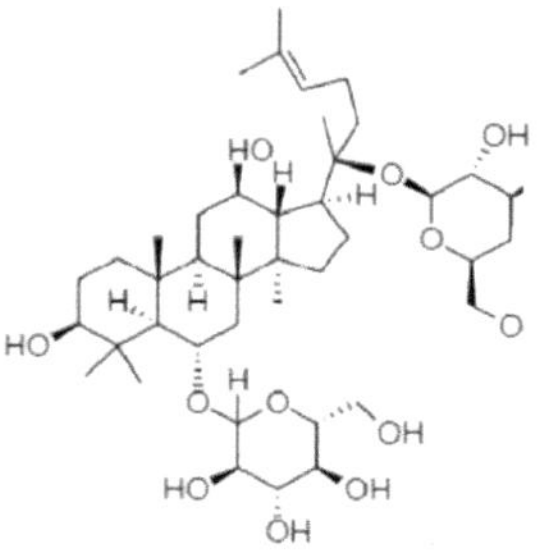

v.Ginsenosides

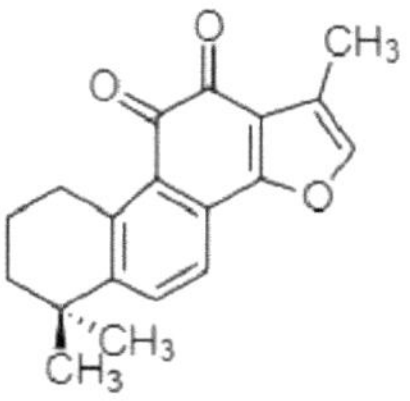

vi.Tanshinone

2.7.4 Alkaloids

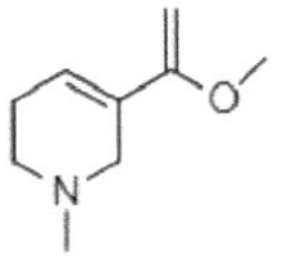

i. Arecoline

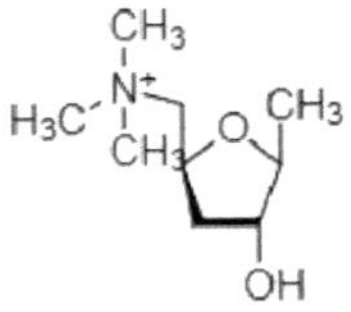

ii. Muscarine

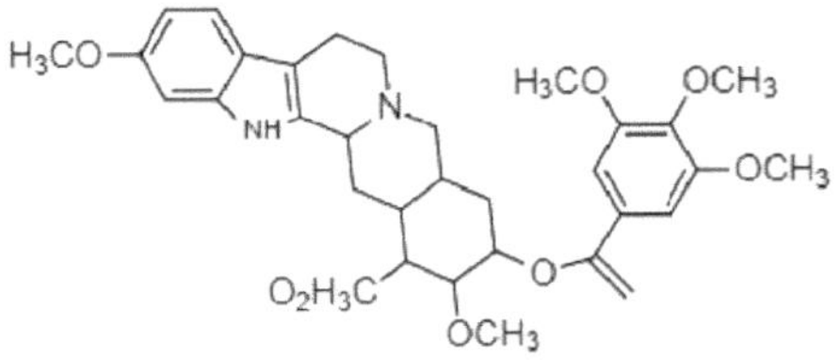

iii. Reserpine

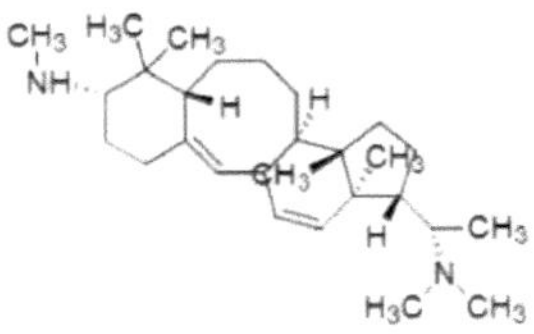

iv. Buxamine-B

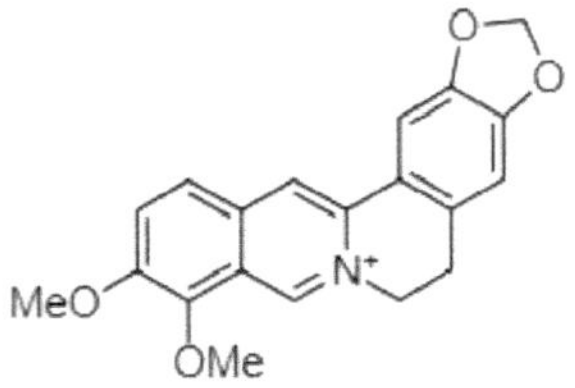

v. Berberine

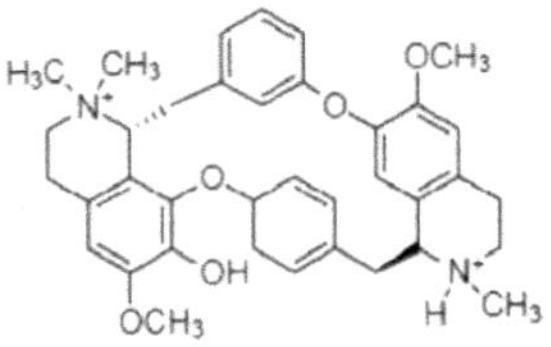

vi. Tubocurarine

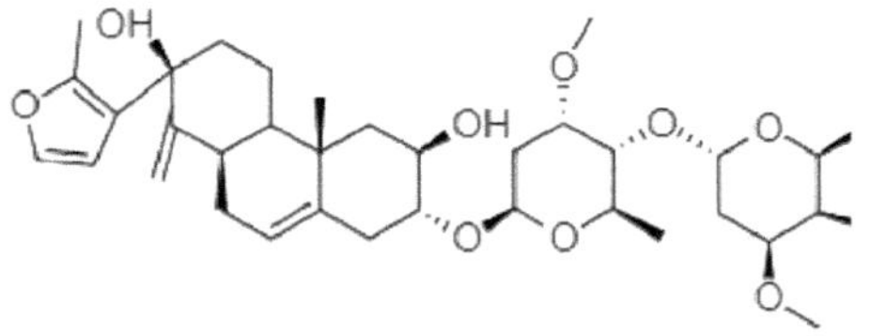

vii. Cynatroside B

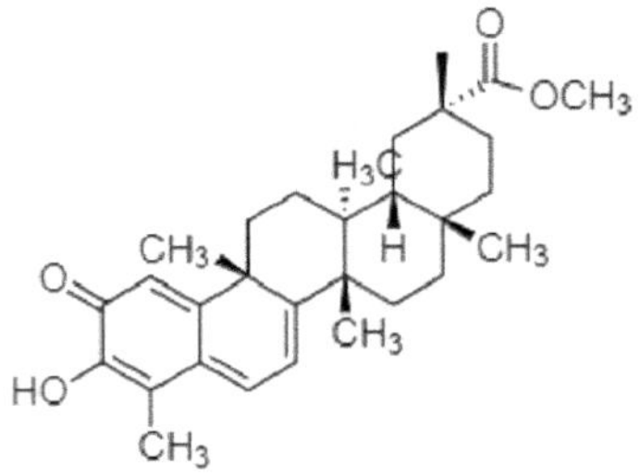

viii. Celastrine

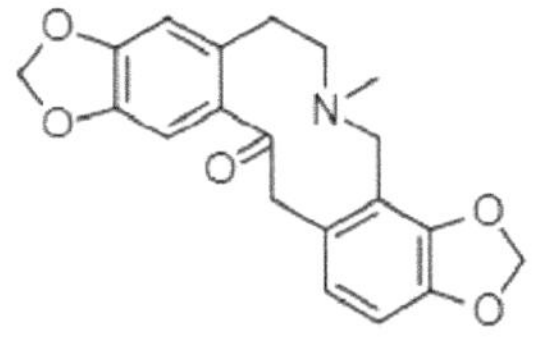

ix. Protopine

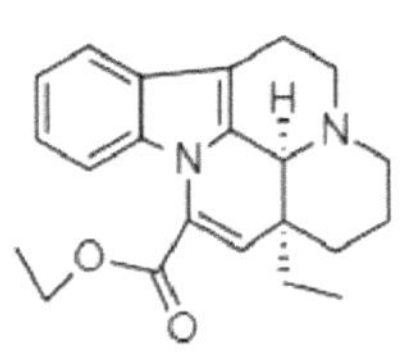

x. Vinpocetine

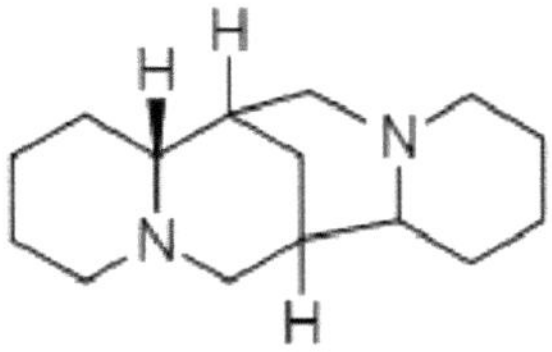

xi. Sparteine

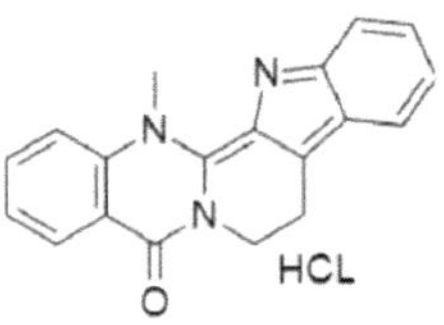

xii. Dehydroevodiamine hydrochloride

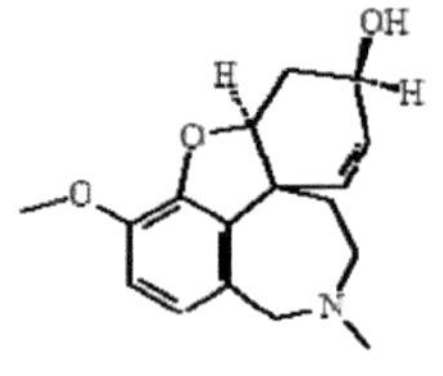

xiii. Galanthamine

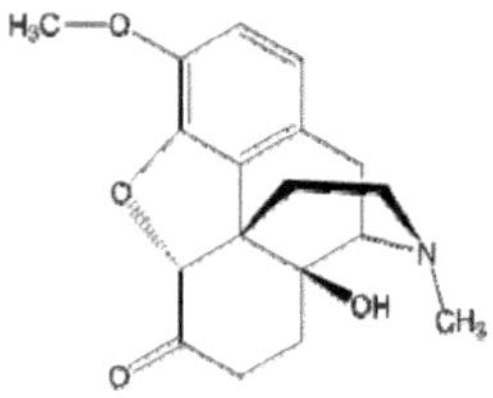

xiv. Huperzine A

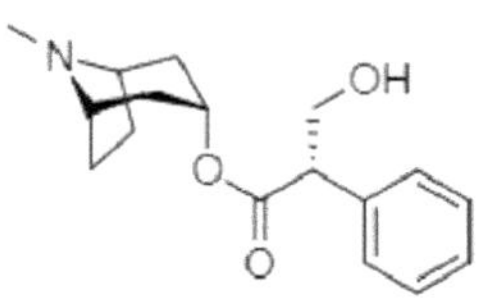

xv. Hyoscyamine

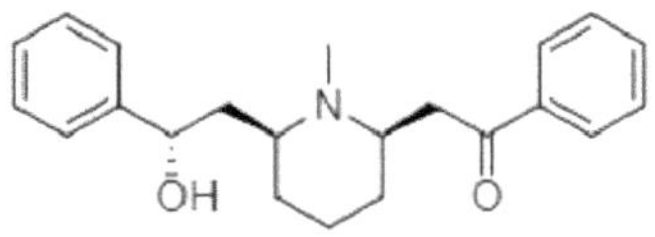

xvi. Lobeline

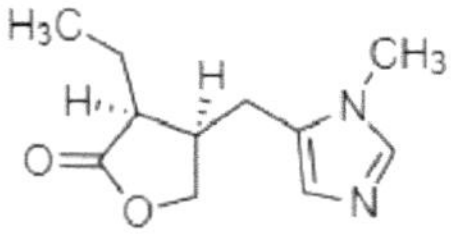

xvii.Pilocarapine

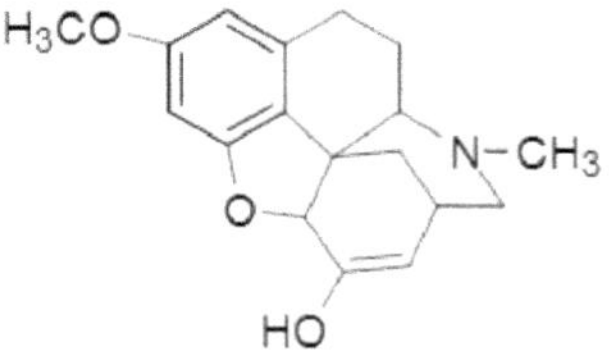

xviii.Codeine

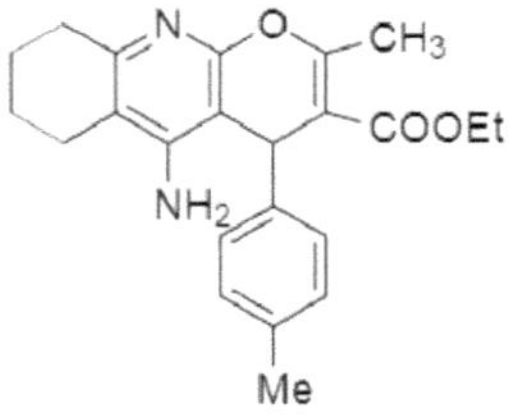

xix. Pyran derivative

2.7.5 Lignans and Lignin

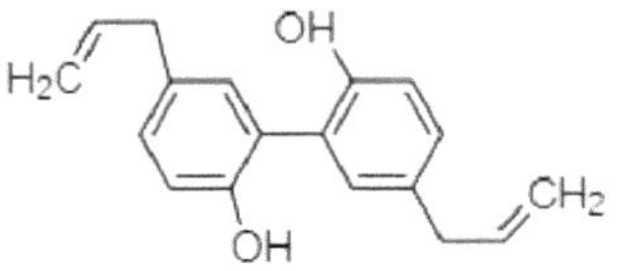

i. Magnolol

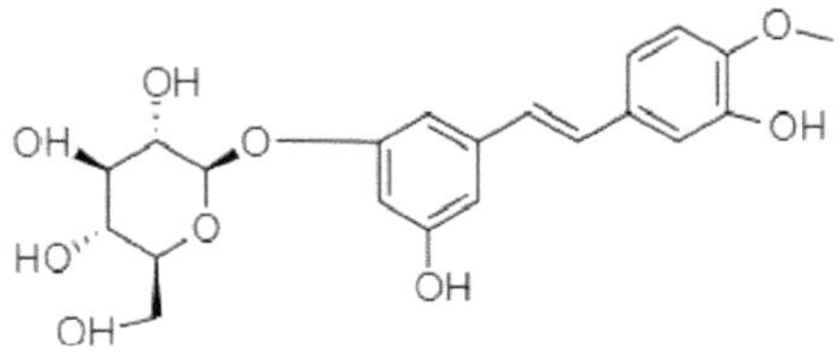

ii.Rhaponticin

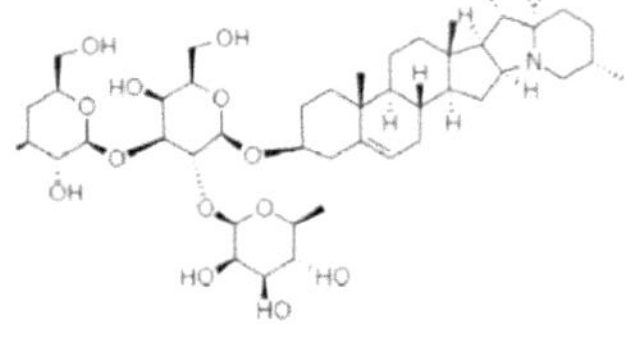

iii. α-Solanine

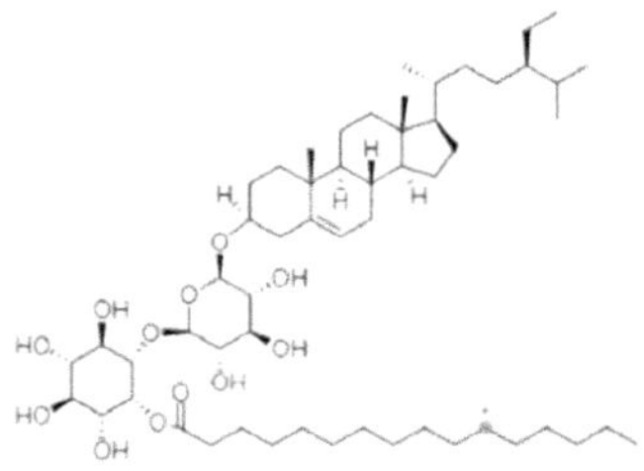

iv. Sitoindosides IX

2.7.6 Organic Compounds

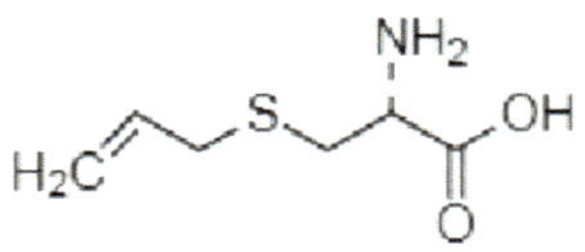

i. S-Allylcysteine

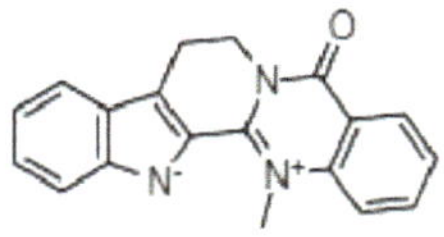

ii. Dehydroevodiamin

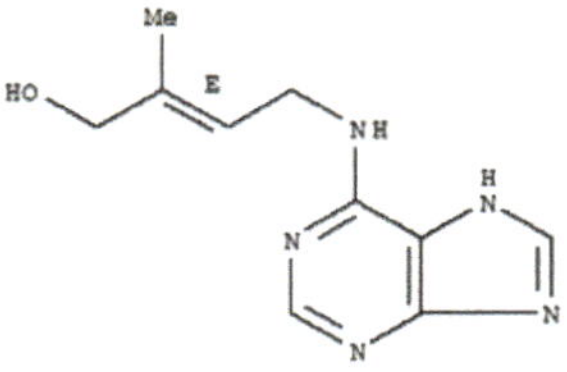

iii. Zeatin

2.8 FDA-APPROVED ANTI-ALZHEIMER'S PHYTOCOMPOUNDS

Currently, most of the drugs approved by the United States Food and Drug Administration (US-FDA) for the treatment of AD are acetylcholinesterase inhibitors (AChEi); for example, huperzine A, an alkaloid found in *Huperzia* spp., and galantamine, a natural alkaloid obtained from *Galanthus* spp., which is an acetylcholinesterase inhibitor commercialized as a dietary supplement for memory support, used to treat AD symptoms. The extent of reporting on the pathology of AD have made it important to identify the mechanism of disease and potential remedial targets. Current research is focused on the medicinal chemistry aspects of new natural products used for the treatment of AD (Salomone, 2011), including the mechanism and the molecular aspects, as well as new strategies for using natural products for AD treatment (Palafoxa et al., 2014) (Figures 2.3 and 2.4; Table 2.3).

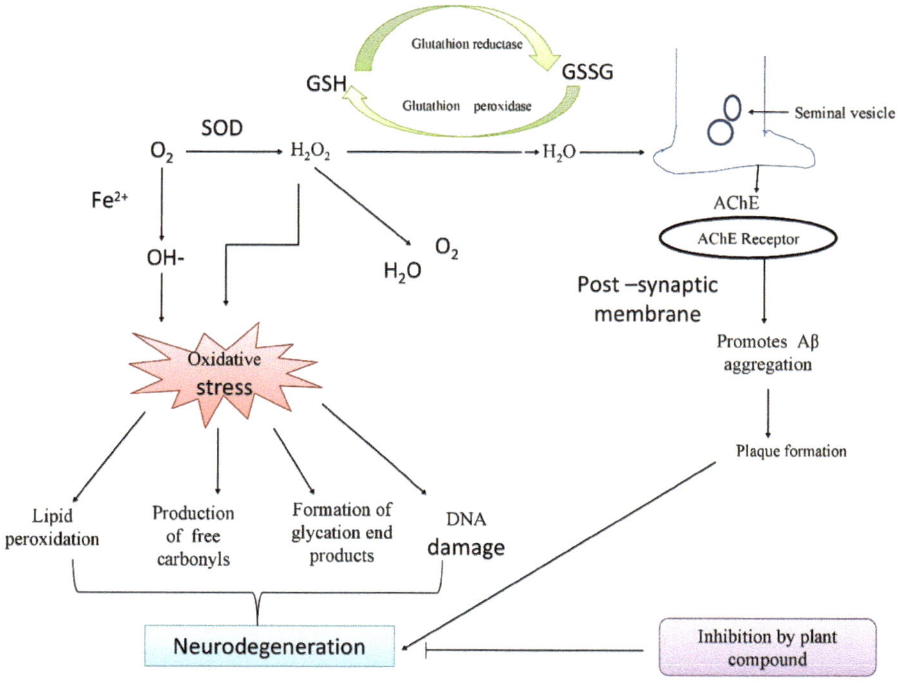

FIGURE 2.3 Mechanism of action of plant-derived compounds against AD (Syad and Devi, 2014).

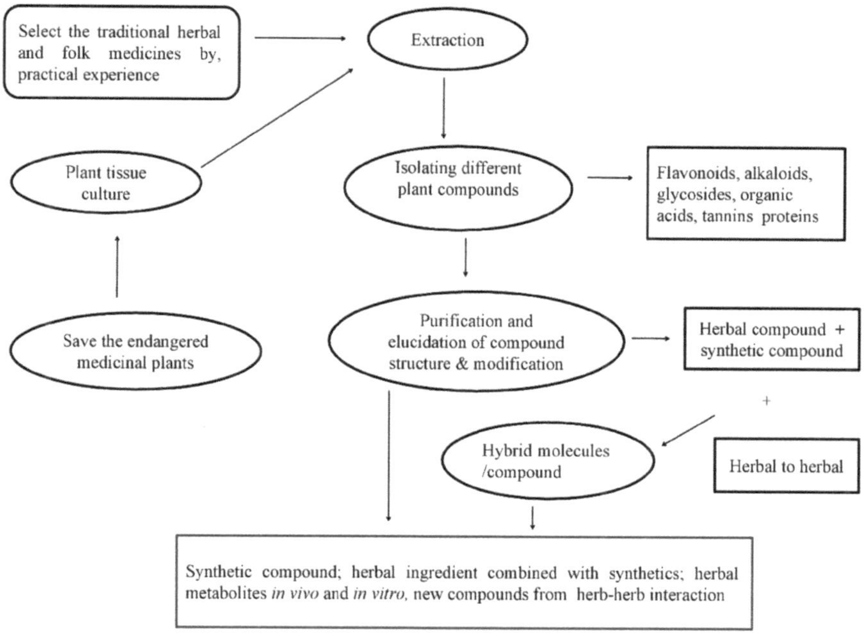

FIGURE 2.4 Recent approaches for drug discovery from herbal medicines (modified Pan et al., 2013).

2.9 LIMITATIONS OF HERBAL DRUGS

The approach of making use of herbal drugs as a different strategy for treating AD is growing nowadays, because of the inefficiency of conservative medicines and the side effects of synthetic drugs (Anand and Mahdi, 2014). But herbal drugs may also produce harsh side effects, such as hepatic failure, as a result of the use of highly concentrated preparations of herbal drugs, which leads to toxicity. Furthermore, (Kelley and Knopman, 2008). For AD, use of herbal drugs should have a wider range of targets like fibrillation, Aβ production, Aβ-mediated oxidative stress, and neuroinflammation (Izzo and Capasso, 2007). One other key limitation is the poor ability of many active principles to cross the BBB. The herbal drugs must reach the brain in the biologically active form to exert their positive effects. One of the most important challenges in developing therapeutic agents (herbal drugs) from natural products is obtaining the bioactive compounds in large enough quantities (Anekonda and Reddy, 2005). Some evidence shows that herbal drugs and their preparations are marketed without any close adherence to Good Manufacturing Practice (GMP) guidelines. Some external factors, like inconsistent environmental conditions at the cultivation site, may also affect the activity of herbal drug preparations. Hence, the use of herbal drugs by physicians and regulators should be performed with caution. Appropriate scientific evidence for the claimed clinical benefits should be mandatory worldwide, and the standards for production and safety monitoring should abide by established standards for chemically defined products (Kumar et al., 2017).

2.10 FUTURE PROSPECTS FOR PHYTOMEDICINES

Currently, FDA-approved drugs (donepezil, galantamine, rivastigmine) are available for the treatment of AD. These are suggestive and do not prevent the development of the AD disease (Herrmann, 2011). Herbal extracts contain one or two active principles. On the contrary, the holistic approach

TABLE 2.3
FDA-Approved Herbal Drugs

Sl.no	Plant Name	Active Compound	Biological Activity	Clinical Trials	FDA Approval (Year)	Reference
1.	*Physostigma venenosum*	Rivastigmine	Inhibits AChE in the cortex and hippocampus region.	-	2000	Mauricio et al., 2014; Bentham, 2014
2.	*Lycoris radiata*	Galantamine	Reversible inhibition of AChE and allosteric potentiation of nicotinic ACh receptors	-	2001	Mauricio et al., 2014
3.	*Cytisus laburnum*	Varenicline	Acetylcholine receptor	Phase 3	2006	Mauricio et al., 2014
4.	*Huperzia* spp.	Huperzine A	AChEi (acetylcholinesterase inhibitor) commercialized as a dietary supplement for memory support, used to treat AD symptoms in China.	Phase 3	-	Mauricio et al., 2014; Bentham, 2014
5.	*Curcuma longa*	Curcumin	Antiamyloidogenic, anti-inflammatory, antiChE, antiβ-secretase	Phase 3	-	Mauricio et al., 2014
6.	*Vitis vinifera*	Resveratrol	Prevents cognitive impairments and associated oxidative stress by reducing plaque formation	Phase 3	-	Mauricio et al., 2014
7.	*Astragalus membranaceus*	Cycloastragenol	Antiaging	-	2014	Mauricio et al., 2014

of multi-target therapy using multicomponent plant extracts, based on network interactions and synergy concepts, can be more effective.

Before the development of novel therapeutic drugs for AD treatment, the mechanisms underlying AD have to be thoroughly investigated. It is very important to understand the relationship between Aβ, AChE, and the tau proteins, and to build up successful modifications in anti-AD drugs. AD treatment is currently effective only in the preliminary stage of the disease. There are few AD drugs which have shown any benefits in middle stage of moderate AD (Galimberti and Scarpini, 2011; Hawes et al., 2013).

The expansion of remedial interventions for preventing AD has been hopeful, although numerous therapeutic drugs have proved to be unsuccessful at different stages of clinical trials. The lack of success is mostly attributed to the fact that the majority of these therapeutic drugs obstruct only one of the several pathways controlling AD. In other words, AD has a complex pathophysiology. AD involves the dysfunction of several different and key molecular pathways, and successful drug design must take into account the combination of multiple disease pathways. In addition to focusing on preventing Aβ and tau aggregation by using natural products, small molecules, and peptidomimetics, researchers have to focus on the growth of multifunctional drugs for AD patients. With such types of drug, AD patients must be capable of preventing Aβ and tau aggregation in the brain, inhibition of β- and α-secretase, and also inhibition of kinase activity. Presently targeting these enzymes (β- and α-secretase enzymes) has revealed some adverse side effects, which were attributed to their crucial role in various biological processes in the brain. Thus, we propose the design of molecular clamps that bind to the targeting sites, like APP and specific phosphorylation sites in Tau, and consequently avoid the undesirable specific activities of the enzymes. Such advanced designs of therapeutic drugs may yield potentially powerful therapeutic drugs for AD patients that may inhibit key enzymatic activity successfully without interfering with the other biological functions of the enzymes. The AD drugs which target the cholinergic system, inflammation, and enzyme inhibition systems have provided indicative relief, although AD drugs can be formulated in combination with multifunctional therapeutic drugs that target the pathology of AD. AD has complex molecular and pathophysiological mechanisms, and treatment is very limited in spite of the large amount of research literature available.

The actual cause and realistic molecular targets need to be discovered and validated on the basis of existing and new knowledge. We are hopeful that researchers will be able to discover multifunctional herbal drugs and develop successful diagnostic and therapeutic interventions for AD in the future.

2.11 CONCLUSIONS

Up to the 21st century, almost every known human civilization has been using herbal medicines as effective medications for the prevention and treatment of multiple health conditions, such as fever, skin infections, asthma, cancer, diabetes, aging, mental illness, and many more. It is primarily because of the general belief that herbal drugs are cheap, without any side effects, and freely available in nature, that they have attracted such interest over the millennia. Medicinal plants are rich in phytochemicals, which are likely to be flavonoids, polyphenols, alkaloids, lignans, sterols, tannins, etc. (Rao et al., 2012). Some medicinal plants with a strong therapeutic efficacy against AD have been investigated. These plants inhibit acetylcholinesterase (AChE) and oxidative stress-related damage, and are capable of protecting the affected neurons. Besides inhibiting AChE, these plants and their constituents also promote acetylcholine synthesis, that improves the ill effects associated with dementia (Jivad and Rabiei, 2014). As a consequence of increasing demand for herbal products, there are also rising concerns about the safety, standardization, efficacy, quality control, accessibility (Steinbach and Chen, 1995), and commercialization of herbal products by policymakers and health professionals, as well as by the common public. Obviously, there is an urgent need for coordinated efforts to conduct the necessary clinical trials to analyse the efficacy and safety of herbal medicines. The recent introduction of cutting-edge analytical techniques and research methodologies has resulted in evaluation and validation of herbal medicinal use according to the standard of modern drugs. Due to the incorporation of improved quality control and regulatory measures, it is foreseen that, in the near future, herbal medicine will be integrated into conventional medical systems, as the "herbal age is about to come" (Mohamed et al., 2012; Srivastava et al., 2016, 2019).

ACKNOWLEDGMENT

The authors are grateful to Mangalore University for the support provided.

REFERENCES

Abascal K and Yarnell E. Alzheimer's Disease. Part 2 – A Botanical Treatment Plan. *Alternative and Complementary Therapies* 2004; 10: 67–72.

Abbott A. Dementia. A Problem for Our Age. *Nature* 2011; 475: S2–S4. 10.1038/475s2a [Pubmed].

Abe F and Yamauchi T. Tanegosides A, B, and C. Lignan Glycosides from *Trachelospermum liukiuense*. *Chemical and Pharmaceutical Bulletin* 1990; 38(8): 2143–2145.

Agarwal NT, Shah RC, and Bennett DA. Alzheimer's Disease: Unique Markers for Diagnosis and New Treatment Modalities. *The Indian Journal of Medical Research* 2015; 142(4): 369–382.

Agrawal AD. Pharmacological Activities of Flavonoids. *A Review IJPSN* 2011; 4(2): 1394–1398.

Ahmad R, Taher SM, Low C, Noor NM, Sillapachaiyaporn C, Chuchawankul S, and Sarachana T. Polygonumins A, A Newly Isolated Compound from the Stem of *Polygonum Minus* Huds with Potential Medicinal Activities. *Scientific Report* 2018; (8): 4042.

Alagha K, Palot A, Sofalvi T, Pahus L, Gouitaa M, Celine T, et al. Long-Acting Muscarinic Receptor Antagonists for the Treatment of Chronic Airway Diseases. *Therapeutic Advances in Chronic Disease* 2014; 5(2): 85–98.

Ali AA, Ahmed HI, and Khaleel SA. Comparative Study on the Influence of Cocoa and/or Vinpocetine against Development of Alzheimer's Disease in Rats: Focus on Social Isolation Associated with Disease Progression. *Alzheimer's and Dementia* 2018; 13(7): 618.

Ali MH, Nesrine S, Hossam MA, and Salah R. Dine Protective Effects of Gingerol on Streptozotocin-Induced Sporadic Alzheimer's Disease: Emphasis on Inhibition of B-Amyloid, Cox-2, Alpha-, Beta-Secretases and Aph1a. *Scientific Report* 2017; (7): 2902.

Anand R, Gill KD, and Mahdi AA. Therapeutics of Alzheimer's Disease: Past, Present, and Future. *Neuropharmacology* 2014; 76: 27.

Anekonda TS and Reddy PH. Can Herbs Provide a New Generation of Drugs for Treating Alzheimer's Disease? *Brain Research Reviews* 2005; 50: 361–376.

Aniszewski T. *Alkaloids – Secrets of Life Book*. Elsevier, 2007.

Ansari M and Khodagholi F. Natural Products as Promising Drug Candidates for the Treatment of Alzheimer's Disease: Molecular Mechanism Aspect. *Current Neuropharmacology* 2013; 11(4): 414–429.

Aquilano K, Baldelli S, Rotilio G, and Ciriolo MR. Role of Nitric Oxide Synthases in Parkinson's Disease: A Review on the Antioxidant and Anti-Inflammatory Activity of Polyphenols. *Neurochemical Research* 2008; 33(12): 2416–2426.

Asa K, Wattmo C, and Minthon L. Galantamine Treatment in Alzheimer's Disease: Response and Long-term Outcome in a Routine Clinical Setting. *Neuropsychiatric Disease and Treatment* 2011; 7: 1–12.

Bais S, Kumari R, and Prashar Y. Ameliorative Effect of *Trans*-Sinapic Acid and Its Protective Role in Cerebral Hypoxia in Aluminium Chloride Induced Dementia of Alzheimer's Type. *CNS and Neurological Disorders Drug Targets* 2018; 17(2): 144–154.

Balez R, Steiner N, Engel M, Muñoz SS, Lum JS, Wu Y, and Wang D. Neuroprotective Effects of Apigenin against Inflammation, Neuronal excitability and Apoptosis in an induced Pluripotent Stem Cell Model of Alzheimer's Disease. *Scientific Report* 2016; 6: 31450.

Battineni JK, Koneti PK, Bakshi V, and Boggula N. Triterpenoids: A Review. *RJIF* 2018; 3(2): 91–96.

Bertram L and Tanzi RE. Thirty Years of Alzheimer's Disease Genetics: The Implications of Systematic Meta-Analyses. *Nature Reviews Neuroscience* 2008; 9: 768–778.

Bhattacharjee A. Anticholinesterase Potential of Phytoextracts and Their Bioactive Compounds: A Promising Therapeutic Agent Against Alzheimer's Disorder. *Tumor Research* 2018; 1(2): 84–88.

Bishayee A, Ahme S, Brankov N, and Perloff M. Triterpenoids as Potential Agents for the Chemoprevention and Therapy of Breast Cancer. *NIH Public Access* 2011; 1(16): 980–996.
Bossy-Wetzel E, Schwarzenbacher R, and Lipton SA. Molecular Pathways to Neuro Degeneration. *Nature Medicine* 2004; 10 Supplement: S2–S9.
Bribi N. Pharmacological Activity of Alkaloids: A Review. *Asian Journal of Botany* 2018; 8(1): 1–8.
Bui TT and Nguyen TH. Natural Product for the Treatment of Alzheimer's Disease. *Journal of Basic and Clinical Physiology and Pharmacology* 2017; 28(5): 413–423.
Canevari L and Clark JB. Alzheimer's Disease and Cholesterol: The Fat Connection. *Neurochemical Research* 2007; 32: 739–750.
Chao WW and Lin BF. Bioactivities of Major Constituents Isolated from *Angelica sinensis* (Danggui). *Chinese Medicine* 2011; 6: 29.
Chen JH, Lin KP, and Chen YC. Risk Factors for Dementia. *Journal of the Formosan Medical Association* 2009; 108: 754–764.
Chen L, Xin X, Zhang H, and Yuan Q. Phytochemical Properties and Antioxidant capacities of Commercial Raspberry Varieties. *Journal of Functional Foods* 2013; 5(1): 508–515.
Choi RJ, Roy A, Jung H, Ali MD, Min BS, Park CH, et al. BACE1 Molecular Docking and Anti-Alzheimer's Disease Activities of Ginsenosides. *Journal of Ethnopharmacology* 2016; 22(190): 219–230.
Chudzik M, Korzonek-Szlacheta I, and Wojciech K. Triterpenes as Potentially Cytotoxic Compounds. *Molecules* 2015; 20: 1610–1625.
Coelho F and Birks J. Physostigmine for Alzheimer's Disease. *Cochrane Database of Systematic Reviews* 2001; (2): Cd001499.
Corder EH, Saunder AM, Strittmatter WJ, Schmechel DE, Gaskell PC, Small GW, et al. Gene Dose of Apo Lipoprotein E Type 4 Allele and The Risk of Alzheimer's Disease in Late Onset Families. *Science Magazine* 1993; 261: 921–923.
Crozier A, Jaganath IB, and Clifford MN. Phenols, Polyphenols, and Tannins: An Overview. *CROZ: "Chap01"* 2006; 4(25): 26–18.
Daly JW. Nicotinic Agonists, Antagonists, and Modulators from Natural Sources. *Cellular and Molecular Neurobiology* 2005; 25(3): 513–552.
De La Monte SM and Wands JR. Review of Insulin and Insulin-Like Growth Factor Expression, Signalling, and Malfunction in the Central Nervous System: Relevance to Alzheimer's Disease. *Journal of Alzheimer's Disease* 2005; 7: 45–61.
Decker MW, Majchrzak MJ, and Arnerić SP. Effects of Lobeline, A Nicotinic Receptor Agonist, on Learning and Memory. *Pharmacology Biochemistry & Behavior* 1993; 45(3): 571–576.
Deka P, Kumar A, Nayak BK, and Eloziia N. Some Plants as a Source of Acetyl Cholinesterase Inhibitors: A Review. *International Research Journal of Pharmacy* 2017; 8(5): 5–13.
Du GH and Zhang JT. Protective Effects of Salvianolic Acid A Against Impairment of Memory Induced by Cerebral Ischemia-Reperfusion in Mice. *Acta Pharmaceutica Sinica* 1995; 30(3): 184–190.
Dzubak P, Hajduch M, Vydra D, Hustova A, Kvasnica AM, Biedermann D, et al. Pharmacological Activities of Natural Triterpenoids and their Therapeutic Implications. *Natural Product Reports* 2005; 22: 487.
Esposito E, Impellizzeri D, Mazzon E, Paterniti I, and Cuzzocrea S. Neuroprotective Activities of Palmitoylethanolamide in an Animal Model of Parkinson's Disease. *PLoS One* 2012; 7(8): e41880.
Evans M. *A Guide to Herbal Remedies.* Orient Paperbacks, New Delhi, India, 1994.
Fanny CF, Ip AD, Pong Y, Ng HJ, Dai AAY, Pang ACHA, et al. *Cycloastragenolis* a Potent Telomerase Activator in Neuronal Cells: Implications for Depression Management. *Neurosignals* 2014; 22: 52–63.
Ferdousy S, Rahman MA, Al-Amin MM, Aklima J, and Chowdhury JKH. Antioxidative and Neuroprotective Effects of *Leea macrophylla* Methanol Root Extracts on Diazepam-Induced Memory Impairment in Amnesic Wistar Albino Rat. *Clinical Phytoscience* 2016; 2(1): 17.
Galimberti D and Scarpini E. Disease-Modifying Treatments for Alzheimer's Disease. *Therapeutic Advances in Neurological Disorders* 2011; 4: 203–216.
Gokare AR and Akula R. *Serotonin and Melatonin: Their Functional Role in Plants, Food, Phytomedicine, and Human Health.* Taylor & Francis, CRC Press, USA, 2010, p. 582. ISBN 9781498739054 – CAT# K26621.
Han N and Bakovic M. Biologically Active Triterpenoids and Their Cardio-Protective and Anti-Inflammatory Effects. *Journal of Bioanalysis & Biomedicine* 2015; 01: S12.
Hawes UW, Abou El-Kassem LT, Awad HM, and Taie HAA. Anti-Alzheimer, Antioxidant Activities and Flavonol Glycosides of *Eryngium campestre* L. *Current Chemical Biology* 2013; 7: 188–195.

Heo HJ, Hong SC, Cho HY, Hong B, Kim HK, Kim EK, and Shin DH. Inhibitory Effect of Zeatin, Isolated from *Fiatoua villosa*, on Acetylcholinesterase Activity from Pcl2 Cells. *Molecular Cells* 2002; 13(1): 113–117.

Herrmann N, Chau S, Kircanski I, and Lanctôt K. Current and Emerging Drug Treatment Options for Alzheimer's Disease: A Systematic Review. *Drugs* 2011; 71: 2031–2065.

Houghton PJ and Howes MJ. Natural Products and Derivatives Affecting Neurotransmission Relevant to Alzheimer's and Parkinson's Disease. *Neurosignals* 2005; 14: 6–22.

Howes MJ, Perry NS, and Houghton PJ. Plants with Traditional Uses and Activities, Relevant to the Management of Alzheimer's Disease and Other Cognitive Disorders. *Phytotherapy Research* 2003; 17: 1–18.

Iriti M, Vitalini S, Fico G, and Faoro F. Neuroprotective Herbs and Foods from Different Traditional Medicines and Diets. *Molecules* 2010; 15: 3517–3555.

Izzo AA and Capasso F. Herbal Medicines to Treat Alzheimer's Disease. *Trends in Pharmacological Sciences* 2007; 28(2): 47.

Jae SC, Nurul MD, Ali Y, Kim YM, Park HJ, Sohn HS, et al. The Effects of C-Glycosylation of Luteolin on its Antioxidant, Anti-Alzheimer's Disease, Anti-Diabetic, and Anti-Inflammatory Activities. *Archives of Pharmacal Research* 2014; 37(10): 1354–1363.

Jivad N and Rabiei Z. A Review Study on Medicinal Plants Used in the Treatment of Learning and Memory Impairments. *Asian Pacific Journal of Tropical Medicine* 2014; 4(10): 780–789.

Kaur R and Arora S. Alkaloids – Important Therapeutic Secondary Metabolites of Plant Origin. *Journal of Critical Reviews* 2018; 2(3): 1–8.

Kelley BJ and Knopman DS. Alternative Medicine and Alzheimer's Disease. *Neurologist* 2008; 14: 299.

Kennedy DO and Wightman EL. Herbal Extracts and Phytochemicals. Plant Secondary Metabolites and the Enhancement of Human Brain Function. *Advances in Nutrition* 2011; 2: 32–50.

Khan H. Brilliant Future of Phytomedicines in the Light of Latest Technological Developments. *The Journal of Phytopharmacology* 2015; 4(1): 58–60.

Khan MSA and Ahmad I. Herbal Medicine: Current Trends and Future Prospects. *New Look to Phytomedicine*, 2019. doi:10.1016/B978-0-12-814619-4.00001-X.

Kim CS, Subedi L, Choi SY, Kim KH, and Lee KR. Lignan Glycosides from the Twigs of *Chaenomeles sinensis* and Their Biological Activities. *Journal of Natural Products* 2015; 78(5): 1174–1178.

Kim MH, Kim SH, and Yang WM. Mechanisms of Action of Phytochemicals from Medicinal Herbs in the Treatment of Alzheimer's Disease. *Planta Medica* 2014; 80: 1249–1258.

Kim SR, Hwang SY, Jang YP, Park MJ, Markelonis GJ, Oh TH, and Kim YC. Protopine from Corydalis Ternata has Anticholinesterase and Antiamnesic Activities. *Planta Medica* 1999; 65(03): 218–221. https://doi.org/10.1055/s-1999-13983

Kim SR, Hwang SY, Pyo Y, Park MJ, and Hawan GT. Coumarins Isolated from *Angelica gigas* Inhibit Acetylcholinesterase: Structure–Activity Relationships. *Journal of Natural Products* 2001; 64(5): 683–685.

Kolarova M, Ia-Sierra FG, Janricny A, and Band RD. Structure and Pathology of Tau Protein in Alzheimer Disease. *International Journal of Alzheimer's Disease* 2012; 2012: 13.

Kumar A, Singh A, and Agarwal A. Therapeutic Potentials of Herbal Drugs for Alzheimer's Disease – An Overview. *Indian Journal of Experimental Biology* 2017; 55: 63–73.

Kumar GP and Khanum F. Neuroprotective Potential of Phytochemicals. *Pharmacognosy Reviews* 2012;6(12): 81.

Kumar S and Pandey AK. Chemistry and Biological Activities of Flavonoids: An Overview. *The Scientific World Journal* 2013; 2013: 16.

Kumar V. Potential Medicinal Plants for CNS Disorders: An Overview. *Phytotherapy Research* 2006; 20: 1023–1035.

Lazarov O, Robinson J, Tang YP, Hairston IS, Korade-Mirnics Z, Lee VM, et al. Environmental Enrichment Reduces Amyloid Beta Levels and Amyloid Deposition in Transgenic Mice. *Cell* 2005; 120: 701–713.

Lee KY, Yoon JS, Kim E, Kang SY, and Kim YC. Anti-Ache and Anti-Amnesic Activities of a Preganane Glycoside, Cynatroside B from *Cynanchum atratum*. *Planta Medica* 2005; 71: 7–11.

Lee M, Yuk DY, Kim TI, Kim YH, Kim KI, Kim KH, et al. Protective Effect of The Ethanol Extract of *Magnolia officinalis* and 4-*O*-Methylhonokiol on Scopolamine-Induced Memory Impairment and the Inhibition of Acetylcholinesterase Activity. *Journal of Natural Medicines* 2009; 63(3): 274–282.

Leslie TND. *Plant Based Drugs and Medicines*. Raintree Nutrition, 2000.

Li J, Wang G, Liu J, Zhou L, Dong M, Wang R, et al. Puerarin attenuates Amyloid-Beta-Induced Cognitive Impairment through Suppression of apoptosis In Rat Hippocampus *In Vivo*. *The European Journal of Pharmacology* 2010; 649(1–3): 195–201.

Lily YL, Changa B, Lowea J, Ardilesc A, Lima J, Angus C, et al. Alzheimer's Disease in The Human Eye. Clinical Tests That Identify Ocular and Visual Information Processing Deficit as Biomarkers. *Alzheimer's & Dementia* 2013; 10: 1–11.

Lin D, Xiao M, Zhao J, Li Z, Xing B, Li X, et al. An Overview of Plant Phenolic Compounds and Their Importance in Human Nutrition and Management of Type 2 Diabetes. *Molecules* 2016; 15(10): 21. Pii: E1374(Pub-Med).

Lin HY, Chang TC, and Chang ST. A Review of Antioxidant and Pharmacological Properties of Phenolic Compounds in Acacia Confuse. *Journal of Traditional and Complementary Medicine* 2018; 8: 1–8.

Liu JB, Zhou L, Zhongwang Y, Wang X, Zhou Y, Zhe W, et al. Neuroprotective Activity of (–)-Epigallocatechin Gallate Against Lipopolysaccharide-Mediated Cytotoxicity. *Journal of Immunology* 2016; 4962351. doi:10.1155/2016/4962351.

Mandel EM and Andelkow K. Tau Protein and Alzheimer's Disease. *Neurobiology of Aging* 1994; 15: 585–586.

Manyam BV. Dementia in Ayurveda. *The Journal of Alternative and Complementary Medicine* 1999; 5: 81–88.

Mishra LC, Singh BB, and Dagenais S. Scientific C. Basis for the Therapeutic Use of *Withania somnifera* (*Ashwagandha*): A Review. *Alternative Medicine Review* 2000; 5: 334–346.

Misiti F, Martorana GE, Nocca G, Di Stasio E, Giardina B, and Clementi ME. Methionine 35 Oxidation Reduces Toxic and Pro-Apoptotic Effects of the Amyloid B-Protein Fragment (31–35) on Isolated Brain Mitochondria. *Neuroscience* 2004; 126: 297–303.

Mohamed A, Shuid B, Borhanuddin N, and Fozi A. The Application of Phytomedicine in Modern Drug Development. *The Internet Journal of Herbal and Plant Medicine* 2012; 1(2): 1–9.

Mosihuzzaman M and Choudhary MI. Protocols on Safety, Efficacy, Standardization, and Documentation of Herbal Medicine. *Pure and Applied Chemistry* 2008; 80(10): 2195–2230.

Nana DU, Liu Y, Zhang X, Jixia W, He JJ, and Zhou H. Discovery of New Muscarinic Acetylcholine Receptor Antagonists from *Scopolia tangutica. Scientific Report* 2017; 7: 460–467.

Nday CM, Eleftheriadou D and Jackson G. Shared Pathological Pathways of Alzheimer's Disease with Specific Comorbidities: Current Perspectives and Interventions. *Journal of Neurochemistry* 2018; 144(4): 360–389. https://doi.org/10.1111/jnc.14256

Ohta H, Ni JW, Matsumoto K, Watanabe H, and Shimizu M. Paeony and Its Major Constituent, Paeoniorin Improve Radial Maze Performance Impaired by Scopolamine in Rats. *Pharmacology Biochemistry & Behavior* 1993; 45: 719–723.

Oksana S, Marian B, Rai M, and Bol SH. Plant Phenolic Compounds for Food, Pharmaceutical and Cosmetics Production. *Journal of Medicinal Plants Research* 2012; 6(13): 2526–2539.

Padma Kumar A, Sharma BA, and Bakshi N. Biological Activity of Alkaloids from *Solanum dulcamara* L. *Natural Product Research* 2009; 23(8), 20: 719–723.

Palafoxa MA, Morenob PP, Ortuñosorianob CI, José L, Cerroc PD, Rincónc CM, et al. Research Strategies Developed for The Treatment of Alzheimer's Disease. Chapter 8. Published by Elsevier Inc. All Rights Reserved. *Frontiers in Drug Design & Discovery* 2014; 6(3): 426–477.

Pan SY, Zhou SF, Gao SH, Yu ZL, Zhang SF, Tang MK, et al. New Perspectives on How to Discover Drugs from Herbal Medicines: CAM's Outstanding Contribution to Modern Therapeutics. *Evidence-Based Complementary and Alternative Medicine* 2013; 2013(1): 627375.

Panche AN, Diwan AD, and Chandra SR. Flavonoids: An Overview. *Journal of Nutritional Science* 2016; 5(47): 1–15.

Panossian AG. Trends in Phytomedicine and Phytotherapy Research: From Traditional Herbal Medicine to Novel Pharmaceuticals Based on the Synergy Concept. *Clinical and Experimental Pharmacology* 2016; 6(Suppl): 2. doi:10.4172/2161-1459.C1.011.

Papandreou MA, Kanakis CD, Polissiou MG, Efthimiopoulos S, Cordopatis P, Margarity M, and Lamari F. Inhibitory Activity on Amyloid-β Aggregation and Antioxidant Properties of *Crocus sativus* Stigmas Extract and its Crocin Constituents. *Journal of Agricultural and Food Chemistry* 2006; 54: 8762–8768.

Parmar SK, Sharma TP, Airao VB, Bhatt R, Aghara R, Chavda S, Rabadiya SO, and Gangwal AP. Neuropharmacological Effects of Triterpenoids. *Phytopharmacology* 2013; 4(2): 354–372.

Paula A, Murraya B, Belén M, Faraonia C, Castroa MJ, and Cavallaro NPA. Natural AChe Inhibitors from Plants and Their Contribution to Alzheimer's Disease Therapy. *Current Neuropharmacology* 2013; 11: 388–413.

Perry EK, Pickering AT, Wang WW, Houghton PT, and Perry NSL. Medicinal Plants and Alzheimer's Disease: From Ethnobotany to Phytotherapy. *Journal of Pharmacy and Pharmacology* 1999; 51: 527–534.

Peters R, Peters J, Warner J, Beckett N, and Bulpitt C. Alcohol, Dementia and Cognitive Decline in the Elderly: A Systematic Review. Oxford University Press on Behalf of The British Geriatrics Society. *Age Ageing* 2008; 37: 505–512.

Peterson J, Dwyer J, Adlercreutz H, Scalbert A, Jacques P, and Mccullough ML. Dietary Lignans: Physiology and Potential for Cardiovascular Disease Risk Reduction. *Nutrition Reviews* 2015; 68(10): 571–603.

Pratap GK, Ashwini S, and Manjula S. Alzheimer's Disease: A Challenge in its Management with Certain Medicinal Plants – A Review. *International Journal of Pharmaceutical Sciences & Research* 2017; 8(12): 4960–4972.

Pravina K, Ravindra KR, Goudar KS, Vinod DR, Joshua AJ, Wasim P, et al. Safety Evaluation of Becoming in Healthy Volunteers: A Phase I Study. *Phytomedicine* 2007; 14: 301–308.

Qiu WQ and Folstein FM. Insulin, Insulin-Degrading Enzyme and Amyloid-B Peptide in Alzheimer's Disease: Review and Hypothesis. *Neurobiology of Aging* 2006; 27: 190–198.

Ramakrishna A, Giridhar P, and Ravishankar GA. Phytoserotonin: A Review. *Plant Signaling & Behavior* 2011; 6: 800–809.

Ramakrishna A, Giridhar P, Udaya Sankar K, and Ravishankar GA. Melatonin and Serotonin Profiles in Beans of *Coffea* spp. *Journal of Pineal Research* 2012; 52: 470–476.

Rao BV, Srikumar BN, and Rao, BSS. Herbal Remedies to Treat Anxiety Disorders. In: *Different Views of Anxiety Disorders*. InTech, 2011. doi:10.5772/23511.

Rao RV, Descamps O, Varghese J, and Bredesen DE. Ayurvedic Medicinal Plants for Alzheimer's Disease: A Review. *Alzheimer's Research & Therapy* 2012; 4: 22.

Reddy PH and Beal MF. Are Mitochondria Critical in The Pathogenesis of Alzheimer's Disease? *Brain Research Reviews* 2005; 49: 618–632.

Richard F and Amouyel P. Genetic Susceptibility Factors for Alzheimer's Disease. *European Journal of Pharmacology* 2001; 412(1): 1–12.

Rinaldia MVN, Díazb IEC, Suffredinib IB, and Morenoc PRH. Alkaloids and Biological Activity of Beribá (*Annona hypoglauca*). *Revista Brasileira De Farmacognosia* 2017; 27: 77–83.

Rodgers AB. *Alzheimer's Disease: Unravelling the Mystery*. U.S. Department of Health and Human Services, NIH Publication #: 08-3782, 2008.

Seiguer E. *Alzheimer's Disease: Research Advances and Medical Reality*. Commonwealth Fund Pub., 2005. https://Www.Cmwf.Org.

Selamoglu Z. Polyphenolic Compounds in Human Health with Pharmacological Properties. *Journal of Traditional Medicine and Clinical Naturopathy* 2017; 6: 4.

Selkoe DJ. Alzheimer's Disease: Genes, Proteins, and Therapy. *Physiological Reviews* 2001; 81: 741–766.

Sen S, Chakraborty R, Sridhar C, Reddy Y, and De B. Free Radicals, Antioxidants, Diseases and Phytomedicines: Current Status and Future Prospect. *International Journal of Pharmaceutical Sciences Review and Research* 2010; 3(1): 91–100.

Sharma DK. Pharmacological Properties of Flavonoids Including Flavonolignans – Integration of Petrocrops with Drug Development from Plants. *Journal of Scientific & Industrial Research* 2006; 65: 477–484.

Shashank D, Rajendra SV, and Anamika M. An Overview of Phytoconstituents and Pharmacological Activities of *Celastrus paniculatus*. *World Journal of Pharmaceutical Research* 2017; 16(4): 307.

Sigurd D, Samantha S, Reiberb H, and Tumania H. Tau Protein in Cerebrospinal Fluid (CSF): A Blood CSF Barrier Related Evaluation in Patients with Various Neurological Diseases. *Neuroscience Letters* 2001; 300: 95–98.

Singh AK, Gupta A, Mishra AK, Gupta V, Bansal P, and Kumar S. Review on Medicinal Plant for Curing Alzheimer's Disease. *International Journal of Pharmaceutical & Biological Archives* 2010; 1(2): 108–114.

Singh N, Pandey BR, and Verma P. An Overview of Phytotherapeutic Approach in Prevention and treatment of Alzheimer's Syndrome & Dementia. *International Journal of Pharmaceutical Sciences and Drug Research* 2011; 3(3): 162–172.

Singhal AK, Naithani V, and Bangar OP. Medicinal Plants with a Potential to Treat Alzheimer and Associated Symptoms. *International Journal of Nutrition, Pharmacology, Neurological Diseases* 2012; 2(2): 84–91.

Soheili M and Taviranand Salami M. Clearance of Amyloid Beta Plaques from Brain of Alzheimeric Rats by *Lavandula angustifolia*. *Neuroscience & Medicine* 2012; 3: 362–367.

Soncrant TT, Raffaele KC, Asthana S, Berardi A, Morris PP, and Haxby JV. Memory Improvement Without Toxicity During Chronic, Low Dose Intravenous Arecoline In Alzheimer's Disease. *Psychopharmacology* 1993; 112: 421–427.

Srivastava P and Yadav RS. Efficacy of Natural Compounds in Neurodegenerative Disorders. In: *The Benefits of Natural Products for Neurodegenerative Diseases*. Springer, 2016, pp. 107–123.

Steinbach JH and Chen Q. Antagonist and Partial Agonist Actions of D-Tubocurarine at Mammalian Muscle Acetylcholine Receptors. *Journal of Neuroscience* 1995; 15(11): 230–240 (Pub-Med).

Subash S, Essa MM, Al-Adawi S, Memon MA, Manivasagam T, and Akbar M. Neuroprotective Effects of Berry Fruits on Neurodegenerative Diseases. *Neural Regeneration Research* 2014; 9(16): 15–57.

Syad AN and Devi KP. Botanics: a potential source of new therapies for Alzheimer's disease? Dove Medical Press is a member of the OAI. *Botanics: Targets and Therapy* 2014; 4: 11–26.

Tanzi RE and Bertram L. Twenty Years of the Alzheimer's Traditional Disease States: Menopause. *American Family Physician* 2005; 66: 129–134.

Tewari D, Stankiewicz AM, Mocan A, Sah AN, Nikolay T, Huminiecki L, et al. Ethnopharmacological Approaches for Dementia Therapy and Significance of Natural Products and Herbal Drugs. *Frontiers in Aging Neuroscience* 2018; 10: 3.

Tungmunnithum D, Thongboonyou A, Pholboo A, and Yangsabai A. Flavonoids and Other Phenolic Compounds from Medicinal Plants for Pharmaceutical and Medical Aspects: An Overview. *Medicines* 2018; 5: 93.

Vyawahare N, Ambikar D, Patil G, Kamble P, and Chitte N. Phytomedicines for Neuroprotection. *Electronic Journal of Pharmacology and Therapy* 2008; 1: 15.

Wang H, Wang H, Cheng H, and Cheng Z. Ameliorating Effect of Luteolin on Memory Impairment in an Alzheimer's Disease Model. *Molecular Medicine Reports* 2016; 13(5): 4215–4220.

Wang X, Kim JR, Lee SB, Kim YJ, Jung MY, Kwon HW, et al. Effects of Curcuminoids Identified in Rhizomes of *Curcuma longa* On Bace-1 Inhibitory and Behavioral Activity and Lifespan of Alzheimer's Disease Drosophila Models. *Complementary and Alternative Medicine* 2014; 14: 88.

Wang YT and Bi QLIK. Bioactive Flavonoids in Medicinal Plants: Structure, Activity and Biological Fate. *Asian Journal of Pharmaceutical Science* 2018; 13: 12–23.

Wink M. Modes of Action of Herbal Medicines and Plant Secondary Metabolites. *Medicines* 2010; 2(3): 251–286.

Wirasathien L, Boonarkart C, Pengsuparp T, and Suttisri R. Biological Activities of Alkaloids from *Pseuduvaria setosa*. *Pharmaceutical Biology* 2006; 44(4): 274–278.

Yina F, JianhuiLiua B, Xiuhong J, Wang YB, Zidichouskib J, and Silibinin JZ. A Novel Inhibitor of a Beta Aggregation. *Neurochemistry International* 2011; 58: 399–403.

Yoo KY and Park SY. Terpenoids as Potential Anti-Alzheimer's Disease. *Therapeutics Molecules* 2012; 17(3): 3524–3538.

Zhao C, Nagatsu AB, Hatano BK, Shirai N, Kato BS, and Ogihara Y. New Lignan Glycosides from Chinese Medicinal Plant, *Sinopodophillum emodi*. *Chemical and Pharmaceutical Bulletin* 2003; 51(3): 255–261.

Zhoua YQ, Li BW, Xua L, and Chen L. *Salvia miltiorrhiza* Phenolic Acids Possess Protective Properties Against Amyloid-Induced Cytotoxicity, Tanshinones Act as Acetylcholinesterase Inhibitors. *Environmental Toxicology and Pharmacology* 2011; 31: 443–452.

Zurita R, Palomares FR, Salguero EG, Peragón L, Medina J, Parra P, et al. Maslinic Acid, A Natural Triterpene, Induces A Death Receptor-Mediated Apoptotic Mechanism in Caco-2 P53-Deficient Colon Adenocarcinoma Cells. *PloS One* 2016; 31: 16.

3 Phytotherapeutic Potential For the Treatment of Alzheimer's Disease

Muhammad Akram, Atanu Bhattacharjee, Naveed Munir, Naheed Akhter, Fozia Anjum, Abida Parveen, Samreen Gul Khan, Muhammad Daniyal, Muhammad Riaz, Fahad Said Khan, Rumaisa Ansari, and Umme Laila

CONTENTS

ABBREVIATIONS

AD	Alzheimer's Disease
ADAS	Alzheimer Disease Assessment Scale
βAPP	Beta-Amyloid Precursor Protein
CDR-SB	Clinical Dementia Rating-Sum of the Boxes
CNS	Central Nervous System
COX-1	Cyclooxygenase-1
GLUT-1	Glucose Transporter-1

3.1 INTRODUCTION

Alzheimer's disease (AD) is defined as a profound loss of memory that may disturb a person's occupational and social life, or even the simple daily tasks. AD was first described by German physician Alois Alzheimer in 1906. It occurs mostly in old age, and 50–60% cases of dementia present with AD (Francis, Palmer et al. 1999). It affects 5% of the population, according to the Center for Disease Control and Prevention. AD is a condition in which the patient presents with episodes of memory loss and it leads to dementia. This occurs because the temporal lobe of the brain becomes atrophied, after it has spread to the frontal, temporal and parietal lobes completely (Klunk, Engler et al. 2004). In the brain, amyloid-beta neuritic plaques are found with neurofibrillary tangles, and amyloid-beta protein also accumulates in vessels of the cortex and meninges (Perl 2010). AD is a neurodegenerative, progressive, and multifactorial disorder that occurs largely in old age, with 50–60% of cases of AD occurring in patients over 65 years of age (Francis, Palmer et al. 1999; Adams, Gmünder et al. 2007). A decrease in the level of neurotransmitter chemical acetylcholine, due to neural degeneration, is a neuro-pathological feature (Howes and Houghton 2003; Zhang 2004). AD occurs in both sporadic and familial forms. Mutations occur in the genes encoding amyloid precursor proteins and presenilin 1 and 2 (Selkoe 2001). The familial disease consists of 2–3% cases of AD (Selkoe and Schenk 2003), whereas sporadic AD occurs in the majority of elderly patients with AD aged above 65 years, and the cause is unknown (Selkoe 2001). The sporadic disease is associated with many factors, including aging (Selkoe 2001), defects in mitochondria (Bertram and Tanzi 2008), and diabetes mellitus (Reddy, Mani et al. 2005; Tanzi and Bertram 2005). It is also triggered by certain environmental factors (de la Monte and Wands 2005). Sporadic AD can be induced by diet (Lazarov, Robinson et al. 2005; Qiu and Folstein 2006). The familial disease, on the other hand, is due to gene mutations which accelerate its development (Selkoe 2001). In the sporadic disease, cellular changes control the disease and do not occur as a result of gene mutations (Reddy, Mani et al. 2005). Studies of the cellular, molecular, and histopathological features of AD shows that it is due to multiple reasons (Reddy and Beal 2005). It is caused by amyloid plaque formation, neurofibrillary tangles, and disturbance in the levels of neurotransmitter chemicals (Selkoe 2001).

Familial and sporadic AD have similar pathological conditions (Selkoe 2001). Sporadic AD shows pathological symptoms later than the familial form (Reddy and Beal 2005; Holmes 2002; Selkoe 2002; Kitazawa, Yamasaki et al. 2004; Manczak, Park et al. 2004; Reddy, McWeeney et al. 2004; Reddy and Beal 2005; Hashimoto, Zielke et al. 1997; Tanzi and Bertram 2005). AD occurs due to abnormality of the amyloid precursor protein (Selkoe and Schenk 2003; Bertram and Tanzi 2008). Brain cells appear to be abnormal, due to the oxidation of proteins, lipids, and DNA, because free radicals damage the amyloid proteins and cause amyloid-mediated neuronal damage (Butterfield, Drake et al. 2001). Amyloid precursor proteins involved in proteolytic cellular processes produce beta proteins, which have neurotoxicity (Yankner 1996; Behl 1997). Amyloid-beta proteins of 39–43 amino acids in senile plaques play a role in progressive pathology (Selkoe 2001). Imbalance between amyloid production and excretion results in plaques (Selkoe 2001). Amyloid beta protein acts as a reactive oxygen species (ROS). It also generates the ROS hydrogen peroxide, that is potentiated by iron and copper ions (Morgan, Diamond et al. 2000; Cotman and Berchtold

2002).When it oxidizes lipids, it impairs ATPase, glutamate transporter proteins and GTP-binding proteins (Mattson 1997), resulting in disturbance of cellular homeostasis, whereas low levels of membrane-associated oxidative stress cause neuronal toxicity and apoptosis. Synapses degenerate and amyloid-induced oxidative stress occurs, impairing functions of ion transport and mitochondrial functions (Hsieh, Lin et al. 2000).

AD is one of the most common causes of memory loss, and is also known as dementia in the elderly, and is the fourth most common cause of death in old people. Younger people below 65 years of age can also be affected by the disease (Francis, 1999). It was known simply as age-related memory loss or senile dementia until research in the 1970's and 1980s on dementia in young and old people uncovered a similar mechanism underlying memory loss in the two age groups (Geldmacher, 1997). The frequency of the disease varies between different age groups and is found to increase with age. Whereas the frequency of AD in people aged 65 to 74 years is only 3% percent, it increases to up to 47.2% at the age of 85 years (Wernicke, 1994; Williams, 2003). Researchers have concluded that the frequency of cases of AD may increase three fold in the next 30 to 40 years (Geldmacher, 1997).

The human brain consists of billions of nerve cells, known as neurons. Neurons work together to form a communication system that receives the messages and constructs the required responses, helping in a number of human functions. Some of our neurons are linked with our cognition, involving actions such as learning, thinking, and memory, while still other neurons are involved in regulating our senses of seeing, hearing, and smell, among others. Disturbance in these neurons ultimately disturbs their respective functions as well, which then present among the symptoms of various brain-related diseases, the commonest of them being AD (Singhal, 2012).

Studies have identified the presence of beta-amyloid protein plaques between the neurons, that may involve neurites, leading to the formation of paired helical filaments or PHF, consisting of over-phosphorylated proteins (Selkoe, 1991).

3.2 CAUSES AND RISK FACTORS OF AD

The causes and factors affecting the triggering of AD have been investigated in different areas of different regions of the world. AD can be caused by genetic factors or environmental factors, that play a role in the progress of the disease. It can be due to exposure to silicon and aluminum (Shin 1997) or may be due to exposure to toxins and free radicals (Rösler, Retz et al. 1998). AD may be triggered by disturbed levels of biometal ions, such as the occurrence of imbalances of copper, zinc, and iron concentrations, and stress to the brain as a result of free radicals, causing AD (Kastenholz 2011). AD can be due to antacids, aluminum cooking pots and foil, beverage cans, and antiperspirants. Others have suggested the inclusion of diabetes, high blood pressure, and elevated cholesterol as factors that can cause dementia.

Mainly, AD is caused by genetic factors, but some other factors, such as environmental agents and aging, are also involved (Munoz and Feldman 2000). AD occurs due to the deposition of beta-amyloid, a brain protein fragment, which accumulates in the brain, becoming the main component of amyloid plaques. Due to this formation of plaque in the brain tissues, microfiber tangles form, causing loss of cells and damage to vessels, which result in loss of memory. The production of beta-amyloid occurs due to gene mutations.

Apolipoprotein E is also a causative agent in the development of AD. Different form of apolipoprotein E are present, like apolipoproteins E2, 3, and 4. Glial cells of the brain, which are also called astrocytes, produce these proteins. The risk of developing AD is greater in the presence of higher apolipoprotein E4 concentrations (Aaronson, Van Den Eeden et al. 2017). If the level of this protein increases, then the probability of death is also increased (Harris, Brecht et al. 2003). AD is also associated with E693G mutations in a gene encoding an amyloid precursor protein (Nilsberth, Westlind-Danielsson et al. 2001). Furthermore, AD is caused by oxidative stress because, in this situation, demand by the brain for oxygen is increased (Butterfield and Lauderback 2002). AD is also associated with some pathogens like *Chlamydia pneumoniae*, which enter the brain tissue and damage brain cells (Harris, Brecht et al. 2003). AD is more common in females, smokers, obese people, patients with high blood pressure or a high level of cholesterol, whereas previous trauma, changes in sleep pattern, and Down syndrome can all increase the risk of AD (Simonson 2018).

3.3 SIGNS AND SYMPTOMS

The hallmark of AD is memory loss and impaired function of the brain. It is recognized by the occurrence of anxiety, depression, disturbed behavior, and hallucinations.

The first stage of AD continues for 2–4 years, presenting with forgetfulness, confusion, disorientation, memory loss, and mood disorder.

The second stage can last for 2–10 years and presents with memory loss, hallucinations, restlessness, muscle spasm, reduced logic, and increased inability.

The third stage lasts for 1–3 years, with symptoms such as aging, injury, dysphagia, skin infections, and seizures (Kuller 1996).

3.4 DIAGNOSIS

AD is diagnosed by completing the following examination:

1. A complete medical and psychiatric history of the patient
2. Neurological examination of the patient
3. Mental state assessment
4. Talking with the family
5. Mini-Cog test to diagnose the patient
6. Urinalysis to determine whether there may be a urinary cause.
7. Mild cognitive impairment test
8. Visual clues for dementia testing
9. Lumbar puncture test
10. Mental state mini examination
11. Electroencephalogram

Memory loss is the most common feature of this disease, according to the results of a worldwide study of more than 24 million people suffering from AD (Penido, De Morais et al. 2017). As this disease progresses, the patient suffers an increasing number of problems, such as loss of memory, problems in walking and working, and may also suffer personality disorders, like changes in behavior, and have reduced ability to think (Jivad and Rabiei 2014). All these problems occur because cells of the brain are damaged. Inflammation of brain tissues, involvement of free radicals, and deficiency of acetylcholine are factors which play important roles in the development of AD. Acetylcholine is an important neurotransmitter, which is required for the prevention of mental illness and for good memory. AD progresses when the concentration of this neurotransmitter is decreased (Penido, De Morais et al. 2017). AD occurs as a result of the destruction of this neurotransmitter; for the prevention of disease symptoms, we inhibit the activity of those enzymes which degrade these neurotransmitters (Singhal, Naithani et al. 2012), such as cholinesterase and acetylcholinesterase. In AD, plaque formation occurs in the damaged part of the brain (Kim and Oh 2012). The hippocampus, which is the part of the brain where memory formation occurs, is affected first. Due to this connection between the nerve cells, they are destroyed, and the patient suffers from AD (Beard 2004). For AD, no proper treatment is available, but many herbal drugs are used for the prevention of symptom development associated with this disease, because of their fewer side effects as compared with allopathic medicines. Extracts from herbal plants have shown antioxidant activities which prevent symptom development from this disease. Cereals and fruits are rich sources of antioxidant activity. Flavonoids, selenium, vitamin C and E are good antioxidants which are present in our food. Those herbal plants which have antioxidant, anti-inflammatory and anticholinergic activity are effective in the treatment of AD. These herbal drugs also treat memory loss, which is a major problem for patients suffering from this disease (Penido, De Morais et al. 2017).

3.5 PATHOPHYSIOLOGY AND ETIOLOGY OF AD

Two main features of AD occur: one is the formation of plaque outside the cell, and the other is tangles formation inside the cell (Braak and Braak 1990). In AD, β-amyloid peptides play important roles in its pathology. Mutations occur in the precursor of amyloid protein (Schenk, Barbour et al. 1999). Amyloid precursor protein (APP) has many functions, such as maintaining normal activity of neurons and aiding synaptic functions. If the APP is deficient, then structural and neuronal functional problems occur (Dong, Duan et al. 2012). Due to gene mutations, a 42-amino acid peptide forms, which is an important peptide present in the plaques of beta-amyloid in the brains of people with AD. In this condition, an amino acid at the original valine position is replaced by phenylalanine (Schenk, Barbour et al. 1999). Amyloid plaque interacts with synapse activity, causing loss of function inside the neurons, and ultimately apoptosis occurs. Levels of norepinephrine and serotonin become deficient due to loss of neurons and raphe nuclei present in the brainstem; due to this abnormal activity, loss of memory occurs, which is a major feature of AD. Vascular damage and a decrease in supply of blood to the brain are the initial features which cause impairment of memory, and the brain does not use glucose properly, resulting in damage to the neurons (Farkas and Luiten 2001). Usually, at an initial stage, when the cell cycle has been completed, differentiation of neurons occurs. In case of AD, however, at the G2 stage, progression of the cell cycle continues, and neuron differentiation may result in AD or neuron death (Nagy, Esiri et al. 1998). AD progression occurs as a result of mutations on chromosomes 1, 21, and 14 (Cummings, Vinters et al. 1998).

Different hypotheses suggest the operation of different mechanisms underlying the etiology of AD. However, it has been established that, at the histological and molecular level, the main abnormalities occurring are the extracellular formation of amyloid β-peptide (AβP) and the formation of neurofibrillary tangles inside the cells, ultimately leading to an extensive loss of cholinergic neurons in the hippocampus, cerebral cortex, and other areas of brain that are mainly involved in memory and cognition (Rui Wang, 2006).

Amyloid is basically an insoluble form of protein, that is formed as a result of abnormal folding of polypeptides which are normally present. The precursor of amyloid is called Beta-Amyloid Precursor Protein (βAPP) that ultimately gives rise to amyloid proteins (Yuhai Zhao, 2014).

β-APP is encoded by a gene present on the 21q chromosome arm. Due to gene mutations, structural rearrangements, or even deletions, an increase in the number of genetically altered mRNAs encoding βAPP are produced in some specific tissues or cells. The abnormal βAPP polypeptides are formed which, when presented for proteolytic processing, are cleaved, mostly at residue 687 of the βAPP, thus preventing the formation of AβP. This is what normally happens but, sometimes, overuse of alternate proteolytic pathways leads to the production of large amounts of AβP contained in C-terminal fragments. This AβP is then accumulated in several brain regions, forming the amyloid plaques. The microglia and astrocytes at the site of these abnormal plaques are activated and some AβP-associated proteins are also attracted to accumulate in said plaques. These plaques cause degeneration of the in-contact neurons of cortical and subcortical regions of the brain. Many neurons are affected but studies have associated the clinical signs and symptoms of AD with the loss of cholinergic neurons in the cerebral cortex and hippocampus. The degenerative changes in the neurons start by the formation of the neurofibrillary tangles, that are formed by the hyperphosphorylation of the tau proteins that are normally involved in the formation of microtubules inside neurons. As a result, microtubule formation is disturbed, leading to impaired communication and loss of neuronic function. All these changes occur over several years, to ultimately result in the clinical manifestation of AD (Selkoe, 1991).

The decrease in the number of cholinergic neurons was the first indicator of AD discovered in the struggle to uncover the mechanism of the disease. Because these neurons are associated with keeping the short-term memory intact, it was established that the loss of short-term memory that occurs in AD was associated with the loss of these neurons. The degenerative process is seen to start in the entorhinal cortex and nucleus basalis. In advanced AD, the loss of cholinergic neurons may reach up to 90%, leading to the symptoms of dementia. In patients with AD, the concentrations of acetylcholinesterase and choline acetyltransferase were found to be low, and continued to decline further with the advancement of the disease. Recent pharmacotherapy aims to compensate for the loss of these cholinergic function losses by increasing concentrations of the neurotransmitter acetylcholine by introducing cholinesterase inhibitors, precursors of acetylcholine or agonists of nicotinic and muscarinic receptors (Abbasi, 2006), but, because multiple neurons are affected and not just those of the cholinergic types, only management of the symptoms of dementia associated with the disease is achieved, and the patients cannot find complete relief (Selkoe, 1991).

3.6 CLINICAL FEATURES

In AD, the main symptom which appears in patients is loss of memory and it occurs due to damage to brain tissue. Initially, patients have problems remembering those events which occurred recently; after this, slow progression of the disease occurs, and it becomes more severe. Some other problems, like loss of thinking, e.g. remembering numbers, are very difficult for a patient. Patients cannot carry out more than one task at a time, and also have difficulties in remembering the names of their family members, with problems also occurring in decision making, judgment calls, etc. A major issue is changes in personality, such as social withdrawal, not wanting to meet with other people, and remaining sad and depressed all the time (Simonson 2018). Patients also have difficulty with speech and reading, and their writing skills are also affected (Seshadri, Drachman et al. 1995). Patients can also have problem with sleeping, whereas language problems initially occur (Wint and Tavee 2014).

3.7 EPIDEMIOLOGY

In epidemiological studies, it is observed that dementia occurs as part of this disease. It is an age-related disease, mostly affecting people after the age of 60 years, and the proportion of the population with this disease is increasing every five years. Many factors are involved in the progress of this disease, namely educational factors, drugs, genetic, and environmental factors. If patient had a previous head injury, then this can also trigger AD (Dong, Duan et al. 2012). Females are more commonly affected than males (Wint and Tavee 2012).

3.8 HERBAL TREATMENT

Many synthetic medicines are available which have effective roles in the management of dementia. So far, the treatment of AD has been carried out by using cholinesterase inhibitors, a strategy which is approved by the Food and Drug Administration of the US. Other chemicals, such as vitamin E, anti-inflammatory drugs, and selegiline (an enzyme blocker which slows the breakdown of some neurotransmitters), have been studied for their usage but their use is still not fully approved. Many herbal plants have been tested for the treatment of AD. Extracts from these plants can prevent this disease. Many herbal plants have important chemical constituents which have pharmacological roles, and these constituents can act in inhibitory or excitatory ways. Several plants are being trialed for the treatment of AD and these are discussed in the rest of this chapter (Geun Kim and Sook Oh 2012).

3.9 MEDICINAL PLANTS WITH ANTI-ALZHEIMER'S DISEASE POTENTIAL

3.9.1 *Hypericum perforatum* (St. John's Wort)

H. perforatum plant is a herb, and the height of this plant is up to 80 cm. The shape of the leaves of this plant is like a spoon. The most important constituents of this plant are choline, hypericin, hyperforin, flavonoids, tannins, and essential oils, obtained from the leaves of this plant. All the constituents of the plant have important role in the treatment of brain diseases, because they have properties to treat anxiety and depression, and to achieve relief from inflammation. Quercitrin and quercetin are both important flavonoids obtained from this plant which have antioxidant activity, inhibiting the oxidation of lipids. Thirty minutes before giving an injection of 1.4 mg/kg body-weight scopolamine to induce oxidative stress, the patients were first treated with *H. perforatum* extract at dosages of 4 mg/kg, 8 mg/kg, or 12 mg/kg, which proved to be effective in the treatment of oxidative stress. Hyperforin has been used to treat memory loss, and this plant can play an important role in the treatment of AD (Jivad and Rabiei 2014).

3.9.2 *Curcuma longa* (Turmeric)

C. longa, also commonly known as Haldi in Urdu, belongs to the ginger family Zingiberaceae, and is known as a powerful antioxidant and anti-inflammatory (Singhal 2012). Studies to uncover the underlying mechanism of AD have established the presence of activated microglia and astrocytes surrounding the beta-amyloid plaques, indicating that amyloid plaques are the sites of chronic inflammation (Selkoe 1991). *C. longa* acts as an anti-inflammatory, thus lowering the inflammation associated with AD. Moreover, free radicals in the body are identified to be one of the reasons behind the gene mutations, leading to production of abnormal AβP in the brain. Being a powerful antioxidant, turmeric can lower the oxidative stress inside the body, thus preventing or suppressing development of the disease.

Curcumin from *C. longa* rhizomes, also known as diferuloyl methane, has shown anti-inflammatory effect, whereas polyphenolic components obtained from turmeric have also shown beneficial effects in the treatment of AD. In AD, plaque is formed and this amyloid plaque can be removed by treatment with curcumin, which stimulates macrophages to remove foreign particles. Macrophages are a part of our immune system and have the tendency to remove abnormally formed plaque. By removing this plaque, it may be possible to prevent AD (Geun Kim and Sook Oh 2012).

3.9.3 *Prunella vulgaris* (Self-Heal)

Self-heal is a traditional herbal plant used to treat AD. It has anti-inflammatory, antimicrobial and antioxidant activities. It is also used to treat depression and anxiety and improves the loss of memory, all symptoms associated with AD. Patients with AD, who are treated with self-heal extracts at a dose of 25 mg/kg or 50 mg/kg, exhibit marked improvements against this disease (Jivad and Rabiei 2014).

3.9.4 *Bacopa monnieri* (Brahmi, Water Hyssop)

This species belongs to the family Plantaginaceae. It contains reserpine and chloromazine in aerial parts of plant, which have potential to treat AD (Zhang 2004; Misra, Lal et al. 2008). *B. monnieri* is an important herb, used for the treatment of anxiety, a symptom which appears in AD patients. This herb is important for the treatment of memory loss and for improvement of learning ability. The active components include saponins (e.g. bacopasides I–XII), D-mannitol, and alkaloids, including herpestine. Beta-sitosterol, betulic acid, and bacosides play important roles in the prevention of AD

(Geun Kim and Sook Oh 2012). *Bacopa* extracts are used to enhance memory, learning, to control epilepsy, protect the brain, and treat anxiety (Simpson, Pase et al. 2015). Aging causes degenerative changes in the body and contributes to hormone deficiencies with resultant oxidative damage, because normal functions require adequate concentrations of neurotransmitter chemicals. *Bacopa* contain alkaloids such as asbrahmine, hersaponin, monnierin, and herpestine, and terpenes such as stigmasterol, betulic acid, bacosides and bacopasaponins (Aguiar and Borowski 2013). *Bacopa* extracts repair neuron actions by inducing neuronal synthesis, synaptic activity, and kinase activity (Mathur, Goyal et al. 2016).

B. monniera extract has been shown to exert improvements in Alzheimer's patients, as observed in various study models. The plant is generally also known as brahmi in India and has been used in Ayurvedic medicine for a long time (Jesky, 2011). A recent study was performed in India to observe the effects of the plant extract on AD patients. In the study, the plant extract was used at a dose of 300 mg/d in normal and healthy adults for a period of 15 d, with no mortality or serious side effects. After 15 d, the dosage was enhanced to 450 mg/d, which was still concluded to be a safe dosage of the extract, with only mild to moderate gastrointestinal symptoms (Pravina 2007).

Another study was performed in the United States recently, in which the plant extract was administered at a dose of 300 mg/d to 24 subjects, resulting in positive effects on cognition, with no adverse effects on mood, behavior, or blood pressure being observed, deeming the plant extract to be useful in relieving symptoms associated with AD, although some gastrointestinal side effects were still observed. Further studies may still be required to acquire a dosage free of any side effects or to identify any obscure adverse effects related to the ingestion of the plant and still to be uncovered (Calabrese 2008).

3.9.5 *Ginkgo biloba* (Maidenhair Tree)

This tree belongs to family Ginkgoaceae. Leaf extracts contain the flavonoid kaempferol, which has been used to treat AD (Smith and Luo 2004; Luo 2006). *G. biloba* extract is used for the treatment of AD. The extract obtained from this plant has proven effectiveness in treating memory loss. *G. biloba* extracts have been used for thousands of years in Chinese traditional medicine to treat a variety of ailments. Studies have shown that the plant extract can be used to slow down the progression of AD and to improve the symptoms of the disease. *G. biloba* extract has been found to be most effective in treating AD at an early stage of the disease, as the plant extract has been found to enhance oxygen and blood flow to the brain, thereby enhancing memory and overall brain function. In a trial performed on 309 patients with mild dementia, the extract was given at a dose of 120 mg daily for up to a year. Of the patients, 27% showed moderate improvement as determined using various cognitive tests after a period of six months usage of the extract (Kanowski 2003). Similarly, another study was carried out on a group of 112 patients who suffered chronically from cerebral insufficiency. When the extract was supplied at a dose of 120 mg/d, there was an increase in the blood flow and oxygen supply to the brain of the patients, enhancing overall brain health and improving the memory of the patients (Le Bars 1997). Earlier studies had shown that the G. *biloba* extract normalized the abnormal acetylcholine receptors found in the brains of old animals (Feudis, 1991). *G. biloba* extract has also been shown to increase the activity of cholinergic neurons and to improve other signs and symptoms associated with AD (Kleijnen 1992). A study performed to confirm the medical benefits of the plant extract used a dose of 240 mg daily in 216 patients. The study confirmed that the plant extract improved the clinical presentations of the disease better than did a corresponding placebo (Wettstein 2000).

G. biloba has been sold in Europe in the form of EGb761. Studies were performed to compare the effectiveness of EGb761 with synthetic drugs for AD treatment, such as donepezil and rivastigmine, with the results that EGb761 was just as effective as the drugs but was more natural and protective to the human body. EGb761 is taken in a dose of 80 to 120 mg/d (Dore, Bastianetto et al. 1999), and has been shown to prevent the spread of toxic effects of beta-amyloid plaque to the surrounding brain cells, which is a characteristic typical of the development of disease (Kanowski, 2003).

Care should be taken not to take *G. biloba* extract in conjunction with anticoagulant drugs and it should be administered only under with the advice of a physician. Although treatment with *G. biloba* extract has resulted in improvements in overall brain function, as well as in cognition, the exact mechanism by which the extract acts is not well known, and acetylcholinesterase inhibitors are still preferred over the *Ginkgo* extract to treat AD (Kurz 2004).

3.9.6 *Withania somnifera* (Ashwagandha)

W. somnifera has been shown to be effective in boosting memory and cognitive skills. Beta-amyloids are toxic to the brain when they accumulate (Prasansuklab and Tencomnao 2013). Administration of ashwagandha root extract to mice eliminated amyloid plaques in the cortex and hippocampus (Sehgal, Gupta et al. 2012) Sitoindosides VII-X and withaferin A are active phytophenols that increase the cortical muscarinic acetylcholine capacity and cholinergic functions (Misra, Lal et al. 2008). It is an important phenolic compound which overcomes memory loss and helps in the treatment of AD; if ashwagandha is taken for 14 d, then AD can be prevented (Geun Kim and Sook Oh 2012).

3.9.7 *Cyperus rotundus* (Common Nut Sedge)

C. rotundus is an important plant and the components of the abundant oil from this plant include an alcohol, isociprol, and the terpenes cineole and pinene. These components of the extract have antiacetylcholinergic activity. Treatment of patients with the extract of *C. rotundus* at a dose of 100 mg or 200 mg daily enhances the memory and treats AD symptoms (Jivad and Rabiei 2014).

3.9.8 *Huperzia serrata* (Toothed Clubmoss)

The Chinese medicinal plant *H. serrata* belongs to the family Lycopodiaceae and extracts contain the alkaloid huperzine A, which plays important roles in the treatment of memory loss and other symptoms associated with AD (Ott and Owens 1998; Chiu and Zhang 2000; Galvão, Marques et al. 2002). This herb also has anticholinergic effect. Chinese scientists selected 450 subjects who suffered from AD. Those given huperzine A showed significant improvement, suggesting that this herb can prevent AD (Akhondzadeh, Sabet et al. 2010). For best results, this drug needs to be given for twelve weeks (Tian, Shi et al. 2010).

H. serrata has been used in China for centuries as part of traditional medicine for the treatment of diseases such as schizophrenia, strains, and contusions. Huperzine A is a selective and reversible cholinesterase inhibitor and the duration of its inhibitory effect compares favorably with some of the other, commonly used drugs, such as donepezil, galantamine, rivastigmine, and tacrine. The plant has been studied for its effects on improvements in Alzheimer's patients in China, with the establishment that the plant improves cognitive function and enhances memory in patients with AD and vascular dementia. Extracts of the plant have been found not to cause any noticeable side effects (Rui Wang 2006).

A study was performed, comparing the inhibitory effects of huperzine A with other commonly used inhibitors, with the result that huperzine A was more potent in inhibiting acetylcholinesterase activity but less potent in inhibiting butyrylcholinesterase activity, compared with rivastigmine, galantamine, physostigmine, and tacrine. The study was based on half-maximal inhibitory concentration (Rui Wang 2006).

In other studies, the effect of huperzine A was observed on the levels of βAPP and protein kinase C-alpha (PKC-alpha), to establish whether the alkaloid has neuroprotective properties. The study identified that huperzine A changed the disturbances in amyloid precursor proteins and PKC-alpha, as observed in the HEK293sw cell line as well as in rats (Zhang, 2004). Levels of both βAPP and PKC-alpha decreased in the presence of beta-amyloid protein but, following the administration of huperzine A, the changes were reversed or reduced to a great extent. Because amyloid precursor proteins are known to be neuroprotective, it was established that huperzine A has neuroprotective properties (Rui Wang 2006).

3.9.9 *Panax ginseng* (Korean Ginseng)

It belongs to the family Araliaceae, and crude extracts contain the saponins ginsenosides Rg1, Rg2, and Rg3 (Chen, Eckman et al. 2006; Joo, Yoo et al. 2008). Also known as Korean ginseng, this plant has been used in traditional Korean medicine to prevent memory loss. The plant not only enhances memory (Reid 1986) but has also been observed to increase cholinergic activity in rats' brains (Nitta 1995; Salim 1997), while also exhibiting a neuroprotective effect (Wen 1996; Lim 1997). *Panax* saponins are the important active components of this plant, which is effective in treating AD. Administration of this extract resulted in improved memory and learning. It also decreased the level of beta-amyloid in the brain and normalized cholinesterase activities (Tian, Shi et al. 2010).

P. ginseng root powder was taken at a dosage of 4.5 g/d for 12 weeks in a study performed with 97 subjects with AD, who showed improvement in cognition in response. Similarly, a study was performed with a dosage of 4.5 or 9 g/d of Korean red ginseng powder for a period of 12 weeks, and the AD patients showed improvements in cognitive clinical presentation. Improvement was assessed using the Alzheimer Disease Assessment Scale (ADAS) for the lower dose, whereas the Clinical Dementia Rating (CDR) was used for the study performed at the higher dose (Hyo Geun Kim, 2012).

3.9.10 *Spatholobus suberectus* (*Caulis spatholobi*)

This plant is a member of the Fabaceae family, and contains epigallocatechin gallate present in the whole herb (Lin, Ho et al. 2008). A dose of 9 μg/ml of an ethanolic extract of *S. suberectus* stem showed an inhibitory effect on acetylcholinesterase. An aqueous extract was prepared by soaking 10g of *caulis spatholobi* herb in 10 ml of water, and showed 77.74% inhibition of acetylcholinesterase activity, whereas an ethanolic extract, prepared by soaking 10 g of herb in 50 ml of pure ethanol twice overnight, gave an inhibition percentage of 64.68 (Lin 2008).

3.9.11 *Salvia miltiorrhiza* (Red Sage)

This plant is a part of traditional Chinese medicine and has been used in decoctions for insomnia. Ethanolic extracts of the roots have been studied and found to inhibit acetylcholinesterase activity at a dose of 5 μg/ml. The inhibitory effect was found to be due to the presence of two triterpenoids. Aqueous and ethanolic extracts were prepared as described in 3.9.10 and caused percentage inhibition of acetylcholinesterase activity of 46.07% and 72.17%, respectively (Lin 2008).

3.9.12 *Paeonia alba* (White Peony)

Radix *Paeoniae alba*, at a dose of 8 μg/ml of extracts have been studied for the inhibition of acetylcholinesterase activity. Aqueous and ethanolic extracts were prepared as described in 3.9.10 and caused percentage inhibition of acetylcholinesterase activity of 58.51% and 78.74%, respectively (Lin 2008).

3.9.13 *Melissa officinalis* (Lemon Balm)

M. officinalis is an important medicinal herb, used for many years for the treatment of cognitive problems. The mechanism underlying such effects of the plant has been studied, showing that the plant has cholinergic activities as it has acetylcholine receptor-binding activities of both the muscarinic and nicotinic types (Perry 1998,1999). The plant extract is seen to improve AD symptoms in subjects at only mild to moderate stages of the disease, whereas studies have revealed that the plant improves cognition and mood in even healthy and young people (Kennedy 2002).

Another study was performed recently to assess the effects of the plant extract on cognition and mood. The study was placebo controlled and involved a total of 42 patients suffering from mild to moderate AD treated with the plant extract or a placebo, for a period of four months. Different cognition tests performed after 16 weeks showed a marked difference in the extent of improvement between the two groups, with the group treated with the plant extract showing higher scores in cognition tests compared with the placebo group. The patients treated with the plant extract were also less agitated and were calmer than subjects in the group receiving the placebo treatment. The cognition tests used include Clinical Dementia Rating-Sum of the Boxes (CDR-SB) and (ADSC-cog) AD Assessment Scale (ADSC-cog) (Akhondzadeh 2003).

3.9.14 *Salvia officinalis* (Sage)

S. officinalis is also studied for its effects on cognition in Alzheimer's patients, with the recognition that the plant extract, like that of *M. officinalis*, enhances cognition and lowers AD-induced agitation in the patients after usage for sixteen weeks in a placebo-controlled study. The results were assessed using the CDR-SB and ADSC-cog tests and scores were compared for both groups, where the higher the score, the better which clearly shows greater improvement of cognition in the extract-treated group (Akhondzadeh 2003).

An important active component of *Salvia officinalis* is rosmarinic acid, which has a number of important features, like antioxidant effects, preventing peroxidation of lipids. Patients treated with rosmarinic acid for sixteen weeks showed improvements in their health (Tian, Shi et al. 2010).

3.9.15 *Codonopsis pilosula* (Poor Man's Ginseng)

Two types of extracts were prepared of the *Radix codonopsis* herb, one being the aqueous extract (prepared by soaking 10 g of herb in 10 ml of water) while the other is the ethanol extract (prepared by soaking 10 g of herb in 50 ml of pure ethanol twice overnight). The aqueous extract showed inhibition of acetylcholinesterase activity by 6.54%, whereas the ethanolic extract exhibited 26.31% inhibition (Lin 2008).

3.9.16 *Scutellaria baicalensis* (Baikal Skullcap)

The aqueous extract is prepared by soaking the 10g of the *Radix scutellariae* herb in 10 ml of water, and exhibited 27.09% inhibition of acetylcholinesterase activity, whereas the ethanolic extract is prepared by soaking 10 g of herb in 50 ml of pure ethanol twice overnight, and caused 40.21% inhibition (Lin 2008).

3.9.17 *Pinellia ternata* (Crow Dipper)

The aqueous extract is prepared by soaking 10g of the *Rhizoma pinelliae* herb in 10 ml of water and showed 4.80% inhibition of acetylcholinesterase activity, whereas the ethanolic extract is prepared by soaking 10 g of the herb in 50 ml of pure ethanol twice overnight, giving a 9.74% inhibition (Lin 2008).

3.9.18 *Centella asiatica* (Indian Pennywort, Gotu Kola)

This is a medicinal plant where the leaves have been used in Ayurvedic medicine as an agent of medhyarasayna, to decrease brain stress (Ray and Ray 2015). The major active compounds are triterpenoid saponins and sapogenins (Kulkarni, Girish et al. 2012), such as hydrocotylin and hersaponin, that have been used to treat AD (Anekonda 2005; Veerendra Kumar and Gupta 2003). Its mechanism of action is not known.

3.9.19 *Allium sativum* (Garlic)

It belongs to the family Amaryllidaceae, and contains S-allyl cysteine in the bulb, which has potential to treat AD (Anekonda 2005).

3.9.20 *Angelica sinensis* (Female Ginseng)

This plant belongs to the family Apiaceae. It contains z-ligustilide, 11-angeloylsenkyunolide F, coniferyl ferulate, and ferulic acid in the roots, which have potential to treat AD (Hsieh, Lin et al. 2000; Hsieh, Tsai et al. 2002; Zhang 2004; Ho, Kumaran et al. 2009).

3.9.21 *Astragalus* spp. (Milk Vetch)

These plants belongs to the family Fabaceae, and contain cycloastragenol in roots, which could be used to treat AD (Jiankang and Akitane 1993; Hong, Qin et al. 1994; Toda, Yase et al. 2000; Zhang 2004).

3.9.22 *Platycladus orientalis* (Chinese Thuja)

This tree belongs to the family Cupressaceae, and contains pinusolides in the seeds, which are suggested to treat AD (Nishiyama, Chu et al. 1995; Zhang 2004).

3.9.23 *Rosmarinus officinalis* (Rosemary)

R. officinalis belongs to the family Lamiaceae, and exhibits strong antioxidant and anti-inflammatory properties. Studies have shown the plant to be a natural inhibitor of cycloxygenase-1 (COX-1). The constituents present in the plant that inhibit COX-1 include the terpenes carvacrol, apigenin, eugenol, ursolic acid, oleanolic acid, and thymol (Singhal 2012). Since COX-1 promotes inflammatory processes occurring in amyloid plaques, its inhibition could relieve AD-associated symptoms.

3.9.24 *Matricaria chamomilla* (German Chamomile)

This plant belongs to the family Asteraceae and it can be used to obtain relief from the mood swings associated with AD, as the chamomile decoction helps in calming the nerves, and treating insomnia and anxiety (Singhal 2012).

3.9.25 *Camellia sinensis* (Chinese Tea)

This shrub belongs to the family Theaceae, and contains epigallocatechin gallate in the leaves, that has the potential to treat AD (Anekonda 2005).

3.9.26 *Celastrus paniculatus* (Intellect Plant)

It belongs to the family Celastraceae, and contains several phytoconstituents like alkaloids, triterpenoids, esters, carbohydrates, vitamin C, monounsaturated and polyunsaturated fats, saturated fats, proteins, minerals and sesquiterpene polyolest with potential to treat AD as well as other brain disorders (Nalini, Karanth et al. 1995; Zhang 2004; Kumar and Khanum 2012).

3.9.27 *Schisandra chinensis* (Magnolia Vine)

A member of the Magnoliaceae family, it contains schizandrin present in the fruit that can treat AD (Sinclair 1998; Zhang 2004).

An aqueous extract, prepared by soaking 10 g of herb in 10 ml of water) caused 1.49% inhibition of acetylcholinesterase activity, whereas an ethanolic extract, prepared by soaking 10 g of herb in 50 ml of pure ethanol twice overnight, resulted in 5.76% inhibition (Lin 2008).

3.9.28 *Clitoria ternatea* (Asian Pigeonwings)

This plant belongs to the family Fabaceae, and contains tannins, phlobatannin, carbohydrates, saponins, triterpenoids, phenols, flavanoids, flavonol glycosides, proteins, alkaloids, antharaquinone, anthocyanins, cardiac glycosides, Stigmast- 4-ene-3,6-dione, volatile oils and steroids in the roots that could treat AD (Zhang 2004).

3.9.29 *Coptis chinensis* (Goldthread)

This plant belongs to the family Ranunculaceae, and contains the alkaloid berberine present in the whole plant to treat AD (Asai, Iwata et al. 2007).

3.9.30 *Dipsacus asper* (Japanese Teasel)

It belongs to the family Caprifoliaceae, and contains dipsacus saponins in the roots that are used to treat AD (Qian, Liu et al. 2002; Zhang 2004).

3.9.31 *Tetradium ruticarpum* (*Euodia ruticarpa*) (Euodia)

It belongs to the family Rutaceae, and contains the alkaloid dehydroevodiamine in the fruits (Park, Kim et al. 1996; Zhang 2004).

3.9.32 *Gastrodia elata* (Tianma)

It belongs to the family Orchidaceae and contains *p*-hydroxybenzyl alcohol and gastrodin in the rhizomes that can be used to treat AD (Zhang 2004).

3.9.33 *Heteropterys aphrodisiaca*

It belongs to the family Malpighiaceae and contains quercetin in the roots to treat AD (Smith and Luo 2004; Zhang 2004).

3.9.34 *Indigofera tinctoria* (True Indigo)

It belongs to the family Apiaceae, and contains indirubins present in the plant-based herbal powder (*Indigo naturalis*) that treats AD (Leclerc, Garnier et al. 2001).

3.9.35 *Lycium barbarum* (Wolfberry)

This plant belongs to the family Solanaceae, and contains lyceum barbarum polysaccharide in the fruit to treat AD (Peila, Rodriguez et al. 2002; Yu, Leung et al. 2005; Yu, Lai et al. 2007; Chang and So 2008; Kalaria, Maestre et al. 2008; Ho, So et al. 2010).

3.9.36 *Lycoris radiata* (Red Spider Lily)

It belongs to the family Amaryllidaceae and contains galantamine in the whole plant, that is used to treat AD (Bores, Huger et al. 1996; Howes and Houghton 2003).

3.9.37 *Nicotiana tabacum* (Tobacco)

This plant belongs to the family Solanaceae and contains nicotine which is present in leaves, and is used to treat AD (Nordberg, Hellström-Lindahl et al. 2002).

3.9.38 *Ophiopogon japonicus* (Mondograss)

It belongs to family Asparagaceae, and contains nicotine present in the tubers that is used to treat AD (Ichikawa, Wang et al. 2003; Zhang 2004).

3.9.39 *Polygala tenuifolia*

It belongs to the family Polygalaceae, and contain tenuifolin in the roots to treat AD (Park, Kim et al. 1996; Jia, Jiang et al. 2004; Zhang 2004).

3.9.40 *Paeonia lactiflora* (Chinese Peony)

This plant belongs to the family Ranunculaceae. An ethanol extract of the whole herb is used to treat AD (Lin, Wu et al. 2003). An aqueous extract, prepared by soaking 10 g of herb in 10 ml of water, caused 77.54% inhibition of acetylcholinesterase activity, whereas an ethanolic extract, prepared by soaking 10 g of herb in 50 ml of pure ethanol twice overnight, gave 65.92% inhibition (Lin 2008).

3.9.41 *Acorus tatarinowii*

It belongs to the family Acoraceae, and contains eugenol present in leaves that can treat the AD (Irie and Keung 2003). The ethanolic extract is prepared by soaking 10 g of herb in 50 ml of pure ethanol twice overnight, giving an acetylcholinesterase inhibition of 55.76 (Lin 2008).

3.9.42 *Tripterygium wilfordii* (Thunder God Vine)

It belongs to the family Celastraceae, and contains celastrol in the whole plant that can treat AD (Sassa, Takaishi et al. 1990; Allison, Cacabelos et al. 2001).

3.9.43 *Uncaria tomentosa* (Cat's Claw)

It belongs to the family Rubiaceae, and it contains uncarine E in the aerial part of the plant that can be used to treat AD (Sassa, Takaishi et al. 1990; Zhang 2004).

3.9.44 *Vitis vinifera* (Grapevine)

This plant belongs to the family Vitiaceae and the fruit skins and seeds contain resveratrol, that is used to treat AD (Sharma and Gupta 2002; Russo, Palumbo et al. 2003).

3.10 HERBAL PREPARATIONS AND PHYTOCHEMICAL CONSTITUENTS WITH ANTI-ALZHEIMER'S DISEASE POTENTIAL

3.10.1 *Radix bupleuri*

An aqueous extract, prepared by soaking 10 g of herb in 10 ml of water, shows 6.31% inhibition of acetylcholinesterase activity, whereas an ethanolic extract, prepared by soaking 10 g of herb in 50 ml of pure ethanol twice overnight, achieves 51.34% inhibition (Lin 2008).

3.10.2 *Radix etrhizoma glycyrrhizae*

An aqueous extract, prepared by soaking 10 g of herb in 10 ml of water, causes 5.74% inhibition of acetylcholinesterase activity, whereas an ethanolic extract, which is prepared by soaking 10 g of herb in 50 ml of pure ethanol twice overnight, causes 8.65% inhibition (Lin 2008).

3.10.3 *Radix polygonimultiflori*

An aqueous extract, prepared by soaking 10 g of herb in 10 ml of water, shows 59.88% inhibition of acetylcholinesterase activity, whereas an ethanolic extract, prepared by soaking 10 g of herb in 50 ml of pure ethanol twice overnight, shows 47.24% inhibition (Lin 2008).

3.10.4 *Fructus gardenia*

An aqueous extract, prepared by soaking 10 g of herb in 10 ml of water, shows 33.62% inhibition of acetylcholinesterase activity, whereas an ethanolic extract, prepared by soaking 10 g of herb in 50 ml of pure ethanol twice overnight, causes 56.44% inhibition (Lin 2008).

3.10.5 Ganoderma

An ethanolic extract is prepared by soaking 10 g of herb in 50 ml of pure ethanol twice overnight, and caused 33.87% inhibition of acetylcholinesterase activity (Lin 2008).

3.10.6 Vinpocetine

This is an active component, which is obtained from the African periwinkle plant seeds and leaves. It has a role in the treatment of AD because it has the capability to improve neurological problems. Cavinton is another name of this drug, which is used in Europe.

3.10.7 Resveratrol

This is a phytophenol with antioxidant properties, found in red grapes. Peripheral administration of resveratrol into the CNS protects neurons and the spinal cord from injury (Kumar and Khanum 2012). In rats, it has been observed that resveratrol protects rats from ischemic damage of the spinal cord and cerebrovascular system (Arteaga, Revuelta et al. 2015). It also provides protection from nitric oxide-mediated oxidative stress, that cause death of cultured neurons (Singh, Agrawal et al. 2013). It also protects neurons from the beta-amyloid peptide and helps in its elimination (Mathur, Goyal et al. 2016).

3.10.8 *Narcissus confuses*

It is derived from a member of the family Amarylidaceae, which contains galantamine present in the crude bulb extract that is used to treat AD (Ott and Owens 1998; López, Bastida et al. 2002).

3.10.9 *Corni fructus*

An aqueous extract is prepared by soaking 10 g of herb in 10 ml of water and the extract shows 45.45% inhibition of acetylcholinesterase activity, whereas the ethanolic extract, prepared by soaking 10 g of herb in 50 ml of pure ethanol twice overnight, causes 29.55% inhibition (Lin 2008).

3.10.10 *Bombyx batryticatus*

The ethanolic extract is prepared by soaking 10 g of the preparation in 50 ml of pure ethanol twice overnight, causing 17.55% inhibition of acetylcholinesterase activity (Lin 2008).

3.10.11 *Cordyceps*

An ethanolic extract is prepared by soaking 10 g of the fungal preparation in 50 ml of pure ethanol twice overnight, and exhibits 14.03% inhibition of acetylcholinesterase activity (Lin 2008).

3.10.12 *Fructus alpiniae oxyphyllae*

An aqueous extract, prepared by soaking 10 g of herb in 10 ml of water, shows 21.30% inhibition of acetylcholinesterase activity, whereas an ethanolic extract, prepared by soaking 10 g of herb in 50 ml of pure ethanol twice overnight, causes 4.94% inhibition (Lin 2008).

3.10.13 *Fructus ligustri lucidi*

An ethanolic extract is prepared by soaking 10 g of herb in 50 ml of pure ethanol twice overnight, giving a 24.52% inhibition of acetylcholinesterase activity (Lin 2008).

3.10.14 *Ramulus uncariae cum*

An aqueous extract is prepared by soaking 10 g of herb in 10 ml of water and showed 55.23% inhibition of acetylcholinesterase activity, whereas an ethanolic extract, prepared by soaking 10 g of herb in 50 ml of pure ethanol twice overnight, caused 19.58% inhibition (Lin 2008).

3.10.15 *Rhizoma dioscoreae*

An aqueous extract, prepared by soaking 10 g of herb in 10 ml of water, caused 7.62% inhibition of acetylcholinesterase activity, whereas an ethanolic extract, prepared by soaking 10 g of herb in 50 ml of pure ethanol twice overnight, caused 20.73% inhibition (Lin 2008).

3.10.16 Caprylic Acid and Coconut Oil

Caprylic acid, which is a triglyceride and an important component of Axona, which is obtained from the oil of coconut, has important features for the treatment of AD. As the disease progresses, the AD brain does not properly use glucose, resulting in the appearance of neurological signs and symptoms that slowly lead to AD. Glucose transporter-1 (GLUT-1) is the carrier that transports glucose across the blood–brain barrier and cell membrane. AD progresses when GLUT-1 function is reduced (Winkler, Nishida et al. 2015). Using caprylic acid, the brain damage can be prevented because caprylic acid has the ability to be converted into keto bodies, which act as an alternative energy source (Geun Kim and Sook Oh 2012).

3.10.17 Galantamine

Galantamine is derived from members of the family Amaryllidaceae, which contain galantamine in crude bulb extracts that can be used to treat AD (Ott and Owens 1998). Galantamine, which is obtained from daffodils in Europe, is an important alkaloid which has anticholinergic activity. It acts on the receptors of cholinesterase. If galantamine is given for six months at a dose of 24 mg/d, it enhances the short-term memory, with this alkaloid being very effective for the treatment of AD (Akhondzadeh, Sabet et al. 2010).

Galantamine is an alkaloid derived originally from *Galanthus nivalis*, known commonly as snowdrops (Perry 1999), and is used as a cholinesterase inhibitor. It not only inhibits cholinesterase activity but also alters the nicotinic acetylcholine receptors. The drug is metabolized by cytochrome P450 (CYP-450) enzymes and has a half-life of 5 to 6 h (Abbasi 2006). Clinical trials have not shown any hepatic toxicity of galantamine (Raskind 2000). Four trials, performed on patients with mild AD, have shown that galantamine is effective at improving cognition and memory at a specific dose of 24 mg/d for a duration of up to six months. These trials proved that the patients with mild AD can get relief from their symptoms using galantamine at the specific doses described (Akhondzadeh 2002; Raskind 2000).

3.10.18 *Radix et rhizome rhei*

An aqueous extract, prepared by soaking 10 g of herb in 10 ml of water, shows 80.97% inhibition of acetylcholinesterase activity, whereas an ethanolic extract, prepared by soaking 10 g of herb in 50 ml of pure ethanol twice overnight, caused 75.26% inhibition (Lin 2008).

3.10.19 *Radix Rehmanniae species*

An ethanolic extract, prepared by soaking 10 g of herb in 50 ml of pure ethanol twice overnight, caused 23.77% inhibition of acetylcholinesterase activity (Lin 2008).

3.10.20 *Radix polygalae*

An aqueous extract is prepared by soaking 10 g of herb in 10 ml of water, exhibiting 24.44% inhibition of acetylcholinesterase activity (Lin 2008).

3.11 CONCLUSION

AD is a neurodegenerative disease that can severely impair cognitive functions of the brain, ultimately resulting in loss of memory, intellectual ability, disturbance in daily life routine, insomnia, anxiety, and depression due to self-consciousness. Herbal drugs used for the treatment of diseases have pharmacological actions with not well reported side-effects. Several herbs have been used to treat AD. Phytochemicals are present in herbs that prevent the degeneration of proteins, lipids, and neurons. Some herbs contain alkaloid compounds, that are active toward the central nervous system, and which can reduce the oxidative stress of the brain and prevent brain aging. Many research studies have been performed on herbs and it has attracted physicians to use herbs for treatment of diseases because of their beneficial effects. Herbal drugs are successful in providing symptomatic relief while minimizing side effects associated with the administration of synthetic drugs. This chapter concludes that the herbal drugs are not only a more natural way of treatment, but they can be just as effective, if not more so, than the synthetic drugs, but with minimal or no side effects. Medicinal plants, which we discussed above, have antioxidant and anti-inflammatory activities, which play pivotal roles in the treatment of AD. Herbal plants can show significant improvement in cognitive functions in AD patients within six months. The use of appropriate herbal remedies should be encouraged within the specific dosages of the plants approved by the Food and Drug Administration and related regulatory bodies.

REFERENCES

Aaronson, D. S., S. Van Den Eeden, et al. (2017). "Physicians' perceptions of factors influencing the treatment decision-making process for men with low-risk prostate cancer." *Value Health* **20**(10): 1345–1354.

Adams, M., F. Gmünder, et al. (2007). "Plants traditionally used in age related brain disorders—a survey of ethnobotanical literature." *Journal of Ethnopharmacology* **113**(3): 363–381.

Aguiar, S. and T. Borowski (2013). "Neuropharmacological review of the nootropic herb Bacopa monnieri." *Rejuvenation Research* **16**(4): 313–326.

Akhondzadeh, S., M. Noroozian, et al. (2003). Melissa officinalis extract in the treatment of patients with mild to moderate Alzheimer's disease: a double blind, randomised, placebo controlled trial. *Journal of Neurology, Neurosurgery & Psychiatry* **74**(7): 863–866.

Akhondzadeh, S., M. S. Sabet, et al. (2010). "A 22-week, multicenter, randomized, double-blind controlled trial of Crocus sativus in the treatment of mild-to-moderate Alzheimer's disease." *Psychopharmacology* **207**(4): 637–643.

Allison, A. C., R. Cacabelos, et al. (2001). "Celastrol, a potent antioxidant and anti-inflammatory drug, as a possible treatment for Alzheimer's disease." *Progress in Neuro-Psychopharmacology and Biological Psychiatry* **25**(7): 1341–1357.

Anekonda, T. S. and R. P. Hemachandra. (2005). Can herbs provide a new generation of drugs for treating Alzheimer's disease? *Brain Research Reviews* **50**: 361–376.

Arteaga, O., M. Revuelta, et al. (2015). "Pretreatment with resveratrol prevents neuronal injury and cognitive deficits induced by perinatal hypoxia-ischemia in rats." *PloS One* **10**(11): e0142424.

Asai, M., N. Iwata, et al. (2007). "Berberine alters the processing of Alzheimer's amyloid precursor protein to decrease Aβ secretion." *Biochemical and Biophysical Research Communications* **352**(2): 498–502.

Beard, R. L. (2004). "Advocating voice: organisational, historical and social milieux of the Alzheimer's disease movement." *Sociology of Health & Illness* **26**(6): 797–819.

Behl, C. (1997). "Amyloid β-protein toxicity and oxidative stress in Alzheimer's disease." *Cell and Tissue Research* **290**(3): 471–480.

Bertram, L. and R. E. Tanzi (2008). "Thirty years of Alzheimer's disease genetics: the implications of systematic meta-analyses." *Nature Reviews Neuroscience* **9**(10): 768.

Bores, G. M., F. P. Huger, et al. (1996). "Pharmacological evaluation of novel Alzheimer's disease therapeutics: acetylcholinesterase inhibitors related to galanthamine." *Journal of Pharmacology and Experimental Therapeutics* **277**(2): 728–738.

Braak, H. and E. Braak (1990). "Alzheimer's disease: striatal amyloid deposits and neurofibrillary changes." *Journal of Neuropathology & Experimental Neurology* **49**(3): 215–224.

Butterfield, D. A., J. Drake, et al. (2001). "Evidence of oxidative damage in Alzheimer's disease brain: central role for amyloid β-peptide." *Trends in Molecular Medicine* **7**(12): 548–554.

Butterfield, D. A. and C. M. Lauderback (2002). "Lipid peroxidation and protein oxidation in Alzheimer's disease brain: potential causes and consequences involving amyloid β-peptide-associated free radical oxidative stress1, 2." *Free Radical Biology and Medicine* **32**(11): 1050–1060.

Calabrese, E. J. (2008). Hormesis: why it is important to toxicology and toxicologists. *Environmental Toxicology and Chemistry: An International Journal* **27**(7): 1451–1474.

Chang, R. C.-C. and K.-F. So (2008). "Use of anti-aging herbal medicine, Lycium barbarum, against aging-associated diseases. What do we know so far?" *Cellular and Molecular Neurobiology* **28**(5): 643–652.

Chen, F., E. A. Eckman, et al. (2006). "Reductions in levels of the Alzheimer's amyloid β peptide after oral administration of ginsenosides." *The FASEB Journal* **20**(8): 1269–1271.

Chiu, H. F. K. and M. Zhang (2000). "Dementia research in China." *International Journal of Geriatric Psychiatry* **15**(10): 947–953.

Cotman, C. W. and N. C. Berchtold (2002). "Exercise: a behavioral intervention to enhance brain health and plasticity." *Trends in Neurosciences* **25**(6): 295–301.

Cummings, J. L., H. V. Vinters, et al. (1998). "Alzheimer's disease etiologies, pathophysiology, cognitive reserve, and treatment opportunities." *Neurology* **51**(1 Suppl 1): S2–S17.

de la Monte, S. M. and J. R. Wands (2005). "Review of insulin and insulin-like growth factor expression, signaling, and malfunction in the central nervous system: relevance to Alzheimer's disease." *Journal of Alzheimer's Disease* **7**(1): 45–61.

Dong, S., Y. Duan, et al. (2012). "Advances in the pathogenesis of Alzheimer's disease: a re-evaluation of amyloid cascade hypothesis." *Translational Neurodegeneration* **1**(1): 18.

Dore, S., S. Bastianetto, et al. (1999). "Protective and rescuing abilities of IGF-I and some putative free radical scavengers against β-amyloid-inducing toxicity in neurons." *Annals of the New York Academy of Sciences* **890**(1): 356–364.

Farkas, E. and P. G. Luiten (2001). "Cerebral microvascular pathology in aging and Alzheimer's disease." *Progress in Neurobiology* **64**(6): 575–611.

Francis, P. T., A. M. Palmer, et al. (1999). "The cholinergic hypothesis of Alzheimer's disease: a review of progress." *Journal of Neurology, Neurosurgery & Psychiatry* **66**(2): 137–147.

Galvão, S., L. Marques, et al. (2002). "Heteropterys aphrodisiaca (extract BST0298): a Brazilian plant that improves memory in aged rats." *Journal of Ethnopharmacology* **79**(3): 305–311.

Geldmacher, D. S. and P. J. Whitehouse. (1997). Differential diagnosis of Alzheimer's disease. *Neurology* **48**(5 Suppl 6): 2S–9S.

Geun Kim, H. and M. Sook Oh (2012). "Herbal medicines for the prevention and treatment of Alzheimer's disease." *Current Pharmaceutical Design* **18**(1): 57–75.

Harris, F. M., W. J. Brecht, et al. (2003). "Carboxyl-terminal-truncated apolipoprotein E4 causes Alzheimer's disease-like neurodegeneration and behavioral deficits in transgenic mice." *Proceedings of the National Academy of Sciences* **100**(19): 10966–10971.

Hashimoto, E., B. Zielke, et al. (1997). "Oxidative-stress associated parameters (lactoferrin, superoxide dismutases) in serum of patients with Alzheimers's disease." *Life Sciences* **60**: 13–19.

Ho, C. C., A. Kumaran, et al. (2009). "Bio-assay guided isolation and identification of anti-Alzheimer active compounds from the root of Angelica sinensis." *Food Chemistry* **114**(1): 246–252.

Ho, Y.-S., K.-F. So, et al. (2010). "Anti-aging herbal medicine—how and why can they be used in aging-associated neurodegenerative diseases?" *Ageing Research Reviews* **9**(3): 354–362.

Holmes, C. (2002). "Genotype and phenotype in Alzheimer's disease." *The British Journal of Psychiatry* **180**(2): 131–134.

Hong, G., W. Qin, et al. (1994). "Memory-improving effect of aqueous extract of Astragalus membranaceus (Fisch.) Bge." *Zhongguo Zhong yao za zhi = Zhongguo zhongyao zazhi = China Journal of Chinese Materia Medica* **19**(11): 687–688, 704.

Howes, M.-J. R. and P. J. Houghton (2003). "Plants used in Chinese and Indian traditional medicine for improvement of memory and cognitive function." *Pharmacology Biochemistry and Behavior* **75**(3): 513–527.

Hsieh, M.-T., Y.-T. Lin, et al. (2000). "Radix Angelica Sinensis extracts ameliorate scopolamine-and cycloheximide-induced amnesia, but not p-chloroamphetamine-induced amnesia in rats." *The American Journal of Chinese Medicine* **28**(02): 263–272.

Hsieh, M.-T., F.-H. Tsai, et al. (2002). "Effects of ferulic acid on the impairment of inhibitory avoidance performance in rats." *Planta Medica* **68**(08): 754–756.

Ichikawa, H., X. Wang, et al. (2003). "Role of component herbs in antioxidant activity of shengmai san—a traditional Chinese medicine formula preventing cerebral oxidative damage in rat." *The American Journal of Chinese Medicine* **31**(04): 509–521.

Irie, Y. and W. M. Keung (2003). "Rhizoma acori graminei and its active principles protect PC-12 cells from the toxic effect of amyloid-β peptide." *Brain Research* **963**(1–2): 282–289.

Jia, H., Y. Jiang, et al. (2004). "Tenuigenin treatment decreases secretion of the Alzheimer's disease amyloid β-protein in cultured cells." *Neuroscience Letters* **367**(1): 123–128.

Jiankang, L. and M. Akitane (1993). "Antioxidant and pro-oxidant activities of p-hydroxybenzyl alcohol and vanillin: effects on free radicals, brain peroxidation and degradation of benzoate, deoxyribose, amino acids and DNA." *Neuropharmacology* **32**(7): 659–669.

Jivad, N. and Z. Rabiei (2014). "A review study on medicinal plants used in the treatment of learning and memory impairments." *Asian Pacific Journal of Tropical Biomedicine* **4**(10): 780–789.

Joo, S. S., Y. M. Yoo, et al. (2008). "Prevention of inflammation-mediated neurotoxicity by Rg3 and its role in microglial activation." *Biological and Pharmaceutical Bulletin* **31**(7): 1392–1396.

Kalaria, R. N., G. E. Maestre, et al. (2008). "Alzheimer's disease and vascular dementia in developing countries: prevalence, management, and risk factors." *The Lancet Neurology* **7**(9): 812–826.

Kanowski, S. and R. Hoerr. (2003). Ginkgo biloba extract EGb 761® in dementia: intent-to-treat analyses of a 24-week, multi-center, double-blind, placebo-controlled, randomized trial. *Pharmacopsychiatry* **36**(06): 297–303.

Kastenholz, B. (2011). "Phytopharmaceuticals in the therapy of younger Alzheimer patients." *Webmed Central Aging* **2**(7):WMC002011.

Kennedy, D. O., A. B. Scholey, and K. A. Wesnes. (2002). Modulation of cognition and mood following administration of single doses of Ginkgo biloba, ginseng, and a ginkgo/ginseng combination to healthy young adults. *Physiology & behavior* **75**(5): 739–751.

Khalifa, A. E. (2001). "Hypericum perforatum as a nootropic drug: enhancement of retrieval memory of a passive avoidance conditioning paradigm in mice." *Journal of Ethnopharmacology* **76**(1): 49–57.
Kitazawa, M., T. R. Yamasaki, et al. (2004). "Microglia as a potential bridge between the amyloid β-peptide and tau." *Annals of the New York Academy of Sciences* **1035**(1): 85–103.
Kleijnen, J. and P. Knipschild. (1992). Ginkgo biloba for cerebral insufficiency. *British Journal of Clinical Pharmacology* **34**(4): 352–358.
Klunk, W. E., H. Engler, et al. (2004). "Imaging brain amyloid in Alzheimer's disease with Pittsburgh compound-B." *Annals of Neurology* **55**(3): 306–319.
Kulkarni, R., K. Girish, et al. (2012). "Nootropic herbs (Medhya Rasayana) in Ayurveda: an update." *Pharmacognosy Reviews* **6**(12): 147.
Kuller, L. H. (1996). "Hormone replacement therapy and its potential relationship to dementia." *Journal of the American Geriatrics Society* **44**(7): 878–880.
Kumar, G. P. and F. Khanum (2012). "Neuroprotective potential of phytochemicals." *Pharmacognosy Reviews* **6**(12): 81.
Kurz, A. and D. Van Baelen. (2004). Ginkgo biloba compared with cholinesterase inhibitors in the treatment of dementia: a review based on meta-analyses by the cochrane collaboration. *Dementia and Geriatric Cognitive Disorders* **18**(2): 217–226.
Lazarov, O., J. Robinson, et al. (2005). "Environmental enrichment reduces Aβ levels and amyloid deposition in transgenic mice." *Cell* **120**(5): 701–713.
Le Bars, P. L., M. M. Katz, et al. (1997). A placebo-controlled, double-blind, randomized trial of an extract of Ginkgo biloba for dementia. *JAMA* **278**(16): 1327–1332.
Leclerc, S., M. Garnier, et al. (2001). "Indirubins inhibit glycogen synthase kinase-3β and CDK5/P25, two protein kinases involved in abnormal tau phosphorylation in Alzheimer's disease a property common to most cyclin-dependent kinase inhibitors?" *Journal of Biological Chemistry* **276**(1): 251–260.
Lim, J. H., T. C. Wen, et al. (1997). Protection of ischemic hippocampal neurons by ginsenoside Rb1, a main ingredient of ginseng root. *Neuroscience Research* **28**(3): 191–200.
Lin, H. Q., M. T. Ho, et al. (2008). "Anti-acetylcholinesterase activities of traditional Chinese medicine for treating Alzheimer's disease." *Chemico-Biological Interactions* **175**(1–3): 352–354.
Lin, Y.-C., C.-R. Wu, et al. (2003). "The ameliorating effects of cognition-enhancing Chinese herbs on scopolamine-and MK-801-induced amnesia in rats." *The American Journal of Chinese Medicine* **31**(04): 543–549.
López, S., J. Bastida, et al. (2002). "Acetylcholinesterase inhibitory activity of some Amaryllidaceae alkaloids and Narcissus extracts." *Life Sciences* **71**(21): 2521–2529.
Luo, Y. (2006). "Alzheimer's disease, the nematode Caenorhabditis elegans, and ginkgo biloba leaf extract." *Life Sciences* **78**(18): 2066–2072.
Manczak, M., B. S. Park, et al. (2004). "Differential expression of oxidative phosphorylation genes in patients with Alzheimer's disease." *Neuromolecular Medicine* **5**(2): 147–162.
Mathur, D., K. Goyal, et al. (2016). "The molecular links of re-emerging therapy: a review of evidence of Brahmi (Bacopa monniera)." *Frontiers in Pharmacology* **7**: 44.
Mattson, M. P. (1997). "Cellular actions of beta-amyloid precursor protein and its soluble and fibrillogenic derivatives." *Physiological Reviews* **77**(4): 1081–1132.
Misra, L., P. Lal, et al. (2008). "Selective reactivity of 2-mercaptoethanol with 5β, 6β-epoxide in steroids from Withania somnifera." *Steroids* **73**(3): 245–251.
Morgan, D., D. M. Diamond, et al. (2000). "Aβ peptide vaccination prevents memory loss in an animal model of Alzheimer's disease." *Nature* **408**(6815): 982.
Munoz, D. G. and H. Feldman (2000). "Causes of Alzheimer's disease." *CMAJ* **162**(1): 65–72.
Nagy, Z., M. Esiri, et al. (1998). "The cell division cycle and the pathophysiology of Alzheimer's disease." *Neuroscience* **87**(4): 731–739.
Nalini, K., K. Karanth, et al. (1995). "Effects of Celastrus paniculatus on passive avoidance performance and biogenic amine turnover in albino rats." *Journal of Ethnopharmacology* **47**(2): 101–108.
Nilsberth, C., A. Westlind-Danielsson, et al. (2001). "The 'Arctic' APP mutation (E693G) causes Alzheimer's disease by enhanced Aβ protofibril formation." *Nature Neuroscience* **4**(9): 887.
Nishiyama, N., P. Chu, et al. (1995). "Beneficial effects of Biota, a traditional Chinese herbal medicine, on learning impairment induced by basal forebrain-lesion in mice." *Biological and Pharmaceutical Bulletin* **18**(11): 1513–1517.
Nordberg, A., E. Hellström-Lindahl, et al. (2002). "Chronic nicotine treatment reduces β-amyloidosis in the brain of a mouse model of Alzheimer's disease (APPsw)." *Journal of Neurochemistry* **81**(3): 655–658.
Ott, B. R. and N. J. Owens (1998). "Complementary and alternative medicines for Alzheimer's disease." *Journal of Geriatric Psychiatry and Neurology* **11**(4): 163–173.

Park, C. H., S.-H. Kim, et al. (1996). "Novel anticholinesterase and antiamnesic activities of dehydroevodiamine, a constituent of Evodia rutaecarpa." *Planta Medica* **62**(05): 405–409.

Peila, R., B. L. Rodriguez, et al. (2002). "Type 2 diabetes, APOE gene, and the risk for dementia and related pathologies: The Honolulu-Asia Aging Study." *Diabetes* **51**(4): 1256–1262.

Penido, A. B., S. M. De Morais, et al. (2017). "Medicinal plants from northeastern Brazil against Alzheimer's disease." *Evidence-Based Complementary and Alternative Medicine* **2017**: 1753673.

Perl, D. P. (2010). "Neuropathology of Alzheimer's disease." *Mount Sinai Journal of Medicine* **77**(1): 32–42.

Perry, R. J. and J. R. Hodges. (1999). Attention and executive deficits in Alzheimer's disease: A critical review. *Brain* **122**(3): 383–404.

Prasansuklab, A. and T. Tencomnao (2013). "Amyloidosis in Alzheimer's disease: the toxicity of amyloid beta (Aβ), mechanisms of its accumulation and implications of medicinal plants for therapy." *Evidence-Based Complementary and Alternative Medicine* **2013**: 413808.

Qian, Y.-H., Y. Liu, et al. (2002). "The effects of the total saponin of Dipsacus asperoides on the damage of cultured neurons induced by β-amyloid protein 25–35." *Anatomical Science International* **77**(3): 196–200.

Qiu, W. Q. and M. F. Folstein (2006). "Insulin, insulin-degrading enzyme and amyloid-β peptide in Alzheimer's disease: review and hypothesis." *Neurobiology of Aging* **27**(2): 190–198.

Ray, S. and A. Ray (2015). "Medhya rasayanas in brain function and disease." *Medicinal Chemistry* **5**(12): 505–511.

Perry, R. J. and J. R. Hodges. (1999). Attention and executive deficits in Alzheimer's disease: A critical review. *Brain* **122**(3): 383–404.

Raskind, M. A., E. R. Peskind, et al. (2000). Galantamine in AD: a 6-month randomized, placebo-controlled trial with a 6-month extension. *Neurology* **54**(12): 2261–2268.

Reddy, P. H. and M. F. Beal (2005). "Are mitochondria critical in the pathogenesis of Alzheimer's disease?" *Brain Research Reviews* **49**(3): 618–632.

Reddy, P. H., G. Mani, et al. (2005). "Differential loss of synaptic proteins in Alzheimer's disease: implications for synaptic dysfunction." *Journal of Alzheimer's Disease* **7**(2): 103–117.

Reddy, P. H., S. McWeeney, et al. (2004). "Gene expression profiles of transcripts in amyloid precursor protein transgenic mice: up-regulation of mitochondrial metabolism and apoptotic genes is an early cellular change in Alzheimer's disease." *Human Molecular Genetics* **13**(12): 1225–1240.

Rösler, M., W. Retz, et al. (1998). Free radicals in Alzheimer's dementia: currently available therapeutic strategies. Alzheimer's Disease—From Basic Research to Clinical Applications, Springer: 211–219.

Russo, A., M. Palumbo, et al. (2003). "Red wine micronutrients as protective agents in Alzheimer-like induced insult." *Life Sciences* **72**(21): 2369–2379.

Sassa, H., Y. Takaishi, et al. (1990). "The triterpene celastrol as a very potent inhibitor of lipid peroxidation in mitochondria." *Biochemical and Biophysical Research Communications* **172**(2): 890–897.

Schenk, D., R. Barbour, et al. (1999). "Immunization with amyloid-β attenuates Alzheimer-disease-like pathology in the PDAPP mouse." *Nature* **400**(6740): 173.

Sehgal, N., A. Gupta, et al. (2012). "Withania somnifera reverses Alzheimer's disease pathology by enhancing low-density lipoprotein receptor-related protein in liver." *Proceedings of the National Academy of Sciences* **109**(9): 3510–3515.

Selkoe, D. J. (1991). The molecular pathology of Alzheimer's disease. *Neuron* **6**(4): 487–498.

Selkoe, D. J. (2001). "Alzheimer's disease: genes, proteins, and therapy." *Physiological Reviews* **81**(2): 741–766.

Selkoe, D. J. (2002). "Alzheimer's disease is a synaptic failure." *Science* **298**(5594): 789–791.

Selkoe, D. J. and D. Schenk (2003). "Alzheimer's disease: molecular understanding predicts amyloid-based therapeutics." *Annual Review of Pharmacology and Toxicology* **43**(1): 545–584.

Seshadri, S., D. A. Drachman, et al. (1995). "Apolipoprotein E ε4 allele and the lifetime risk of Alzheimer's disease: What physicians know, and what they should know." *Archives of Neurology* **52**(11): 1074–1079.

Sharma, M. and Y. Gupta (2002). "Chronic treatment with trans resveratrol prevents intracerebroventricular streptozotocin induced cognitive impairment and oxidative stress in rats." *Life Sciences* **71**(21): 2489–2498.

Shin, R.-W. (1997). "Interaction of aluminum with paired helical filament tau is involved in neurofibrillary pathology of Alzheimer's disease." *Gerontology* **43**(Suppl. 1): 16–23.

Simonson, W. (2018). "Slow progress towards prevention and treatment of Alzheimer's disease." *Geriatric Nursing* **39**(5): 597–598.

Simpson, T., M. Pase, et al. (2015). "Bacopa monnieri as an antioxidant therapy to reduce oxidative stress in the aging brain." *Evidence-Based Complementary and Alternative Medicine* **2015**: 9.

Sinclair, S. (1998). "Chinese herbs: a clinical review of Astragalus, Ligusticum, and Schizandrae." *Alternative Medicine Review* **3**: 338–344.
Singh, N., M. Agrawal, et al. (2013). "Neuroprotective properties and mechanisms of resveratrol in in vitro and in vivo experimental cerebral stroke models." *ACS Chemical Neuroscience* **4**(8): 1151–1162.
Singhal, A. K., V. Naithani, et al. (2012). "Medicinal plants with a potential to treat Alzheimer and associated symptoms." *International Journal of Nutrition, Pharmacology, Neurological Diseases* **2**(2): 84.
Smith, J. and Y. Luo (2004). "Studies on molecular mechanisms of Ginkgo biloba extract." *Applied Microbiology and Biotechnology* **64**(4): 465–472.
Tanzi, R. and L. Bertram (2005). "Twenty years of the Alzheimer's traditional disease states: menopause." *American Family Physician* **66**: 129–134.
Tian, J., J. Shi, et al. (2010). "Herbal therapy: a new pathway for the treatment of Alzheimer's disease." *Alzheimer's Research & Therapy* **2**(5): 30.
Toda, S., Y. Yase, et al. (2000). "Inhibitory effects of astragali radix, crude drug in Oriental medicines on lipid peroxidation and protein oxidative modification of mouse brain homogenate by copper." *Phytotherapy Research* **14**(4): 294–296.
Veerendra Kumar, M. and Y. Gupta (2003). "Effect of Centella asiatica on cognition and oxidative stress in an intracerebroventricular streptozotocin model of Alzheimer's disease in rats." *Clinical and Experimental Pharmacology and Physiology* **30**(5–6): 336–342.
Wang, R., H. Yan and X. C. Tang. (2006). Progress in studies of huperzine A, a natural cholinesterase inhibitor from Chinese herbal medicine. *Acta Pharmacologica Sinica* **27**(1): 1–26.
Wettstein, A. (2000). "Cholinesterase inhibitors and Ginkgo extracts—are they comparable in the treatment of dementia?: comparison of published placebo-controlled efficacy studies of at least six months' duration." *Phytomedicine* **6**(6): 393–401.
Williams, B. R., A. Nazarians and M. A. Gill. (2003). A review of rivastigmine: a reversible cholinesterase inhibitor. *Clinical Therapeutics* **25**(6): 1634–1653.
Winkler, E. A., Y. Nishida, et al. (2015). "GLUT1 reductions exacerbate Alzheimer's disease vasculo-neuronal dysfunction and degeneration." *Nature Neuroscience* **18**(4): 521.
Wint, D. and J. Tavee (2014). "Alzheimer Disease." Cleveland Clinic [Internet]. http://www.clevelandclinicmeded.com/medicalpubs/diseasemanagement/neurology/alzheimers-disease/
Yankner, B. A. (1996). "Mechanisms of neuronal degeneration in Alzheimer's disease." *Neuron* **16**(5): 921–932.
Yu, M.-S., C. S.-W. Lai, et al. (2007). "Characterization of the effects of anti-aging medicine Fructus lycii on β-amyloid peptide neurotoxicity." *International Journal of Molecular Medicine* **20**(2): 261–268.
Yu, M.-S., S. K.-Y. Leung, et al. (2005). "Neuroprotective effects of anti-aging oriental medicine Lycium barbarum against β-amyloid peptide neurotoxicity." *Experimental Gerontology* **40**(8–9): 716–727.
Zhang, Z.-J. (2004). "Therapeutic effects of herbal extracts and constituents in animal models of psychiatric disorders." *Life Sciences* **75**(14): 1659–1699.
Zhao, Y., J. M. Hill, et al. (2014). Aluminum-induced amyloidogenesis and impairment in the clearance of amyloid peptides from the central nervous system in Alzheimer's disease. *Frontiers in Neurology* **5**(5): 167.

4 Cognitive Improvement, Neuroprotective, and Nootropic Effect of *Medhya Rasāyana* Drugs in Alzheimer's Disease

Rinki Kumari, Jasmit Singh, Bhargawi Mishra, Anamika Tiwari, and Abaidya Nath Singh

CONTENTS

4.1 INTRODUCTION

Alzheimer's disease (AD) is a chronic neurodegenerative disease of undetermined etiology, seen in the elderly, but rarely in people younger than 60 years old, except in its familial form, where its inheritance is autosomal dominant. It is an irreversible, progressive brain disorder that slowly destroys memory and thinking skills and, eventually, the ability to carry out the simplest tasks (Ballard et al., 2011; Ryman et al., 2014). AD is associated with accumulations of specific proteins in areas of brain tissue, represented by plaques and tangles, and loss of connections between neurons in the brain. The combined presence of amyloid-beta (Aβ) and tau (τ) proteins stands out as the hallmark of progressive AD and is the target of most disease-modifying therapies (Scheltens et al., 2016; Akiyama, 2016). Other features include atrophy of certain parts of the brain, inflammation, production of free radicals, and mitochondrial dysfunction. Advances in brain imaging techniques, such as the iDISCO visualization method and Raman imaging, allow sharp images to be obtained of these affected areas and to see the development and spread of abnormal amyloid and tau proteins in the living brain, as well as changes in brain structure and function. The most common cause of dementia among older adults, initial clinical symptoms of AD include short-term memory loss, subsequently followed by the impairment of recent memory which is followed by impairment of cognitive abilities, vocabulary, and concepts or executive dysfunction, confusion, agitation, and behavioral disturbance, to the most severe stage, when the person has to depend completely on others for the basic activities of daily living (Markowitsch and Staniloiu, 2012).

Short-term memory loss is due to involvement of the median temporal lobe and hippocampus, which control recent memory; consequently, involvement of other areas of brain may manifest as sleep disturbances, problems in judgment, psychological alterations, pyramidal and extrapyramidal motor signs and symptoms (Scoville and Milner, 1957; Alzheimer's Association, 2010).

Currently, AD is ranked as the sixth leading cause of death in the United States, but recent estimates indicate that the disorder may rank third, just behind heart disease and cancer, as a cause of death for older people. AD was first identified more than 100 years ago, but more than 70 years passed before it was recognized as the most common cause of dementia, as well as a major cause of death (Katzman, 1976). Alzheimer's and other dementias are the major cause of disabilities in later life. AD represents the most common neurodegenerative dementia, amounting to 50–75% of all dementias and the incidence of AD is expected to increase threefold by 2050, and about 36 million people have dementia all over the world (Alzheimer's Association, 2015; Götz et al., 2006). According to a 2019 report, nearly 50 million people have a type of neurodegenerative disease. Only one in four people with AD have been diagnosed. AD and dementia are most common in western Europe, whereas AD is least prevalent in sub-Saharan Africa.

According to the World Alzheimer's Report 2015, the prevalence of dementia increases day by day and rose from 30 million (2010) to 46.8 million in 2015, in the United States. The expenditure on dementia rose from US$ 604 million (2010) to US$ 818 million (2015). Report has also declared that ADis the only disease in the ten leading causes of deaths in the United States that cannot be cured, prevented, or slowed. Statistical evaluation reported that 1 in 10 Americans over the age of 65 ha sAD. Between 2017 and 2025, every state is expected to see at least a 14% rise in the prevalence of dementias. The proportion of the US population with AD by age is 85+ years (38%), 75–84 years (44%), 65–74 years (15%), and <65 years (4%). According to a report in the US in 2016, 15.9 million family caregivers provided an estimated 18.2 billion hours, valued at $230 billion, to people with dementia, and, in 2017, the cost to the United States was $259 billion. In India, the prevalence of dementia was 33.6 in every 1,000 people, of which 54% were cases of AD (WHO, 2015).

It is estimated that, by the year 2020, approximately 70% of the world's population aged 60 and above will be living in developing countries, with 14.2% in India (WHO, 1998). The reported incidence rates for AD has been lower in Asian countries than in the industrialized world (Zhang et al., 1998; Chen et al., 2011). Although AD prevalence studies are available from Asian countries, including India (Chiu et al., 1998; Vas et al., 2001), there is a dearth of incidence data (Zhang et al., 1998; Chen et al., 2011). However, these data are from prospective long-term studies, which means there is not a full understanding of the mechanism as of yet.

The pathogenesis of AD is still not completely understood. There are three potential mechanisms that are involved in the causation of AD:

1. deposition of Aβ proteins;
2. deposition of τ proteins in cytoplasm of neurons;
3. neuronal degeneration due to the two above components (Masliah et al., 1993).

Numerous studies have identified some genes involved in the pathogenesis of AD and determined that mutation in these genes decided the stage of AD, such as presenelin-1 (PS1), amyloid precursor protein (APP), presenelin-2 (PS2), and apolipoprotein E (APOE). *APP* and *PSEN1* gene mutations result in early-onset AD, with the *APOE* mutation being implicated in late-onset AD, whereas PS2 has a more variable onset effect (Selkoe, 2001).

There are two types of PSEN gene involved in the pathogenesis of AD, *PSEN1* and *PSEN2*. The *PSEN1* gene is located on chromosome 14q and regulates intracellular Ca^{2+} signaling and trafficking of membrane proteins, and is involved in the regulation of the stabilization of β-catenin. Studies reported that any type of mutation in the *PSEN1* gene results in the formation of Aβ peptides of varying lengths, due to cleavage at different sites by γ-secretase. These peptides are highly fibrillogenic, causing increased aggregation of Aβ plaques in the brain (Brunkan and Goate, 2005). The second presenilin gene, *PSEN2*, is located on chromosome 1q and encodes the PS2 transmembrane protein, isoform 2 of which is found in the brain. *PSEN2* mutations cause accumulation of the Aβ42 protein, which is the hallmark of AD (Cai et al., 2015).

Another gene, the amyloid precursor protein gene (*APP*), is present on chromosome 21q and synthesizes the protein, APP. APP is present in the plasma membrane as a transmembrane protein, and has both intracellular and extracellular parts. Normally, cleavage by α-secretase is followed by cleavage by γ-secretase, which results in the formation of soluble proteins. Alpha- and β-secretase cleavage sites are present on the surface of the cell, whereas γ-secretase has a cleavage site in the intra-membrane region of the protein. In an AD patient, β-secretase carries out the first cleavage, which is followed by cleavage by γ-secretase, resulting in the generation of the Aβ protein, which becomes aggregated and is deposited in various parts of the brain to cause neuronal degeneration (Priller et al., 2006). Aβ protein is also deposited in the walls of the blood vessels, where it weakens them, resulting in amyloid angiopathy.

Studies have reported that the *APOE* gene produces the Apo-E protein, which normally helps in the removal of Aβ proteins as well as protecting neurons from damage. There are three variants of Apo-E proteins, namely ε2, ε3, and ε4. The mutant oxidized form of ε4 binds readily to Aβ protein and results in deposition as amyloid plaques, as well as decreasing cholinergic activity in the brain (Poirier et al., 1995).

Normally, τ proteins provide stability to the microtubules but, in AD, they undergo hyperphosphorylation, becoming aggregated and forming neurofibrillary tangles in the cytoplasm of the neurons (Chaudhari et al., 2017).

Numerous reports have shown that aggregation of amyloid plaques in the brain, causing high amyloid signals, is among the earliest AD indications, while brain atrophy and detectable cognitive changes are more dynamic later. The amyloid signal is more frequently related to cognition in AD patents and causes neurodegeneration. By the time AD processes have progressed enough to cause cognitive decline, the amyloid plaque may have promoted other mechanisms that influence cognition, such as toxicity caused by neurofibrillary tangles, inflammation, or Aβ oligomers (Braskie et al., 2013).

Many studies have shown that, at an early stage of AD, the level of brain amyloid rises rapidly, but may plateau as cognitive decline progresses. Cognitive impairment and other AD biomarkers, such as hippocampal atrophy, may continue to progress while the deposition of brain amyloid may not, resulting in a disconnection between amyloid and cognitive performance later in AD. In addition, in AD patients and those at increased risk of AD, brain amyloid may influence cognition directly or indirectly, through neurodegenerative processes. Other measures of brain health, such as vascular health and individual differences in brain structure and its connectivity throughout a lifetime, may be associated with cognitive changes. Several longitudinal studies and studies with imaging biomarkers from multiple modalities provide valuable insights into cognitive deficits in AD (Braskie et al., 2013). Therefore, AD involves a progressive, inexorable loss of cognitive function, associated with the presence of senile plaques in the hippocampal area of the brain.

In short, the neuropathological process of AD consists of neuronal loss and atrophy, principally in the temporo-parietal and frontal cortices, with an inflammatory response to the deposition of amyloid plaques. An abnormal aggregation of protein fragments and neurofibillary tangles causes AD.

4.2 *ĀYURVEDIC* APPROACH OF ALZHEIMER'S DISEASE

Āyurveda is considered the *Upaveda* of *Atharva Veda*, being the oldest recorded wisdom of the earth. *Rasāyana* has been considered as a form of rejuvenative recipes, dietary regimens and special health-promoting conduct and behavior i.e. *Medhya Rasāyana*, *Ācāra-Rasāyana*, etc. This therapy helps the individual to attain longevity, memory, intelligence, freedom from disorder, youthful age, excellence of luster, complexion, and voice, optimum strength of physique and sense organs, successful words, respectability, and brilliance. *Āyurveda* cures human diseases through establishment of equilibrium in the different elements of human life, the body, the mind, the intellect, and the soul (Ven et al., 2010).

The ancient *Āyurvedic* approach to disease prevention involves therapeutic measures to arrest or delay aging and to achieve rejuvenation and whole functional dynamics of the body system. According to *Āyurveda,* the homeostasis of the body is maintained by *Doṣas* that regulate all the metabolic processes: (a) *Vāta* regulates the transportation (movements in the whole body, tissues, cells, and elsewhere), (b) *Pitta* governs the process of nutrient assimilation into tissues (catabolism), and (c) *Kapha* stimulates synthesis of newer tissues (anabolism).

The revitalization and rejuvenation approach of *Āyurveda* is known as the "*Rasāyana cikitsā*" (rejuvenation therapy), one of the eight specialized branches of *Āyurveda.* It aims to achieve enhancement in strength, immunity, *ojus*, vitality, willpower, and determination of the body, longevity, memory, intelligence, excellence of luster, complexion and voice, and optimum strength of physique and sense organs.

4.3 ACCORDING TO THE ANCIENT TEXT, THERE ARE MANY CAUSATIVE FACTORS OF *MANOVIKĀRAS*

1. Improper diet
2. Actions committed in this life,
3. Bad deeds done in the past life,
4. Physical illnesses and overindulgence.
5. Severe mental or physical stress
6. Unfavorable personal, familial, or social environments, etc.

4.4 *ĀYURVEDA* ALSO SAYS THAT NEGATIVE FEELINGS ARE EMOTIONAL TOXINS

If they are not driven out of body within a stipulated time, such toxins give rise to chronic mental disorders like anxiety, neurosis, depression, etc. If this is further ignored, it turns into permanent mental disorders like *Unmāda* (unreasonable and irrational state of mind, such as hysteria) and *Apasmāra* (epilepsy).

4.5 MENTAL DISORDERS IN *ĀYURVEDA*

1. *Unmāda*: insanity
2. *Apasmāra*: epilepsy
3. *Avasāda*: depression
4. *Citto-udvega*: anxiety neurosis

5. *Manasa Mandatā*: mental retardation
6. *Atatvā-abhinevisa*: obsessive disorders.
7. *Madātyaya*: intoxication etc.

4.6 GENERAL PRINCIPLES OF MANAGEMENT

1. *Daiva vyapāsraya cikitsā* (chanting of *Mantras*, *Homa*; spiritual healing, religious rites, etc.)
2. *Yukti vyapāsraya cikitsā* (medicines i.e. *Śodhana* and *Śamana*, psychotropic drugs and diet)
3. *Satvāvajaya cikitsā* (psychotherapy)

In short, *Āyurvedic* texts deal with the nervous system and disorders associated with it. Nervous system disorders, called '*Vātavyādhi*' in *Sanskṛata*, were thought to be brought on by imbalances of *Vāta*, the biological air humor, the energy that moves through the brain, and the nerves (the ancients considered nerve impulses to be a kind of wind or air traveling through the body), controling both voluntary and involuntary functions. Hence, *Vāta* derangements always involve some weakness, disturbance, or hypersensitivity of the nervous system. Included in these texts are direct references to age-associated memory loss, preventive care, and therapeutic interventions.

Despite extensive research efforts, AD-based research has suffered major setbacks, as no new drugs have been discovered in the past decade, and pathological mechanisms are still not clearly understood. Transgenic animal models show Aβ-amyloids, neuritic plaques, and neurofibrillary tangles (NFTs) as well as synaptic and degenerative changes, but do not show the typical AD phenotypic features. Therefore, the treatment that works in these models may fail in humans. A meteoric rise in the global burden of AD is predicted, whereas the few available medications remain unchanged and are associated with major side effects (Hanaa et al., 2014).

Globally, herbal medications receive widespread acclaim from more than 90% of the world population, due to their higher biosafety profile relative to synthetic drugs. Their scientific and commercial significance also appear to be gathering momentum in health-relevant areas. These plant-derived products are carefully standardized, and their efficacy and safety for a specific application have been demonstrated. Products extracted from plant species and their derivatives have neuroprotectant effects *in vitro* and *in vivo*. In addition to neuroprotection, natural products also exhibit biological effects that target biochemical pathways underlying associated symptoms of neurodegenerative disorders, that include cognitive impairments, energy/fatigue, mood, and anxiety (Rao et al., 2012).

Āyurvedic medicine is a system of traditional medicine native to India, and *Āyurvedic* practitioners have developed a number of medicinal preparations called herbal formulations. *Āyurveda* texts explain the use of several herbs and their qualities and energetics for nervous system disorders, including memory loss typically seen in older adults, but only recently have there been mechanistic studies on the role of these herbs in nervous system disorders and dementias, including dementia associated with AD. A number of scientific studies have described the use of various *Āyurvedic* medicinal plants termed "nervines" and their constituents to strengthen the functional activity of the nervous system and to achieve restoration of memory. They have also helped to nourish blood, lymph, flesh, adipose tissue, and semen, and are involved in the prevention of chronic degenerative diseases. These medicinal plants have various essential phyto-chemicals such as lignans, flavonoids, tannins, polyphenols, triterpenes, sterols, and alkaloids, that show a wide spectrum of pharmacological activities, including anti-inflammatory, antiamyloidogenic, anticholinesterase, hypolipidemic, and antioxidant effects (Abascal et al., 2004; Bredesen, 2009; Alzheimer's Association, 2010; Rao et al., 2012).

In this chapter, we will extensively review the literature of different herbal nootropic drugs related to *Medhya Rasāyana*, with its aim of enhancing strength, immunity, *ojus*, vitality, willpower and determination of the body, longevity, memory, intelligence, excellence of luster, complexion and voice, and optimum strength of physique and sense organs (Chaudhari and Murthy, 2014).

Ācārya Caraka classified all the herbal drugs into three different groups, with different modes of action, as follows:

1. *Doṣa Praśamana*, which pacifies the vitiated *doṣas*;
2. *Dhātu Praduṣaṇa*, which vitiates *Dhātus*; and
3. *Swasthavṛattakara*, which maintains proper health.

Rasāyana drugs are considered to promote nutrition through the following modes of actions:

1. direct enrichment of the nutritional quality of *Rasa Dhātu* (nutritional plasma) as *Śatāvarī*, *Dugdha* (cow's milk) and *Gṛata*.
2. improvement of *Agni* (digestion and metabolism) as *Bhallātaka*, *Pippalī*.
3. promotion of the competence of *Srotas* (microcirculatory channels in the body) as *Guggulu* etc.

In the classical Indian text, *Rasāyanīs* is the achievement of the finest quality of *Rasādidhātu* (body tissues), which increases life span, improves *medhya* (intelligence), cures disease, stabilizes youthfulness, improves luster, complexion, and voice, and improves body and senses, making them strong and healthy, etc. *Ācārya Caraka* has explained that the equilibrium of *Agni* of *Dhātu* (*Dhātvāgni*), *Vāyu*, and *Srotas* (microchannels of the body) are the most important things for maintaining normal health, comparing it with strength, color, and prolonged existence of the body and *Medhā* (*Dhī, Dhṛati* and *Smṛati*). *Medhya* provide some important mental faculties, are interrelated with each other and with different capabilities of the brain, such as *Grahaṇa Śakti* (Power of Grasping), *Dhāraṇa Śakti* (Power of Retention), *Viveka Śakti* (Power of Discrimination), and *Smṛati* (Power of Recollection) (Singh et al., 2014).

There are different *Rasāyana* drugs, which act as:

a. immunomodulator, used to help regulate or normalize the immune system;
b. adaptogen, used in herbal medicine for the purported stabilization of physiological processes and promotion of homeostasis, or increasing the ability of an organism to adapt to its environmental factors e.g., *Aśwagandhā, Tulasī, Haridrā, Pippalī, Āmalakī, Guḍūcī, Śatāvarī* etc;
c. antioxidant, that inhibits oxidation, especially when used to counteract the deterioration of stored food products or circumvent the damage caused by oxygen free radicals. Here, we are focused on the nootropic drugs under the *Medhya Rasāyanas* text of *Āyurveda*;
d. nootropic, also known as a smart drug and cognitive enhancer. These drugs act as supplements to other substances that may improve cognitive function, particularly executive functions, memory, creativity, or motivation, in healthy individuals, or promote intelligence and functions of brain e.g. *Medhya Rasāyana* drugs (namely *Maṇḍūkaparṇī, Guḍūcī, Yaṣṭhīmadhu* and *Śankhpuṣpī*) (Ray and Ray, 2015).

4.7 *ĀYURVEDIC* PRACTITIONERS HAVE DEVELOPED TWO TYPES OF FORMULATION OF *MEDHYA RASĀYANA*

1. *Śīta Vīrya* and *Madhura Vipāka* – they promote *Kapha* and enhance "*Dhāraṇa Karma*" (i.e. retention of cognition) e.g. *Yaṣṭhīmadhu, Brāmhī, Śankhpuṣpī*, etc.
2. *Uṣṇa Vīrya* and *Tikta Rasa* – they promote *Pitta* and enhance *Grahaṇa* and *Smaraṇa* (i.e. grasping power and memory) e.g. *Guḍūcī, Vacā, Jyotiṣmatī*, etc.

These ***Medhya Rasāyana*** act at different levels of *prakṛiti*:

1. at the level of *Rasa*
2. by stimulating and improving the function of *Agni*;
3. by improving circulation of *Rasa* by opening and cleaning the microchannels and thus improving *Medhya* function.

4.8 GENERAL MECHANISM OF *MEDHYA RASĀYANA* DRUGS IN THE TREATMENT OF NEUROLOGICAL DISEASES

In *Āyurveda*, *Medhya rasāyana* drugs play an essential role in the treatment of psychiatric and psychosomatic diseases, with a safe mode of action. The mechanism of this therapy involves the individual attaining calmness, tranquility, or a stimulation of activities of the brain. Based on different research, both experimental and clinical, these drugs exert varying degrees of psychotropic action and are known to exhibit antidepressant, sedative, and tranquilizing action. *Medhya Rasāyana* drugs are used for prevention and treatment of mental disorders in all age groups. These drugs promote the intellect (*Dhī*) retention power (*Dhṛati*) and memory (*Smṛiti*). In fact, they produce neuronutrient effects by improving cerebral metabolism. These drugs are known to have a specific effect on mental performance by promoting the functions of "*Buddhi*" and "*Manas*" and by correcting the disturbances of "*Rājasa*" and "*Tāmasa*". This helps the patient to get relief from stress, anxiety, and depression.

As mentioned in the *Āyurveda* text, "*Medhya Rasāyanas*" has originated from the *Sanskṛata* words "*medhya*", meaning intellect or cognition, and "*Rasāyan*"', meaning rejuvenation. There are so many medicinal plants under the *Medhya Rasāyanas Āyurvedic* system that they are known as "*Medhya Rasāyanas*" drugs. These drugs act as a nootropic agents, brain tonics or rejuvenators. Numerous studies defined various neurological and psychiatric disorders which are generally associated with loss of memory, cognitive deficits, impaired mental function, etc. so we need such a *Medhya Rasāyanas* drugs to improve the intellect e.g., *Brāhmī Aindrī* (*Bacopa monnieri*), *Maṇḍūkaparṇī* (*Centella asiatica*), *Āmalakī* (*Emblica officinale*), *Vacā* (*Acorus calamus*), *Aśwagandhā* (*Withania somnifera*), *Śankhapuṣpī* (*Convolvulus pluricaulis*), *Jyotiṣmatī (Celastrus paniculatus*), *Jaṭāmānsī* (*Nardostachys jatamansi*), *Tagara* (*Valeriana wallichii*), *Yaṣṭimadhu* (*Glycyrrhiza glabra*), *Guḍūcī* (*Tinospora cordifolia*), and *Kuṣmāṇḍa* (*Benincasa hispida*), Table 4.1 describes the drugs having the *Medhya Rasāyana* property.

4.8.1 *Brāhmī*

Brāhmī is widely used as '*Medhya Rasāyana*' in *Āyurveda*. Two species are considered to be *Brāhmī*, namely *Aindrī (Bacopa monnieri)* and *Maṇḍūkaparṇī (Centella asiatica)*.

4.8.2 *Aindrī (Bacopa monnieri)*

Bacopa monniera has been classified under "*Medhya rasāyana*", i.e. medicinal plants rejuvenating intellect and memory (Rai et al., 2003). The name *Brāhmī* is derived from the word *'Brahma'*, the mythical 'creator' in the Hindu pantheon. Because the brain is the center for creative activity, any compound that improves brain health is called *Brāhmī* (Figure 4.1).

B. monnieri, belonging to the family Plantaginaceae, is a small, creeping herb with numerous branches, small, oblong leaves, and light small purple or white flowers, with four or five petals. The leaves are succulent, relatively thick, and oblanceolate, and are arranged oppositely on the stem.

Compounds responsible for the pharmacological effects include alkaloids, saponins, and sterols. Detailed investigations first reported the isolation of the alkaloid "brahmine" (Bose and Bose, 1931).

TABLE 4.1
The *Medhya Rasāyana* Drugs Involved in the Treatment of Alzheimer's Disease and Improvement of Intellectual Properties

		Properties			
***Medhya* Drugs**	**Synonyms**	***Rasa***	***Guṇa***	***Vīrya***	***Vipāka***
Aindrī (*Bacopa monnieri* (Linn.) Pennell.)	*Brāhmī, Sarasvatī, Kapota vankgā, Somavallī*	*Tikta*	*Laghu*	*Uṣṇa*	*Kaṭu*
Maṇḍūkaparṇī (*Centella asiatica* Linn.)	*Māṇḍukī, Divyā, Mahauṣadhī, Brāhmī, Tvāṣṭrī*	*Tikta*	*Laghu*	*Śīta*	*Madhura*
Āmalakī (*Embelica officinale*)	*Dhātrī, Vayasyā, Jātiphalarasā, Śiva, Vṛaṣyā, Amṛatā, Amṛata phala, Sriphala, Tiṣyaphalā*	*Panca rasa,lavaṇa rahita*	*Guru, Rukṣa, Śīta*	*Śīta*	*Madhura*
Aśwagandhā (*Withania somnifera*)	*Vajigandhā, VaradÁ, GokarÆÍ, Hayagandhā, Turagí, VanajÁ, VÁjinÍ, Varāhakarṇī, BalyÁ,*	*Madhura Kaṣāya, Tikta,*	*Laghu, Snigdha*	*Uṣṇa*	*Madhura*
Śankhapuṣpī (*Convolvulus pluricaulis* Chois.)	*Kṣīrpuṣpī, Māngalyakusuma*	*Tikta*	*Snigdha Picchila*	*Śīta*	*Madhura*
Jyotiṣmatī (*Celastrus paniculatus* Willd.)	*Kaṭabhī, Jyotishka, Kangunī, Pārāvatpadī, Pinya, Latā, Kākāndaī, Mālakanganī*	*Kaṭu, Tikta*	*Tikṣṇa*	*Uṣṇa*	*Kaṭu*
Jaṭāmānsī (*Nardostachys jatamansi* DC.)	*Bhūtjaṭā, Jaṭilā, Tapasvinī, Mānasī*	*Tikta, Kaṣāya Madhura*	*Laghu, Snigdha*	*Śīta*	*Kaṭu*
Tagara (*Valeriana wallichii*)	*Nata, Vakra, Kuṭila, Nahuṣa*	*Tikta, Kaṭu, Kaṣāya*	*Laghu, Snigdha*	*Uṣṇa*	*Kaṭu*
Yaṣṭimadhu (*Glycyrrhiza glabra* Linn.)	*Yaṣṭimadhuka, Klītaka*	*Madhura*	*Guru, Snigdha*	*Śīta*	*Madhura*
Guḍūcī (*Tinospora cordifolia* Willd. Miers.)	*Amṛatā, Madhuparṇī, Chinnamulā, Cakra-lakṣaṇīkā, Amṛatavallī, Chinnā, Chinnodhbhava, Vatsādanī, Jivantī, Tantrikā, Soma, Somavallī, Kuṇḍalī, Dhīra, Viśalyā, Rasāyanī, Candrahāsā, Vayasthā, Maṇḍalī,*	*Tikta, Kaṣāya*	*Guru, Snigdha*	*Uṣṇa*	*Madhura*
Kuṣmāṇḍa (*Benincasa hispida* Thunb. Cogn.)	*Puṣpaphalā, Pītapuśpā, Bṛahatphalā*	*Madhura*	*Laghu, Snigdha*	*Śīta*	*Madhura*
Vacā (*Acorus calamus* Linn.)	*Vaca, Ugragandhā, Ṣaḍagranthā, Golomī, Śatparvikā, Khudra-patrī, Māngalyā, Jaṭilā, Ugra, Lomaśā,*	*Kaṭu, Tikta*	*Laghu, Tikṣṇa*	*Uṣṇa*	*Kaṭu*
Bhangā (*Cannabis sativa*)	*Ganjā, Mātulānī, Mādinī, Vijayā, Jayā*	*Tikta*	*Laghu, Tikṣṇa*	*Uṣṇa*	*Kaṭu*
Ahiphena (*Papaver somniferum*)	*Khasaphala Kṣīra, Āphūka, Ahiphenaka*	*Tikta, Kaṣāya*	*Laghu, Rukṣa*	*Uṣṇa*	*Kaṭu*

Later, other alkaloids, like nicotine and herpestine, have also been reported (Chopra, 1956). Subsequently, the isolation of D-mannitol, and a saponin, hersaponin, and potassium salts were reported (Sastri et al., 1959).

The major chemical entity shown to be responsible for neuropharmacological effects and the nootropic action or antiamnestic effect of *Brāhmī* is bacoside A, classified as 3-(α-L-arabinopyranosyl)-*O*-β-D-glucopyranoside-10, 20-dihydroxy-16-keto-dammar-24-ene (Chatterji et al., 1965).

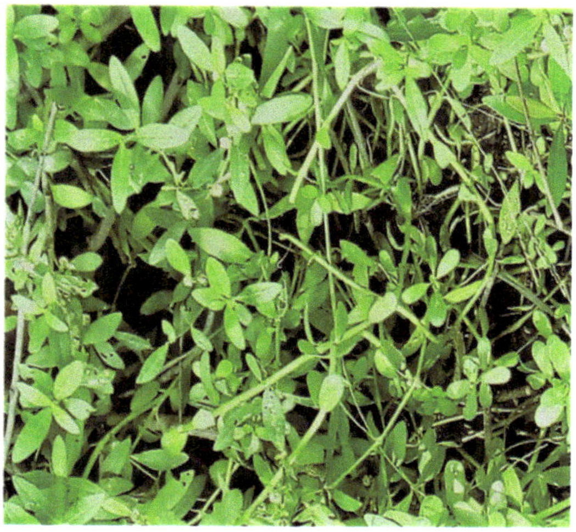

FIGURE 4.1 *Brahmi* (*Bacopa monnieri*).

Sedative and tranquillizing properties were effected by the saponin glycosides' (Malhotra and Das, 1959). Cognitive deficits were induced by intracerebro ventricularly administered colchicine and the injection of ibotenic acid into the nucleus basalis magnocellularis (Bhattacharya et al., 1999). For anxiety, it had been demonstrated that Brahmi contains 25% bacoside. Bacoside reduces anxiety without inducing amnesia, the side effect associated with lorazepam, but instead has a memory-enhancing effect (Bhattacharya and Ghosal, 1998; Shankar and Singh, 2000).

The antidepressant potential of Brāhmī had been evaluated in an earlier study wherein it showed a significant antidepressant activity in the most commonly used behavior paradigms in animal models of depression, namely the forced swim test and the learned helplessness test (Sairam et al., 2002; Kumari et al., 2016). Brāhmī has been indicated as a remedy for epilepsy in *Āyurvedic* medicine (Shanmugasundaram et al., 1991).

4.8.3 *Maṇḍūkaparṇī (Centella asiatica)*

It has been used as a medicine in the *Āyurvedic* tradition of India for thousands of years and is listed in the historic *Susṛuta Samhitā*, *Caraka Samhitā* and other *Āyurvedic* ancient texts. In China, known as *Gotukola*, it is one of the reported "miracle elixirs of life", known for more than 2000 years ago.

Maṇḍūkaparṇī (Figure 4.2) is a perennial herbaceous creeper, having small fan-shaped green leaves with white or light purple-to-pink or white flowers and bears small oval fruit. It belongs to the family Apiaceae and is found throughout India in moist places up to an altitude of 1800 m in tropical and subtropical regions in swampy areas.

Maṇḍūkaparṇī contains saponins (also called triterpenoids), including asiaticosides, in which a trisaccharide moiety is linked to the aglycones asiatic acid, madecassoside, and madasiatic acid (Singh and Rastogi, 1969). These include brahmoside and brahminoside, which are postulated to be responsible for CNS and uterorelaxant actions, but these effects have yet to be confirmed by clinical studies. A crude extract that contained the glycosides isothankuniside and thankuniside showed antifertility action in mice.

Maṇḍūkaparṇī has CNS effects described in Indian literature, such as stimulatory-nerve tonic, rejuvenator, sedative, tranquilizer, and intelligence-promoting properties (Kumar, 2006; Gupta et al., 2003). It increases the cerebral levels of γ-amino butyric acid (GABA), which explains its traditional use as an anxiolytic and an anticonvulsant. It is known that GABA and its agonists inhibit the central cholinergic action by affecting the turnover rate of acetylcholine in the rat brain. The

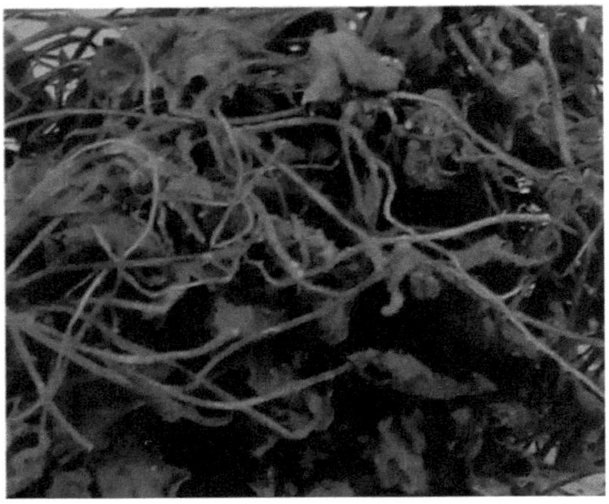

FIGURE 4.2 *MAṆḌŪKAPARṆĪ (Centella asiatica).*

isolated steroids from the plant have been used to treat epilepsy (Hausen, 1993). Therefore, by acting on behavior as well as being neuroprotective, brain-growth promoters inhibit the memory impairment induced by scopolamine through the inhibition of AChE.

4.8.4 *AŚVAGANDHĀ (WITHANIA SOMNIFERA)*

Withania somnifera (family Solanaceae) (Figure 4.3) is a highly esteemed medicinal herb in *Āyurveda* and is mostly known as *Aśvagandhā*, although other common names include the King of *Āyurveda*, Indian ginseng (although it is not related to *Panax ginseng*) and winter cherry. The herb is classified as *rasāyana* in *Āyurvedic* medicine due to its being a general tonic, and, in modern terms, it is called an adaptogen for similar reasons, and is also classified as *balya* (increases strength) and *vajikara* (aphrodisiac) (Ven Murthy et al., 2010).

The name *Aśvagandhā* comes from the translation "Smell of Horse", which is thought to be due to two main reasons: the root itself smells like a horse, and the root is supposed to imbibe you with the strength and virility of a horse. It produces *Kāmaśakti* like a horse in humans, and the plant does smell like a horse. In addition to those uses, it has been traditionally used as an analgesic, astringent,

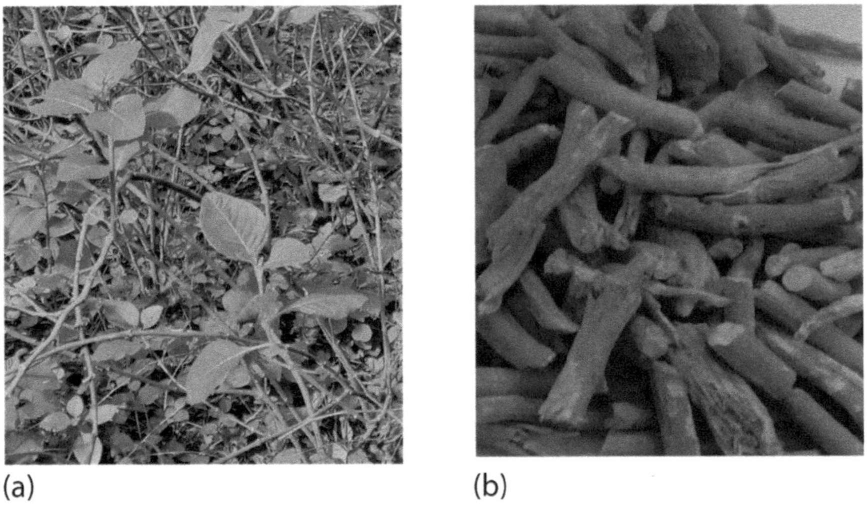

FIGURE 4.3 (a) *AŚVAGANDHĀ (Withania somnifera)* (fresh form). (b) *AŚVAGANDHĀ (W. somnifera)* (dry form).

and antispasmodic, whereas it is also used to treat inflammation, cancer, stress, fatigue, diabetes, and cardiovascular complications, whereas its adaptogenic usage is emphasized by its use to treat stress-related insomnia, debility, and nervous exhaustion. *Aśvagandhā* has also been reported to be an immunostimulant compound, with particular emphasis for treating stress-related suppression of immunity (Mishra et al., 2000; Kumar et al., 2015; Kumari et al., 2016).

Aśvagandhā is a highly esteemed medicinal plant in traditional Indian medicine for a wide variety of ailments but usually focused on stress, immune support (with regard to stress), anxiety, and depression (again, with respect to stress), and the treatment of cancer and inflammation. Historically, it boasts low toxicity when consumed as the root extract at the same time as food (Kumari et al., 2016).

4.8.5 *Bhangā (Cannabis sativa)*

Bhānga (Figure 4.4) has been used in India since Vedic time, and is an integral part of North Indian culture. *Sadhus* and *Sufis* use bhang to boost meditation and to achieve transcendental states. Using a mortar and pestle, the buds and leaves of cannabis are ground into a paste (Fuller, 2000). The *bhānga* base is now ready to be made into a heavy drink, an alternative to alcohol, which is also used as a stupefying agent (Fuller, 2000).

It is grown on the Indian sub-continent, Iran, Siberia, Pakistan and Nepal; it is also the name of a weed that can be seen on any piece of waste ground. It is an herbaceous annual plant; the rough, angular, branched stems reach a height of 3–10 feet and bear opposite (alternate toward the top) palmate leaves with 5–7 narrow, lanceolate, coarsely serrate, pointed leaflets. The flowers are small and green, the male flowers growing on one plant in axillary panicles, the female on a separate plant in spike-like clusters from August to October. The fruit is a small, ash-colored achene (Appendino et al., 2008; Andre et al., 2016).

Bhānga is used as a psychotropic drug, a pain reliever for sufferers of arthritis, gout, neuralgia, rheumatism, delirium tremens, insanity, infant convulsions and insomnia. It produces exhilaration, but also hallucinations, and is known in the East as the 'leaf of delusion', 'increaser of pleasure,' 'cementer of friendship' (Bao et al., 2014).

4.8.6 *Śankhapuṣpī (Convolvulus pluricaulis)*

There are two species regarded as *Śankhapuṣpī* i.e. *Convolvulus pluricaulis* and *Clitoea ternata*, but *C. pluricaulis* is usually regarded as *Śankhapuṣpī* (Figure 4.5) (Acharya, 2002).

Śankhapuṣpī (*C. pluricaulis*) is a perennial, prostrate or suberect, spreading, hairy herb, found throughout India. The recommended therapeutic form is a fine paste of the whole plant. It is highly regarded as *Medhya* (intellect promoter). Important chemical principles are microphyllic acid,

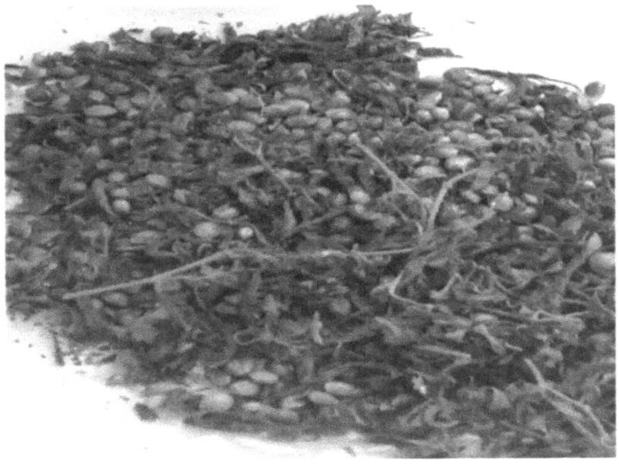

FIGURE 4.4 *BHĀNGA (Cannabis sativa)* (dry form).

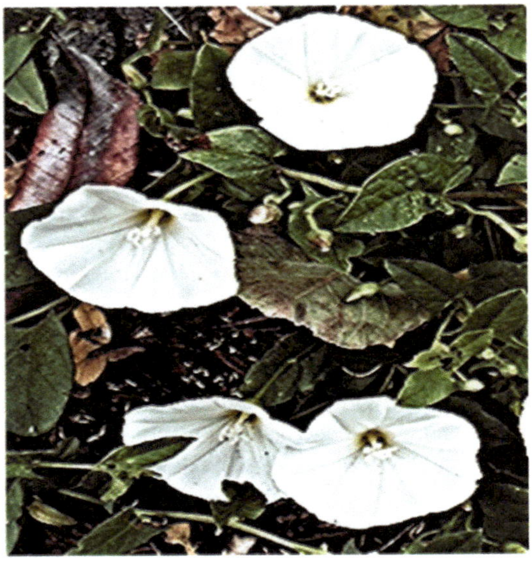

FIGURE 4.5 *ŚANKHAPUṢPĪ* (*Convolvulus pluricaulis*).

shankhapushpin, kaempferol, kaempferol-3-glucoside, 3,4-dihydroxycinnamic acid, and sitosterols. Neuroprotective and intellect-promoting activities are associated with free radical scavenging and antioxidant properties. BR-16A (Mentat), a polyherbal combination containing *Śankhapuṣpī*, significantly reversed the social-isolation stress-induced prolongation of the onset and decrease in pentobarbitone-induced sleep, increased total motor activity and stress-induced antinociception in an experimental model. Ayushman-8 (containing *Śankhapuṣpī*, *Brāhmī* and *Vacā*) is reported to be effective on *Mānasa-mandatā* (mental impairment) (Goyal and Singh, 2005).

Śankhapuṣpī composite, containing *Śankhapuṣpī*, *Sarpagandhā*, and *Gokṣura* in equal quantities, has been shown to be effective in treating *Cittodvega* (anxiety disorders). *Sanjay Parsania* reported *Śankhapuṣpī* to be effective at relieving signs and symptoms of *Cittodvega*. Herbalists believe that *Śankhapuṣpī* calms the nerves by regulating the body's production of the stress hormones, adrenaline and cortisol. Several investigations have reported that *Śankhapuṣpī* has potent depressive action in mice. *C. pluricaulis* whole plant extract shows the highest inhibitory activity against *Helicobacter muridarum*. Its effectiveness in treating *Cittodvega* (anxiety disorders) reverses the social isolation stress-induced prolongation of onset and decrease in pentobarbitone-induced sleep, increased total motor activity and stress-induced antinociception in an experimental model (Hetal et al., 2014).

4.8.7 *Ahiphena* (*Papaver somniferum*)

Opium (Figure 4.6) has been eaten, drunk, and smoked for centuries. The poppy, from which opium is derived, is not known from the wild; it has been domesticated for its seeds, which are used for oil and food, and for its dried sap, which produces opium, A common method of preparing opium was to dissolve it in alcohol, and this tincture (infusion, extraction, or solution), later known as laudanum, became a popular medication for centuries. Medications at that time were administered not so much to heal as they were to simply alleviate pain (Yilmaz and Emir, 2017; Marciano et al., 2018).

It is a very powerful hypnotic and narcotic, with powerful analgesic properties. Morphine is the most abundant component of opium, ranging from 4 to 21% by weight. Morphine is still unsurpassed in its ability to deaden pain. It is considered the most powerful naturally occurring analgesic. It is a general central nervous system (CNS) depressant and, in overdose, can lead to death by completely suppressing the respiratory center of the brain. The study of opium led to the discovery of the first alkaloid, morphine, and the study of morphine led to the discovery of the brain's own

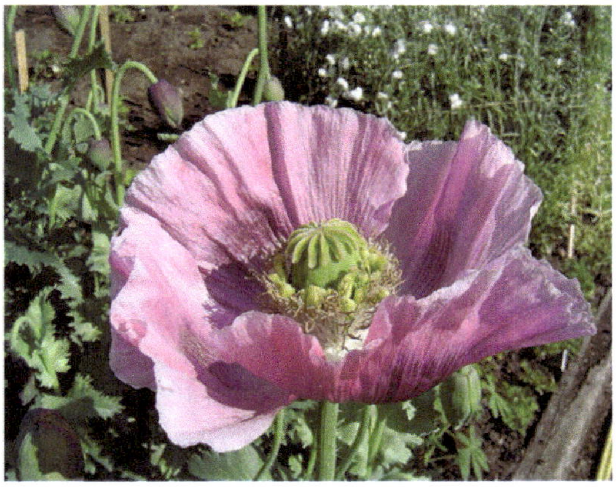

FIGURE 4.6 *AHIPHENA (Papaver somniferum).*

painkillers, the endorphins, perhaps the most important advance in neurochemistry of the past half-century (Avijeet et al., 2011; Karandikar et al., 2013; Srivastava et al., 2017).

4.8.8 Guḍūcī (Tinospora cordifolia)

Tinospora cordifolia (Figure 4.7) is also known as "*Guḍucī*" in Sanskṛata, and belongs to the family Menispermaceae. It is a genetically diverse, large, deciduous, climbing shrub with greenish-yellow typical flowers, found at high altitude. Numerous studies have shown a variety of phytoactive molecules isolated from different parts of the plant, including the root, stem, and whole plant, such as alkaloids, steroids, diterpenoid lactones, aliphatics, and glycosides. Due to the presence of various photochemicals, it possesses different pharmacological activities, such as antidiabetic, antiperiodic, antispasmodic, anti-inflammatory, antiarthritic, antioxidant, antiallergic, antistress, antileprotic, antimalarial, hepatoprotective, immunomodulatory, and antineoplastic activities (Saha and Ghosh, 2012).

Research has reported that it exhibits learning- and memory-enhancing properties, antioxidant and anti-stress activities, and enhances cognition in normal and cognition-deficit animals in behavioral tests. It is useful for treatment of *bhrama* (vertigo), in improving behavior disorders, mental deficit and IQ levels (Saha and Ghosh, 2012).

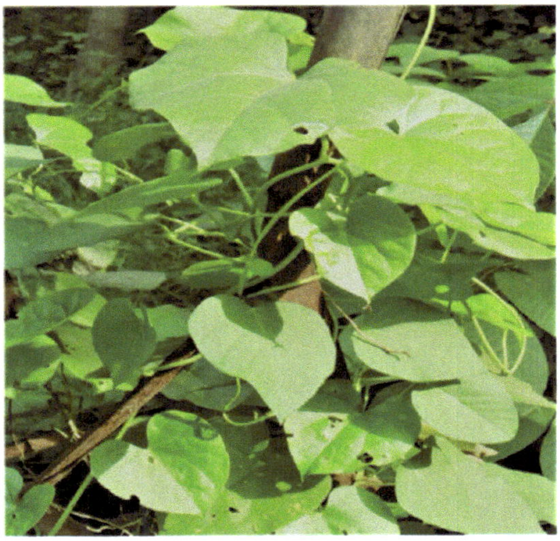

FIGURE 4.7 *GUḌŪCĪ (Tinospora cordifolia).*

Its anti-stress action has been shown to be advantageous in treating depression and in improving cognition and memory in AD subjects. The most likely antidepressant mechanisms involve inhibiting reuptake of amines in the brain. The drugs cause improved levels of norepinephrine (NE), serotonin (5-hydroxytryptamine or 5-HT), and dopamine (DA), and decreased levels of gamma-aminobutyric acid (GABA). It also inhibits the degradation of amines, mainly norepinehphrine and serotonin (Dhingra and Goyal, 2008). GABA-B receptor antagonism, G-protein-mediated signaling, and antioxidant and protective properties all play an important role in improving cognition, concentration, and memory. The ethanol extract of *T. cordifolia* aerial parts has shown neuroprotective activity in a study involving a 6-hydroxy dopamine (6-OHDA)-lesion rat model of Parkinson's disease (PD) (Kosaraju et al., 2014), and was involved in therapy of glioblastomas (Mishra and Kaur, 2013). Its neuroprotective activity involves modulation of the antioxidant system in rat hippocampal slices subjected to oxygen-glucose deprivation, and it also plays an effective role against ischemic brain damage as it attenuates oxidative stress-mediated cell injury during oxygen-glucose deprivation (OGD) in rat hippocampal slices (Rawal et al., 2004). The extract is also involved in the prevention of oxidative stress injury and in the regulation of cytokines, which are possible mechanisms involved in exerting these beneficial effects. *T. cordifolia* works synergistically with many other herbal preparations, which makes it an important component of polyherbal formulations. *T. cordifolia* act as one of the inimitable herbal medicines in the management of depression, AD, and attention-deficit/hyperactivity disorder (Mutalik and Mutalik, 2011).

4.8.9 YAṢṬHIMADHU (*GLYCYRRHIZA GLABRA* LINN.)

In India, this licorice root carries the ancient Sanskrit name of 'Yaṣṭhimadhu' (sweet-stalk) and the plant is also known as *Glycyrrhiza glabra* (Figure 4.8). It has been used worldwide in various systems of medicine such as *Āyurvedic*, allopathic and other traditional systems of medicine, and has been used in the preparation of more than 1250 polyherbal formulations. It has different pharmacological activities, such as anti-inflammatory, antiviral, antimicrobial, antioxidative, anticancer, immunomodulatory, hepatoprotective, and cardioprotective activities, due to the presence of a large number of bioactive components, such as triterpene saponins, flavonoids, isoflavonoids, and chalcones. This herb is mainly used for the treatment of peptic ulcers, hepatitis C, pulmonary diseases, and skin diseases. This herb was used as a special food, served to eliminate excess, as well as to strengthen any deficiencies, and to restore and rejuvenate (Korhalkar et al., 2012).

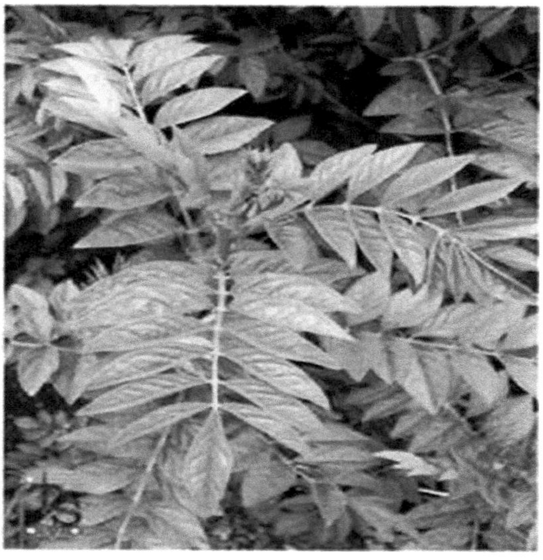

FIGURE 4.8 YAṢṬHIMADHU (*Glycyrrhiza glabra*).

Glycyrrhizin showed a neuroprotective effect due to presence of triterpenes and rhizomes in the kainic acid-induced neuronal cell death in an animal model experiment. This mechanism is mediated *via* suppression of gliosis and induction of proinflammatory markers (cyclooxygenase [COX-2], inducible nitric oxide synthase [iNOS], and tumor necrosis factor-alpha [TNF-α]) (Luo et al., 2014). Further research has also shown similar effects on the brain of the post-ischemic rat after middle cerebral artery occlusion (MCAO), with the mechanism involving the anti-inflammatory, antiexcitotoxic, and antioxidative effects of glycyrrhizin, and, in particular, its anti-inflammatory effect (Kim et al., 2012). Research has shown that 2',2',4'-trihydroxychalcone from *G. glabra* is a novel specific inhibitor of beta-site amyloid precursor protein (APP)-cleaving enzyme 1 (BACE1), that efficiently ameliorates memory impairment in mice (Zhu et al., 2010). The roots of *G. glabra* contain the most important bioactive molecule, glabridin, which increases the circulation into the CNS system, improves learning and memory, and has a neuroprotective effect *via* modulation of multiple pathways associated with apoptosis (Cui et al., 2008; Yu et al., 2008).

Other studies have supported the neuroprotective role of glabridin, related to memory-enhancing properties in exteroceptive and interoceptive behavioral animal models of memory, and also on the learning activity in the mouse brain, due to facilitation of cholinergic transmission (Parle et al., 2004; Dhingra et al., 2004). In mouse models of immobility tests due to presence of bioactive molecules, glabridin showed antidepressant-like properties through regulation of different neurotransmitters in different zones of the brain (Dhingra and Sharma, 2006). In addition, other findings also supported its anticonvulsant property *via* its action on markers of oxidative stress, as shown in pentylenetetrazole (PTZ)-induced seizure in an animal model (Chowdhury et al., 2013). Therefore, the neuroprotective effect of glabridin involved the improvement of cognition and memory in AD patients.

4.8.10 Vacā (Acorus calamus)

Vacā (*Acorus calamus*) (Figure 4.9) is among the rare treatments that finds mention inside the *Vedas*. Latterday *Ācāryas* worked well, not only on the nervous system and the brain, but also on additional parts of the entire body. It has been described for use in Indian and Chinese systems of medicine

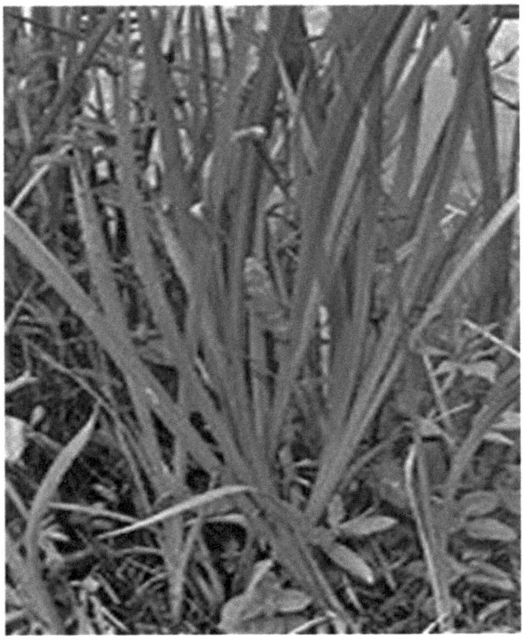

FIGURE 4.9 Vaca (*Acorus calamus*).

for hundreds of years to treat diseases, especially those involving CNS abnormalities. In *Sanskṛata*, *Vacā* literally means 'speaking' as in its use for clearing of the voice, meaning that it is probably used to treat diseases of the CNS, stuttering, and other related disorders. It has been demonstrated to have a strong psycho-pharmacological effect, which has a favorable impact on the memory as well as on the learning process (Bhujbal et al., 2008; Pandy et al., 2009; Balakumbahan et al., 2010).

Vacā is a herb of choice for use in the case of loud eructation. Powder of *vacā* and white sandal makes a very effective face-pack in the treatment of blemishes and pimples. In many Indian homes, *Vacā* is customarily administered in a minute quantity with honey to infants on the 11th and 21st days after birth. It is also used for Swarṇa *prāsana Samskāra* in South India on *Puṣya nakṣatra*, up to the age of 16 years. It is believed that this practice helps the children to be mentally active and vocal (Vengadesh et al., 2009).

4.9 FUTURE PERSPECTIVES

AD is an age-associated, irreversible, progressive, and increasingly common neurodegenerative disease, causing loss of memory, unusual behavior, personality changes, and cognitive impairment, and affecting the quality of life, and it is a major burden on the socio-economic system of the nation. It is an irreversible, progressive brain disease which slowly destroys memory and thinking skills, eventually eroding even the ability to carry out the simplest tasks of daily life. This inescapable loss of cognitive function is associated with the presence of senile plaques in the hippocampal area of the brain, resulting in the gradual decline of a person's memory and the ability to learn, reason, make judgements, and communicate (Ballard et al., 2011; Markowitsch and Staniloiu, 2012; Ryman et al., 2014). AD is becoming more and more frequent in line with the growing population. This disease is a primary neurodegenerative disease, with characteristic neuropathological and neurochemical features, and is also characterized by a reduction in cholinergic neurotransmission and an increase in oxidative stress. Neurofibrillary tangles and neuritic plaques are the two main pathological hallmarks of AD, which spread throughout the brain in stereotypical patterns (Francis et al., 1999; Scheltens et al., 2016; Akiyama, 2016).

Today, it is very unfortunate that, in spite of the advances in modern medicine, its success is very limited with respect to neurological and neurodegenerative diseases, due to the multi-factorial nature of these diseases. Clinically available modern medicines to treat AD are very expensive, and are effective only in a certain proportion of the patients. These drugs are often associated with side effects or adverse effects, such as nausea, vomiting, gastrointestinal discomfort, sexual dysfunction, and weight loss, etc. Occasionally, some patients may experience excitement, anxiety, insomnia, restlessness or seizure, blurred vision, difficulty passing urine, and orthostatic hypotension, hypertensive crisis, insomnia, and restlessness, and these effects collectively affect cognition and behavior (Hanaa et al., 2014).

To obtain better and less expensive therapeutic benefits, with fewer and less severe adverse reactions, the focus of the search should move toward alternative medicines from natural sources i.e. herbal remedies, used traditionally and documented to have a safe profile. These plant-based drugs may be helpful in enhancing memory and improving cognition in AD patients. Our knowledge of medicinal plants helps in the development of drugs for the modern medicine system. Therefore, the concept of modern medicine-based therapy for treatment of such patients may be more effective when based on psychoactive plant-based drugs. Hence, the dissection and analysis of medicinal plants from around the world for improving cognitive function with minimal side effects is essential today, to overcome cognitive-deficit diseases, such as AD (Chaudhari and Murthy, 2014).

These *Āyurvedic* medicinal plants have been the single most-productive source of leads for the development of new herbal and allopathic drugs, with more than one hundred new products being developed and clinically used. Indeed, several scientific studies have demonstrated that various *Āyurvedic* medicinal plants and their bioactive molecules (lignans, flavonoids, tannins, polyphenols, triterpenes, sterols, and alkaloids) are useful in the treatment of AD. The exact mode of action of these drugs is still not clear, with these bioactive molecules showing a wide spectrum of pharmacological activities, including anti-inflammatory, antiamyloidogenic, anticholinesterase, hypolipidemic, and antioxidant effects (Abascal et al., 2004; Bredesen, 2009; Alzheimer's Association, 2010; Rao et al., 2012).

This chapter has gathered research on various *Āyurvedic* medicinal plants that have shown promise in reversing the AD pathology. The information concerning the phytochemistry, biological, and cellular activities, as well as the clinical applications of these various medicinal plants, has been summarized in order to provide sufficient baseline information that could be used in drug discovery campaigns and development processes, thereby providing new functional leads for drugs for the treatment of AD. Therefore, we have critically reviewed various *Medhya Rasāyana* (nootropic drug) herbal medicines derived from extract of *Āyurvedic* medicinal plants. Studies have shown that *Medhya Rasāyana* herbal formulations promote free radical scavenger mechanisms and protect cells in the prefrontal cortex, hippocampus, and striatum against cytotoxicity and DNA damage implicated in AD (Chaudhari and Murthy, 2014).

These *Āyurvedic* drugs protect the cholinergic neurons and reduce anticholinesterase activity. They also reduce β-amyloid deposition and stress-induced hippocampal damage. The neuroprotective effect of *Medhya Rasāyana* drugs are also due to nitric oxide-mediated cerebral vasodilation. These *Āyurvedic* herbal drugs have improved the total memory score in different experimental models. Herbal medicine promises to be a novel agent in AD treatment; however, further human clinical trials are recommended to verify the efficacy and the lack of side effects, as evidenced by the experimental models (Chaudhari and Murthy, 2014).

4.10 CONCLUSIONS

In AD patients, the brain amyloid may influence cognition indirectly, through neurodegenerative processes. In the modern health system, there is no definitive way of preventing amyloid accumulation, of achieving early diagnosis of AD, or of treating AD symptoms effectively. The pharmaceutical industry is facing serious challenges as the drug discovery process for progressive neurodegenerative diseases, such as AD, is becoming extremely expensive, riskier and, most critically, inefficient. Therefore, the demand for new drugs by combining traditional information and modern science, by developing effective disease-modifying drugs, is proving to be a difficult task. These herbal neuroprotective drugs have promise in terms of slowing or preventing neuronal dysfunction, using herbal medicines to alleviate the burden of AD and to promote healthy living. These traditional medicines are regarded as new and promising sources of potential anti-AD drugs. Encouraging results from preclinical and clinical trials suggest that traditional medicines include promising candidates for the treatment of AD. Consequently, the need to explore the applied use of medicinal plants to overcome such cognition-deficient diseases worldwide is of pressing importance today.

REFERENCES

Abascal K, Yarnell E. Alzheimer's disease: part 2—a botanical treatment plan. *Alternative and Complementary Therapies*, 2004;10:67–72.

Acharya YT. *Charaka Samhita*. 7th ed. Varanasi: Chaukhambha Orientalia, 2002, p. 385–542.

Akiyama H. Development of disease-modifying therapy for Alzheimer's disease. *Brain Nerve*, 2016;68:463–472.

Alzheimer's Association. Alzheimer's disease facts and figures. *Alzheimer's Dement*, 2010;6:158–194.

Alzheimer's Association. 2015 Alzheimer's disease facts and figures. *Alzheimer's Dement*, 2015;11:332–384.

Andre CM, Hausman J-F, Guerriero G. *Cannabis sativa*: the plant of the thousand and one molecules. *Frontiers in Plant Science*, 2016;7:19. doi:10.3389/fpls.2016.00019.

Appendino G, Gibbons S, Giana A, Pagani A, Grassi G, Stavri M. Antibacterial cannabinoids from *Cannabis sativa*: a structure-activity study. *The Journal of Natural Products*, 2008;71:1427–1430.

Avijeet C, et al. Impact of mutagenesis on cytological behavior in relation to specific alkaloids in Opium Poppy (*Papaver somniferum* L.). *Caryologia*, 2011;64(1):14–24.

Balakumbahan R, Rajamani K, Kumanan K. *Acorus calamus*: an overview. *The Journal of Medicinal Plants Research*, 2010;4(25):2740–2745.

Ballard C, Gauthier S, Corbett A, Brayne C, Aarsland D, Jones E. Alzheimer's disease. *Lancet*, 2011;377:1019–1031.

Bao Q, Liu H, Fu K, Zhang C, Wang C, Feng Y. *Hemp Bast Fiber Extract with Antibacterial Activity, Preparation Method and Application of Hemp Bast Fiber Extract.* Patent publication number CN104018343A. Washington, DC: U.S. Patent and Trademark Office, 2014.

Bhattacharya SK, Ghoshal A. Anxiolytic activity of a standardized extract of *Bacopa monnieri*: an experimental study. *Phytomedicine*, 1998;5:95–100.

Bhattacharya SK, Kumar A, Ghoshal S. Effect of *Bacopa monnieri* of animal models of Alzheimer's disease and perturbed central markers of cognition in rats. *Research Communications in Pharmacology and Toxicology*, 1999;4:1–12.

Bhujbal SS, Patil MJ, Chitlange SS, Kulkarni PA. Herbal drugs for mental disorders. *Pharmainfo.net*, 2008;6(1).

Bose KC, Bose NK. Observations on the actions and uses of *Herpestis monniera*. *Journal of Indian Medical Association*, 1931;1:60.

Braskie MN, Thompson PM. Understanding cognitive deficits in Alzheimer's disease based on neuroimaging findings. *Trends in Cognitive Sciences*, 2013;17(10):510–516. doi:10.1016/j.tics.2013.08.007.

Bredesen DE. Neurodegeneration in Alzheimer's disease: caspases and synaptic element interdependence. *Molecular Neurodegeneration*, 2009;4:27.

Brunkan AL, Goate AM. Presenilin function and gamma-secretase activity. *Journal of Neurochemistry*, 2005;93:769–792.

Cai Y, An SS, Kim S. Mutations in presenilin 2 and its implications in Alzheimer's disease and other dementia-associated disorders. *Clinical Interventions in Aging*, 2015;10:1163–1172.

Chatterji N, Rastogi RP, Dhar ML. Chemical examination of *Bacopa monniera* Wettst.: parti-isolation of chemical constituents. *Indian Journal of Chemistry*, 1965;3:24–29.

Chaudhari K, Murthy ARV. Effect of rasayana on mental health – a review study. *International Journal of Ayurveda and Alternative Medicine*, 2014;2:1–7.

Chaudhari KS, Tiwari NR, Tiwari RR, Sharma RS. Neurocognitive effect of nootropic drug *Brahmi* (*Bacopa monnieri*) in Alzheimer's disease. *Annals of Neurosciences*, 2017;24(2):111–122. doi:10.1159/000475900.

Chen R, Hu Z, Wei L, Ma Y, Liu Z, Copeland JR. Incident dementia in a defined older Chinese population. *PLoS One*, 2011;6(9):e24817.

Chiu HF, Lam LC, Chi I, Leung T, Li SW, Law WT, Chung DW, Fung HH, Kan PS, Lum CM, Ng J, Lau J. Prevalence of dementia in Chinese elderly in Hong Kong. *Neurology*, 1998;50(4):1002–1009.

Chopra RN, Nayar L, Chopra IC. *Glossary of Indian Medicinal Plants.* New Delhi: Council of Scientific and Industrial Research, 1956, 32.

Chowdhury B, Bhattamisra SK, Das MC. Anti-convulsant action and amelioration of oxidative stress by Glycyrrhiza glabra root extract in pentylenetetrazole-induced seizure in albino rats. *The Indian Journal of Pharmacology*, 2013;45:40–43.

Cui YM, Ao MZ, Li W, Yu LJ. Effect of glabridin from Glycyrrhiza glabra on learning and memory in mice. *Planta Medica*, 2008;74:377–380.

Dhingra D, Goyal PK. Evidences for the involvement of monoaminergic and GABAergic systems in antidepressant-like activity of *Tinospora cordifolia* in mice. *The Indian Journal of Pharmaceutical Sciences*, 2008;70:761–767.

Dhingra D, Parle M, Kulkarni SK. Memory enhancing activity of *Glycyrrhiza glabra* in mice. *The Journal of Ethnopharmacology*, 2004;91:361–365.

Dhingra D, Sharma A. Antidepressant-like activity of *Glycyrrhiza glabra* L. in mouse models of immobility tests. *Progress in Neuro-Psychopharmacology & Biological Psychiatry*, 2006;30:449–454.

Francis PT, et al. The cholinergic hypothesis of Alzheimer's disease: a review of progress. *Journal of Neurology, Neurosurgery & Psychiatry*, 1999;66:137–147.

Fuller R. *Stairways to Heaven*. Westview Press, 2000. ISBN 0813366127.

Götz J, Ittner LM, Schonrock N. Alzheimer's disease and frontotemporal dementia: prospects of a tailored therapy? *Medical Journal of Australia*, 2006;185:381–384.

Goyal PR, Singh KP. Shankhpuspi (*Evolvulus alsinoides* Linn) [J] a medicinal herb. *International Journal of Mendel*, 2005;22:124–125.

Gupta YK, Veerendra Kumar MH, Srivastava AK. Effect of *Centella asiatica* on pentylenetetrazole-induced kindling, cognition and oxidative stress in rats. *Pharmacology Biochemistry & Behavior*, 2003;74:579–585.

Hanaa H, Ahmeda AM, Zaazaab, Bosy A, Motelpb AE. *Zingiber officinale* and Alzheimer's disease: evidences and mechanisms. *International Journal of Pharmaceutical Sciences* Review, 2014;27:142–152.

Hausen BM. *Centella asiatica* (Indian pennywort), an effective therapeutic but a weak sensitizer. *Contact Dermatitis*, 1993;29:175–179.

Hetal A, Rohit S, Mahesh V, Prajapatil PK, Kartar D. Shankhapushpi (*Convolvulus pluricaulis* Choisy): validation of the Ayurvedic therapeutic claims through contemporary studies. *International Journal of Green Pharmacy*, 2014;4(8):193–198.

Joshi KS, Bhonde R. Insights from Ayurveda for translational stem cell research. *The Journal of Ayurveda and Integrative Medicine*, 2014;5:4–10.

Karandikar YS, Bhagat VA, Mate VH. Comparative study of CNS effects of opium in homeopathic potencies with pentazocine in mice. *International Journal of Advanced Ayurveda, Yoga, Unani, Siddha and Homeopathy*, 2013;2:105–111.

Katzman R. The prevalence and malignancy of Alzheimer disease: a major killer. *Archives of Neurology*, 1976;33:217–218.

Kim SW, et al. Glycyrrhizic acid affords robust neuroprotection in the postischemic brain via anti-inflammatory effect by inhibiting HMGB1 phosphorylation and secretion. *Neurobiology of Disease*, 2012;46:147–156.

Korhalkar A, Deshpande M, Lele P, Modak M. *Global Journal of Research on Medicinal Plants & Indigenous Medicine*, 2012;1(12):687–693.

Kosaraju J, et al. Neuroprotective effect of *Tinospora cordifolia* ethanol extract on 6-hydroxy dopamine induced Parkinsonism. *Indian Journal of Pharmacology*, 2014;46:176–180.

Kumar A, et al. Homocysteine- and cysteine-mediated growth defect is not associated with induction of oxidative stress response genes in yeast. *Biochemical Journal*, 2006;396(1):61–69.

Kumar V, Dey A, Hadimani M, Marcović T, Emerald M. Chemistry and pharmacology of *Withania somnifera*: an update. *TANG Humanitas Medicine*, 2015;5:1–13.

Kumari R, Agrawal A, Singh KP, Singh GPI, Dubey GP. Chapter 28 *Regulation of Serotonin in Depression: Efficacy of Ayurvedic Plants.* 6000 Broken Sound Parkway NW, Suite 300, Boca Raton, FL 33487–2742: Taylor & Francis Group, CRC Press, 2016, 397–420.

Luo L, Jin Y, Kim ID, Lee JK. Glycyrrhizin suppresses HMGB1 inductions in the hippocampus and subsequent accumulation in serum of a kainic acid induced seizure mouse model. *Cellular and Molecular Neurobiology*, 2014;34:987–997.

Malhotra CK, Das PK. Pharmacological studies of *Herpestis monniera* Linn (Brahmi). *The Indian Journal of Medical Research*, 1959;47:294–305.

Marciano MA, et al. Development of a method to extract Opium Poppy (*Papaver somniferum* L.) DNA from heroin. *Scientific Reports*, 2018;8.

Markowitsch HJ, Staniloiu A. Amnesic disorders. *Lancet*, 2012;380:1429–1440.

Masliah E, et al. Re-evaluation of the structural organization of neuritic plaques in Alzheimer's disease. *The Journal of Neuropathology & Experimental Neurology*, 1993;52:619–632.

Mishra LC, Singh BB, Dagenais S. Scientific basis for the therapeutic use of *Withania somnifera* (ashwagandha): a review. *Alternative Medicine Review*, 2000;5:334–346.

Mishra R, Kaur G. Aqueous ethanolic extract of *Tinospora cordifolia* as a potential candidate for differentiation based therapy of glioblastomas. *PLoS One*, 2013;8:e78764.

Mutalik M, Mutalik M. *Tinospora cordifolia*: role in depression, cognition and memory. *Australian Journal of Medical Herbalism*, 2011;23:4.

Pandy V, Jose N, Subhash H. CNS activity of methanol and acetone extracts of *Acorus calamus* leaves in mice. *Journal of Pharmacology and Toxicology*, 2009;4(2):79–86.

Parle M, Dhingra D, Kulkarni SK. Memory-strengthening activity of *Glycyrrhiza glabra* in exteroceptive and interoceptive behavioral models. *Journal of Medicinal Food*, 2004;7:462–466.

Poirier J, et al. Apolipoprotein E4 allele as a predictor of cholinergic deficits and treatment outcome in Alzheimer disease. *Proceedings of the National Academy of Sciences of the United States of America*, 1995;92:12260–12264.

Priller C, Bauer T, Mitteregger G, Krebs B, Kretzschmar HA, Herms J. Synapse formation and function is modulated by the amyloid precursor protein. *Journal of Neuroscience*, 2006;26:7212–7221.

Rai D, Bhatia G, Palit G, Pal R, Singh S, Singh HK. Adaptogenic effect of *Bacopa monniera* (Brahmi). *Pharmacology Biochemistry & Behavior*, 2003;75:823–830.

Rao JS, Kellom M, Kim HW, Rapoport SI, Reese EA. Neuroinflammation and synaptic loss. *Neurochem. Res.* 2012;37:903–910.

Rawal AK, Muddeshwar MG, Biswas SK. *Rubia cordifolia*, *Fagonia cretica* linn and *Tinospora cordifolia* exert neuroprotection by modulating the antioxidant system in rat hippocampal slices subjected to oxygen glucose deprivation. *BMC Complementary and Alternative Medicine*, 2004;4:11.

Ray S, Ray A. Medhya Rasayanas in brain function and disease. *Medicinal Chemistry*, 2015;5:505–511.

Ryman DC, et al. Symptom onset in autosomal dominant Alzheimer disease: a systematic review and meta-analysis. *Neurology*, 2014;83:253–260.

Saha S, Ghosh S. *Tinospora cordifolia*: one plant, many roles. *Ancient Science of Life*, 2012;31(4):151–159. doi:10.4103/0257-7941.107344.

Sairam K, Rao CHV, Agarwal VK, Joshi VK, Goel RK. Effect of *Bacopa monniera* Linn on gastric ulceration and secretion. *The Indian Journal of Pharmacology*, 2000;32:81.

Sastri MS, Dhalla NS, Malhotra CL. Chemical investigation of *Herpestis monniera* Linn (Brahmi). *The Indian Journal of Pharmacology*, 1959;21:303–304.

Scheltens P, Blennow K, Breteler MM, de Strooper B, Frisoni GB, Salloway S, Van der Flier WM. Alzheimer's disease. *Lancet*, 2016;388:505–517.

Scoville WB, Milner B. Loss of recent memory after bilateral hippocampal lesions. *The Journal of Neurology, Neurosurgery, and Psychiatry*, 1957;20:11–21.

Selkoe DJ. Alzheimer's disease: genes, proteins, and therapy. *Physiological Reviews*, 2001;81:741–766.

Shanker G, Singh HK. Anxiolytic profile of standardized Brahmi extract. *The Indian Journal of Pharmacology*, 2000;32:152.

Shanmugasundaram ER, Akbar GK, Shanmugasundaram KR. Brahmighritham, an Ayurvedic herbal formula for the control of epilepsy. *Journal of Ethnopharmacology*, 1991;33:269–276.

Singh AK, Gupta AK, Manish Singh PK. Rasayana therapy: a magic contribution of Ayurveda for healthy long life. *International Journal of Research in Ayurveda and Pharmacy*, 2014;5:41–47.

Singh B, Rastogi RP. A reinvestigation of the triterpenes of *Centella asiatica*. *Phytochemistry*, 1969;8:917–921.

Srivastava A, et al. *Ageratum enation virus* infection induces programmed cell death and alters metabolite biosynthesis in *Papaver somniferum*. *Frontiers in Plant Science*, 2017;8: 1172.

Vas CJ, Pinto C, Panikker D, Noronha S, Deshpande N, Kulkarni L, Sachdeva S. Prevalence of dementia in an urban Indian population. *International Psychogeriatrics*, 2001;13(4):439–450.

Ven Murthy MR, Ranjekar PK, Ramassamy C, Deshpande M. Scientific basis for the use of Indian ayurvedic medicinal plants in the treatment of neurodegenerative disorders: Ashwagandha. *Central Nervous System Agents in Medicinal Chemistry*, 2010;10:238–246.

Vengadesh Prabu K, et al. Neuromodulatory effect of *Acorus calamus* leaves extract on dopaminergic system in mice. *International Journal of PharmTech Research*, 2009;1(4):1255–1259.

5 Prevention and Treatment of Alzheimer's Disease in the Light of Ayurveda

Vinayak Majhi, Bishnu Choudhury, and Sudip Paul

CONTENTS

ABBREVIATIONS

AD Alzheimer's Disease
BBB Blood–Brain Barrier
CNS Central Nervous System
WHO World Health Organization

5.1 INTRODUCTION

Alzheimer's disease (AD) is a complex neurodegenerative disorder, with major clinical hallmarks of memory loss, dementia, and cognitive impairment (Bekris et al. 2010). The cognition effects include memory orientation and judgment. AD was initially thought to represent a relatively uncommon form of pre-senile dementia, but it later became clear that it could occur at any decade of adulthood. More than 90% of cases of AD are sporadic and occur in individuals older than 60 years of age (Bertram and Tanzi 2004).

There are many symptoms common to all AD patients, although the progress of AD is different for each patient. Early symptoms are often mistakenly thought to be merely 'age-related' concerns or manifestations of stress (Essa et al. 2016). AD is characterized by memory impairment as a prominent and early feature, and more advanced AD presents as profound cognitive impairment, which leads to the patient becoming totally dependent (Tarawneh and Holtzman 2012). In the early stages, the most common symptom is difficulty in remembering recent events, commonly known as short-term memory loss. When the disease becomes more severe, many other symptoms, like confusion, irritability, aggression, mood swings, trouble with language, and long-term memory loss also become more prominent (Akula et al. 2011; Burns and Iliffe 2009; Ramakrishna et al. 2012; Ravishankar and Ramakrishna 2016).

5.2 SIGNIFICANCE

AD is one of the most-deadly diseases worldwide at present. In 2006, the worldwide incidence of AD was 26.6 million. By 2050, this figure will have quadrupled, by which time 1 in 85 persons worldwide will be suffering from the disease (Wimo et al. 2003). It is estimated that 43% of AD patients need a higher level of care (Brookmeyer et al. 2007). AD incidence rates increase exponentially with increasing age. On average, the number of AD patients has doubled every 5.5 years from its initial count. The doubling times in North America and Europe are 6.0 and 5.8 years, respectively, whereas the doubling times in all other parts of the world are 5.0 years (Ziegler-Graham et al. 2008). It is estimated that, by the year 2020, approximately 70% of the world's population aged 60 and above will be living in developing countries, with 14.2% living in India (Kalache 1999). The WHO report showed that people of high or upper-middle income economies are most affected group by AD, as shown in Figure 5.1 and Figure 5.2. The incidence of this disease is increasing at such a high rate but it is still incurable at present. Early detection can only control AD at the primary stage. There is no proper treatment for AD in modern medicine (WHO 2018).

5.3 ETIOPATHOGENESIS

The cause of AD is unknown, but both environmental and genetic risk factors combine to trigger a pathophysiological cascade, throughout the life span of the patient, leading to Alzheimer's pathology and dementia (Santos et al. 2017).

5.3.1 Risk Factors

The role of genetic factors is understood to play a part in the development of the disorder in around 40% of patients who have a family history of AD (Blazer and Hernandez 2006; Tsuang et al. 2004). Mutations in genes such as the amyloid precursor protein gene on chromosome 21 or the presenilin-1 gene on chromosome 14 or the presenilin-2 gene on chromosome 1 unequivocally cause early-onset autosomal dominant AD. Although so many risk factors for AD have been identified, the age-related risk factor causes early, progressive disease, and is related to glial dysfunction. Glial dysfunction and myelin breakdown occur as early as midlife and progress over the next 30–40 years. Midlife hypertension is another established risk factor (Bekris et al. 2010).

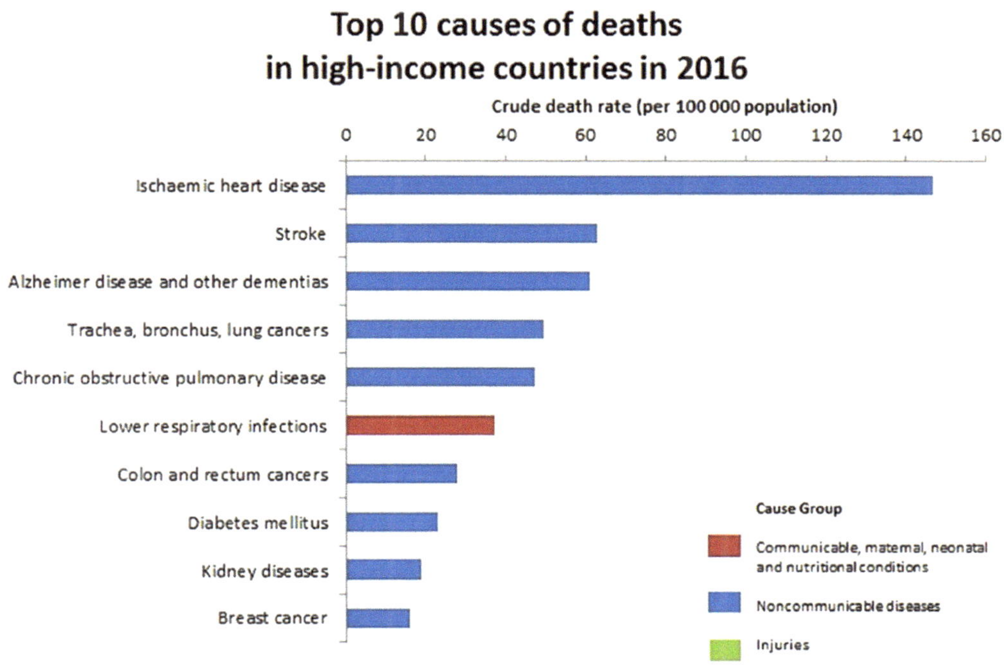

FIGURE 5.1 WHO report of causes of death in high-income economics (WHO 2018).

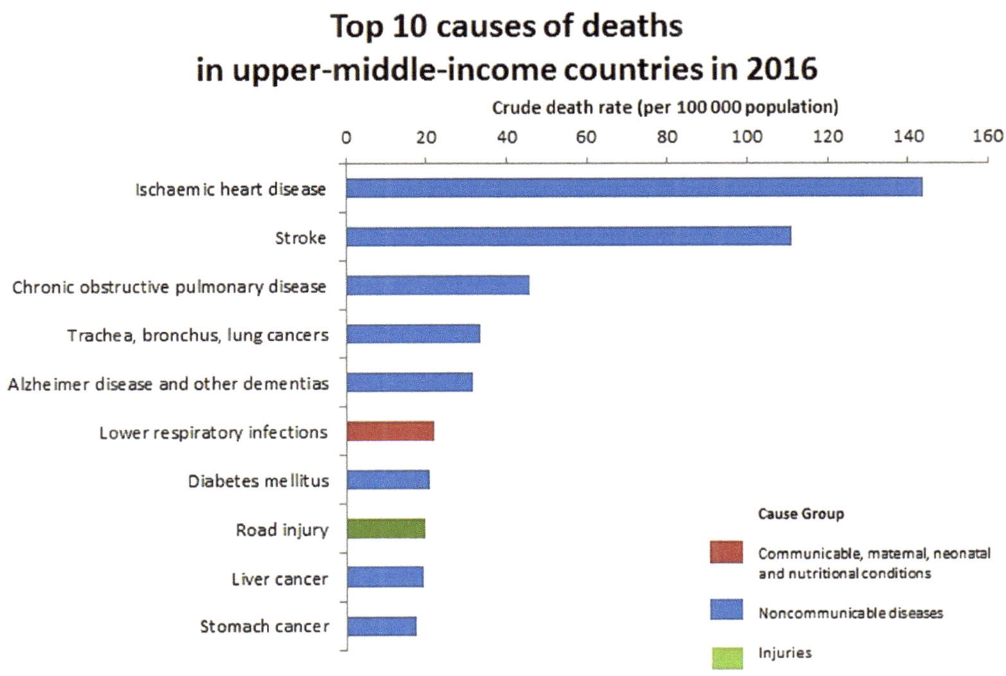

FIGURE 5.2 WHO report of causes of death in upper-middle-income economics countries (WHO 2018).

5.3.2 Pathophysiology

In AD, both pathophysiological symptoms and the aging problem have equal relevance (Jack et al. 2013). The three processes, communication, metabolism, and repair, which are key to keeping a neuron healthy, are most affected in AD. Pathologically, in AD, the secondary enlargement of the ventricular system is affected by the gross diffuse atrophy of the cerebral cortex (Serrano-Pozo et al. 2011). Senile plaques, neurofibrillary tangles, neuronal loss (particularly in the cortex and hippocampus), synaptic loss, and granulovascular degeneration in the cortex are found under microscopic analysis. Microscopic plaques develop in the hippocampus and in other areas of the cerebral cortex that are involved in thinking and decision making, where the hippocampus is the main structure, deep in the brain, that helps to encode memories. But the cause of AD occurrence is unknown, as we cannot say whether the plaques themselves cause AD or they are a by-product of the AD process (Mangalasseri and Chandran 2017).

5.4 PREVENTIVE MEASURES FOR AD

AD has multiple risk factors. Some factors cannot be controlled, such as aging or genetics. But other trigger factors can be controlled by changing daily habits and lifestyle (Smith et al. 2018).

5.4.1 Exercise

Regular moderate physical exercise for 150 minutes each week helps to prevent AD or slows the development of the disease in those who are at the preliminary stage (Ahlskog et al. 2011).

5.4.2 Social Engagement

Social contact and regular meetings, like joining a club, meeting weekly with friends, or connecting with other people *via* social networks, can prevent AD (Anderson et al. 2012).

5.4.3 Healthy Diet

A healthy diet, which includes fresh vegetables and fruits, whole grains, nuts, fish, eggs, dairy, and a moderate amount of wine, is highly relevant for people who have a greater risk of developing AD (Hu et al. 2013).

5.4.4 Mental Stimulation

People who regularly do exciting activities, learn something new, practice memorization, or solve puzzles, have less risk of suffering from AD (Anderson et al. 2012).

5.4.5 Quality Sleep

It is suggested that at least 8 h sleep is needed for adults to prevent AD, because poor sleep at night may decrease your thinking ability or impair your memory (Anderson et al. 2012).

5.4.6 Stress Management

Chronic stress can cause brain shrinkage, hampering nerve cell growth. To reduce stress, people should practice regular meditation, prayer, having fun, or keeping their sense of humor, to defer the onset of AD (Khalsa 2015).

5.5 AD: AN AYURVEDIC VIEW

There is no condition, as defined in Ayurveda, which can be clinically associated with AD. But in the Ayurvedic classic texts, Smṛtināsha (loss of memory) is specified as being among the prodromal symptoms of jarā (aging). In Jarāvasthā (old age), starting from 60 years of age, according to Charaka (one of the principal contributors to Ayurveda), Smṛti and other mental capabilities gradually deteriorate naturally. According to Vāgbhaṭa (As.Sam.Sha 8/25) and Sharṅgadhara (Prathama Khaṇḍa 6/20), the functions of Manas (mind, psyche) and Buddhi (intellect) start declining from the ninth decade of life. Mental function declines at the 11th decade of life, as described by Sharṅgadhara. Furthermore, Smṛtibhramsha (disturbed memory) is described as a symptom where Smṛti (memory) is vitiated by rajas (passion) and tamas (obscurity). Thus, dementia can be explained as Jarājanya Smṛtibhramsha, according to Ayurvedic principles (Nishteswar et al. 2014).

AD is often termed "Smrti Nasha" in Ayurveda and is caused by the exhaustion of dhatus (tissues) and by deterioration of Satva Guna (the attribute of the mind that represents purity and consciousness) by rajas (the attribute of the mind that typically represents energy and dynamism) and tamas (the attribute of mind representing passivity and ignorance) (Tiwari and Tripathi 2013).

When the Manovaha srotas (channels carrying cyclic impulses, mainly liable for memory) are affected with Vata dosha, the person is affected and there is a run-down of mental activities (Sharma et al. 2018).

This condition is not considered to be a disease entity in the different chapters of the Ayurvedic classics, but is regarded as a natural phenomenon; however, the sign and symptoms of dementia are often understood in terms of Ayurvedic concepts. In order to know the etiopathogenesis of dementia in the light of Ayurvedic literature, it is necessary to review the overall physiology of Manas and Buddhi. Before discussing the etiology and psychopathology of Smritibuddhihrass, it is worthwhile considering the relationships of Mana, Buddhi, Medha, Dhriti, and Smriti with one another. In terms of knowledge, mental capability, which determines the nature, merits, and demerits of an object of knowledge, is Buddhi. Buddhi and Mana are connected with Karya Karana Sambandh as in the method of evolution; Buddhi is the first entity (Tatva), which is accountable for additional development of Indriyas and Manas (Tiwari and Tripathi 2013).

According to Ayurveda, Mana and Indriyas are Panchabhautic, and this idea considers the anatomical aspect of Mana in particular. Acharya Bhela was the primary person who finally stopped the controversy regarding the location of Manas and declared that it is present between Shira and Talu, i.e. within the Mastishka. Now, it is very clear that all restrictive and cognitive functions are accomplished by activity of the brain, and human beings are totally different from other developed animals in that they have a larger brain. It is essential to discuss Mastishka and the view of Ayurveda about this (Tiwari and Tripathi 2013).

5.5.1 Brain (Mastishka) in Classics

According to the Ayurvedic concept, the Mastishka or Mastulunga is derived from Majja Dhatu and is like a semisolid Ghrita, viz.

- Shirastho Majja
- Mastulunga Shirso Baladhanam Styanaghritakaram Mastulungamuchyate
- Ardhavilina Ghritakaromastaka Majja

In Ayurveda, disease involving mental capability has been loosely classified into two categories, those affecting intellectual capacities (buddhinasa) and those affecting consciousness (sanja nasa). The persons who are usually predisposed to having avarsara (inferior quality) of Majja (bone marrow) and Satwa (quality of mind) are at increased risk of AD (Mangalasseri and Chandran 2017).

According to Ayurveda, learning or acquisition of information may be a result of consecutive and complicated interactions and coordination of Atma (soul), Indriyas (cognitive organs), Mana (psyche), and Indriyartha (sense organs). The functioning of those factors is ruled by Tridosha (Vata, Pitta, and Kapha) and Triguna (Satwa, Rajas and Tamas) as a result of specific coordination and balance. Any disturbance in these Tridosha and Triguna can cause disordered functioning of Indriya (cognitive and motor organs), Mana (psyche), and Buddhi (intellect), resulting in impaired memory (Sharma et al. 2012).

When explaining the consequences of aging according to the different decades, Ayurveda describes the loss of Medha (cognitive ability) by the end of the fourth decade, and loss of Manasakti (mental strength) and Buddhi (intelligence) by the end of the ninth decade. Medha is the capability to understand or accumulate new knowledge for storage. Mana (mind) and Buddhi (intellect) are terms for intellectual capacities. The ancient Ayurvedic scholar represented the psychological changes after sixty years of age as a weakening of the body tissues, the strength of the sense organs, energy, power of understanding, retention, and memorizing and analyzing facts, that substantiate the aging theory in AD (Banth and Talwar 2012).

Six cognitive domains, that are commonly disturbed in AD, are memory, executive functioning, language, visual functioning, attention, and affection. Of these, memory impairment is the central problem, especially short-term/ working memory. Memory impairment is of two types: the ability to learn new information and the ability to recall previously learned information. The mechanism of memory is achieved by a comprehensive physiology of indriyas (sensorium), mana (mind) and atma (soul). Atma perceives information using mana (mind), buddhi (intellect), jnana and karmendriya (cognitive sense organs). The collective information is stored by smaskara (processing) in the form of smriti (memory). Smriti is explained as a remembrance of things directly perceived, heard, or experienced earlier, which is the property of atma (soul). Indriyas are controlled by mana, and mana is itself under the control of Vata. The mental activity is being kept under control and moved forward by Vata. Vata also harmonized all the senses and established the relations with the objects that are sensed. On aging, Vata (body humor) becomes vitiated, which leads to improper functioning of mental properties, leading to humility and delirium. With the vitiation of vata dosha, alpasmriti (impaired memory) develops (Gold and Budson 2008).

5.5.2 Tridosha and Cognitive Functions

Doshas play important roles in maintaining cognitive functions. Any factors that impair the Shareerika bhava (physical factors) can also have an effect on the Manashika bhava (mental factors). Vata regulates the proper functioning of the Buddhi (intellect), Indriya (cognitive and motor organs), and Mana (psyche), whereas pitta enhances Medha (intellect) and Kapha nurtures dhee (intelligence), dhriti (fortitude), and Smriti (memory). Therefore, the normalcy of Tridosha is important for maintaining cognitive functions (Kundu et al. 2010; Deole et al. 2012).

Lack of Smriti will be attributed to the samvarana swabhava (obscuring nature) of Tamas. Rajas, Tamas, and Satwa are the qualities of mind, the proportion, and their interaction, which confirm the character of a person. Buddhinirodha (impaired cognitive functions) is additionally a tamasik quality. There is an eternal union between the rajas and tamas. Tamas cannot manifest its actions without rajas. Vata is represented as rajobahula (excessive rajas); once the functioning of Vatavaha sira (vata functioning channels) is clear, buddhikarmas (intellectual functioning) becomes effective. On aging, vata accumulates within the body, compared with other doshas, that leads to comparative rajovriddhi (increased rajas) in the mind. Because of the eternal union nature of both psychic doshas, tamas becomes imbalanced by rajovriddhi. Pathologically, rajotamovriddhi (increased rajas and tamas) and subsequent avarana (obstruction) of buddhi hampers cognitive functions of various sense organs as well as of memory (Deole et al. 2012).

Neuropsychological disturbance and deterioration in intelligence could also be due to the connection of rajas and tamas, which are liable for smritibhramsha. Moreover, dementia of the AD type, which may be explained in terms of disturbance within the function of Sadhakapitta, also represents a damaged condition of dhi, dhriti, and smriti (Kulatunga et al. 2012).

5.5.2.1 *Dhivibhramsha*

Dhivibhramsha means disorder of understanding, of the eternal and the non-eternal (Nityanitya), or good and bad (Hitahita), which are mistaken for one another; for true understanding, always identify things in their proper perspective (Tiwari and Tripathi 2013).

5.5.2.2 *Dhritivibhransha*

In the crisis of the disturbance of the will (Dhriti), the psyche (Sattva), which is always reaching out for its favorable objects, is ineffective at being discrete from unwanted objects, for the will (Dhriti) is the monitor and regulator (Tiwari and Tripathi 2013).

5.5.2.3 *Smritivibhransha*

When, on account of the psyche (Manas) being clouded by passion and deception, i.e. Rajomohavritatmanah, the confinement of true knowledge is broken down. The state is called the disorder of memory (Smriti), for, indeed, memorable things live in the memory.

In dementia, memory (Smriti) impairment is usually early and apparent, but is not anatomically localized; it may reflect disturbed registration (frontotemporal interactions), encoding (mesial temporal lobe), or retrieval systems (frontal lobe) (Kulatunga et al. 2012).

5.5.3 Drug Management

In Ayurvedic classics, there is much information regarding the drugs and compounds which are indicated to treat various realms of cognitive deficits and aging. Panchakarma (Penta bio-purification and rejuvenation) therapy, especially Nasya, Sirodhara, Matra Vasti (medicated enema), and Mridu Virechana (mild purgation) give outstanding results. Nasya and Sirodhara are the most efficient techniques with which to treat AD (Sharma 2003; Ramteke et al. 2016; Nakanekar et al. 2015; Shah et al. 2010; Kadus and Vedpathak 2017).

The Ayurvedic classics identified the relevance of higher faculties concerned with memory and introduced a separate group of drugs namely Medhya Rasayanas. Regular intake of such drugs is beneficial for a patient to resist the premature onset of degenerative change in the brain. Ayurveda can play an important role in controling such geriatric conditions (Jara) (Raghu et al. 2017).

Ayurveda classic texts described four Medhya Rasayana (herbal intellect rejuvenators), which have the quality to boost the higher activities of the brain and to improve the memory. They are Mandukparni (*Centella asiatica*), Shankhpushpi (*Convolvulus pluricaulis*), Madhuyasthi (*Glycyrrhiza glabra*), and Guduchi (*Tinospora cordifolia*), which are particularly specified as intellect-promoting drugs, of which Shankhpushpi is interpreted as the drug *par excellence* for the promotion of Medha (intellect). Additional herbal plants include such as Ashwagandha (*Withania somnifera*), Turmeric (*Curcuma longa*), Brahmi (*Bacopa monnieri*), Jyotishmati (*Celastrus paniculatus*), Jatamansi (*Nardostachys jatamansi*), and *Ginkgo biloba*, used separately or together, which mitigate Vata and help to minimize the degeneration of dhatus (nervous tissue or bone marrow), and support cognitive functions, along with immunity. These drugs are also described for avoidance and management of mental disorders, and for managing the consequences of aging (Raghu et al. 2017).

5.5.4 *Nasya*

According to Ayurveda, Nasya is one of the important therapeutic procedures where the route of drug administration is through the nose. When the drug (powder, juice, decoction, etc.) or medicated oil is administered through the nostrils, the procedure is called Nasya. According to Ayurveda, the nose is the gateway to the head. Nasya Karma is the process which eliminates the vitiated Doshas of the Urdhvanga (supraclavicular region), ensuring the smooth functioning of the CNS as well as rejuvenation of brain cells (Goldman 2006). Figure 5.3 shows the Nasys karma.

Ayurveda has some novel methods of administering herbs, or their preparations, for treating CNS disorders. One novel method of herbal drug delivery, called "Nasya", involves intranasal delivery of dry herbal powders or medicated oils. This is a practical, non-invasive, rapid, and simple method to deliver the therapeutic agents into the CNS. The use of medicated oils for Nasya require that the herbs be cooked in four parts oil and 16 parts water over a low flame until all of the water evaporates. This ensures the transport of lipophilic and lipid-soluble molecules across

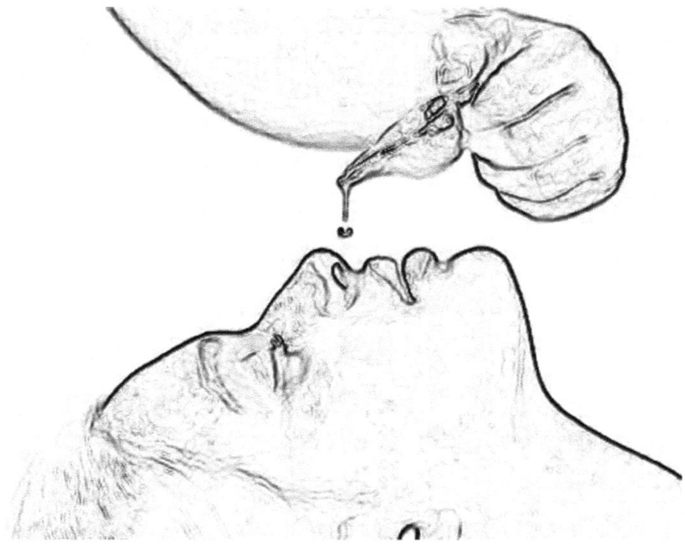

FIGURE 5.3 Nasya Karma.

the Blood–Brain Barrier (BBB) membrane, where hydrophilic compounds exhibit minimal permeation. Intranasal administration offers numerous benefits for drug delivery into the CNS, and interest in this non-invasive route of administration has increased. The delivery is rapid, bypasses the BBB, and directly targets the CNS, thereby reducing systemic exposure and subsequent side effects (Rao et al. 2012).

The nasal route is easily accessible, convenient, and reliable, with a porous, endothelial membrane and a highly vascularized epithelium that provides rapid absorption of compounds into the systemic circulation, avoiding the hepatic first-pass elimination. In addition, intranasal drug delivery enables dose reduction, rapid attainment of therapeutic blood levels, quicker onset of pharmacological activity, and fewer side effects. The nasal delivery seems to be a favorable way to bypass the obstacles of the BBB, allowing direct drug delivery to the biophase of the CNS-active compounds (Jaiswal et al. 2017). The pharmacodynamics of Nasya karma can be explained, in light of modern anatomical and physiological studies as follows:

5.5.4.1 Vascular Pathway

The nasal tissue is highly vascularized, making it an attractive site for rapid and efficient systemic absorption. The rich vascular plexus permits topically administered drugs to rapidly achieve effective blood levels, while avoiding intravenous catheters. Vascular path transportation is possible through the pooling of nasal venous blood into the facial vein, which occurs naturally. The facial vein has no valves, so it communicates freely with the intracranial circulation. It communicates through the pterygoid plexus with the cavernous venous sinus (Prasad et al. 1996).

5.5.4.2 Neurological Pathway

The olfactory nerve is a chemoreceptor in nature. It is known that, through the olfactory pathway, this nerve is connected with the limbic system and hypothalamus, which exert control over endocrine secretions. Moreover, the hypothalamus is considered to be responsible for integrating the functions of the endocrine system and the nervous system. Electrical stimulation of the hypothalamus in animals is capable of inducing secretions in the anterior pituitary, so that drugs administered here stimulate the higher centers of the brain, which acts to regulate the endocrine and nervous system functions (Shankar et al. 2015; Srikanth et al. 2011).

5.5.4.3 Diffusion through the Nasal Mucosa

In the absorption of drugs from the nasal cavity, the first step is passage through the mucus. Large and charged particles may find it more difficult to cross, but small and uncharged particles easily pass through this layer (Srikanth et al. 2011). Mechanisms for absorption of drugs through the nasal mucosa include the following:

- The paracellular route is the first transport mechanism, which is an aqueous route of transport. This is a slow and passive route.
- The transcellular process is the second mechanism of transport, through a lipoidal route, and is responsible for the transport of lipophilic drugs that show an absorption rate dependent on their lipophilicity. Drugs also cross cell membranes by an active transport route *via* carrier-mediated means or transport through the opening of tight junctions.

5.5.5 Shirodhara

Shirodhara is an important therapeutic measure in the Ayurvedic system of medicine, which has attracted worldwide popularity because of its simple administration and efficacy in a variety of lifestyle disorders, including neurological disorders, memory loss, insomnia, etc. Shirodhara is a purifying and rejuvenating therapy, designed to eliminate toxins and mental exhaustion as well as to relieve stress and any ill effects on the CNS. Shirodhara is a unique form of ancient therapy of pouring liquid/oil on the forehead from a specific height and for a specific period, continuously and rhythmically, allowing the liquid/oil to run through the scalp. The liquids used in Shirodhara depend on the condition being treated, but can include oil, milk, buttermilk, coconut water, or even plain water. The duration of Shirodhara treatment may extend from 30 to 45 minutes, depending on the condition of the patient (Akiko et al. 2016). Figure 5.4 shows the Shirodhara.

Shirodhara may begin with a full body massage, known as Abhyangam. Shirodhara also involves a head massage. Shirodhara is thought to work by relaxing the hypothalamus in the brain. It can also normalize the functions of hormones that regulate sleep, emotions, and cognitive functions (Akiko et al. 2016).

Pouring of lukewarm oils stimulates and soothes the hypothalamus, thereby regulating the functions of the pituitary gland and inducing sleep. Shirodhara stimulates Marma's or Vital Points in the head and improves circulation. Shirodhara produces a constant pressure and vibration, which is

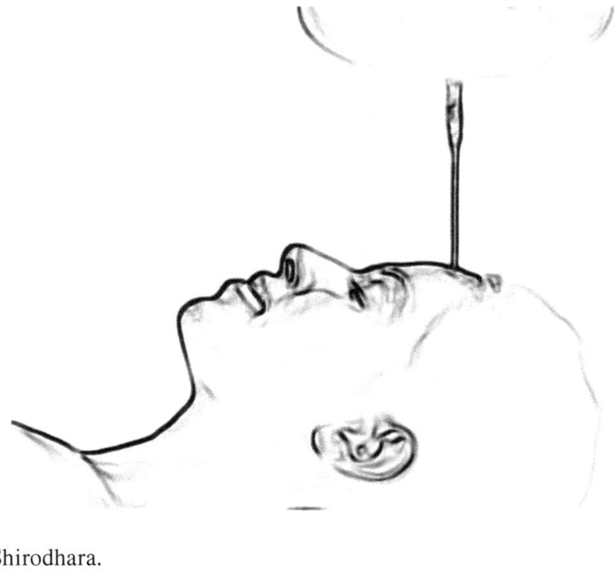

FIGURE 5.4 Shirodhara.

amplified by the hollow sinus present in the frontal bone. The vibration is then transmitted inwards through the fluid medium of the cerebrospinal fluid (CSF). This vibration, along with the slightly elevated temperature, may activate the functions of the thalamus and the basal fore brain, which helps to adjust the amount of serotonin and catecholamine to the normal level. The lukewarm oils used for Shirodhara also cause vasodilatation of all the channels and thereby improve the blood circulation to the brain and rejuvenate the brain cells, boosting memory (Vinjamury et al. 2014).

5.6 CONCLUSION

AD seems to be a Yapyavyadhi (palliative condition) according to Ayurvedic understanding of its pathogenesis. Early detection of the problem and an early start to the treatment is required to prevent the progress of the disease. An Ayurvedic approach to management, with Medhya rasayana and Panchakarma therapy, is useful in the treatment of AD and effective in improving the quality-of-life of the patient. Ayurvedic medications and therapeutic techniques for the management of neurodegenerative diseases, such as AD, are very effective, if used judiciously. AD is, to date, an incurable disease. At present, several medication systems can only give support to prevent the fast-developing nature of this disease. Only symptomatic treatment can be provided to achieve prevention of this disease. If the signs and symptoms can be identified in the early stages of AD, then only the precautionary approach is needed to prevent the AD from developing further. Panchakarma method such as Sirodhara and Nasya along with use of certain Rasayana Herbs (Anti Oxident, Immune and intellect rejuvenating Herbs which helps to minimize the degeneration of nervine tissue) can only prevent AD in the early stages or can halt further development of AD. If we can balance all the physiological and psychological parameters of the patient, then that patient can be cured from AD.

ACKNOWLEDGMENTS

We are sincerely thankful to the institute of the North Eastern Institute of Ayurveda and Homeopathy (NEIAH, Shillong) for giving us the opportunity to acquire the knowledge and practical experience of Nasya karma and Shirodhara. We are also thankful to all the staff of the Department of Kayachikitsa and Panchakarma, NEIAH, for providing us with a practical demonstration of the correct way of preparing herbs for Nasya karma and Shirodhara.

REFERENCES

Ahlskog, J. Eric, Yonas E. Geda, Neill R. Graff-Radford, and Ronald C. Petersen. 2011. "Physical Exercise as a Preventive or Disease-Modifying Treatment of Dementia and Brain Aging." *Mayo Clinic Proceedings* no. 86 (9):876–884. doi:10.4065/mcp.2011.0252.

Akiko, Tokinobu, Yorifuji Takashi, Tsuda Toshihide, and Doi Hiroyuki. 2016. "Effects of Ayurvedic Oil-Dripping Treatment with Sesame Oil vs. with Warm Water on Sleep: A Randomized Single-Blinded Crossover Pilot Study." *The Journal of Alternative and Complementary Medicine* no. 22 (1):52–58. doi:10.1089/acm.2015.0018.

Akula, Ramakrishna, P. Giridhar, and G. A. Ravishankar. 2011. "Phytoserotonin." *Plant Signaling & Behavior* no. 6 (6):800–809. doi:10.4161/psb.6.6.15242.

Anderson, Nicole D., Kelly J. Murphy, and Angela K. Troyer. 2012. *Living with Mild Cognitive Impairment: A Guide to Maximizing Brain Health and Reducing Risk of Dementia*. 1 edition. Oxford University Press.

Banth, S., and C. Talwar. 2012. "Anasakti, the Hindu Ideal, and its Relationship to Well-Being and Orientations to Happiness." *Journal of Religion and Health* no. 51 (3):934–946. doi:10.1007/s10943-010-9402-3.

Bekris, Lynn M., Chang-En Yu, Thomas D. Bird, and Debby W. Tsuang. 2010. "Genetics of Alzheimer Disease." *Journal of Geriatric Psychiatry and Neurology* no. 23 (4):213–227. doi:10.1177/0891988710383571.

Bertram, L., and R. E. Tanzi. 2004. "Alzheimer's Disease: One Disorder, Too Many Genes?" *Human Molecular Genetics* no. 13 Spec No. 1:R135–R141. doi:10.1093/hmg/ddh077.

Blazer, Dan G., and Lyla M. Hernandez. 2006. *Genes, Behavior, and the Social Environment: Moving Beyond the Nature/Nurture Debate*. National Academies Press.

Brookmeyer, R., E. Johnson, K. Ziegler-Graham, and H. M. Arrighi. 2007. "Forecasting the Global Burden of Alzheimer's Disease." Alzheimer's and Dementia no. 3 (3):186–191. doi:10.1016/j.jalz.2007.04.381.

Burns, Alistair, and Steve Iliffe. 2009. "Alzheimer's Disease." *BMJ* no. 338. doi:10.1136/bmj.b158.

Deole, Y. S., A. B. Thakar, H. Chandola, and B. Ravishankar. 2012. "Observational Study on External Social and Lifestyle Related Factors and Their Role in Pathogenesis of Premature Ageing and Stress." *AYU* no. 33 (3):378–386. doi:10.4103/0974-8520.108828.

Essa, M. Mohamed, Mohammed Akbar, and Gilles Guillemin. 2016. *The Benefits of Natural Products for Neurodegenerative Diseases*. Vol. 232. Springer.

Gold, Carl A., and Andrew E. Budson. 2008. "Memory Loss in Alzheimer's Disease: Implications for Development of Therapeutics." *Expert Review of Neurotherapeutics* no. 8 (12):1879–1891. doi:10.1586/14737175.8.12.1879.

Goldman, Ran D. 2006. "Intranasal drug delivery for children with acute illness." *Current Drug Therapy* no. 1 (1):127–130.

Hu, Nan, Jin-Tai Yu, Lin Tan, Ying-Li Wang, Lei Sun, and Lan Tan. 2013. "Nutrition and the Risk of Alzheimer's Disease." *BioMed Research International* no. 2013:524820. doi:10.1155/2013/524820.

Jack Jr., Clifford R., David S. Knopman, William J. Jagust, Ronald C. Petersen, Michael W. Weiner, Paul S. Aisen, Leslie M. Shaw, Prashanthi Vemuri, Heather J. Wiste, and Stephen D. Weigand. 2013. "Tracking Pathophysiological Processes in Alzheimer's Disease: An Updated Hypothetical Model of Dynamic Biomarkers." *The Lancet Neurology* no. 12 (2):207–216.

Jaiswal, P. L., A. B. Darekar, and R. B. Saudagar. 2017. "A Recent Review on Nasal Microemulsion for Treatment of CNS Disorder." *International Journal of Current Pharmaceutical Research* no. 9 (4):5–13. doi:10.22159/ijcpr.2017v9i4.20963.

Kadus, P. A., and S. M. Vedpathak. 2017. "Comparative Study of Anuvasana Basti with Constant and Escalating Dose as an Alternative to Snehapana in Purvakarma of Vamana and Virechana." *The Journal of Ayurveda and Integrative Medicine* no. 8 (3):194–199. doi:10.1016/j.jaim.2016.11.001.

Kalache, Alexandre. 1999. "Ageing: A Global Perspective." *Community Eye Health* no. 12 (29):1–4.

Khalsa, Dharma Singh. 2015. "Stress, Meditation, and Alzheimer's Disease Prevention: Where the Evidence Stands." Journal of Alzheimer's Disease no. 48 (1):1–12. doi:10.3233/JAD-142766.

Kulatunga, R. D., A. R. Dave, and M. S. Baghel. 2012. "Clinical Efficacy of Guduchyadi Medhya Rasayana on Senile Memory Impairment." *AYU* no. 33 (2):202–208. doi:10.4103/0974-8520.105239.

Kundu, C., V. D. Shukla, M. A. Santwani, and N. N. Bhatt. 2010. "The Role of Psychic Factors in Pathogenesis of Essential Hypertension and its Management by Shirodhara and Sarpagandha Vati." *AYU* no. 31 (4):436–441. doi:10.4103/0974-8520.82035.

Mangalasseri, Prakash, and Seetha Chandran. 2017. "A Brief Insight Into the Pathogenesis and Management of Alzheimer's Disease in Ayurvedic Parlance." *International Journal of Green Pharmacy* no. 11 (1):S81–S85.

Nakanekar, A., S. Bhople, H. Gulhane, S. Rathod, J. Gulhane, and P. Bonde. 2015. "An Ayurvedic Approach in the Management of Guillain-Barre Syndrome: A Case Study." *Ancient Science of Life* no. 35 (1):52–57. doi:10.4103/0257-7941.164540.

Nishteswar, K., Hemang Joshi, and Rahul Dutt Karra. 2014. "Role of Indigenous Herbs in the Management of Alzheimer's Disease." *Ancient Science of Life* no. 34 (1):3–7. doi:10.4103/0257-7941.150763.

Prasad, Y. V. Rama, Y. S. R. Krishnaiah, and S. Satyanarayana. 1996. "Intranasal Drug Delivery Systems: An Overview." *Indian Journal of Pharmaceutical Sciences* no. 58 (1):1.

Raghu, K. S., B. R. Shamprasad, S. P. Kabekkodu, P. Paladhi, M. B. Joshi, M. S. Valiathan, K. P. Guruprasad, and K. Satyamoorthy. 2017. "Age Dependent Neuroprotective Effects of Medhya Rasayana Prepared from *Clitoria ternatea* Linn. in Stress Induced Rat Brain." *The Journal of Ethnopharmacology* no. 197:173–183. doi:10.1016/j.jep.2016.07.068.

Ramakrishna, Akula, Parvatam Giridhar, Kadimi Udaya Sankar, and Gokare Aswathanarayana Ravishankar. 2012. "Melatonin and Serotonin Profiles in Beans of *Coffea* Species." *Journal of Pineal Research* no. 52 (4):470–476.

Ramteke, R. S., P. D. Patil, and A. B. Thakar. 2016. "Efficacy of Nasya (Nasal Medication) in Coma: A Case Study." *Ancient Science of Life* no. 35 (4):232–235. doi:10.4103/0257-7941.188188.

Rao, Rammohan V., Olivier Descamps, Varghese John, and Dale E. Bredesen. 2012. "Ayurvedic Medicinal Plants for Alzheimer's Disease: A Review." Alzheimer's Research & Therapy no. 4 (3):22–22. doi:10.1186/alzrt125.

Ravishankar, Gokare A., and Akula Ramakrishna. 2016. *Serotonin and Melatonin: Their Functional Role in Plants, Food, Phytomedicine, and Human Health*. CRC Press.

Santos, Cláudia Y., Peter J. Snyder, Wen-Chih Wu, Mia Zhang, Ana Echeverria, and Jessica Alber. 2017. "Pathophysiologic Relationship Between Alzheimer's Disease, Cerebrovascular Disease, and Cardiovascular Risk: A Review and Synthesis." Alzheimer's & Dementia no. 7:69–87. doi:10.1016/j.dadm.2017.01.005.

Serrano-Pozo, A., M. P. Frosch, E. Masliah, and B. T. Hyman. 2011. "Neuropathological Alterations in Alzheimer Disease." *Cold Spring Harbor Perspectives in Medicine* no. 1 (1):a006189. doi:10.1101/cshperspect.a006189.

Shah, M. R., C. S. Mehta, V. D. Shukla, A. R. Dave, and N. N. Bhatt. 2010. "A Clinical Study of Matra Vasti and an Ayurvedic Indigenous Compound Drug in the Management of Sandhigatavata (Osteoarthritis)." *AYU* no. 31 (2):210–217. doi:10.4103/0974-8520.72399.

Shankar, Singh Daya, Jayvindra Singh, and Vijay Kumar. 2015. "Role of Ksheer –Neti in Special Reference of Eye Disease." *World Journal of Pharmaceutical Research* no. 4 (7):1642–1649.

Sharma, A., V. K. Gothecha, and N. K. Ojha. 2012. "Dyslexia: A Solution Through Ayurveda. Evidences from Ayurveda for the Management of Dyslexia in Children: A Review." *AYU* no. 33 (4):486–490. doi:10.4103/0974-8520.110521.

Sharma, Ajay Kumar. 2003. "Panchakarma Therapy in Ayurvedic Medicine." In *Scientific Basis for Ayurvedic Therapies*, 67–86. Routledge.

Sharma, Satyam, Anuradha Balsavar, R. P. Beniwal, Triptish Bhatia, and Smita N. Deshpande. 2018. "A Pilot Study of Correlation between Intelligence Quotient, Social Quotient, and Ayurveda Parameters in Children." *Indian Journal of Psychological Medicine* no. 40 (1):74–79. doi:10.4103/IJPSYM.IJPSYM_227_17.

Smith, Melinda, Lawrence Robinson, and Jeanne Segal. 2018. *Preventing* Alzheimer's Disease. helpguide.org Trusted guide to mental, emotional & social health, September 2018. Available from https://www.helpguide.org/articles/alzheimers-dementia-aging/preventing-alzheimers-disease.htm.

Srikanth, K. Y., V. Krishnamurthy, and M. Srinivasulu. 2011. "Pharmacodynamics of Nasya Karma." *International Journal of Research in Ayurveda and Pharmacy* no. 2 (1):24–26.

Tarawneh, Rawan, and David M. Holtzman. 2012. "The Clinical Problem of Symptomatic Alzheimer Disease and Mild Cognitive Impairment." *Cold Spring Harbor Perspectives in Medicine* no. 2 (5):a006148. doi:10.1101/cshperspect.a006148.

Tiwari, Radhey Shyam, and Jyoti Shankar Tripathi. 2013. "A Critical Appraisal of Dementia with Special Reference to Smritibuddhihrass." *AYU* no. 34 (3):235–242. doi:10.4103/0974-8520.123102.

Tsuang, Ming T., Jessica L. Bar, William S. Stone, and Stephen V. Faraone. 2004. "Gene-Environment Interactions in Mental Disorders." *World Psychiatry* no. 3 (2):73–83.

Vinjamury, S. P., M. Vinjamury, C. der Martirosian, and J. Miller. 2014. "Ayurvedic Therapy (Shirodhara) for Insomnia: A Case Series." *Global Advances in Health and Medicine* no. 3 (1):75–80. doi:10.7453/gahmj.2012.086.

WHO. *The Top 10 Causes of Death*. World Health Organization, 24 May 2018. Available from http://www.who.int/en/news-room/fact-sheets/detail/the-top-10-causes-of-death.

Wimo, A., B. Winblad, H. Aguero-Torres, and E. von Strauss. 2003. "The Magnitude of Dementia Occurrence in the World." *Alzheimer Disease and Associated Disorders* no. 17 (2):63–67.

Ziegler-Graham, K., R. Brookmeyer, E. Johnson, and H. M. Arrighi. 2008. "Worldwide Variation in the Doubling Time of Alzheimer's Disease Incidence Rates." Alzheimer's & Dementia no. 4 (5):316–323. doi:10.1016/j.jalz.2008.05.2479.

6 Medha Rasayana Plants
Ayurvedic Approach to Alzheimer's Disease

Atanu Bhattacharjee and Biplab Kumar Dey

CONTENTS

6.1 INTRODUCTION

Ayurveda (traditional Indian system of medicine) emphasizes the root cause of any disease. According to Ayurveda, there are three different bio-energies (Dosha), namely Vata (all types of Movement), Pitta (Digestive and Metabolic Activities), and Kapha (Growth, Union, Stability, and Composition). There are also seven different body tissues (Dhatu) and three wastes (Mala). which are very significant for maintaining the healthy life of human beings. Among all the Dhatus, the Majja Dhatu (Nervous Tissue or Bone Marrow) is responsible for communication, intelligence, and movement. When there is an imbalance between Dosha and Majja Dhatu, a neurological disorder occurs. Predominance of Vata, which is dry and cold in nature, when combined with Majja Dhatu in the cerebral cortex, results in cortical shrinkage, shrinkage in the hippocampus and formation of amyloid β (Aβ) plaques, which gradually result in various neurological disorders, such as Alzheimer's disease (AD) (Adewusi et al., 2011). AD is a progressive neurodegenerative disorder, characterized by low levels of the neurotransmitter acetylcholine (ACh) in the cerebrum. It is an irreversible, age-related type of dementia that gradually damages the mind and steals away the individual memory and psychological abilities, causing changes in personality and conduct (Amod et al., 2005; Colucci et al., 2012). AD was first described in 1906 by German neuropsychiatrist Prof. Alois Alzheimer. It is a complex, multifactorial, progressive disorder, associated with diminished levels of ACh in the brain (Dwivedi et al., 1978). Normally, ACh is stored in the nerve terminals, in structures called vesicles, and is released from the nerve endings following depolarization of nerve terminals, entering the synapse and binding to the receptor. However, in patients with AD, the ACh which is released has a very short half-life due to the presence of large amounts of the enzymes acetylcholinesterase (AChE) and butyrylcholinesterase (BChE), which are both present in the brain and are detected among the neurofibrillary tangles and neuritic plaques. These enzymes hydrolyze the ester bond of the ACh molecule to choline and acetate, leading to loss of stimulatory activity (Zhang et al., 2015; Anderson, 2002). Two major pathological hallmarks of AD are characterized by deposition of abnormal Aβ protein plaques and the formation of neurofibrillary tangles of tau proteins, resulting in diminished impulse transmission from the end of one neuron to the beginning of another (Doraiswamy, 2002; Lemstra et al., 2003; Gupta et al., 2013).

AD is the main cause of dementia in the elderly, with a period of around nine years between the beginning of clinical side effects and the demise of the patient, and the incidence of AD has increased to become one of the deadliest issues in developed countries. The World Health Organization (WHO) has predicted that, by 2040, around 71% of the dementia cases will happen in developing nations (Atanu et al., 2015). There are considerable financial, social, and emotional burdens associated with caring for patients with this disease. In fact, in the advanced robotic phase of the disease, where life expectancy is long, this disease is a major cause of morbidity, and it imposes severe strains on the social welfare systems. It is estimated that, in the USA alone, more than 5 million people are affected by AD whereas, in the Indian scenario, the disease has already emerged as one of the deadliest threats to mankind, after diabetes, cancer and cardiac disease (Berrino et al., 2002).

One of the major clinical advances in the treatment of AD have been the utilization of AChE and BChE inhibitors to increase ACh levels in the cerebrum, although cholinergic agents with nicotinic and muscarinic agonist properties have also been targeted (Orhan et al., 2007; Rammohan et al., 2012). BChE, primarily associated with glial cells and specific neuronal pathways, cleaves ACh in a manner similar to AChE. Such studies on choline esterase inhibitors, resulting in statistically significantly slower decline in the cognitive performance of dementia patients carrying specific BChE polymorphisms that naturally lower BChE activity, have targeted BChE as a new target with which to intercede in the progression of AD (Vinutha et al., 2007; Adewusi et al., 2011). At present, there are very few drugs available to treat AD and the greater part of the treatment available can only postpone the development of AD indicators and alleviate symptoms over a brief timeframe.

Restorative plants represent a largely undiscovered store of bioactive chemicals and a potential reservoir of AChE inhibitors. The assorted variety of chemicals in medicinal plants makes them an important resource for novel lead mixes for the identification or development of chemicals to treat AD. Consequently, systematic ethnopharmacological screening of these plants may provide valuable leads in the development of new medications for AD treatment.

Approaches to enhancing cholinergic function in AD have included stimulation of cholinergic receptors or extension of the availability of ACh released into the neuronal synaptic cleft by use of agents which restore the level of acetylcholine through inhibition of both AChE and BChE (Harvey. 2008; Dahanukar et al., 2000a). Recent studies indicated that cholinesterase inhibitors hold a key role in not only enhancing cholinergic transmission in the brain but also possibly playing a modulatory role with regard to Aβ plaque deposition and neurotoxic fibril formation *via* suppressing amyloid precursor protein (APP) expression (Rinne et al., 2003; Mahesh et al., 2014). Therefore, AChE and BChE inhibitors have become remarkable alternatives for the treatment of AD. Existing anticholinesterase drugs, such as tacrine, donepezil, physostigmine, galantamine, and heptyl physostigmine, for the treatment of dementia are reported to have several dangerous side effects such as hepatotoxicity, short duration of biological action, low bioavailability, adverse cholinergic side effects in the periphery, and a narrow therapeutic window (Chatellier et al., 1990; Spiegel, 2002; Clegg et al., 2002).

Medicinal plants and their concentrates are assuming an indispensable role in the current treatment of psychological issues, as either the standard drug or as an integral drug, with specific reference to their ethnopharmacological perspectives (George et al., 2011). The history of drug discovery has shown that plants contain active compounds that have become new sources for study by the pharmaceutical industry. Plant constituents may act not only synergistically with other constituents from the same plant but may also enhance the activity of compounds or counteract toxic effects of compounds from other plant species. In traditional practices, numerous plants have been used to treat cognitive disorders, including neurodegenerative diseases and different neuropharmacological disorders (Perry et al., 1999; Vaidya, 1997). Basically, in Ayurveda, these medicinal plants are named "medharasayanas" (Sanskrit: "medha" implies intellect/cognition and "rasayana" implies revival). Medharasayanas incorporate a gathering of four therapeutic plants with multifold benefits, particularly to enhance memory and acumen by Prabhava (specific action) namely Mandukaparni (*Centella asiatica*; family: Apiaceae), Yastimadhu (*Glycyrrhiza glabra*; family: Fabaceae), Guduchi (*Tinospora cordifolia*; family: Menispermaceae), and Shankhapushpi (*Convolvulus pluricaulis*; family: Convolvulaceae) (Rammohan et al., 2012; Manyam, 1999). Traditional Indian medicinal plants, like Ashwagandha (*Withania somnifera*; family: Solanaceae), Brahmi (*Bacopa monnieri*; family: Plantaginaceae), Jyothishmati (*Celastrus paniculatus*; family: Celastraceae), Kushmanda (*Benincasa hispida*; family: Cucurbitaceae), Vacha (*Acorus calamus*; family: Acoraceae), and Jatamamsi (*Nardostachys jatamamsi*; family: Caprifoliaceae), are very highly revered in Ayurveda and other traditional texts as brain tonics and memory enhancers (Mishra et al., 2010; Singh et al., 1978; Anil et al., 2009). Indian turmeric (*Curcuma longa*; family: Zingiberaceae) contains curcumin, a phytochemical with demonstrable cell reinforcement and anticholinesterase activity, and its use to delay the progress of AD is compelling (Rammohan et al., 2012; Ahmed et al., 2009). Yokukansan, a Chinese herbal remedy which is used to treat various neurological states, has been reported as being effective in improving overall health status with no adverse effects (Howes et al., 2003). Furthermore, galantamine, an alkaloid from snowdrop, has been approved by the Food and Drug Administration in the United States for use in the treatment of AD (Rhee et al., 2001). Since AD has become a public health burden, and the commonly available synthetic drugs have undesirable side effects, new treatment strategies based on medicinal plants have become the focus of current research. With this scientific background, the current chapter has been prepared to gather together the up-to-date information about the role of alternative medicine to treat AD.

6.2 ETIOLOGY AND PATHOGENESIS

In patients with AD, the neurons become disabled. At an early stage of AD, the neuron's ability to produce the energy (by metabolism) for efficient coordination between them is blocked. They also lose the ability to repair themselves, which ultimately leads to death of neuron cells. Exactly what interferes with the normal functioning of the neuron is still a mystery, but, with the recent progress of medical science, three pathological hallmarks are being postulated as potential targets.

6.2.1 β-Amyloid Plaques

Tucked into the spaces between neurons are thick and sticky deposits of plaques made up of a protein called β-amyloid (Aβ). These plaques are also surrounded by other protein fragments, neuroremnants, immune cells, namely microglia, which, in turn, digest the damaged neurons and cause neuroinflammation. Aβ, a spontaneously aggregating peptide of 39-43 amino acids, is a fragment snipped from a larger protein called the amyloid precursor protein (APP). APP is an essential component for neuron growth which rests, in part inside and in part outside the cell. Aβ is derived from sequential proteolytic cleavage of the APP by β- and γ-secretases (Roberts, 2002). Initial cleavage by β-secretase (β-site of APP cleaving enzyme; BACE), a membrane-anchored aspartic protease, generates a soluble N-terminal fragment and a membrane-associated C-terminal fragment. The C-terminal fragment then undergoes proteolysis by γ-secretase to generate the Aβ peptides which progressively attach to one another, to be converted into insoluble plaques (Ghosh et al., 2014; Kar et al., 2004). According to the 'β-amyloid cascade', deposition of Aβ plaques triggers the neurotoxic cascade and promotes neuroinflammation, which ultimately results in neurodegeneration (Mahesh et al., 2014) (Figure 6.1).

6.2.2 Neurofibrillary Tangles

One of the pathological hallmarks of AD is the formation of intracellular neurofibrillary tangles, which consists of hyperphosphorylated tau proteins (Prerna et al., 2010). Tau is an axonal protein which binds to microtubules and promotes their assembly and stability. Phosphorylation

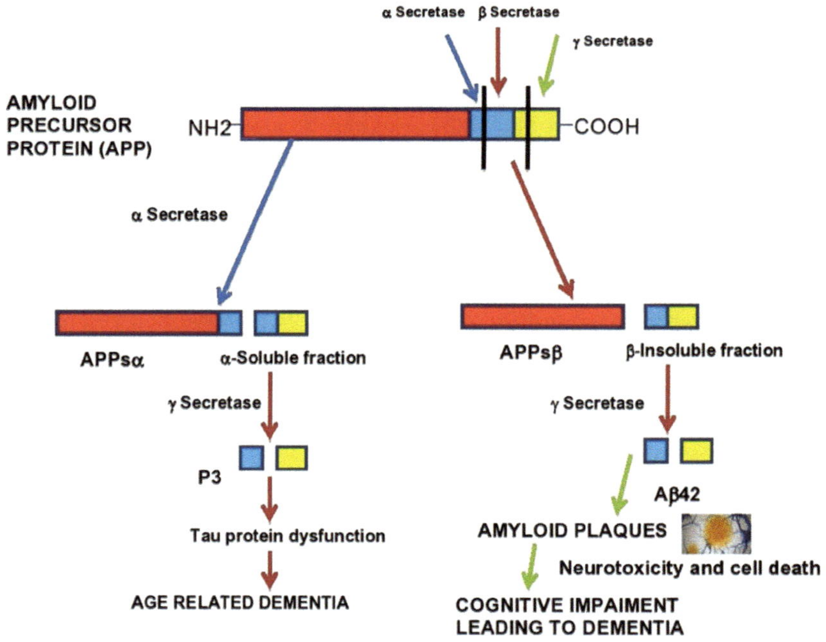

FIGURE 6.1 Modified amyloid cascade hypothesis (adopted and modified from Karren et al., 2016).

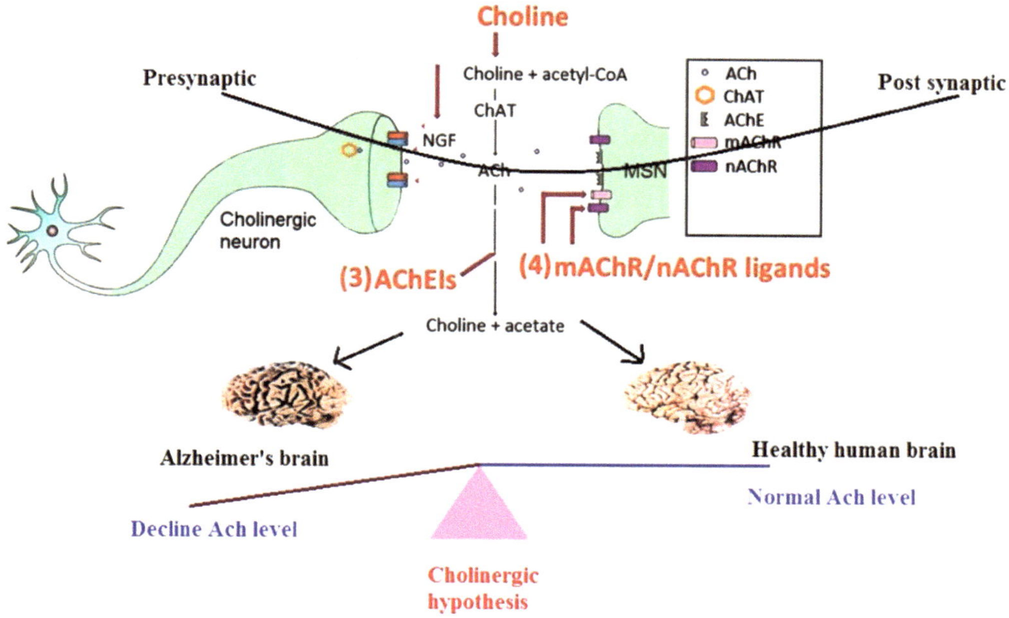

FIGURE 6.2 Possible therapeutic approaches for modulation of cholinergic transmission. 1. Increase in ChAT activity; 2. Inhibition of ACh release; 3. Inhibition of AChE; 4. Promotion of choline transport (adapted and modified from Jian-Zhi et al., 2006).

of tau protein is regulated by the balance between multiple kinases (e.g. glycogen synthetase kinase-3 (GSK3) and cyclin-dependent kinase-5 (CDK5)) and phosphatases (e.g. PP-1 and PP-2A). Hyperphosphorylation of tau proteins leads to the destruction of microtubule-associated proteins, thereby preventing microtubule assembly and impairing axonal transport, and resulting in neuronal death (Zhang et al., 2015; Gelb, 2000; Volloch and Rits, 2018).

6.2.3 Loss of Cholinergic Neurons

The cholinergic hypothesis claims that the decrease in cognitive function during dementia is predominantly related to a decrease in cholinergic neurotransmission. AD leads to selective degeneration of cholinergic neurons in the basal forebrain and results in the decline of cholinergic markers, namely choline acetyltransferase (ChAT) and ACh level and an increase in AChE (Talic et al., 2014; Jemima et al., 2011) (Figure 6.2).

Moreover, it has been postulated that ACh acts as a protein kinase inhibitor and thereby reduces tau phosphorylation. This inhibits intracellular neurofibrillary tangle formation and delays the progression of AD (Prerna et al., 2010).

Formation of extracellular Aβ plaques with a drastic neuronal and synaptic reduction in the cholinergic system of the brain is considered to be a major pathological hallmark of AD. Therefore, restoration of the central cholinergic function would play a significant role in restoring cognitive impairment in patients with AD. There are three principal approaches by which the cholinergic deficit can be addressed: (i) nicotinic receptor stimulation, (ii) muscarinic receptor stimulation, and (iii) inhibition of cholinesterase (AChE & BChE) activity (Vinutha et al., 2007; Puchchakayala et al., 2012; Jivad et al., 2014).

6.3 AYURVEDIC PERSPECTIVE OF AD

As described in Ayurveda, there is no condition which can be clinically equated to AD. But in the Ayurvedic classic texts, Smṛtināsha (loss of memory) is mentioned among the prodromal symptom of jarā (aging). In Jarāvasthā (old age, ≥ 60 years), according to Caraka, Smṛti and other mental coordination properties gradually deteriorate naturally. According to Vagbhaṭa (As.Sam.Sha 8/25) and Sharṅgadhara (Prathama Khaṇḍa 6/20), the functions of mind and Buddhi start declining from the 9th decade of life. Mental function declines at the 11th decade of life, according to Sharṅgadhara. Furthermore, Smṛtibhramsha (disturbed memory) is described as a symptom where Smṛti (memory) is vitiated by rajas (passion) and tamas (obscurity). Thus, senile dementia can be interpreted as Jarājanya Smṛtibhramsha, according to Ayurvedic principles (Singh et al., 1979a; Abhang, 1987).

AD can be termed "Smrti Nasha" in Ayurveda and is caused by the depletion of dhatus (tissues) and impairment of Satva Guna (the attribute of mind which represents purity and consciousness) by rajas (the attribute of mind which usually represents energy and dynamism) and tamas (the attribute of mind representing passivity and ignorance). When the Manovaha srotas (channels carrying cyclic impulses principally responsible for memory) are afflicted with Vata dosha, the person is affected and there is a malfunction of the mental activities (Singh et al., 1979a).

AD is not described as a disease entity in separate chapters of Ayurvedic classics and is considered to be a natural phenomenon, but the signs and symptoms of dementia can be understood in terms of Ayurvedic concepts. In order to understand the etiopathogenesis of dementia in the light of Ayurvedic literature, it is necessary to review the general physiology of *Manas* and *Buddhi*. Before discussing the etiology and psychopathology of *Smritibuddhihrass*, it is worth considering the relation of *Mana*, *Buddhi*, *Medha*, *Dhriti* and *Smriti* with each other (Akhlaq et al., 2018). In the process of knowledge, the mental faculty that determines the nature, merits, and demerits of an object of knowledge is *Buddhi*. *Buddhi* and *Mana* are related with *Karya Karana Sambandh*, as in the process of evolution, *Buddhi* is the first entity (*Tatva*), which is responsible for further development of *Indriyas* and *Manas* (Rammohan et al., 2012).

Conventional drug therapy is based on various theories to locate a viable treatment for and relief of AD symptoms. These therapies include the amyloid cascade and the cholinergic hypothesis. Certain other important aspects, like inflammatory, oxidative cascade, and hormonal pathways also play a vital role in AD (Vaidya, 1997; Bush, 2003). Some other lifestyle-associated possible causes may include a lack of routine exercise, intake of fast foods with high glycemic index and rich in saturated fats, an insufficient intake of plant-based nutrition, antioxidant substances (e.g., phytoestrogens), and seafood rich in ω-3 fatty acids. These may lead to insulin resistance, increased oxidative stress, and homocysteine and estrogen deficiencies (Fernando et al., 2008; Huang et al., 2016).

In a planned investigation of hazard factors, increasing age, absence of instruction, and the apolipoprotein E ε4 allele were observed to be interconnected, with increased risk of AD (Huang et al., 2012). Furthermore, use of non-steroidal anti-inflammatory drugs, wine, and routine daily activity were observed to be associated with diminished risk of AD (Aisen, 2002a; Nillert et al., 2017). Some studies propose that oxidative damage to brain tissue might be associated with pathogenesis, which occurs before the appearance of side effects and the development of Aβ plaques and neurofibrillary tangles (Lindsay et al., 2012).

Hereditable variables may also be included, although the situation with genetic factors for AD has not yet been clarified fully. The identification of pathogenic transformations in the β-amyloid peptide (β-APP) and the presenilin proteins provide a sound foundation for the hereditable theory, on the grounds that Aβ generation and statement add to the causes of AD (Schneider, 1996). Certain scientific investigations have reported that modifications in the lysosomal framework may play a significant role in the progression of neurodegeneration associated with AD. Lysosomal abnormality possibly deals with the generation of free radicals in the cerebrum and increased oxidative stress, which prompt a steady loss of metabolic movement, resulting in reduced life expectancy of the person concerned (Bahr et al., 2002).

6.4 CLINICAL EXAMINATION AND DIAGNOSIS

AD can be considered to be an advanced form of dementia which, in Ayurveda, is termed "Smrti Nasha" (loss of memory). Affliction of Manovaha srotas (retention of sequential events of learning responsible for memory) with Vata dosha may lead to deterioration of mental status of the person suffering from AD. The Ayurvedic system of medicine has developed certain dietary and therapeutic measures to delay aging and for rejuvenating whole functional dynamics of the body organs, which is known as "Rasayana chikitsa" (rejuvenation therapy).

AD is a life-changing disease for both the patient and care giver. At present, treatments are available to provide symptomatic relief from the disease for only a short period of time, if the disease is diagnosed in its early stages. According to Ayurveda, the physician must elaborate a concept about the progression and treatment of AD. In the early stages, Rookshana and Amapachana medicines are prescribed along with Shadangam kashaya, Saddharanam churna. Rookshana and Amapachana help Srotas prepare for the Snehana and Shodhana procedures. Sometime, Langhana (lightning therapy) is advised even before selecting Brihana (nourishing), to induce clarity of senses, expulsion of wastes, and achieve lightness in the body. But care must be taken to prevent aggravation of Vata dosha. Snehana therapy is another effective type of treatment where Pranaavruta Samana and Chatushprakara snehana (four types of unctuous substances, namely ghee, oil, fat, and bone marrow) are being induced. Medicines which are Brimhana (nourishing) and Vatanulomana (downward movement of Vata) should be selected, like Kshirabala, Vatasini, Dhanwantaram, Narayana, or Lakshaditaila. Murdhatailam with Balalakshadi, Kshirabala, or Vatasini can be also used for Snehana. After proper Snehana (oilation) and Swedana (Sudation), Shodhana should be carried out in the form of Vasti or Virechana, with the latter being found to be more effective under Pittanubandha conditions.

6.5 MANAGEMENT

The Ayurvedic system of medicine utilizes remedies from natural sources (extracts of plants, animals, and minerals) for the treatment of various mental disorders, including impaired memory condition. There are two methodologies of treatment: the first is general or aggregate prosperity of health, including mental activities (memory amusements, perusal, card recreations) and reflection; the second methodology specifically targets intellect (medha) and memory (smriti) (Jagdeep et al., 2009; Patel et al., 2014). The patient should be given proper counseling and mental support i.e. nothing but the Satvavajaya Chikitsa, as it is the most appropriate in management of Manovikara (psychological disturbances) This will be very helpful in managing the behavioral symptoms of AD patients, such as agitation, wandering, anxiety, anger, and depression. Rasayana therapy, including Medhya Rasayan and Achara Rasayana, must be planned for AD because it helps us in strengthening the host-defense mechanisms. A regulated lifestyle, wholesome diet, appropriate behavior, and following the ideal code of conduct as quoted in Ayurveda, are best to prevent and manage neurodegenerative diseases in general and AD in particular (Frawley, 1989). Some important medications routinely used to treat cognitive dysfunctions are presented below

6.5.1 Medhya Rasayana or Nootropic Drugs

During the Vedic period, the training framework was conferred by oral guidance, and the understudies held and reviewed this information by repeating recitations. In this way, insight was viewed as being identical to memory, and medications that diminished the time taken to remember the exercises were produced from regular sources. Several Ayurvedic medicines have been exploited for the treatment and management of acute and chronic neurological diseases associated with cognitive dysfunctions. These medicines from natural sources are believed to modulate neuroendocrine-immune systems via antioxidants and anti-inflammatory properties, and thereby to enhance memory and rejuvenate cognitive functions. Some of the traditionally reputed Medhya Rasayana drugs are mentioned below:

i. Decoction of Mandhukparni (*Centella asiatica*)
ii. Powder of Jastimadhu (*Glycyrrhiza glabra*) with milk
iii. Juice of Guduchi (*Tinospora cordifolia*)
iv. Paste of Shankhpushpi (*Convolvulus pluricaulis*) leaves

A significant proportion of medicinal plants of Indian origin are said to have brain tonic and memory-boosting impacts. Generally, these plants are prescribed in combination, as they are believed to provide synergistic effects, achieving substantial relief of the symptoms. Sometimes, the formulations are incorporated with drugs of mineral origins (Satyavati, 1987; Khare, 2007). A list of medicinal plants used as brain tonics is shown in Table 6.1.

TABLE 6.1
Indian Medicinal Plants With Nootropic Effects (adapted and modified from Divya et al., 2007)

Sl. No.	Common Name	Scientific Name	Family
1.	Vacha	*Acorus calamus*	Acoraceae
2.	Bada Ilaichi	*Amomum subulatum*	Zingiberaceae
3.	Shatawar	*Asparagus racemosus*	Asparagaceae
4.	Brahmi	*Bacopa monnieri*	Plantaginaceae
5.	Dhak, Palash	*Butea frondosa*	Fabaceae
6.	Sankha Holi	*Canscora decussata*	Gentianaceae
7.	Dalchini	*Cinnamomum zeylanicum*	Lauraceae
8.	Guggulu	*Commiphora wightii*	Burseraceae
9.	Shankhpushpi	*Convolvulus pluricaulis*	Convolvulaceae
10.	Haldi	*Curcuma longa*	Zingiberaceae
11.	Sedge	*Cyperus rotundus*	Cyperaceae
12.	Jadwar Shireen	*Delphinium denudatum*	Ranunculaceae
13.	Choti Elaichi	*Elettaria cardamomum*	Zingiberaceae
14.	Amla	*Emblica officinalis*	Phyllanthaceae
15.	Vayu Vidang	*Embelia ribes*	Phyllanthaceae
16.	Laung	*Eugenia caryophyllus*	Myrtaceae
17.	Bari Saunf	*Foeniculum vulgare*	Apiaceae
18.	Ginkgo	*Ginkgo biloba*	Ginkoaceae
19.	Hypericum	*Hypericum perforatum*	Hypericaceae
20.	Vidari Kand	*Ipomoea paniculata*	Convolvulaceae
21.	Lavander	*Lavandula officinalis*	Lamiaceae
22.	Maca	*Lepidium meyenii*	Brassicaceae
23.	Jatamansi	*Nardostachys jatamansi*	Caprifoliaceae
24.	Nishoth	*Operculina turpethum*	Convolvulaceae
25.	Uood Saleeb	*Paeonia emodi*	Paeoniaceae
26.	Keora	*Pandanus odoratissimus*	Pandanaceae
27.	Saunf	*Pimpinella anisum*	Apiaceae
28.	Renuka	*Piper aurantiacum*	Piperaceae
29.	Peepal, Pippali	*Piper longum*	Piperaceae
30.	Kava	*Piper methysticum*	Piperaceae
31.	Heal-all	*Prunella vulgaris*	Lamiaceae
32.	Badam	*Prunus amygdalis*	Rosaceae
33.	Gulab	*Rosa damascena*	Rosaceae
34.	Kuth	*Saussurea lappa*	Asteraceae
35.	Bahera	*Terminalia bellirica*	Cobretaceae
36.	Harar, Hareetaki	*Terminalia chebula*	Combretaceae
37.	Giloe	*Tinospora cordifolia*	Menispermaceae
38.	Tagar	*Valeriana wallichii*	Caprifoliaceae
39.	Khas	*Vetiveria zizanioides*	Caprifoliaceae
40.	Ashwagandha	*Withania somnifera*	Solanaceae
41.	Adrakh	*Zingiber officinalis*	Zingiberaceae

In conventional practice, the main medications prescribed at present for the treatment of AD are cholinomimetics. In fact, tacrine was the first clinically established synthetic AChE inhibitor developed to increase ACh levels at the nerve endings. Subsequently, second-generation inhibitors were introduced but the resulting side effects and the cost factor limited their use. Although tacrine provides a positive influence in a low proportions of cases with respect to memory impairment, the extentof the improvement was relatively minor. Furthermore, long-term use has severe side effects include stomachache, sickness, vomiting, and looseness of the bowels, and costs can be economically constraining (Gupta et al., 2013). Significant research is being led in different areas, for example, utilizing particular mitigating drugs (specific cyclooxgenase-2 [COX-2] inhibitors), to decrease forgetfulness of mind, and cancer prevention agents (Aisen, 2002b). Other current therapeutic interventions are antiamyloid procedures (e.g. Aβ vaccination, β-secretase inhibitors), modification of metal chelators (e.g. clioquinol), lipid-lowering drugs, anti-hypertensive drugs, vitamins, and synapse receptors (Das et al., 1984; Huang et al., 2012). Phytoextracts from locally available plant materials with AchE inhibitory properties have shown some promise. Ayurveda has numerous definitions and herbomineral drug formulations are utilized to enhance intellectual capacities. The exact biochemical system underlying the activity of these herbs is not clear. It is likely that cell reinforcement and mitigating properties of these herbs might be responsible for their benefits in the treatment of AD.

6.6 SCIENTIFIC BASIS OF MEDHA RASAYANA DRUGS

6.6.1 Based on Pre-Clinical Studies

Below we describe the various Ayurvedic medicinal nervine herbs that are recommended for AD, and their actions on the brain.

6.6.1.1 *Bacopa monnieri* (Brahmi)

The Central Drug Research Institute (CDRI), Lucknow, and other premier scientific organizations of the Government of India, has conducted a systematic study regarding nootropic effects of *B. monnieri*, and, based on the outcome, a polyherbal preparation, "Mentat", has been successfully marketed. It has been observed that an ethanolic extract of *B. monnieri* facilitated the acquisition, consolidation, and retention of memory *in vivo*, as evaluated by the passive avoidance paradigm and maze tests.

The principal constituents of *B. monnieri* are saponins and triterpenoid bacosaponins, that include bacopasides III to V, bacosides A and B, bacosaponins A, B, and C, and the jujubogenin bisdesmosides, bacopasaponins D, E, and F. Other phytoconstituents include alkaloids, phytosterols, betulic acid, polyphenols, and sulfhydryl compounds that exert strong antioxidant activities. In the hippocampus, *B. monnieri* enhances protein kinase activity that may contribute to its nootropic action. *B. monnieri* also inhibits cholinergic degeneration and thereby displayed a nootropic effect in a rat model of AD. A study with a standardized extract of *B. monnieri* reversed the cognitive deficits induced by intracerebroventricularly administered colchicine and ibotenic acid into the nucleus basalis magnocellularis. Furthermore, it also reversed (a) decrease in acetylcholine (ACh) levels, (b) reduction in choline acetyltransferase (ChAT) activity, and (c) decrease in muscarinic cholinergic receptor binding in the frontal cortex and hippocampus. The extracts protected neurons from Aβ-induced cell death by suppressing cellular AChE activity (Gohil et al., 2010; Ahirwar et al., 2012).

6.6.1.2 *Centella asiatica* (Mandookparni)

Administration of a *C. asiatica* (Family: Apiaceae) aqueous extract resulted in improved learning and memory potential *in vivo*. The extract significantly alleviated oxidative stress by decreasing malondialdehyde (MDA) levels and increasing glutathione levels. Furthermore, it also exhibited AChE inhibitory activity; these multiple effects, in combination, may be associated with its cognition-enhancing efficacy (Anil et al., 2009).

6.6.1.3 *Convolvulus pluricaulis* Chois (Shankhpushpi)

Administration of a *C. pluricaulis* (Family: Convolvulaceae) extract significantly increased ACh, and catechol amine and 5- hydroxy tryptamine (5-HT) levels in the brain (Parul et al., 2014). An *in-vitro* assay showed that anticholinesterase activity of the *C. pluricaulis* extract had a mean ± standard deviation half-maximal inhibitory concentration of IC_{50} 234±38 μg/ml (Maya et al., 2014).

6.6.1.4 *Eugenia caryophyllus* spl. (Laung)

The aqueous extract of *E. caryophyllus* (Family: Myrtaceae) exerted significant AchE inhibitory activity, which may be due to the presence of water-soluble phytoconstituents in the extract. Another research report, studying Chavanprash, an Ayurvedic formulation containing *E. caryophyllus*, showed significant anticholinesterase and antioxidant potential *in vivo* against scopolamine-induced amnesia (Akinrimisi et al., 1975).

6.6.1.5 *Glycyrrhiza glabra* Linn. (Yastimadhu)

The alcoholic extract of *G. glabra* and glabridin, a bioactive component isolated from *G. glabra*, showed both AchE and BChE inhibitory activity in a dose-dependent manner. Furthermore, liquiritin and isoliquirin, flavonoid constituents isolated from the plant, showed a significant antioxidant profile against scopolamine-induced amnesia *in vivo* (Muralidharan et al., 2009).

6.6.1.6 *Lawsonia intermis* Linn. (Mehndi)

The acetone-soluble fraction (100 mg/kg bodyweight) of a petroleum ether extract of *L. intermis* leaves showed a significant ($p \leq 0.001$) nootropic effect *in vivo* in a dose-dependent manner. Furthermore, it also affected 5-hydroxy tryptamine levels and noradrenaline-mediated behavior in experimental animals (Iyer et al., 1998).

6.6.1.7 *Nardostachys jatamansi* DC. (Jatamansi)

Jatamansi is a safe and highly regarded Ayurvedic medicinal plant, used as a sedative. The sedative activity is due to the presence of valeranone, a sesquiterpene, and coumarins. Other terpenoids present include spirojatamol, nardostachysin, jatamols A and B, and calarenol.

An alcoholic extract of this plant, administered to both young and aged mice, significantly improved learning and memory, and also reversed amnesia induced by diazepam and scopolamine. Furthermore, it reversed aging-induced amnesia due to the natural aging of mice, suggesting that the compounds in this plant may prove to be useful in restoring memory in older individuals as well as in patients with age-associated dementia (Habibur et al., 2011).

6.6.1.8 *Pongamia pinnata* (Karanj)

A petroleum ether extract of the seeds of *P. pinnata* was tested for nootropic activity in an experimental model of AD (created by ibotenic acid-induced lesioning of the nuclear basalis magnocellularis). It reversed both the cognitive deficits and the reduction in cholinergic markers after 2 weeks of treatment. Reversal of perturbed cholinergic function was considered to be the possible mechanism (Prachi et al., 2017).

6.6.1.9 *Tinospora cordifolia* F.Vill (Guduchi)

An n-butanolic fraction of an ethanolic extract of *T. cordifolia* stem, which contains saponins, showed significant nootropic reduction in cholinergic markers *in vivo* in a dose-dependent manner. Furthermore, the extract also showed anti-inflammatory activity against lipopolysaccharide-induced neuroinflammation. An ethanolic extract of this plant reduced ACh content in the rat whole brain but increased it in the cortex. These findings may be correlated with its nootropic potential as an anti-Alzheimer's drug (Prakash et al., 2017).

6.6.1.10 *Withania somnifera* Dunal (Ashwagandha)

Ashwagandha, a solanaceous drug, is used extensively in Ayurveda as a nervine tonic, aphrodisiac, and 'adaptogen', helping the body adapt to stress. It is categorized as a rasayana (rejuvenative), and is believed to possess antioxidant activity, free radical scavenging activity, and an ability to support a healthy immune system. Ashwagandha has a calming effect and thus may be particularly indicated in people with AD. A total alkaloid extract of Ashwagandha root exhibited CNS-depressant activity, which is correlated with its relaxation and antidepressant properties. Aqueous extracts of this herb have been found to increase cholinergic activity, including increases in the ACh content and ChAT activity in rats, and this might partly explain the cognition-enhancing and memory-improving effects. Moreover, recent reports suggested that a methanol extract of Ashwagandha caused neurite outgrowth in a dose- and time-dependent manner in human neuroblastoma cells. The levels of two dendritic markers, namely MAP2 and PSD-95, were found to be markedly increased in cells treated with Ashwagandha, suggesting that it stimulates dendrite formation (Bhattacharya et al., 1995; Schiloers et al., 1997; Mishra et al., 2000).

6.6.2 Based on Clinical Studies

The data on clinical examinations on Indian therapeutic plants possessing nootropic nootropic is displayed below.

6.6.2.1 *Bacopa monnieri* Linn. (Brahmi)

A significant increase in intelligent quotient (IQ) scores was seen after treatment for 9 months of 110 boys aged from 10 to 13 years with a suksma (miniaturized scale) medication obtained from *B. monnieri*. Memory (direct) and arithmetic tests were utilized. The medication was endured in single (20 to 300 mg) and different dosage (100 or 200 mg for 4 weeks) measurements in a two-fold visually impaired placebo and stage I clinical trials in human volunteers (Carlo et al., 2008).

6.6.2.2 *Centella asiatica* Linn. (Mandookparni)

Treatment with a *C. asiatica* (Family: Apiaceae) aqueous extract showed improved learning and memory potential *in vivo*. The extract significantly alleviated oxidative stress by decreasing malondialdehyde (MDA) levels and increasing glutathione level. Furthermore, it also showed AChE inhibitory activity which, in combination, may be associated with cognition-enhancing efficacy (Anil et al., 2009). In recent randomized clinical trials, 28 participants (> 61 years of age) were administered different dosages of *C. asiatica* extract (250, 500 or 750 mg/d; per oral (p.o.)) for two months. After two months, patients receiving the 750 mg dose extract showed significant improvement in cognitive function (as assessed by event-related potential and the computerized assessment battery test) and mood (using the BondLader visual analog) (Kashmira et al., 2010; Soumyanath et al., 2012).

6.7 POLYHERBAL FORMULATIONS WITH MEDHA RASAYANA PROPERTIES

6.7.1 Indian Noni

Noni, a polyherbal formulation of *Morinda citrifolia* extract and *Garcinia cambogi*, was tested *in vivo* for its nootropic potential against scopolamine-induced amnesia. The formulation (dose: twice/day for 14 days) showed significant ($p<0.01$) decline in transfer latency compared with the scopolamine-induced amnesia group. Furthermore, Noni significantly inhibited AChE activity in a rat brain homogenate and showed antioxidant properties. These results suggested that the Noni formulation might offer a useful therapeutic choice in either the prevention or the treatment of AD (Uma et al., 2014).

6.7.2 Memorin (Phytopharma)

Memorin is a dietary supplement designed to enhance brain functions. The formulation consists of aqueous juice of seven well-known Ayurvedic medicinal plant, namely *Centella. asiatica* (150 mg), *Convolvulus alsinoides* (150 mg), *Glycyrrhiza glabra* (100 mg), *Acorus calamus* (100 mg), *R. serpentina* (30 mg), *Withania somnifera* (100 mg), and *Saussurea lappa* (50 mg). Pretreatment with the formulation (200 mg/kg/d for 21 d) attenuated electroconvulsive shock (ECS)-induced retrograde amnesia in rats. The evaluation method used was a passive-avoidance test in a shuttle box (Dahanukar et al., 2000b).

6.7.3 Mentat (Himalaya Healthcare)

Mentat, a polyherbal formulation, containing extracts of *C. asiatica*, *B. monneri*, and *W. somnifera* is marketed by Himalaya Pvt. Ltd. *B. monneri* is well known for its nootropic effect. *In-vivo* experimentation revealed that the herb enhances memory and learning processes and also calms restlessness in several mental disorders. *C. asiatica* possesses antiepileptic properties and is commonly used as an adjuvant to epileptic drugs. It balances amino acid levels, which is beneficial in treating depression. It also prevents cognitive impairment. Ashvagandha is used as a mood stabilizer in clinical conditions of anxiety and depression. Withanolides, the chemical constituents present in winter cherry, possess rejuvenating properties. The herb also reduces oxidative stress, which can cause mental fatigue (Kulkarni et al., 1994; Handa et al., 1997).

6.7.4 Shankhpushpi Syrup (Baidyanath)

Shankhpushpi syrup is an Ayurvedic remedy for memory and intellect. It is beneficial in treating mental weakness, forgetfulness, memory loss, low retention power, etc. The formulation consists of *C. alsinoids* (200 mg), Brahmi (50 mg), sugar (8000 mg), and citric acid (6 mg). Shankhpushpi is traditionally used as a brain tonic. Brahmi calms the mind and reduces anxiety, mental stress, work-related stress, and depression. The formulation showed excellent nootropic activity *in vivo* in normal and scopolamine-induced amnesic models. At a dose >40 ml/kg p.o., it also showed significant anticholinesterase activity but showed moderate effects on other neurotransmitter concentrations in whole brain tissue (Sharma et al., 2005).

6.7.5 Trasina (Dey's Pharmaceuticals)

Trasina is a polyherbal capsule containing *Ocimum sanctum* (190 mg) and *W. somnifera* (80 mg). Trasina (one capsule/d for 21 d) showed beneficial effects on mental activity in two *in-vivo* models, namely intracerebroventricular injection of colchicine (15 mg/rat) and ibotenic acid-induced neurotoxicity (10 mg/rat). The drug caused significant reductions in time spent on maze apparatus transfer, and increased levels of cholinergic markers and M1 receptor binding in the rat brain. It also showed significant anticholinesterase activity in a dose-dependent manner (Kulkarni et al., 1994; Handa et al., 1997).

6.7.6 Saraswatarishta (Baidyanath)

Saraswatarishta, a polyherbal Ayurvedic liquid formulation (10 ml), containing juice of *Centella asiatica* (960 mg), *Asparagus racemosus* (240 mg), *Pueraria tuberosa* (240 mg), *Terminalia chebula* (240 mg), *Foeniculam vulgare* (240 mg), *Zingiber officinale* (240 mg), *V. zizanioidis* (240 mg), *Withania fruticosa* (240 mg), *Vitex negundo* (240 mg), *Operculina turpethum* (240 mg), and honey. Saraswatarishta also contains 5–10 % of self-generated alcohol. This alcohol and the water present in the product act as media with which to deliver water- and alcohol-soluble active herbal components to the body. A clinical study in 25 patients treated with Saraswatarishta (20 ml taken two times/d for one year) showed prominent antiepileptic activity; The drug showed nootropic effects against various experimental models *in vivo via* anticholinesterase activity (Kulkarni et al., 1994; Handa et al., 1997).

6.7.7 Vidyarthi Amrit (Maharishi Ayurveda)

Vidyarthi amrit, a polyherbal Ayurvedic liquid formulation, containing juice of *Evolvulus alsinoides, C. asiatica, Valeriana wallichii, Embellica ribes, A. racemosus, W. somnifera, Elettaria cardamomum, Pimpinella anisum*, and *Acorus calamus*. The formulation exhibited significant anticholinesterase and antiglutamate activity and resulted in increases in L-aspartate and GABA levels in whole brain tissue *in vivo*, which may be associated with the nootropic potential of the formulation (Kulkarni et al., 1994; Handa et al., 1997).

6.7.8 Dimagh Pushtak Rasayan (Baidyanath)

Dimagh Pushtak Rasayan is an Ayurvedic Rasayana formulation, composed of *C. alsinoids, W. somnifera, C. asiatica, B. monnieri*, Makaradhwaj (sulfide of mercury), and *N. jatamansi*. This drug exhibited nootropic effects in *in-vivo* experimental models. The memory-enhancing effects of the formulation were attributed to cholinergic mechanisms (Kulkarni et al., 1994; Handa et al., 1997).

6.7.9 Geriforte (Himalaya)

Geriforte is an Ayurvedic formulation. Each Geriforte tablet contains Chyavanprash concentrate (100 mg), Himsra (*C. spinosa*) (13.8 mg), Kasani (*Cichorium intybus*) (13.8 mg), Daruharidra (*Berberis aristata*) (10 mg), Vasaka (*Adhatoda vasica*) (10 mg), Kakamachi (*Solanum nigrum*) (6.4 mg), Arjuna (*Terminalia arjuna*) (6.4 mg), Biranjasipha (*Achillea millefolium*) (3.2 mg), Kasamarda (*Celtis occidentalis*) (3.2 mg),

Jhavuka (*Tamarix gallica*) (3.2 mg), Ashvagandha (*W. somnifera*) (30 mg), Shatavari (*Acorus racemosus*) (20 mg), Yashtimadhu (*Glycyrrhiza glabra*) (20 mg), Mandukaparni (*C. asiatica*) (20 mg), Shilajeet (purified) (20 mg), Haritaki (*T. chebula*) (15 mg), Makardhwaj (10 mg), Musali (*A. adscendens*) 910 mg), Udakiryaka (*Caesalpinia digyna*) (10mg), Kapikachchu (*M. pruriens*) (10 mg), Jatiphalam (*M. fragrans*) (10 mg), Pippali (*P. longum*) (10 mg), Jaatipatree (*M. fragrans*) (10 mg), Bhringaraja (*E. alba*) (10 mg), Vriddadaru (*A. speciosa*) (10 mg), Abhrak bhasma (10 mg), Jasad bhasma (10 mg), Kumkuma (*Crocus sativus*) (7 mg), Mandur bhasma (5 mg), Lavanga (*S. aromaticum*) (5 mg), Ela (*E. cardamomum*) (5 mg), Yawani (*C. copticum*) (5 mg), Haridra (*Curcuma longa*) (5 mg), Jyothishmati (*C. paniculatus*) (5 mg), and Loh bhasma (5 mg). The natural ingredients in Geriforte work synergistically to prevent free radical-induced oxidative damage to various organs. The ingredients are natural rejuvenators and cardioprotective agents. As an immunomodulator, Geriforte stimulates the immune system to respond against disease-causing microorganisms. Geriforte is also an adaptogenic which effectively combats stress and fatigue. It also increases stamina and improves overall performance. Clinical psychobiological studies on typical mature subjects, 45 to 50 years of age, were carried out for 3 months, with the test definition. Results demonstrated an increasing feeling of prosperity, physical effectiveness, and enhancement in mental capacities. The treatment diminished uneasiness and achieved better nitrogen maintenance. The medication has all the hallmarks of being a blend of natural substances for early treatment of mental and physical impairments in mature people (Singh et al., 1979b; Boral et al., 1989).

6.8 AYURVEDIC MINERAL COMBINATION WITH MEDHA RASAYANA PROPERTIES

In Ayurveda, minerals are used as therapeutic agents in their calcinated forms. In Ayurvedic preparations like Bhasmas, metals are therapeutically effective and safe for internal use. Several such mineral preparations, associated with learning and memory, are mentioned below.

6.8.1 Siddh Makardhwaja (Mercury)

This medicine is traditionally administered along with milk. The preparation helps in the overall status of experimental animals. It exerts growth-promoting, memory-improving, and carbohydrate-sparing properties without affecting other central nervous system (CNS) parameters in rodents (Vohora et al., 1995).

6.8.2 Swarna Bhasma (Gold)

Swarna Bhasma shows potent antioxidant and free radical scavenging activity. The preparation (25 mg/kg orally for 7 to 10 d) exhibited a nootropic effect *in vivo* compared with *Panax ginseng* tea (350 mg/kg orally for 10 d). The preparation showed significant anticholinesterase activity, which may be associated with beneficial effects on cognitive function (Bajaj et al., 1999, 2000).

6.9 CONCLUSIONS

At present, few pharmaceuticals are available to treat AD, with most of them being used either to postpone the progress of the condition or to alleviate symptoms for a short time. Unfortunately, subsequent adverse reactions, coupled with high economic cost of these medications, have limited their usefulness. As a consequence, it would be beneficial to shift the paradigm from synthetic to natural medicines as the latter are considered to be safer and more economical by the WHO (Perry et al., 2000).

In the field of AD therapy, several developments in the possible role of natural products have already been supported by research. To date, the greatest successes have resulted from discovery programs targeting plant-based AChE inhibitors and antioxidants, which have provided substantial progress in the treatment of AD (Perry et al., 2001). Other approaches include anti-amyloid agents, β-secretase inhibitors, anti-inflammatory drugs, nicotinic and muscarinic receptor agonists, and tau protein inhibitors (Ingkaninan et al., 2006). Currently, investigations into natural products that can act as functional foods is of particular interest, to delay the progression of and symptomatic relief from AD, and to promote other associated health benefits. A significant shift from a single-target to a multi-target drug approach, especially for chronic and complex disease syndromes, is being witnessed in the management of AD. However, cellular level assays to determine the mechanism involved are essential to support the therapeutic claims of these preparations as anti-Alzheimer's drugs. In a recent study, lifestyle modifications, such as a stress-free life, with vacations, adequate spending capacity, and quality time with family members, etc., are found to be beneficial to reducing the risk of dementia. Moreover, yoga and meditation also help to prevent the progress of dementia and AD (Mukherjee et al., 2007; Atanu et al., 2015). If the research develops in a successful manner, the drugs derived from natural sources could be a good substitute for conventional allopathic medicines, as they are readily and economically available.

REFERENCES

Abhang RY. Medhya rasayana: past, present and future. *Deerghayu Int.* 1987; 4: 8–18.

Adewusi EA, Steenkamp V. *In vitro* screening for acetylcholinesterase inhibition and antioxidant activity of medicinal plants from southern Africa. *Asian Pac J Trop Med.* 2011; 5(2): 829–835.

Ahirwar S, Tembhre M, Gour S, Namdeo A. Anticholinesterase efficacy of *Bacopa monnieri* against the brain regions of rat – a novel approach to therapy for Alzheimer's disease. *Asian J Exp Sci.* 2012; 26(1): 65–70.

Ahmed T, Gilani AH. Inhibitory effect of curcuminoids on acetylcholinesterase activity and attenuation of scopolamine-induced amnesia may explain medicinal use of turmeric in Alzheimer's disease. *Pharmacol Biochem Behav.* 2009; 91: 554–559.

Aisen PS. Anti-inflammatory agents in Alzheimer's disease. *Curr Neurol Neurosci Rep.* 2002a; 2: 405–452.

Aisen PS. Evaluation of selective COX-2 inhibitors for the treatment of Alzheimer's disease. *J Pain Symptom Manage.* 2002b; 23 Supplement: S35–S42.

Akhlaq AF, Tahira F, Anil M, Jolin Hwee-Jing O, Wei-Yi O. Ayurvedic medicine for the treatment of dementia: mechanistic aspects. *Evid-Based Complement Altern Med.* 2018; 40(2): 1–11.
Akinrimisi ED, Ainwannde AI. Effect of aqueous extract of *Eugenia caryolphyllus* on brain acetylcholinesterase in rats. *West Afr J Pharmacol Drug Res.* 1975; 2: 127–133.
Amod PK, Laurie AK, Girish JK. Herbal complement inhibitors in the treatment of neuroinflammation. *Ann NY Acad Sci.* 2005; 1056: 413–429.
Anderson RN. Deaths: leading causes for 2000. *Natl Vital Stat Rep.* 2002; 50: 1.
Anil K, Samrita D, Atish P. Neuroprotective effects of *Centella asiatica* against intracerebroventricular colchicine-induced cognitive impairment and oxidative stress. *Int J Alzheimer Dis.* 2009; 9: 1–8.
Anon. *Caraka Samhita*, Shree Gulabkunverba Ayurvedic Society, Jamnagar, India, 5, 490, 1949.
Atanu B, Shastry CS, Saha S. Nootropic activity of *Crataeva nurvala* Buch-ham against scopolamine induced cognitive impairment. *Excli J.* 2015; 14: 335–345.
Ayurvedic Pharmacopoeia of India, Part 1, Vol. 4, Controller of Publications; Ministry of Health and Family Welfare, Govt. of India, Delhi, 2004.
Bahr BA, Bendiske J. The neuropathogenic contributions of lysosomal dysfunction. *J Neurochem.* 2002; 83: 481–492.
Bajaj S, Ahamad I, Fatima M, Raisuddin S, Vohora SB. Immunomadulatory activity of a Unani gold preparation used in Indian system of medicine. *Immunopharmacol Immunotoxicol.* 1999; 21: 151.
Bajaj S, Vohora SB. Anticataleptic, anti-anxiety and anti-depressant activity of gold preparation used in Indian systems of medicine. *Indian J Pharmacol.* 2000; 32: 339.
Berrino F. Western diet and Alzheimer's disease. *Epidemiol Prev.* 2002; 26: 107.
Bhattacharya SK, Kumar A. Effect of glycowithanolides from *Withania somnifera* on an animal model of Alzheimers disease and perturbed central cholinergic markers of cognition in rats. *Phytother Res.* 1995; 9: 110–116.
Boral GC, Gautam B, Anjan B, Das NN, Nandi PS. Geriforte in anxiety neurosis. *Indian J Psychiatr.* 1989 Jul–Sep; 31(3): 258–260.
Bush AI. The metallobiology of Alzheimer's disease. *Trends Neurosci.* 2003; 26(4): 207–214.
Camps P, Munoz-Torrer D. Cholinergic drugs in pharmacotherapy of Alzheimer's disease. *Mini Rev Med Chem.* 2002; 2: 11–17.
Carlo C, William LG, Michael L, Dale K, Kerry B, Barry O. Effects of a standardized *Bacopa monnieri* extract on cognitive performance, anxiety, and depression in the elderly: a randomized, double-blind, placebo-controlled trial. *J Altern Complement Med.* 2008; 14(6): 707–713.
Chatellier G, Lacomblez L. Tacrine (teterahydroaminoacridine; THA) and lecithin in senile dementia of the Alzheimer type: a multicenter trial. *Br J Med.* 1990; 300: 495.
Clegg BJ, Nicholson T, McIntyre L, De Broe S, Gerard K, Waugh N. Clinical and cost effectiveness of donepezil, rivastigmine, and galantamine for Alzheimer's disease: a systematic review. *Int J Technol Assess Health Care.* 2002; 18: 497.
Colucci L, Bosco M, Ziello AR, et al. Effectiveness of nootropic drugs with cholinergic activity in treatment of cognitive deficit: a review. *J Exp Pharmacol.* 2012; 4: 163–172.
Dahanukar SA, Kulkarni RA, Rege NN. Pharmacology of medicinal plants and natural products. *Indian J Pharmacol.* 2000a; 32: S81, 20–30.
Dahanukar SA, Kulkarni RA, Rege NN. Pharmacology of medicinal plants and natural products. *Indian J Pharmacol.* 2000b; 32: 81–88.
Dash B, Kashyap L. *Diagnosis and Treatment of Diseases in Ayurveda, Part 3*, Concept Publishing Company, New Delhi, India, 1984, p. 124.
Dash SC, Tripathi SN, Singh RH. Clinical assessment of medhya drugs in the management of psychosis (unmada). *Ancient Sci Life.* 1983; 3: 77–83.
Divya SV, Lakshmi CM. Alzheimer's disease. *Scientific Basis for Ayurvedic Medicines*, CRC Publishers, New York, NY, 2007.
Doraiswamy PM. Non-cholinergic strategies for treating and preventing Alzheimer's disease. *CNS Drugs.* 2002; 16: 24.
Dwivedi KK, Singh RH. A clinical study of medhya rasayana therapy in the management of convulsive disorder. *J Res Ayurveda Siddha.* 1978; 13: 97.
Fernando GP. Brain foods: the effects of nutrients on brain function. *Nat Rev Neurosci.* 2008; 9(7): 568–578.
Frawley D. *Ayurvedic Healing*, Motilal Banarsidass Publishers, Delhi, India, 1989.
Gelb DJ. Measurement of progression in Alzheimer's disease: A clinician perspective. *Stat Med.* 2000; 19: 1390–1398.

Ghosh AK, Osswald HL. BACE1 (β-Secretase) inhibitors for the treatment of Alzheimer's disease. *Chem Soc Rev.* 2014; 43(19): 6765–6813. doi:10.1039/c3cs60460h.

Gohil KJ, Patel JA. A review on *Bacopa monnieri*: current research and future prospects. *Int J Green Pharm.* 2010; 2: 1–9.

Gupta BM, Bala A. Alzheimer's disease research in India: a scientometric analysis of publications output during 2002–11. *Res Neurol Int J.* 2013; 5(3): 22–31. doi: 10.5171/2013.204542.

Habibur R, Muralidharan P, Anand M. Inhibition of AChE and antioxidant activities are probable mechanism of *Nardostachys jatamansi* DC in sleep deprived Alzheimer's mice model. *Int J PharmTech Res.* 2011; 3(3): 1807–1816.

Handa SS, Bhargava VK. Effect of BR 16-A (Mentat) on cognitive deficits in aluminum treated and aged rats. *Indian J Pharmacol.* 1997; 28: 258–264.

Harvey AL. Natural products in drug discovery. *Drug Discov Today.* 2008; 13: 894–901.

Howes MJ, Houghton PJ. Plants used in Chinese and Indian traditional medicine for improvement of memory and cognitive function. *Pharmacol Biochem Behav.* 2003; 75: 513–527.

Huang W, Zhang X, Chen W. Role of oxidative stress in Alzheimer's disease. *Biomed Rep.* 2016; 4(5): 519–522.

Huang Y, Mucke L. Alzheimer mechanisms and therapeutic strategies. *Cell.* 2012; 148(6): 1204–1222.

Ingkaninan K, Phengpa P, Yuenyongsawad S, Khorana N. Acetylcholinesterase inhibitors from *Stephania venosa* tuber. *J Pharm Pharmacol.* 2006; 58: 695–700.

Iyer MR, Pal SC, Kasture VS, Kasture SB. Effect of *Lawsonia inermis* on memory and behaviour mediated via monoamine neurotransmitters. *Ind J Pharmacol.* 1998; 30: 181–185.

Jagdeep SD, Prasad DN, Avinash CT, Rajiv G. Role of traditional medicine in neuropsychopharmacology. *Asian J Pharm Clin Res.* 2009; 2(2): 72–76.

Jemima J, Bhattacharjee P, Singhal RS. Melatonin – a review on the lesser known potential nutraceutical. *Int J Pharm Sci Res.* 2011; 2(8): 1975–1987.

Jian-zhi W, Ze-fen W. Role of melatonin in Alzheimer-like neurodegeneration. *Acta Pharmacol Sinica.* 2006; 27(1): 41–49.

Jivad N, Rabiei Z. A review study on medicinal plants used in the treatment of learning and memory impairments. *Asian Pac J Trop Biomed.* 2014; 4: 780–789.

Kar S, Slowikowski SPM, Westaway D, Mount HTJ. Interactions between β-amyloid and central cholinergic neurons: Implications for Alzheimer's disease. *J Psychiatr Neurosci.* 2004; 29(6): 427–441.

Karren E, Bard DS. The amyloid cascade hypothesis: are we poised for success or failure? *J Neurichem.* 2016; 139(2) Supplement 2: 237–252.

Kashmira JG, Jagruti P, Anuradha KG. Pharmacological review on *Centella asiatica*: a potential herbal cure-all. *Ind J Pharm Sci.* 2010; 72(5): 546–556.

Khare CP. *Indian Medicinal Plants An Illustrated Dictionary*, Spinger, 2007.

Kulkarni SK, Verma A. BR 16-A (Mentat): a herbal preparation improves learning and memory performance in mice. *Probe.* 1994; 3: 222, 28.

Lemstra AW, Eikelenboom P, Van Gool WA. The cholinergic deficiency syndrome and its therapeutic implications. *Gerontology.* 2003; 49: 55.

Lindsay J, Laurin D, Verreault R, Hebert R, Helliwell B, Hill GB, McDowell I. Risk factors for Alzheimer's disease: A prospective analysis from the Canadian Study of Health and Aging. *Am J Epidemiol.* 2002; 156: 445–452.

Mahesh G, Tasneem S. Biomarker controversies and diagnostic difficulties in Alzheimer's disease. *Am J Phytomed Clin Therap.* 2014; 2(4): 463–468.

Manyam BV. Dementia in Ayurveda. *J Altern Complement Med.* 1999; 5: 81–88.

Maya M, Sarada S. *In vitro* screening for anti-cholinesterase and antioxidant activity of methanolic extracts of Ayurvedic medicinal plants used for cognitive disorders. *Plos One.* 2014; 9(1): e86804.

Mishra LC, Singh BB, Dagenais S. Scientific basis for the therapeutic use of *Withania somnifera* (ashwagandha): a review. *Altern Med Rev.* 2000; 5: 334–346.

Mukherjee PK, Kumar V, Mal M, Houghton PJ. Acetylcholinesterase inhibitors from plants. *Phytomedicine.* 2007; 14: 289–300.

Muralidharan P, Balamurugan G, Venu B. Cerebroprotective effect of *Glycyrrhiza glabra* Linn. root extract on hypoxic rats. *Bangladesh J Pharmacol.* 2009; 4: 60–64.

Nillert W, Pannangrong W, Welbat JU. Neuroprotective effects of aged garlic extract on cognitive dysfunction and neuroinflammation induced by β-amyloid in rats. *Nutrients.* 2017; 9: 24–36.

Orhan I, Kartal M, Naz Q, et al. Antioxidant and anticholinesterase evaluation of selected Turkish Salvia species. *Food Chem.* 2007; 103: 1247–1254.

Parul A, Bhawna S, Amreen F, Sanjay KJ. An update on Ayurvedic herb *Convolvulus pluricaulis* Choisy. *Asian Pac J Trop Biomed.* 2014; 4(3): 245–252.

Pasinetti GM. From epidemiology to therapeutic trials with anti-inflammatory drugs in Alzheimer's disease: the role of NSAIDs and cyclooxygenase in beta-amyloidosis and clinical dementia. *J Alzheimers Dis.* 2002; 4: 435.

Patel VS, Jivani NP, Patel SB. Medicinal plants with potential nootropic activity: a review. *Res J Pharm Bio Chem Sci.* 2014; 5(1): 1–11.

Perry EK, Pickering AT, Wang WW, Houghton PJ, Perry NS. Medicinal plants and Alzheimer's disease: from ethnobotany to phytotherapy. *J Pharm Pharmacol.* 1999; 51: 527–533.

Perry NSL, Houghton PJ, Sampson J, Theolad AE, Hart S, Lis-balchin M. *In vitro* activities of *Salvia lavandulaefolia* (Spanish Sage) relevant to treatment of Alzheimer's disease. *J Pharm Pharmacol.* 2001; 53: 1347–1356.

Perry NSL, Houghton PJ, Theolad AE, Jenner P, Perry EK. *In vitro* inhibition of human erythrocyte acetylcholinesterase by *Salvia lavandulaefolia* essential oil and constituent terpenes. *J Pharm Pharmacol.* 2000; 52: 895–902.

Philomena G. Concerns regarding the safety and toxicity of medicinal plants – an overview. *J Appl Pharm Sci.* 2011; 1(6): 40–44.

Prachi S, Lakshmayya L, Vinod SB. Anti-Alzheimer activity of isolated karanjin from *Pongamia pinnata* (L.) pierre and embelin from *Embelia ribes* Burm.f. *Int Quart J Res Ayurveda.* 2017; 38(1): 76–81.

Prakash R, Sandhya E, Ramya N, Dhivya R, Priyadarshini M, Sakthi Priya B. Neuroprotective activity of ethanolic extract of *Tinospora cordifolia* on LPS induced neuroinflammation. *Transl Biomed.* 2017; 8(4): 135–142.

Prerna U, Vikas S, Mushtaq A. Therapy of Alzheimer's disease: an update. *Afr J Pharm Pharmacol.* 2010; 4(6): 408–421.

Puchchakayala G, Akina S, Thati M. Neuroprotective effects of meloxicam and selegiline in scopolamine-induced cognitive impairment and oxidative stress. *Int J Alzheimer Dis.* 2012; 12: 1–8.

Rammohan VR, Olivier D, Varghese J, Dale EB. Ayurvedic medicinal plants for Alzheimer's disease: a review. *Alzheimer Res Therapy.* 2012; 4(22): 1–12.

Rhee IK, Meent MV, Ingkaninan K, Verpoorte R. Screening for acetylcholinesterase inhibitors from Amaryllidaceae using silica gel thin-layer chromatography in combination with bioactivity staining. *J Chromatogr.* 2001; 915: 217–223.

Rinne JO, Kaasinen V, Jarvenpaa T, et al. Brain acetylcholinesterase activity in mild cognitive impairment and early Alzheimer's disease. *Neurol Neurosurg Psychiatr.* 2003; 74: 113–115.

Roberts SB. Gamma-secretase inhibitors and Alzheimer's disease. *Adv Drug Deliv Rev.* 2002; 54: 1579–1582.

Satyavati GV, Gupta AK, Tandon N, Seth, SD. *Medicinal Plants of India*, Vol. 2, Indian Council of Medical Research, New Delhi, India, 1987.

Schiloers R, Liermann A, Bhattacharya SK, Kumar A, Ghoshal S, Rich V. Systemic administration of defined extracts from *Withania somnifera* (Indian ginseng) and shilajit differentially affects cholinergic but not glutaminergic and gabaergic markers in rat brain. *Neurochem Int.* 1997; 30: 181.

Schneider LS. New therapeutic approaches to Alzheimer's disease. *Psychiatry.* 1996; 57 Supplement 14: 30–36.

Sharma PC, Yelne MB, Dennis TJ. *Database on Medicinal Plants Used in Ayurveda and Siddha*, 1st ed., CCRAS, Dept. of Ayush, Ministry of Health and Family Welfare, Govt. of India, New Delhi, 2005.

Singh RH, Sinha, BN. Clinical and pharmacological studies on the effect of indigenous compound Rasayana drug in apparently normal and aged persons. *J Res Indian Med Yoga Homeopathy.* 1978; 13: 8–17.

Singh RH, Sinha BN. Further studies on the effect of an indigenous compound Rasayana drug on physical and mental disability in aged persons. *J Res Indian Med Yoga Homeopathy.* 1979a; 2(14): 45–51.

Singh RH, Sinha BN, Sarkar FH, Udupa KN. Comparative biochemical studies on the effect of four Medhya Rasayana drugs described by Caraka on some central neurotransmitters in normal and stressed rats. *J Indian Med Yoga Homeopathy.* 1979b; 14: 7–14.

Soumyanath S, Zhong Y, Henson E, et al. *Centella asiatica* extract improves behavioral deficits in a mouse model of Alzheimer's disease: investigation of a possible mechanism of action. *Int J Alzheimers Dis.* 2012; 12: 381–394.

Spiegel R. Rivastigmine: a review of its clinical effectiveness. *Rev Neurol.* 2002; 35: 859.

Talic S, Dragicevic I, Corajevic L, Martinovic BA. Acetylcholinesterase and butyrylcholinesterase inhibitory activity of extracts from medicinal plants. *Bull Chem Technol Bosnia Herzegovania.* 2014; 43: 11–14.

Uma G, Uma Maheswari S. Neuroprotective effects of polyherbal formulation (Indian Noni) on scopolamine-induced memory impairment in mice. *Int J Pharm Pharma Sci.* 2014; 6(1): 354–357.
Vaidya AB. The status and scope of Indian medicinal plants acting on the central nervous system. *Indian J Pharmacol.* 1997; 29: S340, 228–234.
Vinutha B, Prashanth D, Salma K, et al. Screening of selected Indian medicinal plants for acetylcholinesterase inhibitory activity. *J Ethnopharmacol.* 2007; 109: 359–363.
Volloch V, Rita S. Results of beta secretase-inhibitor clinical trials support amyloid precursor protein-independent generation of beta amyloid in sporadic Alzheimer's disease. Med Sci (Basel). 2018; 6(2): 45–58.
Vohora SB, Kim HS, Shah SA, Khanna T, Dandiya PC. CNS and adaptogenic effects of Siddh Makardhwaja: an Ayurvedic mercury preparation. In *Trace Elements in Nutrition and Health*, Jamia Hamdard and Wiley Eastern Ltd., New Delhi, India, 1995.
Zhang F, Jiang L. Neuroinflammation in Alzheimer's disease. *Neuropsychiatr Dis Treat.* 2015; 11: 243–256.

7 Ethnomedicinal Plants Used By The Tribes Of Northeast India To Treat Alzheimer's Disease

Bapi Ray Sarkar

CONTENTS

ABBREVIATIONS

AChE Acetylcholinesterase
AD Alzheimer's Disease
% Percentage
α Alpha
β Beta
p Para
NE North East

7.1 INTRODUCTION

Alzheimer's disease (AD) is an age-related neurodegenerative decline, portrayed clinically by memory deficiencies, hindered psychological capacity, and unseemly behaviour. In developing countries like India and China, AD is largely restricted to older (more than 65 years old) people (Elufioye et al., 2012). It was first described in 1906 by the German doctor Alois Alzheimer. It is the best-known type of dementia and currently affects 24 million individuals around the world. Amid the progression of AD, the damage to brain cells causes a steady increase in memory impairment, a degeneration of scholarly capacity, loss of ability to talk, confusion, and difficulty in walking (Chiu et al., 1997).

Physiological characteristics associated with AD include a lack of acetylcholine, an accumulation of free radicals, and cerebrum tissue aggravation (Akhondzadeh et al., 2003). There is presently no specific remedy for AD, yet a few medications which can defer its progress are available, and new and viable medications are being investigated (Chou et al., 2009). An approach to the treatment of AD is the targeting of characteristic features (Pozen, 2013), such as reduced acetylcholine levels in the brain. Acetylcholine is a synapse neurotransmitter that is fundamental for memory, and psychological wellness issues, including memory impairment, are directly or indirectly associated with low acetylcholine levels. Low concentrations of this neurotransmitter appear to play a critical role in the pathogenesis of AD (Andrieu et al., 2008). As a result, numerous investigations have been undertaken to discover medications to treat memory loss, such as occurs in AD (Prince et al., 2015), centring around increasing the concentrations of acetylcholine (ACh). Acetylcholinesterase inhibitors (AChEIs) constrain acetylcholinesterase, the enzyme in charge of the breakdown of acetylcholine (Avila et al., 2004). Research on medicinal plants with acetylcholinesterase inhibitory action are in progress, with the target of finding new formulations that are effective, less expensive and with fewer unfavourable side effects than synthetic pharmaceuticals (Citron, 2010). Free radicals likewise are involved in numerous ailments, including AD (Arendt, 2009). For instance, lipid peroxidation is a response mediated by free radicals, in which unsaturated fat oxidation happens in cell layers, causing problems with membrane function (Faiyaz et al., 2011). Such oxidative stress can induce conditions such as coronary disease, several types of tumors, cerebrum ischemia, and burning conditions (Bamburg et al., 2009). Some antioxidants can be obtained from plant-derived food, such as phenolics and carotenoids, which constrain lipid peroxidation by means of their free-radical quenching activity (Colpo et al., 2007). Plants which exhibit activities such as acetylcholinesterase inhibition, and cell reinforcement induction are of potential clinical value for the treatment of AD (Andrieu et al., 2008).

The tribal majority states like Arunachal Pradesh, Meghalaya, Mizoram, Nagaland, Assam, and Sikkim in India are all located in the northeast region of the country (Dubey et al., 1994), but less than 10 percent of the total tribal population resides in these areas. Ethnically, the tribes in northeastern India belong to the Mongoloid group (Dastagir et al., 2016). The most important tribal communities in Northeast India are the Lepcha and Bhutia in Sikkim, Rabha and Deori in Assam, Adi, Nyishi, Apatani, Monpa, and Wancho in Arunachal Pradesh, Naga in Nagaland, Garo and Khasi in Meghalaya, the Mizo in Mizoram, some Naga tribes, Mac, and Paite in Manipur, and Tripuri, Riang, and Chakma in Tripura (Das et al., 1999). All these tribes differ in terms of population size, levels of sociocultural and economic development, means of subsistence, religion, and language. However, 90 percent of tribal populations reside in villages (Gurung, 2012). Most of the villagers believe in the traditional system of medicine for their primary health care (The Wealth of India, 2010). Northeast India has great natural resources such as largely unexplored plant species, which is why tribal people of the Northeast rely on plant-based treatments of various diseases by using different plants, types of preparation, and formulations (Asuthosh et al., 2000).

For this chapter, an ethnobotanical review of the principal medicinal plants utilized in the Himalayan region of Northeast India was carried out to identify restorative plants that are potential reservoirs of phytochemicals active against AD (De Caires et al., 2010). Different species were identified and tested for prevention of AD progression (Barrios-Gonzalez et al., 2010). Accordingly, the 100 species that displayed the highest cell reinforcement activities were chosen, and their phenol and flavonoid contents were resolved (Calabrese et al., 2008). The plants that yielded the best outcomes were then exposed to acetylcholinesterase inhibitory tests. The current study surveyed the connections between these properties in the plants, with the point of finding new phytomedicines that could be utilized in the treatment of AD (Amala et al., 2012).

AD represents the most widely recognized type of dementia, which puts an excessive and ever-increasing load on patients, their family-based carers, and society (Prince et al., 2008). Aging is the most important risk factor for dementia, especially AD, and dementia has turned out to be one of the most significant problems in society because of the increasing proportion of older people in the population around the world (Bastos et al., 2007). Areas of the brain associated with learning and memory include the amygdala, the hippocampus, the cerebellum, and the prefrontal cortex, and these regions are diminished in size in AD patients as a consequence of the degeneration of neurotransmitters and the death of neurons (Arendt, 2009). Despite the fact that the fundamental reason for the initiation of AD is as yet still unclear, damage caused by free radicals of oxygen and nitrogen, associated with mitochondrial dysfunction, is found in the brain early in AD pathology (Farokhnia et al., 2014). It was found that most of the ethnomedicinal plants tested show their efficacy against AD due to presence of certain key phytoconstituents (Wimo et al., 2010). Therefore, the vision of this chapter is to create new paradigms for the use of the phytomedicines on a global basis, including new combinations of herbal medicinal plants for the treatment of AD (Chengxuan et al., 2009).

7.2 GLOBAL SCENARIO OF ALZHEIMER'S DISEASE

Neurodegenerative illnesses like AD are among the major health problems of the twenty-first century. The United Nations estimated that the number of individuals experiencing age-related neurodegeneration, especially from AD, will increase exponentially from 25.5 million in 2000 to an expected 114 million in 2050 (Ballard et al., 2011). A number of meta-analyses have identified generally comparable estimates of dementia incidence across different parts of the world. The incidence worldwide of dementia in 2019 in individuals older than 60 years is roughly 3.9%, with 1.6% in Africa, 3.9% in Eastern Europe, 4.0% in China, 4.6% in Latin America, 5.4% in Western Europe, and 6.4% in North America (Bastianetto et al., 2000). The worldwide annual frequency of dementia is estimated to be around 7.5 per 1000 populace, with no significant variation across continents, apart from Africa, where the occurrence rates are estimated to be lower (Barrios-Gonzalez, 2010). The frequency of dementia increases exponentially with age, with comparable rates around the globe. The risk of AD increases exponentially with age in every 5–6 years. For the old people risk of AD increases is more higher compared with young ages (Bastianetto et al., 2000). A great many people with dementia live in developing countries like India. The rates of increase are not uniform across the world; the numbers of dementia sufferers in developed countries are estimated to increase two-fold between 2001 and 2040, whereas the corresponding figure is more than three-fold in India, China, and their south Asian and western Pacific neighbors (Bhanumathy et al., 2010). These worldwide patterns of the incidence of people with dementia as populations age will have enormous ramifications for the general wellbeing, social insurance financing, and conveyance frameworks in the world, particularly in developing countries (Asgarpanah et al., 2012).

As part of this chapter, we have re-assessed our past appraisals of the worldwide frequency, incidence, and cost of dementia. As another element, we have incorporated a precise audit of the proof for and against late patterns in the frequency and rate of dementia after a particular age (Birari et al., 2010). There are approximately 900 million individuals aged 60 years and over living around the world (Bihaqi et al., 2011). The near future will see a rapid increase in this number and is also related to the increasing amounts of incurable ailments like dementia. Between 2015 and 2050, the number of older individuals living in high-income countries is estimated to increase by 56%, compared with 138% in upper/middle-income countries, 185% in lower/middle- income countries, and by 239% (a greater than three-fold higher value than for high-income countries) in low-income countries (Baurle et al.,2009). Older individuals will likewise comprise an increasing proportion of the total population, as a result older population will get effected by AD rapidly in many nations (Bradwejn et al., 2000). Less-fortunate countries will have less financial and human expertise assets to meet the wellbeing and social consideration needs of their rapidly aging population (Cambay et al., 2011). A large number of these nations will face the test of a 'double jeopardy' of constantly high rates of maternal, youth and incurable illnesses, combined with a developing pandemic of incurable non-transmittable diseases (Auddy et al., 2008). With the phenomenal advantages of double-digit increase annual economic growth, rapidly developing countries in Asia and Latin America have attempted to build up far-reaching and powerful frameworks of social security to support older individuals, while neglecting to ensure sufficient income and all-inclusive access to wellbeing and social consideration (Carlo et al., 2008). Generally speaking, economic development at the national level can disguise net imbalances in salary dispersion, with older individuals regularly being the last to profit legitimately from economic growth. In India, more than 4 million individuals have some type of dementia. Around the world, somewhere around 44 million individuals are living with dementia, making the illness a worldwide wellbeing emergency that must be attended to (Cecchini et al., 2012).

7.3 SYMPTOMS OF ALZHEIMER'S DISEASE (AD)

7.3.1 Memory Loss* That Interrupts Daily Life

One of the best-known signs of AD, particularly in the initial stage, is forgetting recently-learned information. Others include forgetting important dates or events, asking the same question repeatedly, and increasingly needing to depend on memory aids (e.g. reminder notes or electronic devices) or relatives for things the patient used to deal with on their own. In some cases, overlooking names or arrangements but recollecting them later is a characteristic sign (Chandrasekaran et al., 2011).

In the event that you or somebody you know is encountering issues with memory or different potential side effects of dementia, please see a specialist. A number of alternative reasons for such manifestations, for example, drug reactions, nutrient deficiencies, and the use of narcotic drugs, etc., are reversible (Ambawade et al., 2009) (Table 7.1 and Table 7.2).

7.3.2 Difficulties in Planning or Solving Problems

Some people living with Alzheimer's may experience changes in their ability to develop and follow a plan, or work with numbers. They may experience difficulties following a familiar recipe or keeping track of monthly bills. They may experience difficulties concentrating, taking much longer to get things done than they did previously. An example of this would be making periodic blunders when adjusting a check book (Chen et al., 2001).

7.3.3 Difficulty Completing Familiar Tasks at Home or Work

People living with Alzheimer's frequently find it difficult to finish daily tasks. Sometimes, they may encounter problems traveling to a familiar location, dealing with a financial plan at work, or remembering the rules of a favorite pastime. This may take the form, for example, of requiring help to use the settings on a microwave or to record a TV program (Choi et al., 2002).

7.3.4 Confusion with Time or Space

Individuals with Alzheimer's can lose track of dates, seasons, and the passage of time. They may experience difficulty understanding something, if it does not happen immediately. Sometimes, people with AD forget where they are or how they got there. Getting confused about the day of the week yet making sense of it later can be a characteristic sign (Christen, 2009).

7.3.5 Trouble Understanding Visual Images and Spatial Relationships

For some people, having vision issues is an indication of Alzheimer's. They may have trouble reading, have problems judging distance, and distinguishing color and shading, which may cause

* **Not all memory loss is brought about by Alzheimer's Disease**

TABLE 7.1
List of Ethnomedicinal Plants Used to Treat Alzheimer's Disease, With Vernacular Name, Used by Tribes, Part Used, and Mode of Preparation

Sl. No.	Scientific Name (With Family)	Vernacular Name	Tribes	Parts Used	Mode of Preparation
1	*Abroma augusta* Linn. (Sterculaceae)	Sano-kapsi	Garo, Khasi and Tripuri	Leaves, root and bark	The decoction of fresh powdered root, bark and leaf juice is effective.
2	*Achyranthus aspera* Linn. (Amaranthaceae)	Apamarg		Root, flower, seeds	Fresh and dried root is ground, and decoction is made with water. Flower powder/seeds and mixed with sugar is used.
3	*Adiantum capillus veneris* Linn. (Pteridaceae)	Sarhaj		Leaves	Dried leaf juice.
4	*Adiantum incisum* Linn. (Pteridaceae)	Phunka		Leaves	Fresh leaf juice.
5	*Amaranthus spinosus* Linn. (Amarathaceae)	Ban lure		Whole plant	Fresh and dried plant, seeds and roots are ground and decoction is made.
6	*Ananas sativus* Linn. (Bromeliaceae)	Anarosh		Leaf	Young leaf is chewed.
7	*Argemone mexicana* Linn. (Papaveraceae)	Sungure Kanra		Seed, leaf, root	All parts are dried and triturated to make pills.
8	*Argyrolobium roseum* Linn. (Fabaceae)	Makhni booti		Whole plant	Decoction of the plants.
9	*Artemisia absinthium* Linn. (Asteraceae)	Jaukay		Whole plant	Decoction of the plants.
10	*Artocarpus chapalasha* Roxb. (Moraceae)	Soh-phan		Fruit	Juice of the ripe fruits
11	*Artocarpus heterophyllus* Linn. (Moraceae)	Rukh Katahar	Lepcha, Bhutia	Fruit, latex	Juice of the ripe fruits and latex after drying.
12	*Asparagus adscendens* Linn. (Asparagaceae)	Musli sufaid.		Rhizome	Water extract.
13	*Asparagus racemosus* Linn. (Asparagaceae)	Kurilo		Tuberous root	Fresh and dried tuber or stem are soaked in a glass of water, then drunk for taken.
14	*Asparagus racemosus* Wild (Asparagaceae)	Shotomuli		Root	Decoction of roots.
15	*Averrhoa carambola* Linn. (Oxalidaceae)	Sohpyrshong		Fruit	Ripe fruit are taken as medicine
16	*Baccaurea ramiflora* Linn. (Euphobiaceae)	Soh ramdieng		Flower	Dried flower parts are used to prepare Gutika.
17	*Bacopa monnieri* Linn. (Plantaginaceae)	Brishmisaag		Whole plant	Paste form of entire plant.
18	*Basella alba* Linn. (Basellaceae)	Poisaag		Tender root and leaf	After boiling, the viscous liquid is taken.
19	*Borreria articularis* Linn. (Rubiaceae)	Phlangbhoi		Leaf	Fresh leaf extract is used
20	*Brassica oleracea* Linn. (Brassicaceae)	Band Gobi		Leaves	Used as a vegetable

(Continued)

TABLE 7.1 (CONTINUED)
List of Ethnomedicinal Plants Used to Treat Alzheimer's Disease, With Vernacular Name, Used by Tribes, Part Used, and Mode of Preparation

Sl. No.	Scientific Name (With Family)	Vernacular Name	Tribes	Parts Used	Mode of Preparation
21	*Bryophyllum calycinum* Linn. (Crassulaceae)	Dawaiein	Rabha, Deori	Leaf	Leaf juice
22	*Cajanus cajan* Linn. (Fabaceae)	Aral sla		Leaf twigs	Extract of leaf twigs is taken.
23	*Calamus erectus* Roxb. (Arecaceae)	Soh thri		Fruit	Fruits are eaten raw.
24	*Camellia sinensis* Linn. (Theaceae)	Chiya		Leaves	Juice of leaves.
25	*Capparis spinosa* Linn. (Capparidaceae)	Baghmukhey		Root bark, flower	Hydro extract of roots and flowers.
26	*Cuscuta reflexa* Roxb (Convolvulaceae)	Man		Entire plant	Whole plant juice
27	*Cassia alata* Linn. (Fabaceae)	Daudraj		Leaf	Decoction of leaves
28	*Castanopsis indica* Linn. (Fagaceae)	Dhalne katush		Stem bark	Stem bark extract
29	*Catharanthus roseus* Linn. (Apocyanaceae)	Sabdabahar	Adi, Nyishi,	Leaves	Hydroalcoholic solution of leaves.
30	*Centella asiatica* Linn. (Apiaceae)	Wangrake	Apatani, Monpa,	Leaf	Decoction of leaves.
31	*Cissampelos pareira* Linn. (Menispermaceae)	Batulepati,	and Wancho	Roots and leaf	Juice of leaf and decoction of roots.
32	*Coelogyne cristala* Lindle (Orchidaceae)	Chandigava		All parts of the plant	Decoction of the desired parts.
33	*Coix lacryma* Linn. (Poaceae)	Sohriew		Seed	Seeds are chewed raw.
34	*Colocasia esculenta* Linn. (Araceae)	Narikel	Naga and Mizo	Stem	Stem decoction
35	*Corchorus aestuans* Linn. (Malv aceae)	Amalthchu		Root	Roots as decoction
36	*Coriandrum sativum* Linn. (Apicaceae)	Dhaniya		Fruit	Mixed with various food preparation.
37	*Croton tiglium* Linn. (Euphorbiaceae)	Runi bih		Fruit	Fresh fruit are eaten
38	*Curcuma amada* Roxb. (Zingiberaceae)	Phacheng		Rhizome	Paste of the rhizome.
39	*Cynodon dactylon* Linn. (Poaceae)	Durba gash		Whole plant	Macerated whole plant.
40	*Desmodium triquetrum* Linn. (Fabaceae)	Yeyjur		Leaf	Crushed leaves.
41	*Desmotachya bipinnata* Linn. (Poaceae)	Kush		Whole plant	Infusion of plant.
42	*Dillenia indica* Linn. (Dilleniaceae)	Soh karbam		Fruit	Decoction of fruit.
43	*Dolichus uniflorus* Linn. (Fabaceae)	Gahat		Seeds	Decoction of dry seed is used.

(Continued)

TABLE 7.1 (CONTINUED)
List of Ethnomedicinal Plants Used to Treat Alzheimer's Disease, With Vernacular Name, Used by Tribes, Part Used, and Mode of Preparation

Sl. No.	Scientific Name (With Family)	Vernacular Name	Tribes	Parts Used	Mode of Preparation
44	*Ephedra saxatilis* Linn. (Ephedraceae)	Ma Houng	Mac and Paite	Flowering tops and stem	Flowering tops and stem in the form of decoction.
45	*Evodia fraxinifolia* Hook (Rutaceae)	Khanakpa		Fruit	Matured fruits are eaten.
46	*Fagopyrum dibotrys* Linn. (Polygonaceae)	Banphapar		Fruits	Matured fruits are eaten.
47	*Ficus racemosa* Linn. (Moraceae)	Jog dumur		Friut	Ripe fruits are used.
48	*Foeniculum vulgare* Hill (Apiaceae)	Sounps		Leaf	Leaf juice.
49	*Gmelina arborea* Roxb. (Verbenaceae)	Khamari		Fruits	Raw fruits are taken.
50	*Helianthus annuus* Linn. (Asteraceae)	Surgi Phool		Seeds	Seeds are separated from fruits and taken in paste form.
51	*Hydrocotyle asiatica* Linn. (Apiaceae)	Golpatta		Leaf	Leaves are mixed with honey and boiled.
52	*Hyptis suaveolens* Linn. (Lamiaceae)	Tokma		Fruit	Fruits are taken ripe.
53	*Impatiens balsamina* Linn. (Balsaminaceae)	Balsam		Flower	Juice of the flower mixed with honey.
54	*Lannea coromandelica* Linn. (Anacardiaceae)	Jiga		Leaf	Decoction of leaves.
55	*Lantana camara* Linn. (Verbenaceae)	Sophangkhlien		Leaf	Crushed leaves.
56	*Luffa acutangula* Linn. (Cucurbitaceae)	Sohprew		Fruit	Unripe fruit is taken as decoction
57	*Lycopodium clavatum* Linn. (Lycopodiaceae)	Naag Beli		Spores	Dried powder of spores are dissolved in sugar solution.
58	*Malvastrum tricuspidatum* Linn. (Malvaceae)	Som zalik		Seeds	Crushed seeds are used.
59	*Melia azedirach* Linn. (Meliaceae)	Bakain		Root	Fresh juice of root is taken.
60	*Mikania micrantha* Linn. (Asteraceae)	Ermapakistan		Leaf	Crushed leaves.
61	*Mimosa pudica* Linn. (Fabaceae)	Lajjaboti	Tripuri and	Root	Decoction of roots.
62	*Momordica charantia* Linn. (Cucurbitaceae)	Daipiat	Chakma	Leaf	Leaves are crushed and taken orally.
63	*Musa paradisiaca* Linn. (Musaceae)	Bichi kola		Fruit	Ripe fruits are taken.
64	*Musa sapientum* Linn. (Musaceae)	Kera		Flower, rhizome	The flowers are crushed to extract juice. The fresh juice of rhizome is also used.

(Continued)

TABLE 7.1 (CONTINUED)
List of Ethnomedicinal Plants Used to Treat Alzheimer's Disease, With Vernacular Name, Used by Tribes, Part Used, and Mode of Preparation

Sl. No.	Scientific Name (With Family)	Vernacular Name	Tribes	Parts Used	Mode of Preparation
65	*Myrsine africana* Linn. (Myrsinaceae)	Khukan		Leaf	Hot juice of the leaves are taken.
66	*Nasturtium fontana* Linn. (Brassicaceae)	Seemrayo		All parts of the plant	Entire plant extract is used.
67	*Ocimum basilicum* Linn. (Lamiaceae)	Babriphul		Flower	Fresh flowers are taken for Infusion.
68	*Ocimum sanctum* Linn. (Lamiaceae)	Lapane		Leaf	Decoction of leaves.
69	*Oxalis corymbosa* Linn. (Oxalidaceae)	Sakhia-palleh		Entire plant	Plant extract taken thrice daily
70	*Panax pseudoginseng* Wall (Araliacae)	Mangan		Root	Extract of roots.
71	*Papaver somniferum* Linn. (Papaveraceae)	Aphim,Poppy phool		Fruit	Incision of the fruits are collected and taken in a very low dose orally.
72	*Persea americana* Mill. (Lauraceae)	Pomsi	Riang, Naga clans	Leaves	Decoction of fresh leaves are used.
73	*Phyllanthus emblica* Linn. (Euphorbiaceae)	Bon bakeri		Fruit	Fruits are used raw form.
74	*Physalis minima* Linn. (Solanaceae)	Jangli phok phokey		Whole plant	Infusion of whole plant used.
75	*Phytolacca acinosa* Roxb. (Phytolaccaceae)	Jaringo		Roots	Roots are dissolved in alcohol for three days, then crushed after drying. Crushed powder is taken orally.
76	*Piper longum* Linn. (Piperaceae)	Pipla		Fruits	Cold macerated solution is taken.
77	*Plantago major* Linn. (Plantaginaceae)	Chhakur-blang		Leaf	Crushed leaves and raw milk mixed.
78	*Polygonum affine* Linn. (Polygonaceae)	Jarian		Leaf	Decoction of leaves.
79	*Polygonum oleracea* Linn. (Polygonaceae)	Jiahusia		Leaf	Leaves as decoction.
80	*Prunus cerasoides* Linn. (Rosaceae)	Paiyun		Stem, fruit	Stem and fruit are crushed and soaked in water.
81	*Psidium guajava* Linn. (Myrtaceae)	Peyara		Leaf	Juice from crushed leaves.
82	*Punica granatum* Linn. (Punicaceae)	Darim		Fruits, flowers	Juice of the fruits and infusion of flowers.
83	*Randia uliginosa* Linn. (Rubiaceae)	Piralu Maidal	Naga clans	Root	Root extract.
84	*Scoparia dulcis* Linn. (Plantaginaceae)	Gymbat-pdyp		Root	Root extract.
85	*Sesamum indicum* Linn. (Pedaliaceae)	Tiil		Seed	Seed oil is used
86	*Smilax zeylandica* Linn. (Smilacaceae)	Kukur dainey		Root	A decoction of root is made with water.

(Continued)

TABLE 7.1 (CONTINUED)
List of Ethnomedicinal Plants Used to Treat Alzheimer's Disease, With Vernacular Name, Used by Tribes, Part Used, and Mode of Preparation

Sl. No.	Scientific Name (With Family)	Vernacular Name	Tribes	Parts Used	Mode of Preparation
87	*Solanum ferox* Linn. (Solanaceae)	Soh-khasi		Fruit	Fresh fruit drink.
88	*Solanum nigrum* Linn. (Solanaceae)	Kalobehi, Kalodatura		Berries	Juice of the fruits.
89	*Sonchus asper* Linn. (Asteraceae)	Jalynniar		Leaf	Leaves as decoction.
90	*Sonchus oleraceus* Linn. (Asteraceae)	Soh lamjew		Fruit	Fruit juice.
91	*Sphaeranthus indicus* Linn. (Asteraceae)	Bandre		Root, seed, flower	Root is powdered and mixed with ghee or honey.
92	*Spilanthes acmella* Linn. (Asteraceae)	Pirazh		Flower bud	Paste form of the flower buds.
93	*Symplocos racemosa* Roxb. (Symplocaceae)	Kharaney		Bark and stem	Infusion of stem and bark is used.
94	*Tamarindus indica* Linn. (Fabaceae)	Tetul		Seed	Expressed juice of the seeds.
95	*Taxus baccata* Linn. (Taxaceae)	Sehblei		Fruit	Fruit juice.
96	*Toona ciliata* (Meliaceae)	Tooni		Bark and flower	Flower is chewed and decoction of bark is given.
97	*Viola serpens* Wall. (Violaceae)	Phul naqsha		Root, leaves, barks	Aqueous extract of all parts.
98	*Withania somnifera* Linn. (Solanaceae)	Aswagandha		Root	Root extract.
99	*Woodfordia fruticosa* Linn. (Lythraceae)	Dhungeri		Dried flower	Dried flower powder with honey is given.
100	*Ziziphus mauritiana* Lam. (Rhamnaceae)	Jujuba		Fruit	Ripe fruits are eaten.

issues with driving. Issues with vision can lead to severe injury to the self as well as other people (Dastmalchi et al., 2009).

7.3.6 New Issues with Words in Speaking or Writing

Individuals with Alzheimer's may experience difficulty following or joining in a conversation. They may stop in the middle of a conversation and have no clue as to how to proceed or they may repeat themselves. They may struggle with vocabulary, having problems finding the correct word, or calling things by the wrong name (e.g. calling a "watch" a "hand-clock") (Dhingra et al., 2004).

7.3.7 Misplacing Things and Losing the Ability to Retrace Your Steps

An individual with Alzheimer's may place things in unusual places, such as an iron in the refrigerator. They may lose things and be unable to retrace their steps to re-discover them once more. Occasionally, they may blame others for taking the items. This may happen more often as the disease progresses. Losing things every now and then and remembering ventures to discover them (Arulselvan et al., 2007)

TABLE 7.2
List of Ethnomedicinal Plants Used to Treat Alzheimer's Disease, with Active Constituents and their Structures

SL. NO.	Scientific Name (With Family)	Active Constituents	Structure
1	*Abroma augusta* Linn. (Sterculiaceae)	Abromine	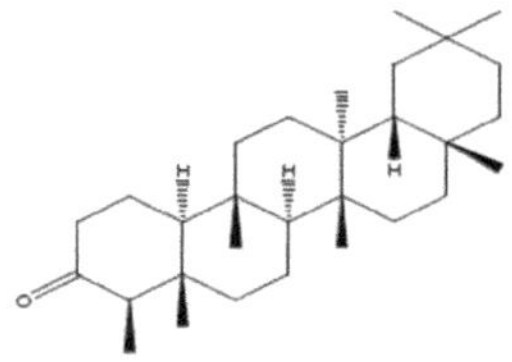
2	*Achyranthus aspera* Linn. (Amaranthaceae)	Oleanolic acid	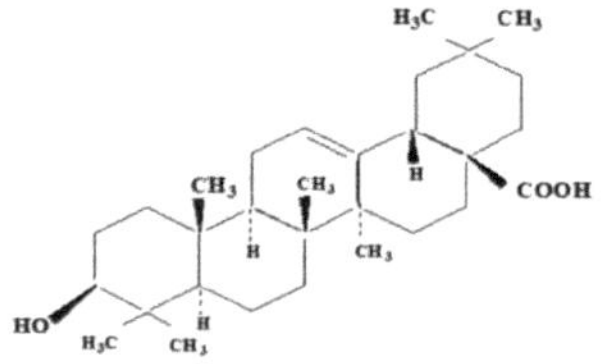
3	*Adiantum capillus-veneris* Linn. (Pteridaceae)	Adiantoxide	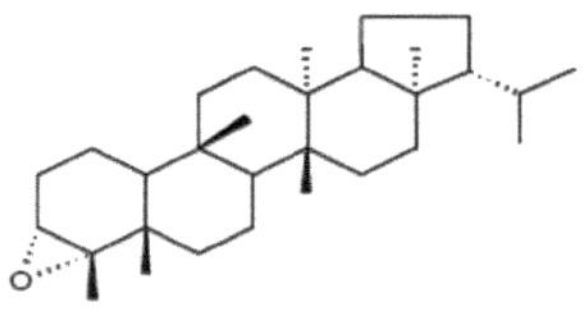
4	*Adiantum incisum* Linn. (Pteridaceae)	Adiantone	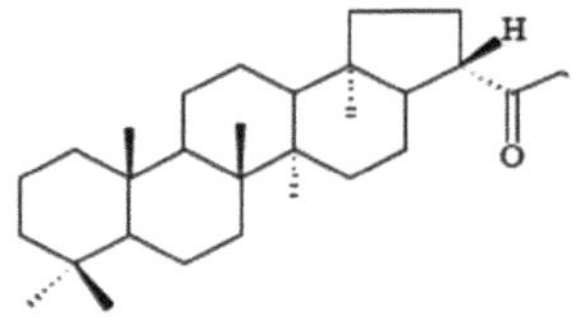
5	*Amaranthus spinosus* Linn. (Amarathaceae)	Betanin and amarathine	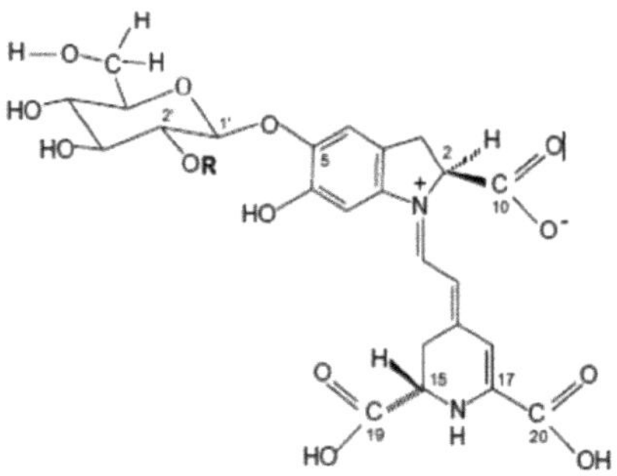 R = H: Betanin R = Glucuronic acid: Amaranthine

(Continued)

TABLE 7.2 (CONTINUED)
List of Ethnomedicinal Plants Used to Treat Alzheimer's Disease, with Active Constituents and their Structures

SL. NO.	Scientific Name (With Family)	Active Constituents	Structure
6	*Ananas sativus* Linn. (Bromeliaceae)	Ascorbic acid	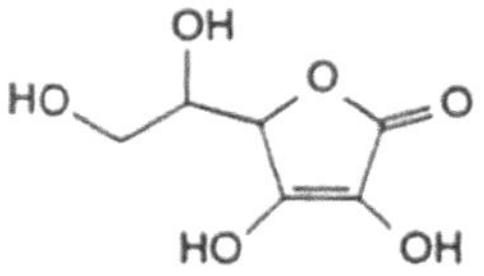
7	*Argemone mexicana* Linn. (Papaveraceae)	Isocorydine	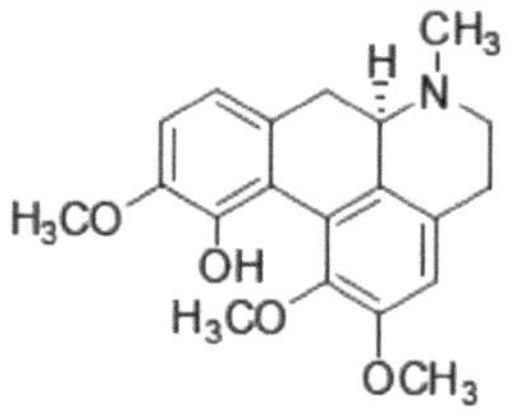
8	*Argyrolobium roseum* Linn. (Fabaceae)	Reticuline	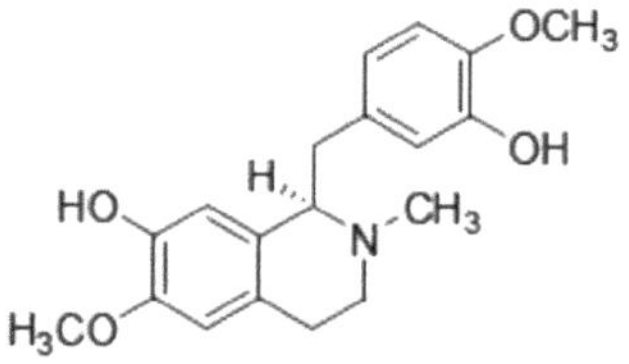
9	*Artemisia absinthium* Linn. (Asteraceae)	Nor-sanguinarine	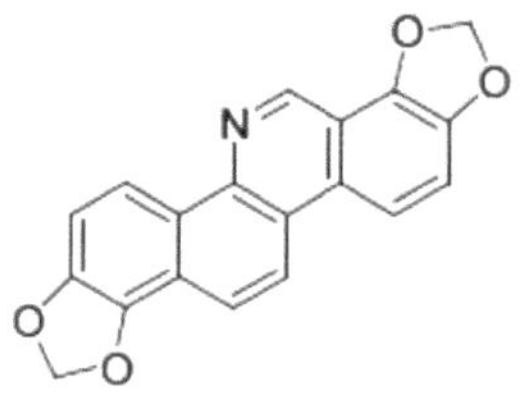
10	*Artocarpus chapalasha* Roxb. (Moraceae)	Artocarpin	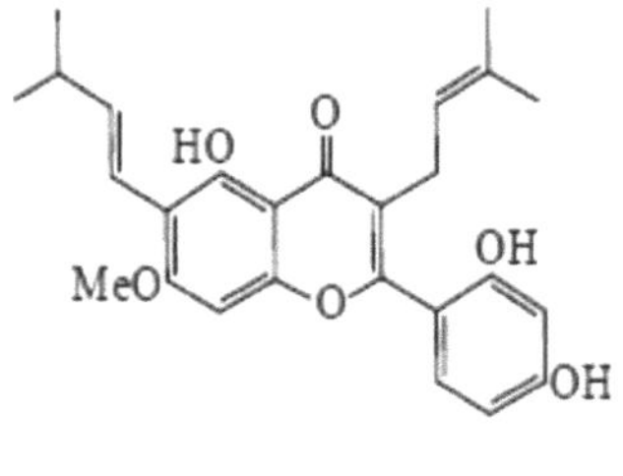
11	*Artocurpus heterophyllus* Linn. (Moraceae)	Heterophyllol	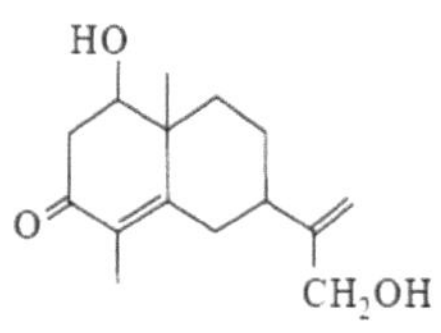

(Continued)

TABLE 7.2 (CONTINUED)
List of Ethnomedicinal Plants Used to Treat Alzheimer's Disease, with Active Constituents and their Structures

SL. NO.	Scientific Name (With Family)	Active Constituents	Structure
12	*Asparagus adscendens* Linn. (Asparagaceae)	Shatavarin	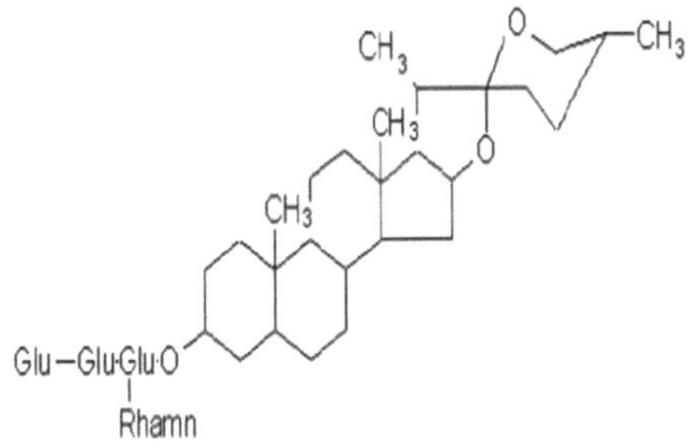
13	*Asparagus racemosus* Linn. (Asparagraceae)	Rutin	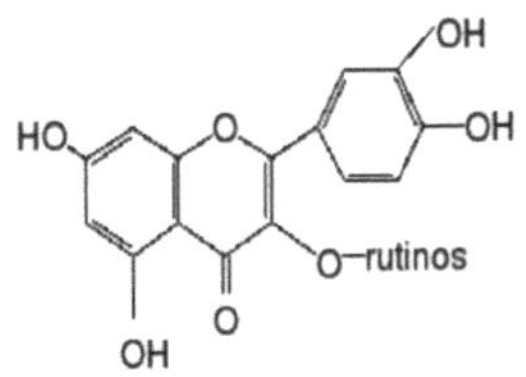
14	*Asparagus racemosus* Wild (Asparagaceae)	Quercetin	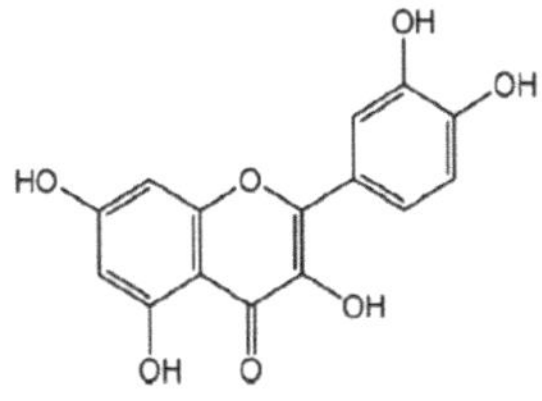
15	*Averrhoa carambola* Linn. (Averrhoaceae)	Ascorbic acid	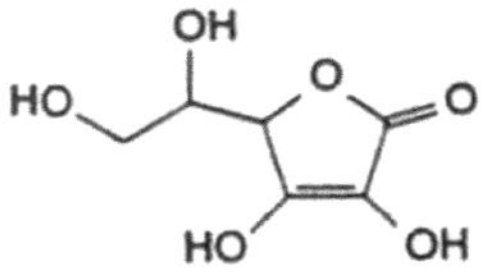
16	*Baccaurea ramiflora* Linn. (Euphobiaceae)	6'-*O*-Vanilloylosotachioside	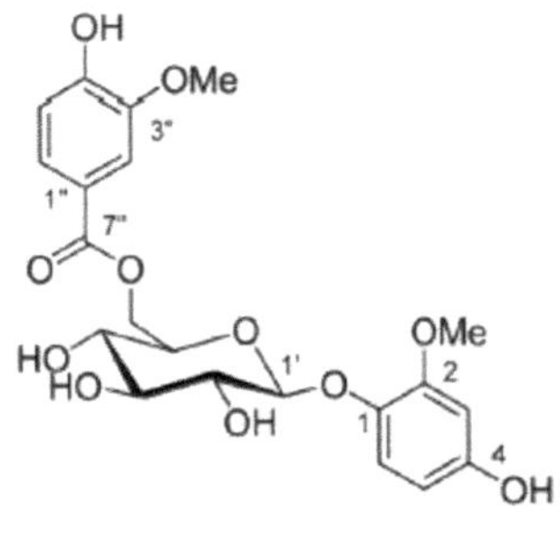

(*Continued*)

TABLE 7.2 (CONTINUED)
List of Ethnomedicinal Plants Used to Treat Alzheimer's Disease, with Active Constituents and their Structures

SL. NO.	Scientific Name (With Family)	Active Constituents	Structure
17	*Bacopa monnieri* Linn. (Plantaginaceae)	Bacoside A and Bacoside B	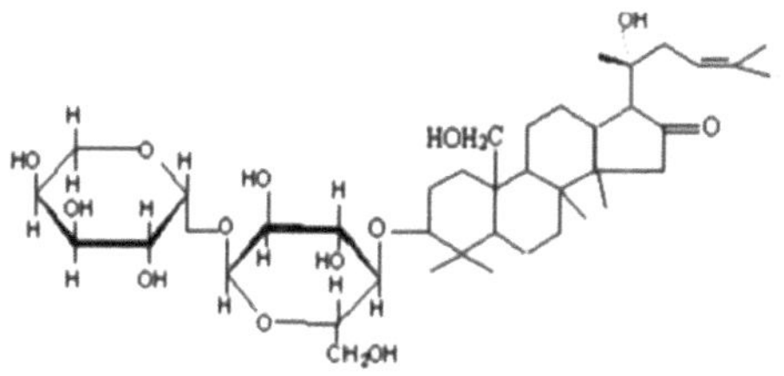 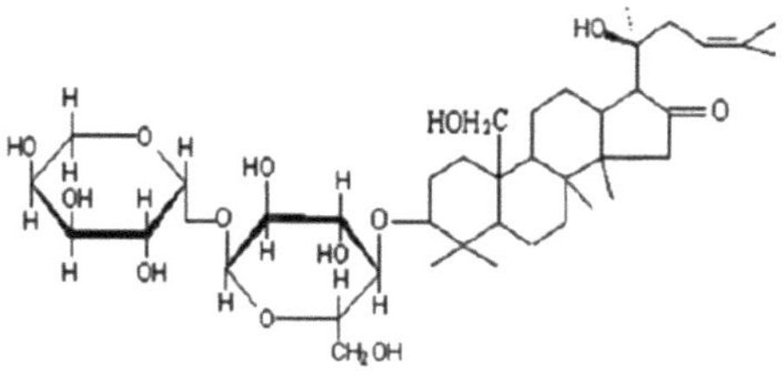
18	*Basella alba* Linn. (Basellaceae)	Retinol	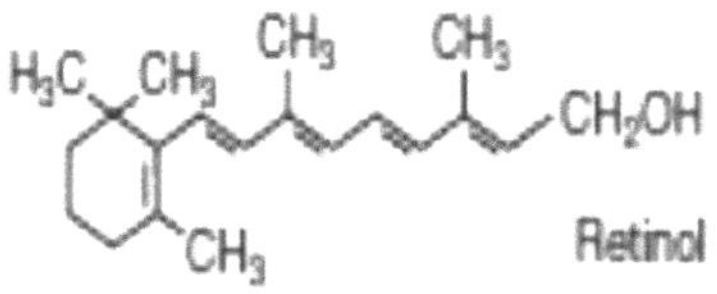
19	*Borreria articularis* Linn. (Rubiaceae)	Terpenoids	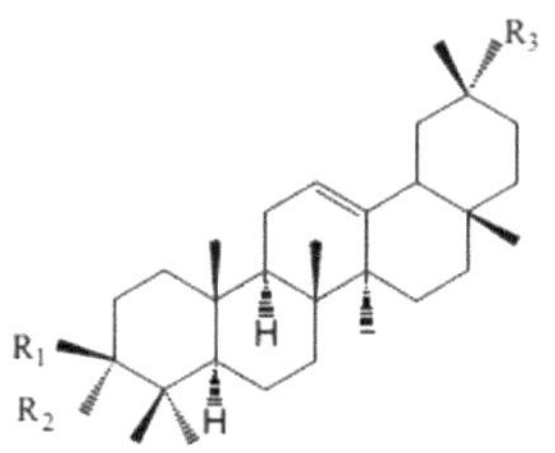 1. R_1=OH, R_2= H, R_3= CH_3 2. R_1=H, R_2= OAc, R_3= COOH 2a. R_1=H, R_2= OH, R_3= COOH 2b. R_1=H, R_2= OH, R_3= $COOCH_3$ 2c. R_1, R_2 = O, R_3= $COOCH_3$
20	*Brassica oleracea* Linn. (Brassicaceae)	Linoleic acid and linolenic acid	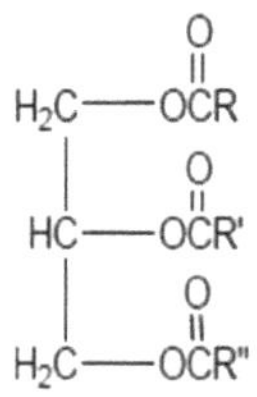 2 R, R', R'' = linoleic acid, linolenic acid

(*Continued*)

TABLE 7.2 (CONTINUED)
List of Ethnomedicinal Plants Used to Treat Alzheimer's Disease, with Active Constituents and their Structures

SL. NO.	Scientific Name (With Family)	Active Constituents	Structure
21	*Bryophyllum calycinum* Linn. (Crassulaceae)	Bryophyllin	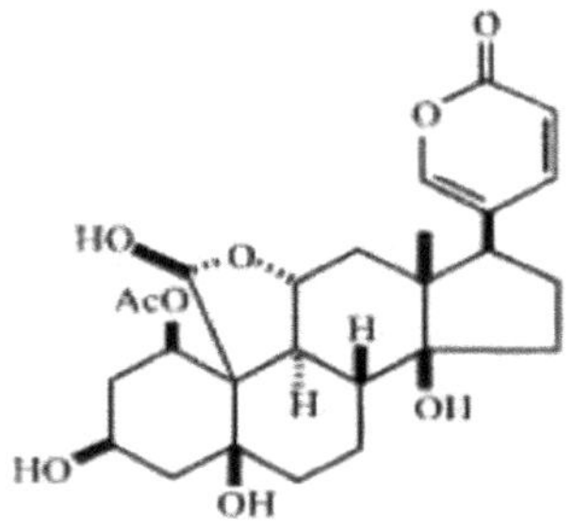
22	*Cajanus cajan* Linn. (Fabaceae)	Luteolin	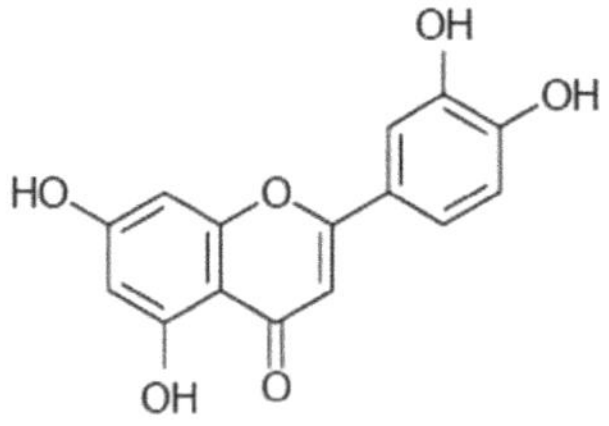
23	*Calamus erectus* Roxb. (Arecaceae)	Apigenin	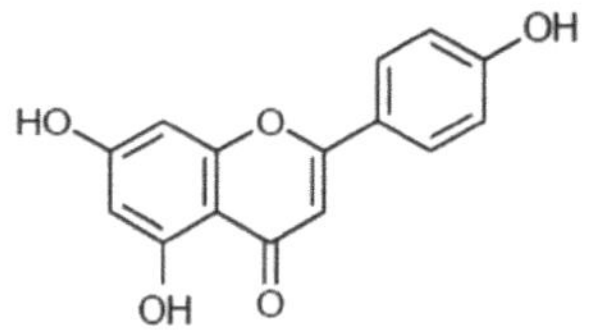
24	*Camellia sinensis* Linn. (Theaceae)	Catechin	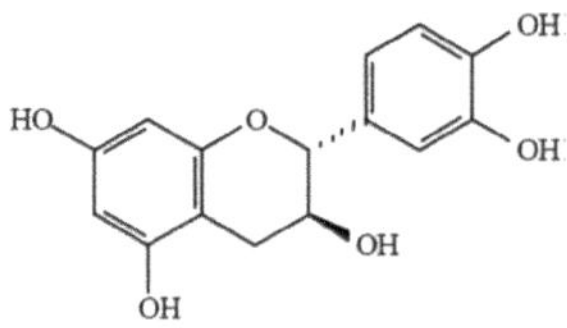
25	*Capparis spinosa* Linn. (Capparidaceae)	Stigmasterol	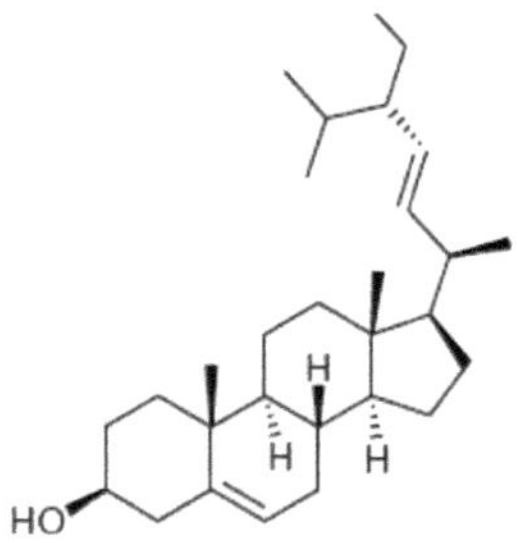

(*Continued*)

TABLE 7.2 (CONTINUED)
List of Ethnomedicinal Plants Used to Treat Alzheimer's Disease, with Active Constituents and their Structures

SL. NO.	Scientific Name (With Family)	Active Constituents	Structure
26	*Cuscuta reflexa* Roxb (Convolvulaceae)	Rhein	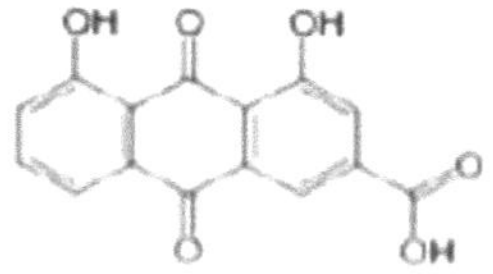
27	*Cassia alata* Linn. (Fabaceae)	Emodin	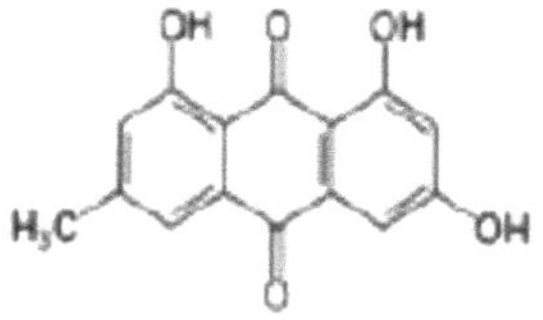
28	*Castanopsis indica* Linn. (Fagaceae)	Tabersonine	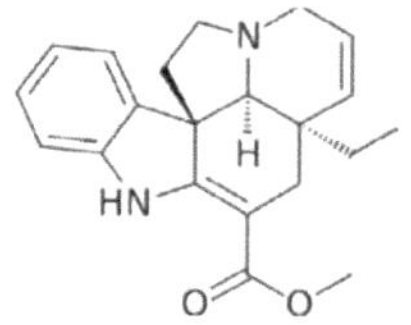
29	*Catharanthus roseus* Linn. (Apocyanaceae)	Vinblastine	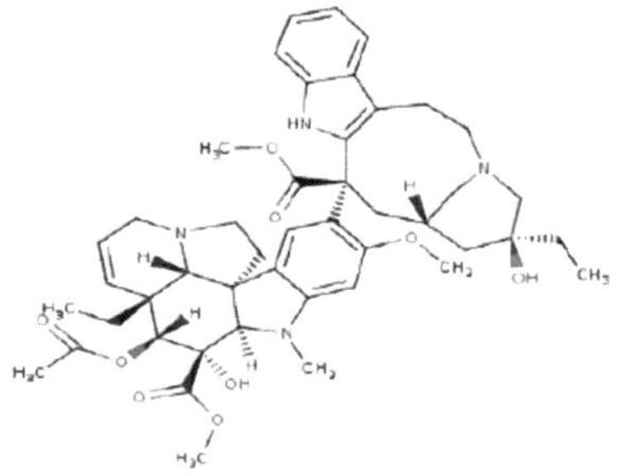
30	*Centella asiatica* Linn. (Apiaceae)	Isoflavonoid phytoalexin	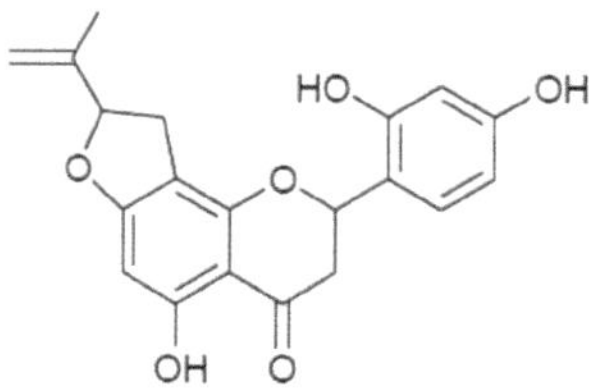
31	*Cissampelos pareira* Linn. (Menispermaceae)	Cajaflavonone	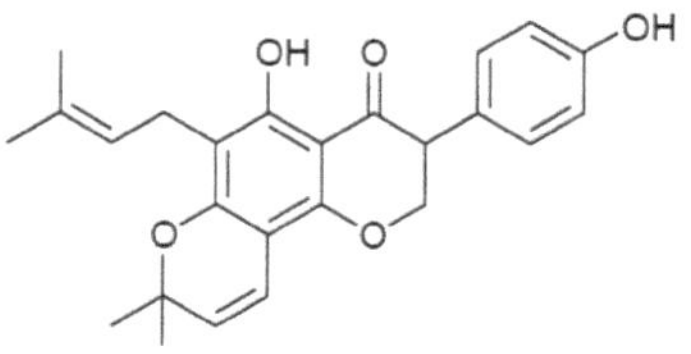

(*Continued*)

TABLE 7.2 (CONTINUED)
List of Ethnomedicinal Plants Used to Treat Alzheimer's Disease, with Active Constituents and their Structures

SL. NO.	Scientific Name (With Family)	Active Constituents	Structure
32	*Coelogyne cristala* Lindle (Orchidaceae)	Squalene	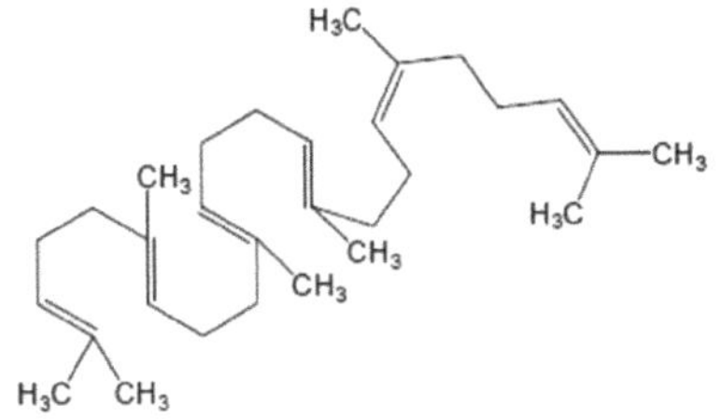
33	*Coix lacryma* Linn. (Poaceae)	Lupane	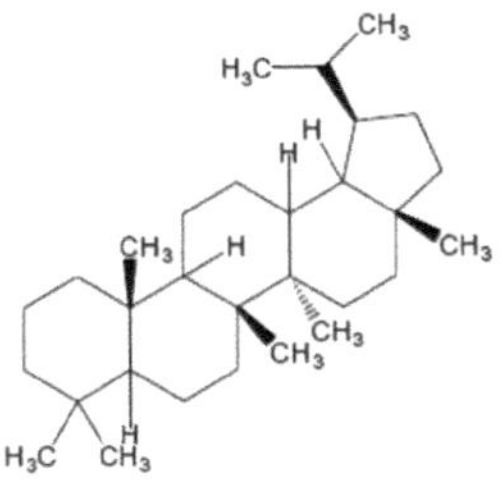
34	*Colocasia esculenta* Linn. (Araceae)	Flavone	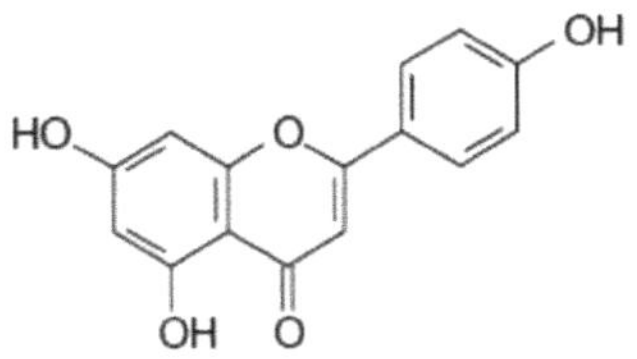
35	*Corchorus aestuans* Linn. (Malvaceae)	Oleanolic acid	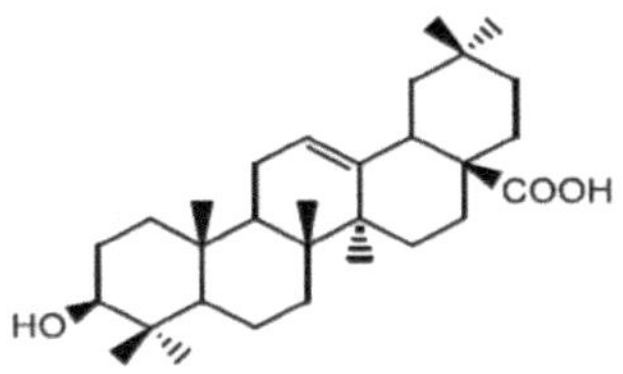
36	*Coriandrum sativum* Linn. (Apiaceae)	Linalool	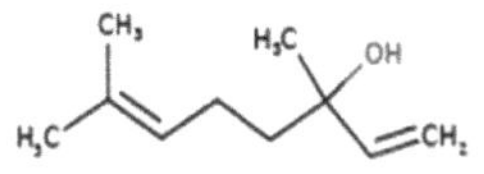
37	*Croton tiglium* Linn. (Euphorbiaceae)	Diterpenoid	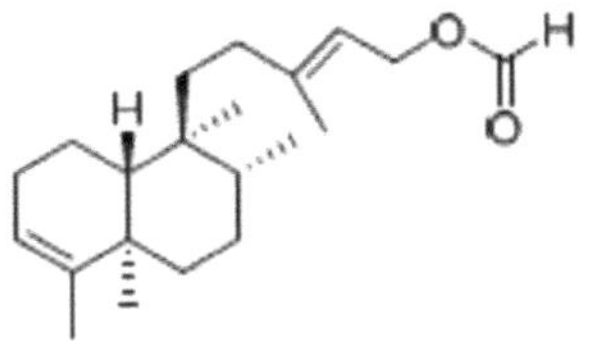

(*Continued*)

TABLE 7.2 (CONTINUED)

List of Ethnomedicinal Plants Used to Treat Alzheimer's Disease, with Active Constituents and their Structures

SL. NO.	Scientific Name (With Family)	Active Constituents	Structure
38	*Curcuma amada* Roxb. (Zingiberaceae)	Curcumin	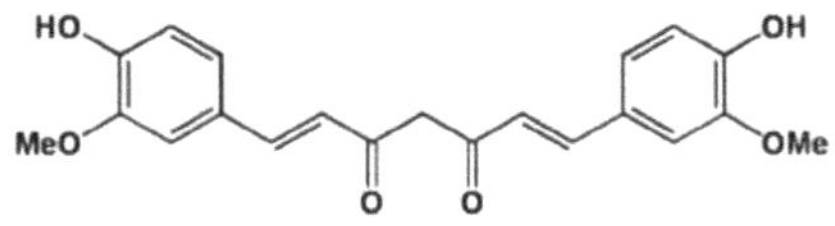
39	*Cynodon dactylon* Linn. (Poaceae)	Vetexin	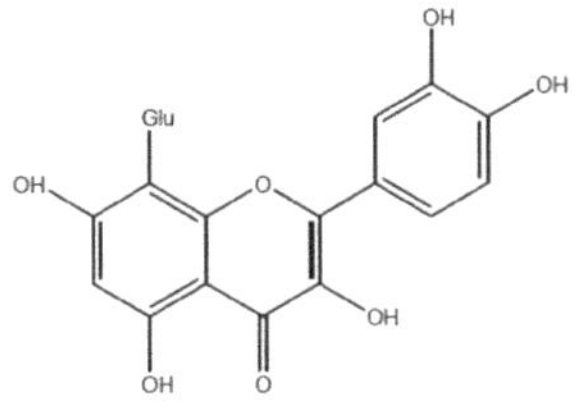
40	*Desmodium triquetrum* Linn. (Fabaceae)	Ferulic acid	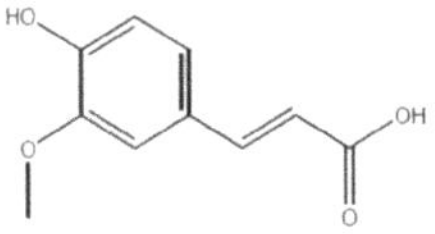
41	*Desmotachya bipinnata* Linn. (Poaceae)	Luteolin	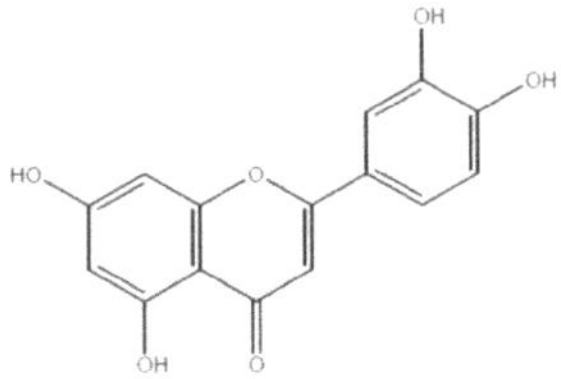
42	*Dillenia indica* Linn. (Dilleniaceae)	Dillenetin	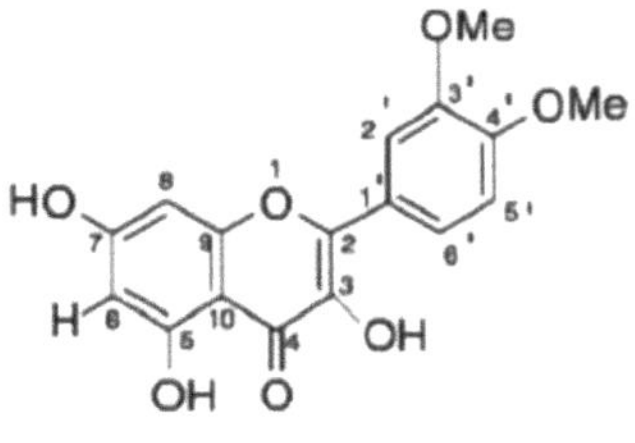
43	*Dolichus uniflorus* Linn. (Fabaceae)	Beta-ionone	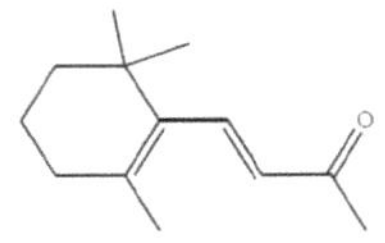
44	*Ephedra sinica* Linn. (Ephedraceae)	(-) Ephedrine	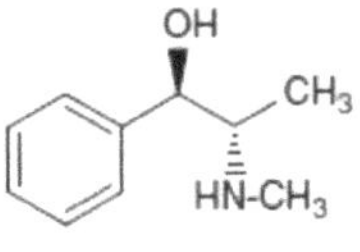

(*Continued*)

TABLE 7.2 (CONTINUED)
List of Ethnomedicinal Plants Used to Treat Alzheimer's Disease, with Active Constituents and their Structures

SL. NO.	Scientific Name (With Family)	Active Constituents	Structure
45	*Tetradium fraxinifolia* Hook (Rutaceae)	Gentisic acid	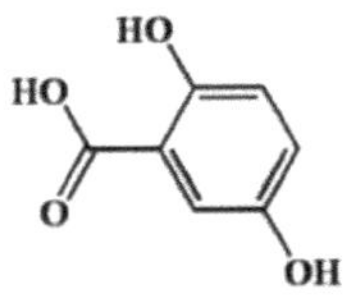
46	*Fagopyrum dibotrys* Linn. (Polygonaceae)	5,7,3',4'-tetrahydroxy flavan-3-ol dimer	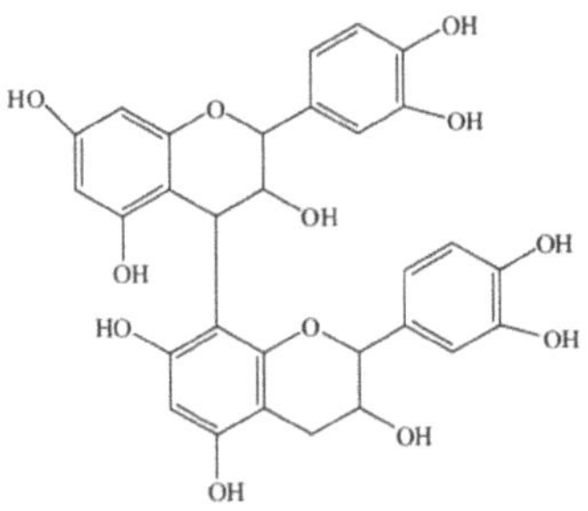
47	*Ficus racemosa* Linn. (Moraceae)	Beta-sitosterol	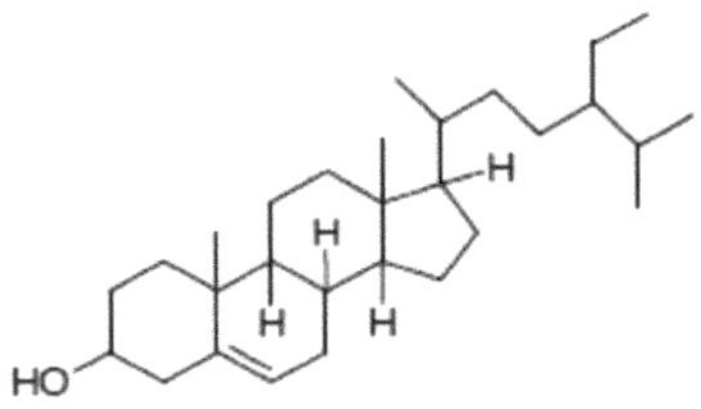
48	*Foeniculum vulgare* Hill (Apiaceae)	Anethole	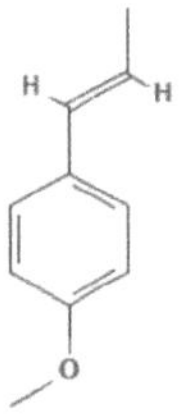
49	*Gmelina arborea* Roxb. (Verbenaceae)	Isoarboreol	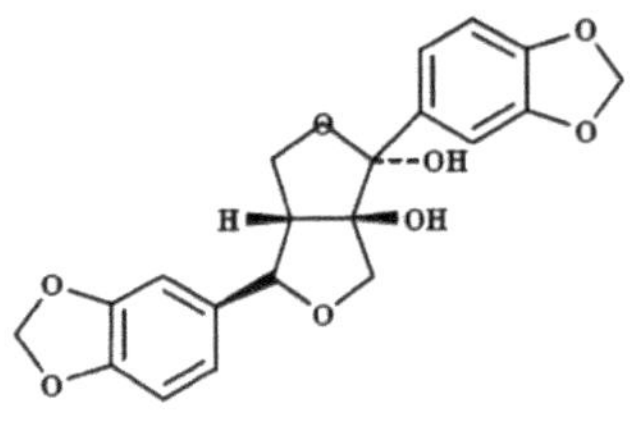

(Continued)

TABLE 7.2 (CONTINUED)
List of Ethnomedicinal Plants Used to Treat Alzheimer's Disease, with Active Constituents and their Structures

SL. NO.	Scientific Name (With Family)	Active Constituents	Structure
50	*Helianthus annuus* Linn. (Asteraceae)	Kaempferol	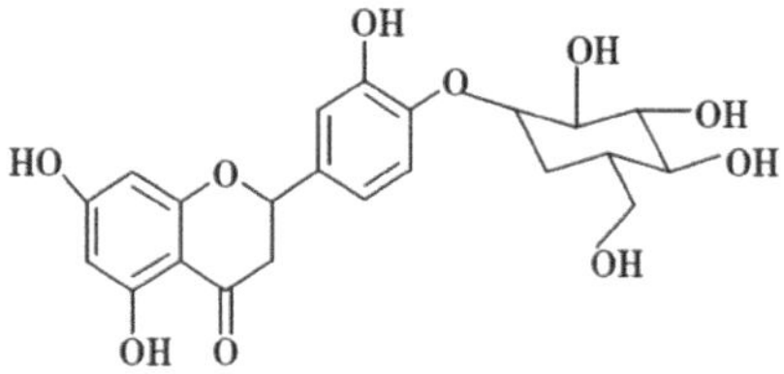
51	*Hydrocotyle asiatica* Linn. (Apiaceae)	Asiatic acid	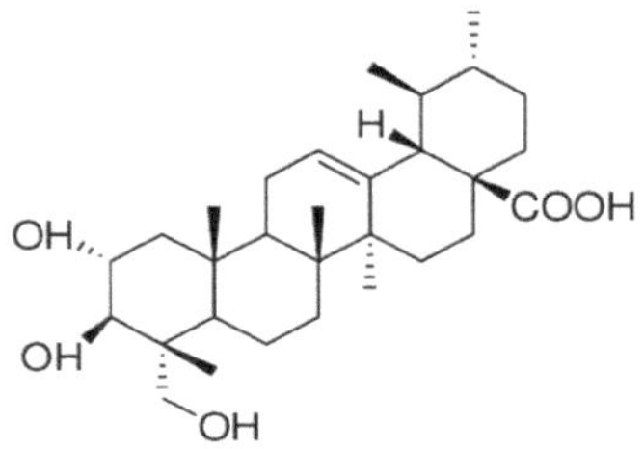
52	*Hyptis suaveolens* Linn. (Lamiaceae)	Sabinene	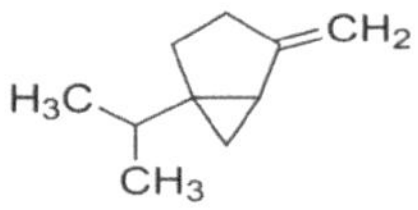
53	*Impatiens balsamina* Linn. (Balsaminaceae)	Lawsone	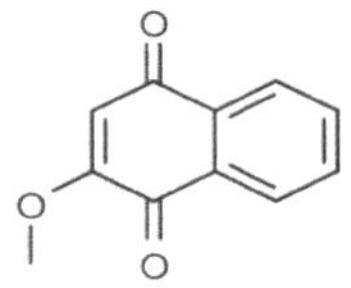
54	*Lannea coromandelica* Linn. (Anacardiaceae)	Quercetin	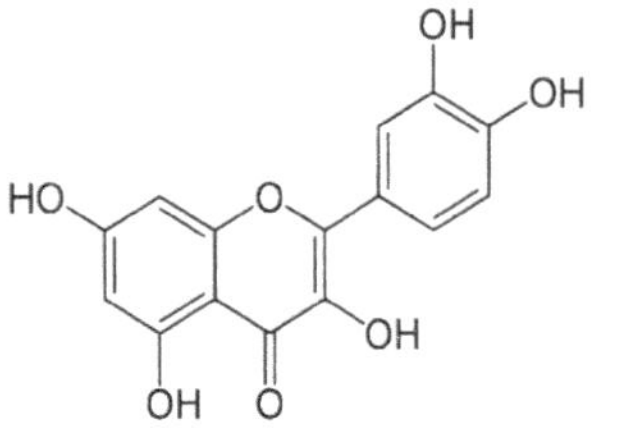
55	*Lantana camara* Linn. (Verbenaceae)	Lantadene	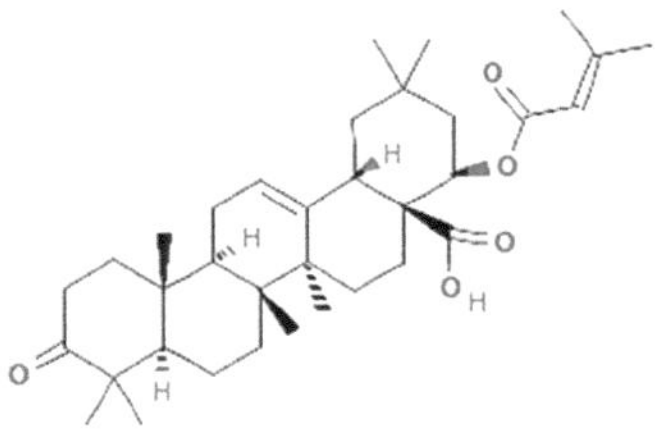

(*Continued*)

TABLE 7.2 (CONTINUED)
List of Ethnomedicinal Plants Used to Treat Alzheimer's Disease, with Active Constituents and their Structures

SL. NO.	Scientific Name (With Family)	Active Constituents	Structure
56	*Luffa acutangula* Linn. (Cucurbitaceae)	Bicyclogermacrene	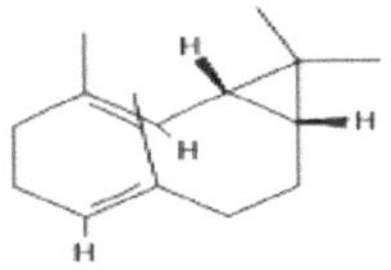
57	*Lycopodium clavatum* Linn. (Lycopodiaceae)	Huperzine A	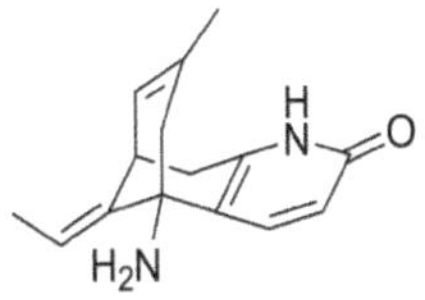
58	*Malvastrum tricuspidatum* Linn. (Malvaceae)	Palmitic acid	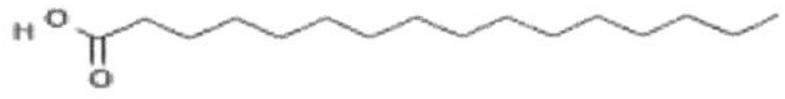
59	*Melia azedirach* Linn. (Meliaceae)	Erucic acid	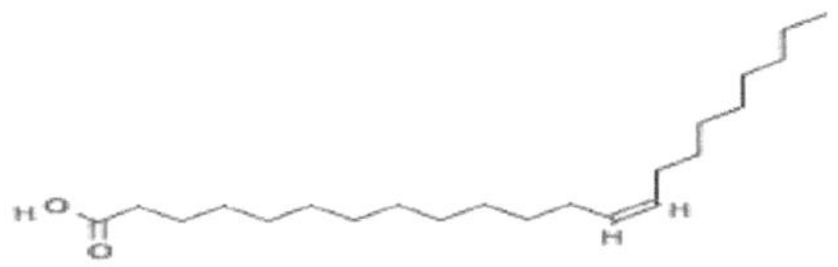
60	*Mikania micrantha* Linn. (Asteraceae)	Eupalitin	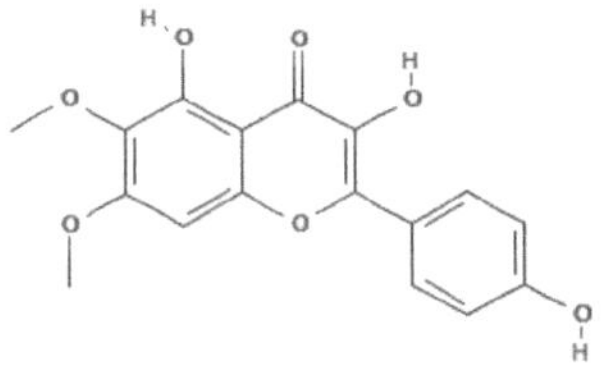
61	*Mimosa pudica* Linn. (Fabaceae)	Mimosine	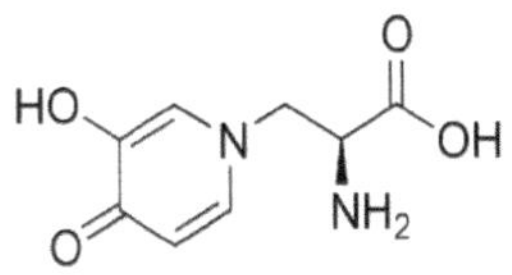
62	*Momordica charantia* Linn. (Cucurbitaceae)	Salicin	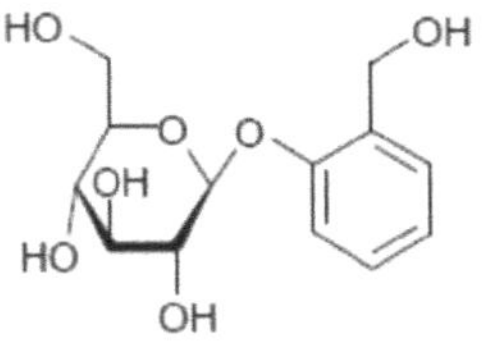

(*Continued*)

TABLE 7.2 (CONTINUED)
List of Ethnomedicinal Plants Used to Treat Alzheimer's Disease, with Active Constituents and their Structures

SL. NO.	Scientific Name (With Family)	Active Constituents	Structure
63	*Musa paradisiaca* Linn. (Musaceae)	Thiophyllin	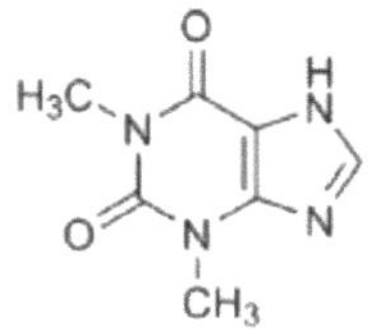
64	*Musa sapientum* Linn. (Musaceae)	Kera	Flower, rhizome
65	*Myrsine africana* Linn. (Myrsinaceae)	Pseudotropine	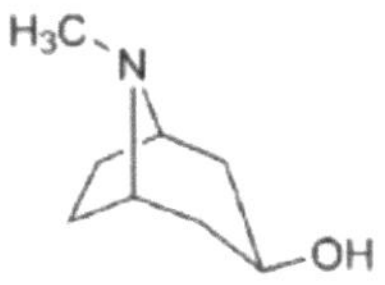
66	*Nasturtium fontana* Linn. (Brassicaceae)	Seemrayo	All parts of the Plant
67	*Ocimum basilicum* Linn. (Lamiaceae)	Methycgonine	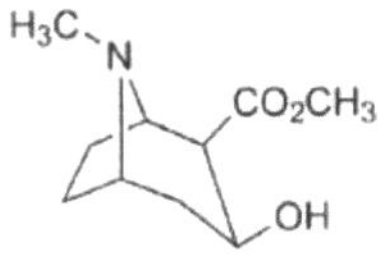
68	*Ocimum sanctum* Linn. (Lamiaceae)	Lupinine	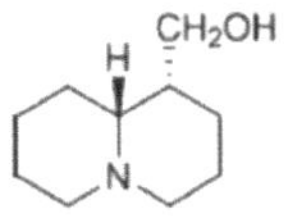
69	*Oxalis corymbosa* Linn. (Oxalidaceae)	Lyconine	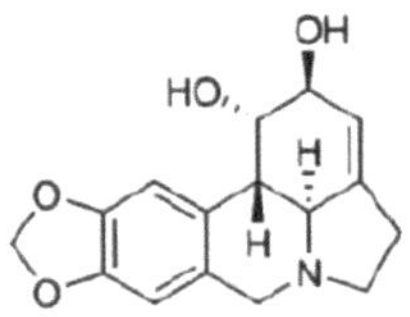

(*Continued*)

TABLE 7.2 (CONTINUED)
List of Ethnomedicinal Plants Used to Treat Alzheimer's Disease, with Active Constituents and their Structures

SL. NO.	Scientific Name (With Family)	Active Constituents	Structure
70	*Panax pseudoginseng* Wall (Araliacae)	Gensenoside	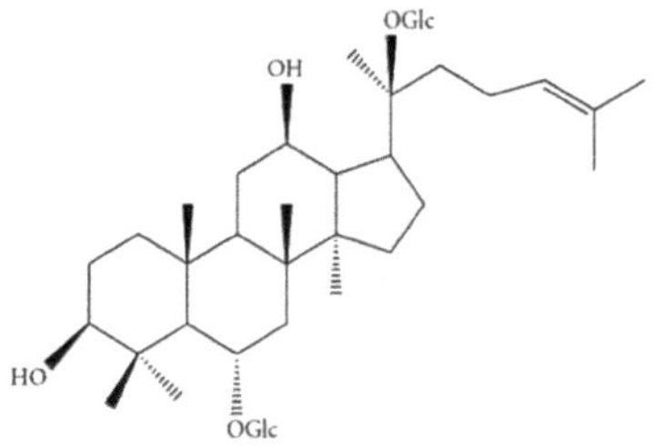
71	*Papaver somniferum* Linn. (Papaveraceae)	Morphine	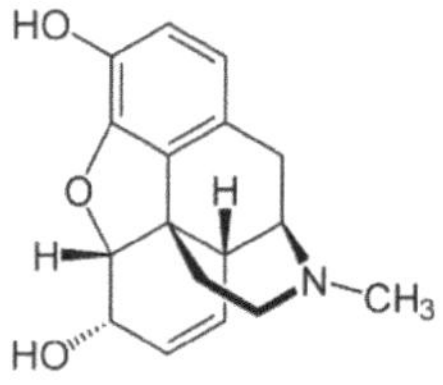
72	*Persea americana* Mill. (Lauraceae)	Linamarin	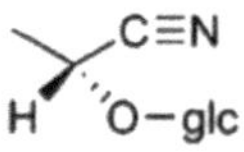
73	*Phyllanthus emblica* Linn. (Euphorbiaceae)	Ethyl gallate	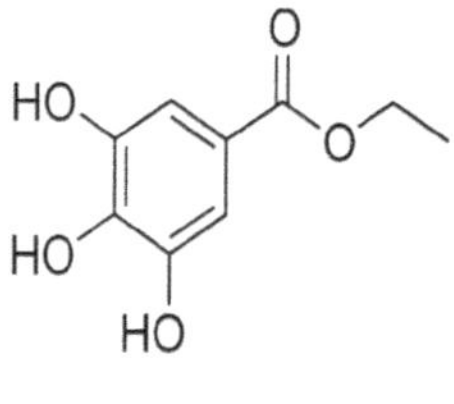
74	*Physalis minima* Linn. (Solanaceae)	*p*-Coumaryl alcohol	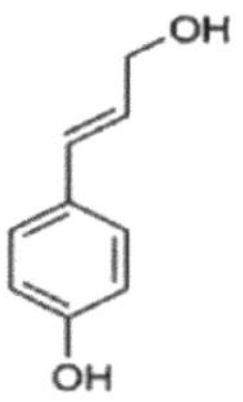
75	*Phytolacca acinosa* Roxb. (Phytolaccaceae)	punicalagin	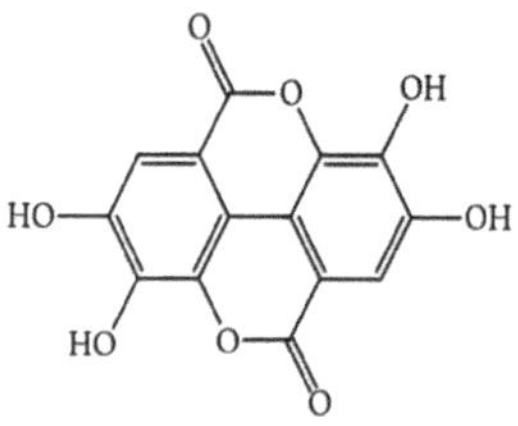

(*Continued*)

TABLE 7.2 (CONTINUED)
List of Ethnomedicinal Plants Used to Treat Alzheimer's Disease, with Active Constituents and their Structures

SL. NO.	Scientific Name (With Family)	Active Constituents	Structure
76	*Piper longum* Linn. (Piperaceae)	Piperine	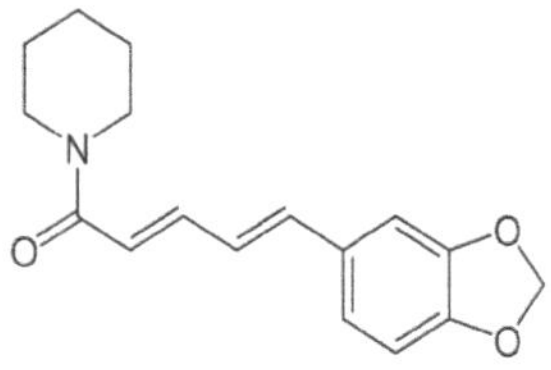
77	*Plantago major* Linn. (Plantaginaceae)	Benzyl acetate	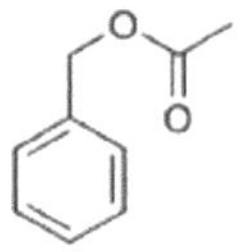
78	*Polygonum affine* Linn. (Polygonaceae)	Rutin	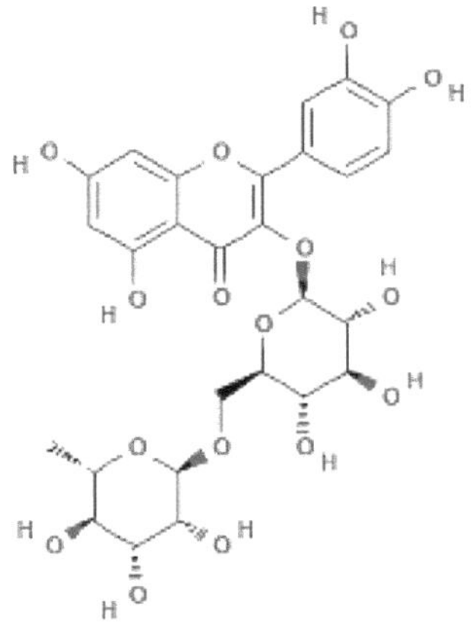
79	*Polygonum oleracea* Linn. (Polygonaceae)	Gallotannin	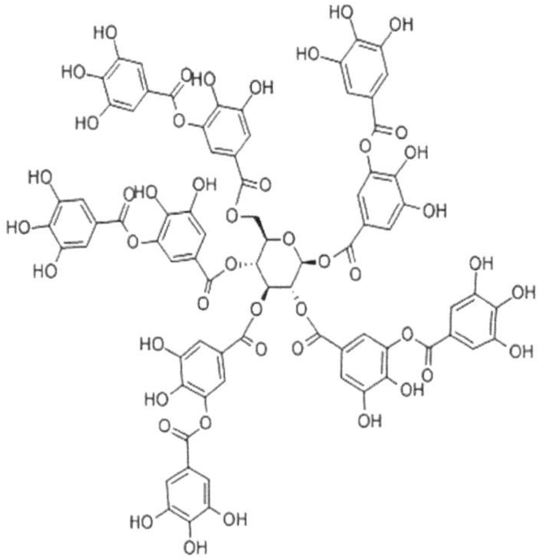

(*Continued*)

TABLE 7.2 (CONTINUED)
List of Ethnomedicinal Plants Used to Treat Alzheimer's Disease, with Active Constituents and their Structures

SL. NO.	Scientific Name (With Family)	Active Constituents	Structure
80	*Prunus cerasoides* Linn. (Rosaceae)	Humulone	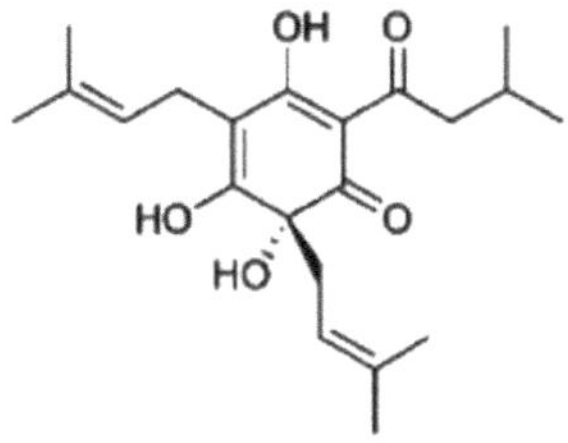
81	*Psidium guajava* Linn. (Myrtaceae)	Ursonic acid	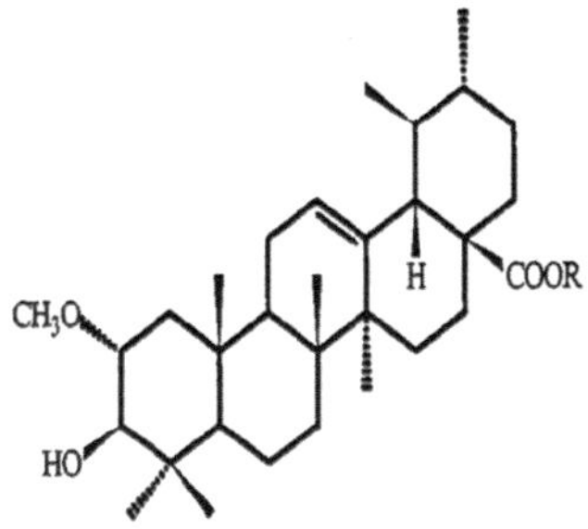
82	*Punica granatum* Linn. (Punicaceae)	Pectin	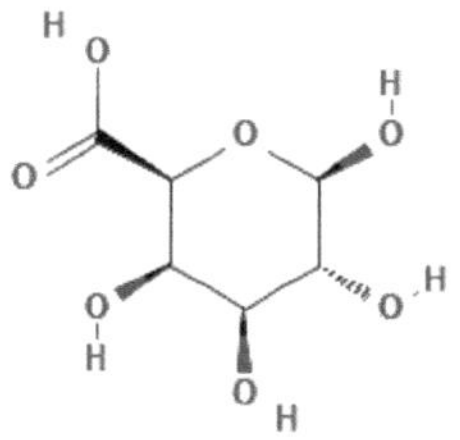
83	*Randia uliginosa* Linn. (Rubiaceae)	Levopimaric acid	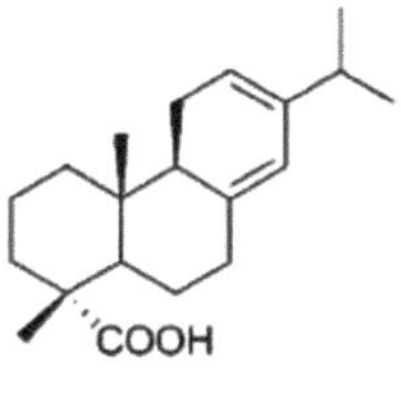

(Continued)

TABLE 7.2 (CONTINUED)
List of Ethnomedicinal Plants Used to Treat Alzheimer's Disease, with Active Constituents and their Structures

SL. NO.	Scientific Name (With Family)	Active Constituents	Structure
84	*Scoparia dulcis* Linn. (Plantaginaceae)	Scoparic acids	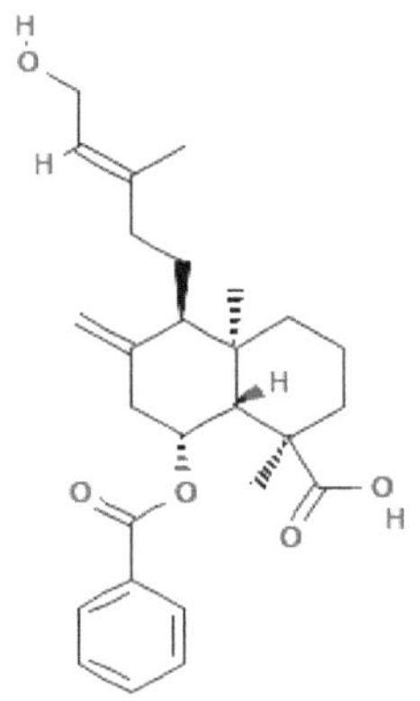
85	*Sesamum indicum* Linn. (Pedaliaceae)	Sesamin oil	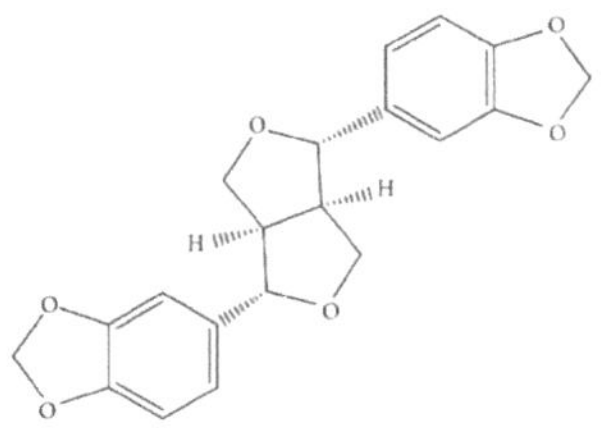
86	*Smilax zeylanica* Linn. (Smilacaceae)	Steroidal saponin	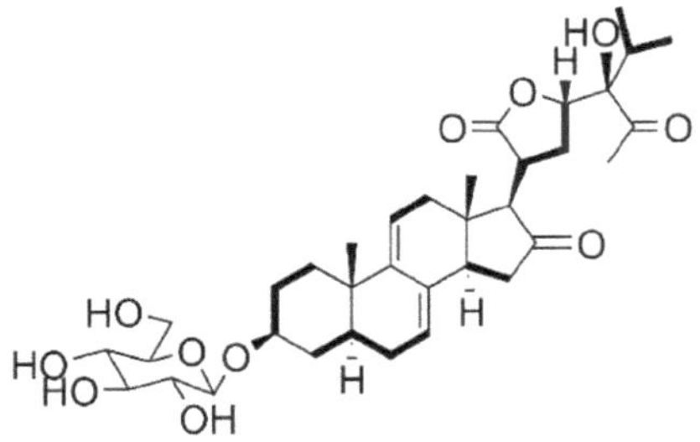
87	*Solanum ferox* Linn. (Solanaceae)	Abietic acid	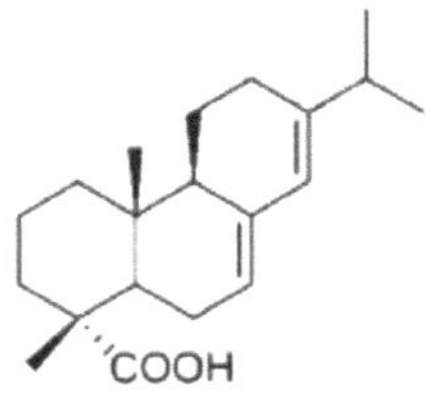

(*Continued*)

TABLE 7.2 (CONTINUED)
List of Ethnomedicinal Plants Used to Treat Alzheimer's Disease, with Active Constituents and their Structures

SL. NO.	Scientific Name (With Family)	Active Constituents	Structure
88	*Solanum nigrum* Linn. (Solanaceae)	Solatriose	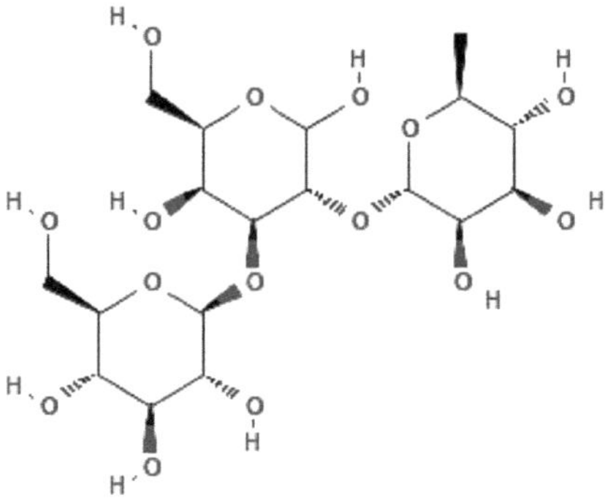
89	*Sonchus asper* Linn. (Asteraceae)	Loganin	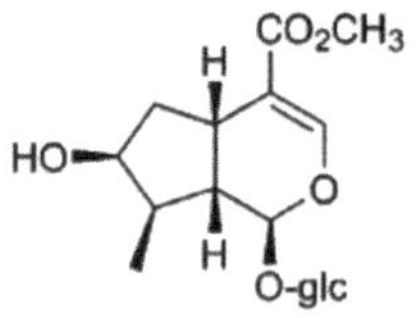
90	*Sonchus oleraceus* Linn. (Asteraceae)	Hyperforin	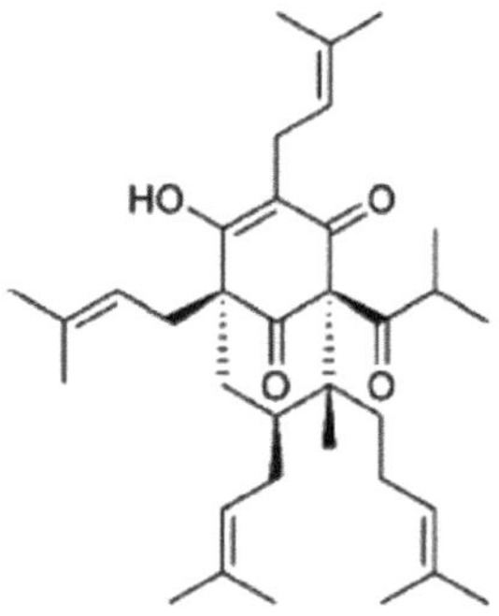
91	*Sphaeranthus indicus* Linn. (Asteraceae)	Parthenolide	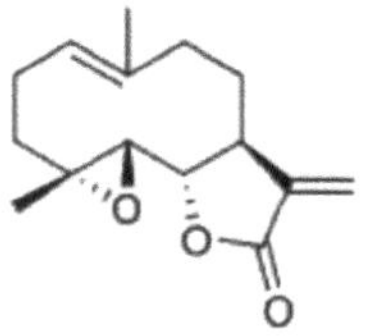

(*Continued*)

TABLE 7.2 (CONTINUED)
List of Ethnomedicinal Plants Used to Treat Alzheimer's Disease, with Active Constituents and their Structures

SL. NO.	Scientific Name (With Family)	Active Constituents	Structure
92	*Spilanthes acmella* Linn. (Asteraceae)	Epicatechin	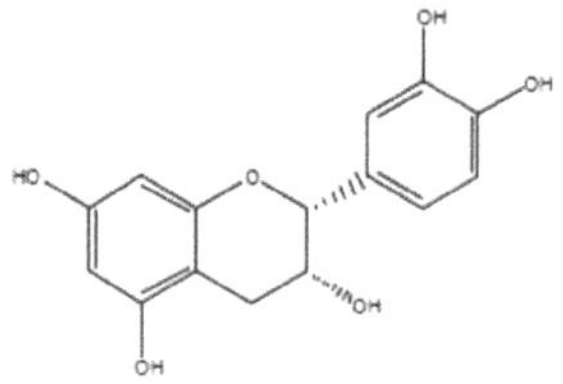
93	*Symplocos racemosa* Roxb. (Symplocaceae)	Scopolatin	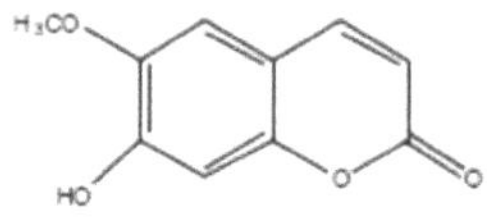
94	*Tamarindus indica* Linn. (Fabaceae)	Methyl gallate	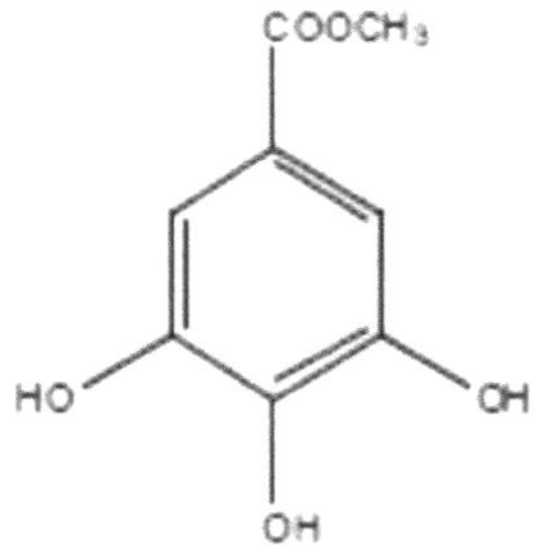
95	*Taxus baccata* Linn. (Taxaceae)	Catechin	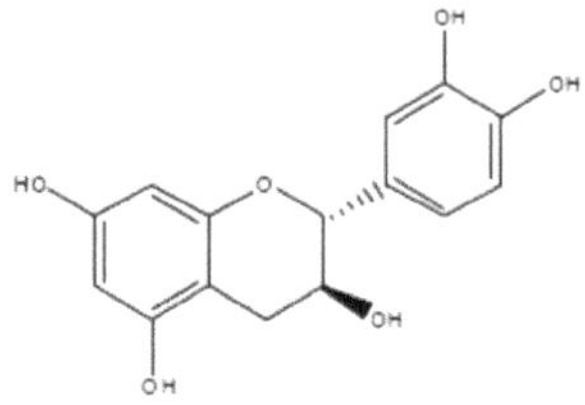
96	*Toona ciliata* Linn. (Meliaceae)	Toonaciliatone A	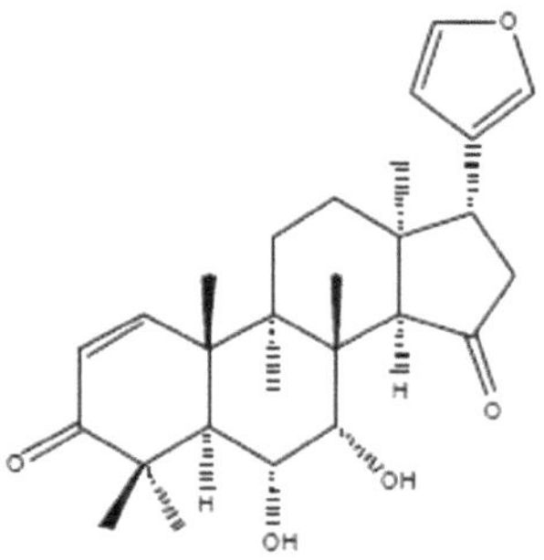

(*Continued*)

TABLE 7.2 (CONTINUED)
List of Ethnomedicinal Plants Used to Treat Alzheimer's Disease, with Active Constituents and their Structures

SL. NO.	Scientific Name (With Family)	Active Constituents	Structure
97	*Viola serpens* Wall. (Violaceae)	Bis-maleate	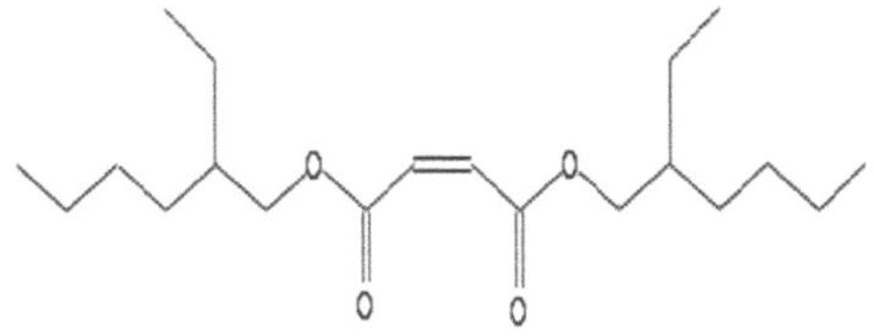
98	*Withania somnifera* Linn. (Solanaceae)	Withasomnine	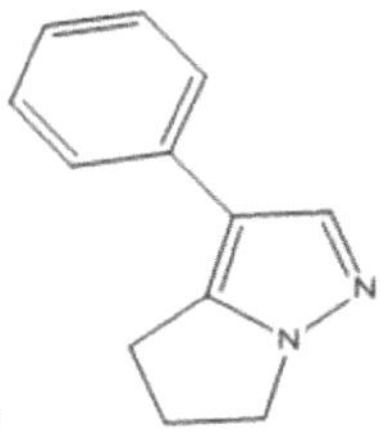
99	*Woodfordia fruticosa* Linn. (Lythraceae)	Beta-sitosterol	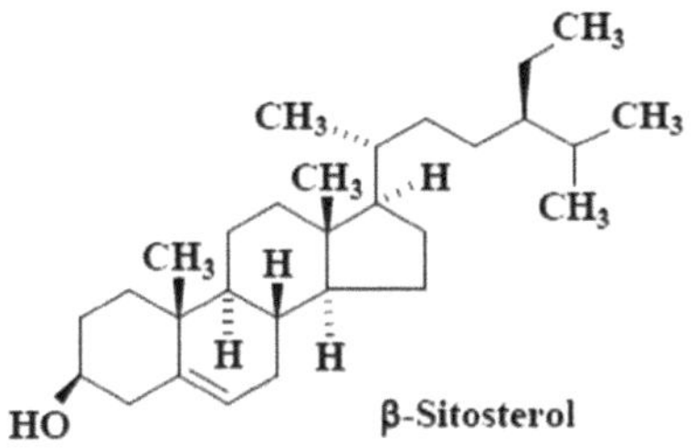
100	*Ziziphus mauritiana* Lam. (Rhamnaceae)	Kaempferol	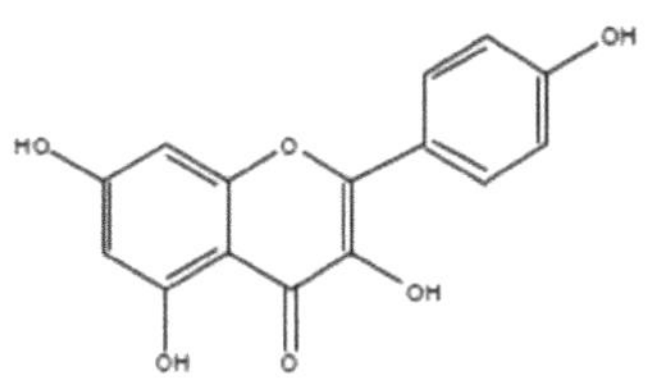

7.3.8 Diminished or Poor Judgment

Individuals with Alzheimer's may exhibit changes in the ability to makes judgments or decisions. For instance, they may show poor judgment when managing cash, such as spending excessively with telemarketers, or making a bad decision (Eidi et al., 2006). They may give less consideration to personal grooming or to keeping themselves clean.

7.3.9 Withdrawal From Work or Social Activities

An individual with Alzheimer's may begin to withdraw themselves from pastimes, social activities, work ventures, or sports. They may experience difficulty following a favorite sports team or recalling the rules of a favorite pastime or hobby. Additionally, they may abstain from being sociable on account of problems they encounter, such as holding a conversation. Some of the time, they may feel disinterested in work, or with respect to family or social commitments (Fan et al., 2015).

7.3.10 Changes in Mood, Temperament, and Personality

The mood and personality of individuals with Alzheimer's can change. They can become confused, suspicious, depressed, fearful, or anxious. They might be easily upset at home, at work, or with friends, or where they are out of their comfort zone. They may develop particular ways of getting things done and become irritable when a routine is upset (Gan, 2013).

7.4 CONCLUSION

AD is portrayed clinically by memory deficiencies, weakened intellectual capacity, and unseemly conduct. Presently, in developing countries like India and China, a subject with AD is typically an old to very old individual. Curative treatment for AD is currently not available, yet symptomatic treatment with ethnomedicinal plants may improve memory loss and other dementia-related issues. Characteristic plant materials have been used as medication with which to treat different human conditions since time immemorial. Northeast India is home to great biodiversity, including a wide assortment of plant species, not many of which have been evaluated for remedial medical usage. Unresearched medicinal plant species have been used as memory enhancers by the local peoples of Northeast India. It was discovered that the vast majority of the ethnomedicinal plants exert their activity toward AD as a reflection of their phytochemical composition. The most significant innate ethnobotanic tribal networks in Northeast India are the Lepcha and Bhutia in Sikkim, Rabha and Deori in Assam, Adi, Nyishi, Apatani, Monpa, and Wancho in Arunachal Pradesh, Naga in Nagaland, Garo and Khasi in Meghalaya, the Mizo in Mizoram, some Naga clans, Mac, and Paite in Manipur, and Tripuri, Riang, and Chakma in Tripura. Every one of these clans varies with respect to population size, degree of sociocultural and economic advancement, methods for subsistence, religion, and language. Northeast India has extraordinary natural assets, such as plant species, which, for the most part, have been untapped. This biodiversity is the reason why individuals of local tribes of the north east depend on plant-based medications to treat different ailments, using various treatments. In this section of this chapter, an ethnobotanical survey of the medicinal plants, used at the different altitudes of the Himalayan region of Northeast India, was coordinated to select helpful plants that are potential reservoirs of therapeutics for administration to treat AD. The present chapter describes the associations between these properties in the plants, with the purpose of finding new phytomedicines that can be used in the treatment of AD. The vision of the chapter is to develop new ideal models for the identification of lead chemicals for phytomedicine on a worldwide premise, including new plant combinations and new preparations and formulations for the treatment of AD.

ACKNOWLEDGMENTS

I offer my sincere gratitude to the almighty God and my beloved Parents, Wife and Daughter. I am thankful to the Head of the Department, Vice-Chancellor, and Registrar of North Bengal University (NBU), West Bengal, India for their moral support.

REFERENCES

Akhondzadeh S., Noroozian M., Mohammadi M., Salvia officinalis extract in the treatment of patients with mild to moderate Alzheimer's disease: a double blind, randomized and placebo-controlled trial. *J Clin Pharm Ther.* 2003; 28:53–59.

Amala S., Yong P., Joseph F., *Centella asiatica* extract improves behavioral deficits in a mouse model of Alzheimer's disease: investigation of a possible mechanism of action. *Int J Alzheimer Dis.* 2012; 38:974–976.

Ambawade S., Kasture V., Kasture S., Anxiolytic activity of *Glycyrrhiza glabra* Linn. *J Nat Remed.* 2009; 2:130–134.

Andrieu S., Ousset P. J., Coley N., Ouzid M., Mathiex-Fortunet H., Vellas B., Guide age study: a 5-year double blind, randomised trial of EGb 761 for the prevention of Alzheimer's disease in elderly subjects with memory complaints. Rationale, design and baseline data. *Curr Alzheimer Res.* 2008; 5:406–415.

Arendt T., Synaptic degeneration in Alzheimer's disease. *Acta Neuropathol.* 2009; 118:167–179.

Arulselvan P., Subramanian S. P., Beneficial effects of *Murraya koenigii* leaves on antioxidant defense system and ultra-structural changes of pancreatic beta-cells in experimental diabetes in rats. *Chem Biol Interact.* 2007; 165:155–164.

Asgarpanah J., Kazemivash N., Phytochemistry and pharmacologic properties of *Myristica fragrans* Hoyutt.: a review. *Afr J Biotechnol.* 2012; 11:12787–12793.

Asuthosh S., Malini K., Bairy M., Effect of *Tinospora cordifolia* on learning and memory in normal and memory deficits rats. *Ind J Pharmacol.* 2000; 34:339–349.

Auddy B., Hazra J., Mitra A., Abedon B., Ghosal S., A standardized *Withania somnifera* extract significantly reduces stress-related parameters in chronically stressed humans: a double-blind randomized, placebo-controlled study. *J Am Nutra Assoc.* 2008; 11:50–56.

Avila J., Lucas J., Pérez M., Hernåndez F., Role of tau protein in both physiological and pathological conditions. *Physiol Rev.* 2004; 84:361–384.

Ballard C., Gauthier S., Corbett A., Brayne C., Aarsland D., Jones E., Alzheimer's disease. *Lancet.* 2011; 377:1019–1031.

Bamburg J. R., Bloom C. S., Cytoskeletal pathologies of Alzheimer's disease. *Cell Motif Cytoskel.* 2009; 66:635–649.

Barrios-Gonzalez J., Miranda R. U., Biotechnological production and applications of statins. *Appl Microbiol Biotechnol.* 2010; 85:869–883.

Bastianetto S., Ramassamy C., Dore S., Christen Y., Poirier J., Quirion R., The *Ginkgo biloba* extract (EGb 761) protects hippocampal neurons against cell death induced by beta-amyloid. *Eur J Neurosci.* 2000; 12:1882–1890.

Bastianetto S., Zheng W. H., Quirion R., The *Ginkgo biloba* extract (EGb 761) protects and rescues hippocampal cells against nitric oxide-induced toxicity: involvement of its flavonoid constituents and protein kinase C. *J Neurochem.* 2000; 74:2268–2277.

Bastos D., Oliveira D., Matsumoto R., Carvalo P., Ribeiro M., Yerba mate (*Ilex paraguariensis*): pharmacological research, research and biotechnology. *Med Plant Aromat Plant Sci Biotechnol.* 2007; 1:37–46.

Baurle P., Suter A., Wormstall H., Safety and effectiveness of a traditional ginkgo fresh plant extract – results from a clinical trial. *Forsch Komplementmed.* 2009; 16:156–161.

Bhanumathy M., Harish M. S., Shivaprasad H. N., Sushma G., Nootropic activity of *Celastrus paniculatus* seed. *Pharm Biol.* 2010; 48:324–327.

Bihaqi S. W., Singh A. P., Tiwari M., In vivo investigation of the neuroprotective property of *Convolvulus pluricaulis* in scopolamineinduced cognitive impairments in Wistar rats. *Ind J Pharmacol.* 2011; 43:520–525.

Birari R., Javia V., Bhutani K. K., Antiobesity and lipid lowering effects of *Murraya koenigii* (L.) Spreng leaves extracts and mahanimbine on high fat diet induced obese rats. *Fitoterapia.* 2010; 81:1129–1133.

Bradwejn J., Zhou Y., Koszycki D., Shlik J., A double-blind, placebo-controlled study on the effects of Gotu Kola (*Centella asiatica*) on acoustic startle response in healthy subjects. *J Clin Psychopharmacol.* 2000; 20:680–684.

Calabrese C., Gregory W. L., Leo M., Kraemer D., Bone K., Oken B., Effects of a standardized *Bacopa monnieri* extract on cognitive performance, anxiety, and depression in the elderly: a randomized, double-blind, placebo-controlled trial. *J Altern Complement Med.* 2008; 14:707–713.

Cambay Z., Baydas G., Tuzcu M., Pomegranate (*Punica granatum* L.) flowers improves learning and memory performances impaired by diabetes mellitus in rats. *Acta Physiol Hung.* 2011; 98:409–420.

Carlo C., William L., Michael L., Effects of a standardized *Bacopa monnieri* extract on cognitive performance, anxiety, and depression in the elderly: a randomized, double-blind, placebo-controlled trial. *J Altern Complement Med.* 2008; 14:707–713.

Cecchini S., Martinez R., *Inclusive Social Protection in Latin America: A Comprehensive, Rights-based Approach*, Santiago, Chile, United Nations, 2012; 5:18–20.

Chandrasekaran K., Mehrabian Z., Spinnewyan B., Drieu K., Kiskum G., Neuroprotective effects of bilobalide, a component of *Ginkgo biloba* extract (EGb 761), in gerbil global brain ischemia. *Brain Res.* 2011; 922:282–292.

Chen Y. L., Lin K. F., Shiao M. S., Chen Y. T., Hong C. Y., Lin S. J., A potent antioxidant from *Magnolia officinalis*, attenuates intimal thickening and MCP-1 expression after balloon injury of the aorta in cholesterol fed rabbits. *Basic Res Cardiol.* 2001; 96:353–363.

Chengxuan Q., Miia K., Eva S., Epidemiology of Alzheimer's disease: occurrence, determinants, and strategies toward intervention. *Clin Neurosci.* 2009; 11:111–128.

Chiu J. H., Ho C. T., Wei Y. H., Lui W. Y., Hong C. Y., In vitro and in vivo protective effect of honokiol on rat liver from per oxidative injury. *Life Sci.* 1997; 61:1961–1971.

Cho I., Effects of Panax ginseng in neurodegenerative diseases. *J Ginseng Res.* 2012; 3:342–353.

Choi B. M., Kim H. J., Oh G. S., Pae H. O., Oh H., Jeong S., Kwon T. O., Kim Y. M., Chung H. T., 1,2,3,4,6-Penta-O-galloyl-beta-d-glucose protects rat neuronal cells (Neuro 2A) from hydrogen peroxide-mediated cell death via the induction of heme oxygenase-1. *Neurosci Lett.* 2002; 328:185–189.

Chou C. H., Gong C. L., Chao C. C., Lin C. H., Kwan C. Y., Hsieh C. L., Leung Y. M., Rhynchophylline from *Uncaria rhynchophylla* functionally turns delayed rectifiers into A-Type K+ channels. *J Nat Prod.* 2009; 72:830–834.

Christen Y., *Ginkgo biloba* and neurodegenerative disorders. *Front Biosci.* 2009; 9:3091–3104.

Citron M., Alzheimer's disease: strategies for disease modification. *Nat Rev Drug Discov.* 2010; 9:387–398.

Colpo G., Trevisol F., Teixeira A., Fachinetto R., Pereira R., Rocha B., *Ilex paraguariensis* has antioxidant potential and attenuates haloperidol-induced orofacial dyskinesia and memory dysfunction in rats. *Neurotox Res.* 2007; 12:171–180.

Das A., Mandal S., Banerjee S., Sinha S., Das J., Studies on antidiarrhoeal activity of *Punica granatum* seed extract in rats. *J Ethnopharmacol.* 1999; 68:205–208.

Dastagir G., Rizvi M., Review – *Glycyrrhiza glabra* L. (Liquorice). *Pak J Pharm Sci.* 2016; 29:1727–1733.

Dastmalchi K., Ollilainen V., Lackman P., Boije af Gennas G., Dorman H. J., Jarvinen P. P., Yli-Kauhaluoma J., Hiltunen R., Acetylcholinesterase inhibitory guided fractionation of *Melissa officinalis* L. *Bioorg Med Chem.* 2009; 17:867–871.

De Caires S., Steenkamp V., Use of Yokukansan (TJ-54) in the treatment of neurological disorders: a review. *Phytother Res.* 2010; 24:1265–1270.

Dhingra D., Parle M., Kulkarni S., Memory enhancing activity of *Glycyrrhiza glabra* in mice. *J Ethnopharmacol.* 2004; 91:361–365.

Dikalov S., Losik T., Arbiser J., Honokiol is a potent scavenger of superoxide and peroxyl radicals. *Biochem Pharmacol.* 2008; 76:589–596.

Dubey G. P., Pathak S. R., Gupta B. S., Combined effect of Brahmi (*Bacopa monnieri*) and Shankhpushpi (*Convolvulus pluricaulis*) on cognitive functions. *Pharmacopsychoecology.* 1994; 7:249–251.

Eidi M., Eidi A., Bahar M., An effect of *Salvia officinalis* leaves on memory retention and its interaction with the cholinergic system in rats. *J Nutr.* 2006; 22:321–326.

Elufioye T., Oladele A., Olutayo C., Agbedahunsi J., Adesanya S., Ethnomedicinal study and screening of plants used for memory enhancement and antiaging in Sagamu, Nigeria. *Europ J Med Plants.* 2012; 2:262–275.

Faiyaz A., Narendra J., Sharath C., Acetylcholine and memory-enhancing activity of *Ficus racemosa* bark. *Pharmacog Res.* 2011; 3:246–249.

Fan Z., Yao J., Li Y., Hu X., Shao H., Tian X., Anti-inflammatory and antioxidant effects of curcumin on acute lung injury in a rodent model of intestinal ischemia reperfusion by inhibiting the pathway of NF-Kb. *Int J Clin Exp Pathol.* 2015; 8:3451–3459.

Farokhnia M., Shafiee S. M., Iranpour N., Gougol A., Yekehtaz H., Alimardani R., Fasrad F., Kamalipour M., Akhondzadeh S., Comparing the efficacy and safety of *Crocus sativus* with memantine in patient with moderate to severe Alzheimer's disease: a double blind randomized clinical trial. *Hum Psychopharmacol.* 2014; 29:351–359.

Gan L., *Income Inequality and Consumption in China*, Texas A&M University, USA and Southwestern University of Finance and Economics, Chengdu, China, 2013; 5:9.

Gurung B., *The Medicinal Plants of Sikkim Himalaya*, Subash Publication, Gangtok, Sikkim, 2012; 3:46–58.

Pozen R. C., *Tackling the Chinese Pension System*, The Paulson Institute, Chicago, 2013:180–189.

Prince M. J., Wu F., Guo Y., Gutierrez Robledo L. M., O'Donnell M., Sullivan R., The burden of disease in older people and implications for health policy and practice. *Lancet.* 2015; 385:5–10.

Prince M., Acosta D., Albanese E., Arizaga R., Ferri C. P., Guerra M., Ageing and dementia in low and middle income countries – using research to engage with public and policy makers. *Int Rev Psychiatr.* 2008; 20(4):332–343.

The Wealth of India. *A Dictionary of Indian Raw Materials and Industrial Products – Raw Materials Series, Publication and Information Directorate*, CSIR, New Delhi, 2010; 1–X1:48–76.

Wimo A., Prince M., *World Alzheimer Report 2010*; *The Global Economic Impact of Dementia*. Alzheimer's Disease International, London, 2010.

World Health Organization. *Dementia*: A Public Health Priority. WHO, Geneva, 2012.

8 Neuroprotective Role of Resveratrol in Alzheimer's Disease

V. S. Dendi and Magisetty Obulesu

CONTENTS

ABBREVIATIONS

Aβ Amyloid-Beta
AD Alzheimer's Disease
ADP Adenosine Diphosphate
AMPK 5' Adenosine Monophosphate Activated Protein Kinase
APP Amyloid Precursor Protein
BBB Blood–Brain Barrier
Bor Borneol
CAT Catalase
COX-2 Cyclooxygenase-2
CSF Cerebrospinal Fluid
DDS Drug Delivery Systems
Fc-β-CD β-Cyclodextrin Nanovalves
FOXO Forkhead Box O
(GSH-Px) Glutathione Peroxidase
HD Huntington's Disease
HO-1 Heme Oxygenase-1
iNOS Inducible Nitric Oxide Synthase
JNK c-Jun N-Terminal Kinase

MCI	Mild Cognitive Impairment
MMP-9	Matrix Metalloproteinase-9
MSe	Mesoporous Nano-Selenium
mTOR	Mammalian Target Of Rapamycin
ND	Neurodegenerative Disease
NFTs	Neurofibrillary Tangles
PC 12	Pheochromocytoma
PCG1-α	Peroxisome Proliferator Activated Receptor Gamma Coactivator 1-alpha
PD	Parkinson's Disease
ROS	Reactive Oxygen Species
RSFC	Resting-State Functional Connectivity
SAMP8	Senescent Accelerated Mouse-Prone
SIRT1	Sirtuin 1
SOD	Superoxide Dismutase

8.1 INTRODUCTION

AD is the most common neurodegenerative disease (ND), affecting millions of people aged more than 65 years in the United States (Esfandiarei et al., 2019). Characteristics of AD include extracellular accumulation of amyloid-β (Aβ), intraneuronal neurofibrillary tangles (NFTs), metal dyshomeostasis, oxidative stress, and apoptosis (Kolarova et al., 2012; Esfandiarei et al., 2019). Increased Aβ accumulation and inflammatory factor levels in the brains of AD patients provoke enhanced production of reactive oxygen species (ROS) by glial cells (Raine, 2000; Hu et al., 2015b; Kwon et al., 2016; Sun et al., 2019). Scant knowledge about the appropriate AD pathogenic factor has markedly impeded the treatment of AD (Kong et al., 2019).

8.2 RESVERATROL

8.2.1 Chemistry

Resveratrol was first isolated and identified from the roots of white hellebore (*Veratrum grandiflorum* O. Loes) in 1940, and functionally classified as a phytoalexin, although it can be structurally categorized in either the stilbene or the polyphenol group (Baur and Sinclair 2006; Delmas et al., 2006; Kores et al., 2019). Despite the discovery of resveratrol in 1940, there were no adequate studies performed on it until the 1990s (Frankel et al., 1993; Pace-Asciak et al., 1996; Blardi et al., 1999; Singh et al., 2019). It has been observed that resveratrol is abundantly available in red wine (Siemann and Creasy, 1992; Lejri et al., 2019). Although resveratrol is available in both *cis* and *trans*-isomeric forms, the *trans* form has been extensively studied due to its incredible health benefits (Borriello et al., 2014; Singh et al., 2019). In addition, the *trans* form is the principal and highly stable form (Gambini et al., 2015; Singh et al., 2019). This polyphenol was found to play a potentially pivotal role in AD treatment (Richard et al., 2011; Lejri et al., 2019). It exhibits antioxidant properties and inhibited oxidative damage by reducing inducible nitric oxide synthase (iNOS) and cyclooxygenase-2 (COX-2) levels (Karuppagounder et al., 2009; Lejri et al., 2019).

8.2.2 Pathways of Protective Efficacy

Polyphenols play a pivotal role in attenuating the AD disease progression in humans (Esfandiarei et al., 2019). Resveratrol (3,5,4 –trihydroxy-*trans*-stilbene) is a phytoalexin abundantly available in grapes, wine, and peanuts, with health benefits such as antioxidant, anti-inflammatory, antiaging, antitumor, and cardioprotective activities (Baur and Sinclair, 2006; Izquierdo et al., 2019). Accordingly, resveratrol offers substantial antioxidant and anti-inflammatory protection against NDs (Renaud and de Lorgeril, 1992; Pervaiz, 2003; de Sa Countinho et al., 2018; Esfandiarei et al., 2019; Obulesu, 2019). Resveratrol shows significant neuroprotection against both AD and Parkinson's disease (PD) (Sun et al., 2010; Gomes et al., 2018; Xia et al., 2019; Izquierdo et al., 2019).

Reveratrol also ameliorates mitochondrial function through its impact on several signaling pathways, antioxidant effects, and the enhancement of Aβ scavenging (Ma et al., 2014; Lejri et al., 2019). Resveratrol shows an impact on the Aβ-induced apoptotic signaling pathway by sirtuin 1 (SIRT-1) activation, involving inhibition of expression of caspase protein-3, the apoptotic regulator bax, c-Jun N-terminal kinase (JNK) activation, Forkhead box O (FOXO), and tumor suppressor protein p53 (Ma et al., 2014; Lejri et al., 2019). Aβ25–35-induced neurotoxicity in PC 12 cells was overcome by resveratrol (20 μM) through tyrosyl tRNA synthetase-poly(ADP ribose) polymerase I and SIRT-1 pathway-dependent autophagy (Deng and Mi, 2016; Lejri et al., 2019).

8.2.3 Combination Treatment and Dietary Supplementation

Exercise training and resveratrol treatment profoundly improved cardiac function and aortic elastin morphology in the 3xTg mouse model of AD (Esfandiarei et al., 2019). A wealth of studies has also shown that the combination of exercise and resveratrol substantially prevented AD-associated cognitive decline (Adlard et al., 2005; Scarmeas et al., 2009; Rayalam et al., 2011; Tou, 2015; Alkhouli et al., 2019). Maternal resveratrol supplementation for two months ameliorated the cognitive deficit in Senescent Accelerated Mouse-Prone (SAMP8) offspring (Izquierdo et al., 2019). In line with this finding, cognitive improvement was confirmed by the novel object recognition and Morris Water Maze tests (Izquierdo et al., 2019). Dietary intake of resveratrol improved cognition and molecular pathways in the hippocampus of normal, aged, and AD mouse models (Rahman, 2008; Porquet et al., 2014; Palomera-Avaloes et al., 2017, 2018; Izquierdo et al., 2019). Based on these findings, considerable attention has been paid toward the elucidation of molecular mechanisms involved in neuroprotection induced by resveratrol (Izquierdo et al., 2019).

8.2.4 Resveratrol Analogs

Modifications to the structure of resveratrol, that affect its biological properties, include the number and position of hydroxyl groups, substitution of hydroxyl groups, intramolecular hydrogen bonds, hosting of extra double bonds, and stereoisomerism (Murias et al., 2004; Ovesna and Horvathova-Kozics, 2005; Li et al., 2014; Savio et al., 2016; Borys et al., 2017; Singh et al., 2019). The more lipophilic nature of methylated resveratrol makes it more bioavailable than resveratrol (Cardile et al., 2007; Singh et al., 2019). Acetylation of resveratrol also improves bioavailability (Colin et al., 2009; Singh et al., 2019). The triple-bond resveratrol analog (3,4',5-trihydroxy-diphenylacetylene) exhibited enhanced anti-inflammatory activity, compared with resveratrol (Antus et al., 2015; Singh et al., 2019). A conjugated phenolic ring system facilitates the conjugation of resveratrol to targets at both deep and/or shallow cavities (Saqib et al., 2018; Singh et al., 2019).

8.2.5 Amyloid–Beta (Aβ)

Mounting evidence has also shown that resveratrol reduces amyloidogenic cleavage of APP, thus mitigating Aβ aggregation (Venkatesan et al., 2009; Hu et al., 2015; Xie et al., 2019). Resveratrol and its glucoside substantially reduced Aβ aggregation (Phan et al., 2019). However, resveratrol enhanced Aβ fibrillation before its inhibitory effect on the aggregation process (Phan et al., 2019). Decreased levels of Aβ were found in resveratrol-treated mouse brains (Karuppagounder et al., 2009; Phan et al., 2019). It has been assumed that Aβ polymerization can be averted using polyphenols, either by directly intervening with Aβ or by binding to its ions (Velander et al., 2017; Phan et al., 2019). Aβ and tau proteins affect mitochondria synergistically, each, in turn, intensifying the toxicity of the other (Ittner and Gotz, 2011; Lejri et al., 2019). Resveratrol reduces Aβ toxicity and attenuates the inflammatory response, as well as showing neuroprotective effects on cells (Baur et al., 2006; Lagouge et al., 2006; Capiralla et al., 2012; Sun et al., 2019). Hypoxia increases total extracellular Aβ1-40 to Aβ1-42 levels, and also increases Aβ1-40 to Aβ1-42 levels in exosomes obtained from APP-overexpressing SH-SY5Y human neuroblastoma cells (Xie et al., 2018, 2019). Resveratrol treatment prevented hypoxia-induced increase in Aβ1-40 to Aβ1-42 levels in the hippocampal lysates and serum-derived exosomes of C57BL/6 mice (Xie et al., 2019).

8.2.6 Metabolism

Resveratrol is swiftly metabolized, primarily into sulfo- and glucuronide forms, which are also removed through urine (Kores et al., 2019). Most of the *trans*-resveratrol and its metabolites are attached to lipoproteins in the plasma (Kores et al., 2019). When orally administered, the concentration of the free resveratrol form was so low that it could not be detected (Cottart et al., 2010; Kores et al., 2019). Free resveratrol mediates cellular processes by inducing vital metabolic proteins like SIRT-1, Peroxisome proliferator-activated receptor gamma coactivator 1-alpha (PCG1-α), and 5' adenosine monophosphate activated protein kinase (AMPK)

(Canto and Auwerx, 2009a, b; Zhou et al., 2018; Lejri et al., 2019). Indeed, the vital neuroprotective ability of resveratrol is based on the activity of SIRT-1 and AMPK, and on the acetylation/phosphorylation status of PGC-1α, which subsequently induces mitochondrial biogenesis, resulting in increased mitochondrial activity (Kulkarni and Canto, 2015; Lejri et al., 2019). Moreover, resveratrol has multiple additional effects, such as increased mitochondrial biogenesis by AMPK activation (Pirola and Frojdo, 2008; Diaz-Gerevini et al., 2016; Price et al., 2012) and decreased autophagy by mammalian target of rapamycin (mTOR) (Park et al., 2016; Izquierdo et al., 2019).

It has also been shown that resveratrol administration substantially decreases cerebrospinal fluid (CSF) concentrations of MMP-9, Aβ40, and Aβ42 (Moussa et al., 2017; Singh et al., 2019). It also showed protective efficacy in animal models of PD and Huntington's disease (HD) (Gerszon et al., 2014; Singh et al., 2019). Resveratrol shows robust antioxidant activity by exhibiting free radical scavenging ability substantially higher than antioxidants such as vitamin E, vitamin C, and propyl gallate, due to the existence of aromatic rings (Soares et al., 2003; Singh et al., 2019). It has also been proven that resveratrol intake improves memory and glucose metabolism, and is capable of enhancing the hippocampal functional link in older people to achieve a healthy aging brain (Witte et al., 2014; Lejri et al., 2019). Conversely, in healthy young people, no influence on cognitive function was observed (Kennedy et al., 2010; Wightman et al., 2014; Lejri et al., 2019).

8.2.7 Resveratrol and Estrogen

Resveratrol's structure resembles the structure of estrogen diethylstilbestrol. It has been observed that AD is associated with lower estrogen levels (Kong et al., 2019). Reduced estrogen levels were found in postmenopausal women. Furthermore, female AD patients showed steeper cognitive decline than did male patients, thus corroborating the role of estrogen in AD pathogenesis (Wei, 2000; Kong et al., 2019). Several lines of evidence have shown that estrogen enhances neuronal activity markedly and inhibits Aβ aggregation, and so can also be used to treat AD (Yang et al., 2012; Kong et al., 2019). Around 15% of women older than 65 suffer from AD, unlike men, where the frequency is approximately 5–6% (Kong et al., 2019). The potential reason for this significant difference is the synthesis of estrogen in the male brain by aromatase-induced catalysis of testosterone or its *de novo* generation by glial cells or neurons (Kong et al., 2019).

8.2.8 Animal Models

Resveratrol improved spatial capabilities, enhancing the expression of glutathione peroxidase (GSH-Px), superoxide dismutase (SOD), catalase (CAT) and hemeoxidase-1 (HO-1), in turn

(Kong et al., 2019). Even at the very low concentration of 0.2 mg/l, resveratrol profoundly blocked Aβ neuropathology and AD-type decline in spatial memory function in Tg2576 mice, which over-express the mutant isoform 695 of APP (Wang et al., 2006; Lejri et al., 2019). In another study, dietary intake of resveratrol (300 mg/kg) reduced Aβ plaque formation in a transgenic mouse model of AD (Tg19959) (Karuppagounder et al., 2009; Lejri et al., 2019). At 5 µg/µl, resveratrol-induced SIRT-1 induction inhbited learning impairment and hippocampal degeneration in the inducible p25 transgenic mouse model of tauopathy and AD (Kim et al., 2007; Lejri et al., 2019). The 3xTg mouse model of AD is susceptible to limb bone fracture, compared with wild-type mice. Resveratrol treatment or exercise, or a combination treatment, ameliorated fracture resistance and cross-sectional geometric indicators of bone strength (Alkhouli et al., 2019).

8.2.9 Human Subjects

Consumption of grapes (containing resveratrol in the skins and seeds) by patients with mild cognitive impairment (MCI) was associated with a protective effect against pathological metabolic deterioration (Lee et al., 2017; Lejri et al., 2019). In another study, conducted on 80 postmenopausal women between 45 and 85 years of age, it was observed that continuous intake of resveratrol (75 mg twice daily) substantially improved cerebrovascular function and reduced the risk of cognitive decline (Evans et al., 2017; Lejri et al., 2019). In another study, resveratrol intake (200 mg/d, 26 weeks) decreased glycated hemoglobin A1c levels, restored hippocampal volume, and increased hippocampal resting-state functional connectivity (RSFC) in 40 well-categorized MCI patients (21 females, 19 males; 50–80 years) (Kobe et al., 2017; Lejri et al., 2019). Further trials are currently in progress (NIH, 2016; Lejri et al., 2019). Turner et al. (2015) showed that resveratrol (at dosages from 500 mg/d to 2 g/d) was well tolerated, inhibited rises in Aβ levels in CSF, but showed no marked effect on cognitive score in AD patients (Lejri et al., 2019). Moreover, recent studies have also shown the role of resveratrol in the regulation of AD biomarker pathways (Sawda et al., 2017; Lejri et al., 2019).

8.2.10 Disadvantages of Resveratrol

Although resveratrol shows appreciable therapeutic efficacy toward several diseases, a few demerits, such as low stability and bioavailability, increased metabolism, low water solubility, and low membrane-spanning ability, impede its potential considerably (Crandall and Barzilai, 2013; Kores et al., 2019).

8.2.11 Nanotechnology

Drug delivery systems (DDS) offer appreciable advantages, such as enhanced systemic circulation, increased drug accumulation in target tissues, and controlled drug release (Zheng et al., 2016; Huang et al., 2017; Sun et al., 2019). Additionally, DDS can be modified to accomplish desired benefits, such as blood–brain barrier (BBB) targeting, initiating a release response. To overcome the shortcomings associated with resveratrol (Section 8.2.10), water-in-oil-in-water emulsions with *trans*-resveratrol (Wang et al., 2017), a soluble galenical form conjugated to chitosan (Amiot et al., 2013), and liposomal formulations are currently in use (Yang et al., 2017; Kores et al., 2019).

Several studies have shown that mesoporous nano-selenium (MSe) can decrease Aβ accumulation and neurotoxicity (Zhang et al., 2014; Zhou et al., 2015; Sun et al., 2019). Recently, a resveratrol-loaded innovative MSe delivery system (MSe-Res/Fc-β-CD/Bor), based on a borneol (Bor) target, β-cyclodextrin nanovalves (Fc-β-CD) were discovered. It has been observed that this delivery system first encounters blood or intracellular esterases and releases Bor, facilitating the entry of the nanosystem through the BBB. Furthermore, the Fc-β-CD is exposed, by the redox (H_2O_2) response, to the release of resveratrol at the target site. This delivery system successfully protected nerve cells and ameliorated memory dysfunction in APP/PS1 mice by attenuating Aβ accumulation, tau hyperphosphorylation, and oxidative stress (Sun et al., 2019).

8.3 CONCLUSION

Despite the profound therapeutic efficacy of resveratrol, the mechanism underlying its neuroprotective effect remains elusive (Izquierdo et al., 2019). The therapeutic ability, safety, and pharmacokinetics of resveratrol have been extensively explored in 244 clinical trials, with a further 27 clinical trials currently in progress (Singh et al., 2019). Despite the lack of clarity on the mechanism, the phytoestrogenic nature of resveratrol probably aids its therapeutic efficacy (Gehm et al., 1997; Singh et al., 2019). A wealth of studies has shown the health benefits of resveratrol and its protective effect against multiple diseases. However, a few studies have shown that its intake induces side effects, such as headache, dizziness, or epididymitis in a few participants (Almeida et al., 2009; Singh et al., 2019). The DDS employed to overcome challenges associated with resveratrol has profoundly improved its efficacy. Therefore, designing more appropriate nanotechnology-based modifications, to enhance the neuroprotective efficacy of such pivotal polyphenols to combat NDs, such as AD, is an urgent need in the field of neuroscience and nanoscience.

REFERENCES

Adlard PA, Perreau VM, Pop V, Cotman CW. Voluntary exercise decreases amyloid load in a transgenic model of Alzheimer's disease. *J Neurosci.* 2005;25:4217–4221.

Alkhouli MF, Hung J, Squire M, Anderson M, Castro M, Babu JR, Al-Nakkash L, Broderick TL, Plochocki JH. Exercise and resveratrol increase fracture resistance in the 3xTg-AD mouse model of Alzheimer's disease. *BMC Complement Altern Med.* 2019;19:39.

Almeida L, Vaz-da-Silva M, Falcao A, Soares E, Costa R, Loureiro AI, Fernandes-Lopes C, Rocha JF, Nunes T, Wright L, Soares-da-Silva P. Pharmacokinetic and safety profile of trans-resveratrol in a rising multiple dose study in healthy volunteers. *Mol Nutr Food Res.* 2009;53 Supplement 1:S7–S15.

Amiot MJ, Romier B, Anh Dao TM, Fanciullino R, Ciccolini J, Burcelin R, Pechere L, Emond C, Savouret JF, Seree E. Optimization of trans-resveratrol bioavailability for human therapy. *Biochimie.* 2013;95:1233–1238.

Antus C, Radnai B, Dombovari P, Fonai F, Avar P, Matyus P, Racz B, Sumegi B, Veres B. Anti-inflammatory effects of a triple-bond resveratrol analog: structure and function relationship. *Eur J Pharmacol.* 2015;748:61–67.

Baur JA, Pearson KJ, Price NL, Jamieson HA, Lerin C, Kalra A, Prabhu VV, Allard JS, Lopez-Lluch G, Lewis K, Pistell PJ, Poosala S, Becker KG, Boss O, Gwinn D, Wang M, Ramaswamy S, Fishbein KW, Spencer RG, Lakatta EG, Le Couteur D, Shaw RJ, Navas P, Puigserver P, Ingram DK, de Cabo R, Sinclair DA. Resveratrol improves health and survival of mice on a high-calorie diet. *Nature.* 2006;444:337.

Baur JA, Sinclair DA. Therapeutic potential of resveratrol: the in vivo evidence. *Nat Rev Drug Discov.* 2006;5:493–506.

Blardi P, De Lalla A, Volpi L, Di Perri T. Stimulation of endogenous adenosine release by oral administration of quercetin and resveratrol in man. *Drugs Exp Clin Res.* 1999;25:105–110.

Borriello A, Bencivenga D, Caldarelli I, Tramontano A, Borgia A, Zappia V, Della Ragione F. Resveratrol: from basic studies to bedside. *Advances in Nutrition and Cancer.* Berlin, Heidelberg: Springer, 2014;159:167–184.

Borys S, Khozmi R, Kranc W, Bryja A, Jeseta M, Kempisty B. Resveratrol and its analogues – is it a new strategy of anticancer therapy? *Adv Cell Biol.* 2017;5:32–42.

Canto C, Auwerx J. Caloric restriction, SIRT1 and longevity. *Trends Endocrinol Metab.* 2009a;20:325–331.

Canto C, Auwerx J. PGC-1α, SIRT1 and AMPK, an energy sensing network that controls energy expenditure. *Curr Opin Lipidol.* 2009b;20:98–105.

Capiralla H, Vingtdeux V, Zhao H, Sankowski R, Al-Abed Y, Davies P, Marambaud P. Resveratrol mitigates lipopolysaccharide- and Aβ-mediated microglial inflammation by inhibiting the TLR4/NF-κB/STAT signaling cascade. *J Neurochem.* 2012;120:461–472.

Cardile V, Chillemi R, Lombardo L, Sciuto S, Spatafora C, Tringali C. Antiproliferative activity of methylated analogues of E-and Z-resveratrol. *Z Naturforsch C.* 2007;62:189–195.

Colin D, Gimazane A, Lizard G, Izard JC, Solary E, Latruffe N, Delmas D. Effects of resveratrol analogs on cell cycle progression, cell cycle associated proteins and 5fluoro-uracil sensitivity in human derived colon cancer cells. *Int J Cancer.* 2009;124:2780–2788.

Cottart CH, Nivet-Antoine V, Laguillier-Morizot C, Beaudeux JL. Resveratrol bioavailability and toxicity in humans. *Mol Nutr Food Res.* 2010;54:7–16.

Crandall JP, Barzilai N. Exploring the promise of resveratrol: where do we go from here? *Diabetes.* 2013;62:1022–1023.

de Sa Coutinho D, Pacheco MT, Frozza RL, Bernardi A. Antiinflammatory effects of resveratrol: mechanistic insights. *Int J Mol Sci.* 2018;19:1812.

Delmas D, Lancon A, Colin D, Jannin B, Latruffe N. Resveratrol as a chemopreventive agent: a promising molecule for fighting cancer. *Curr Drug Targets.* 2006;7:423–442.

Deng H, Mi MT. Resveratrol attenuates Aβ25–35 caused neurotoxicity by inducing autophagy through the TyrRS-PARP1-SIRT1 signaling pathway. *Neurochem Res.* 2016;41:2367–2379.

Diaz-Gerevini GT, Repossi G, Dain A, Tarres MC, Das UN, Eynard AR. Beneficial action of resveratrol: how and why? *Nutrition.* 2016;32:174–178.

Esfandiarei M, Hoxha B, Talley NA, Anderson MR, Alkhouli MF, Squire MA, Eckman DM, Babu JR, Lopaschuk GD, Broderick TL. Beneficial effects of resveratrol and exercise training on cardiac and aortic function and structure in the 3xTg mouse model of Alzheimer's disease. *Drug Des Dev Ther.* 2019;13:1197–1211.

Evans H, Howe P, Wong R. Effects of resveratrol on cognitive performance, mood and cerebrovascular function in post-menopausal women; a 14-week randomized placebo-controlled intervention trial. *Nutrients.* 2017;9:27.

Frankel EN, German JB, Kinsella JE, Parks E, Kanner J. Inhibition of oxidation of human low-density lipoprotein by phenolic substances in red wine. *Lancet.* 1993;341:454–457.

Gambini J, Ingles M, Olaso G, Lopez-Grueso R, Bonet-Costa V, Gimeno-Mallench L, Mas-Bargues C, Abdelaziz KM, Gomez-Cabrera MC, Vina J, Borras C. Properties of resveratrol: in vitro and in vivo studies about metabolism, bioavailability, and biological effects in animal models and humans. *Oxid Med Cell Longev.* 2015;2015:837042.

Gehm BD, McAndrews JM, Chien PY, Jameson JL. Resveratrol, a polyphenolic compound found in grapes and wine, is an agonist for the estrogen receptor. *Proc Natl Acad Sci.* 1997;94:14138–14143.

Gerszon J, Rodacka A, Puchała M. Antioxidant properties of resveratrol and its protective effects in neurodegenerative diseases. *Adv Cell Biol.* 2014;4:97–117.

Gomes BAQ, Silva JPB, Romeiro CFR, Dos Santos SM, Rodrigues CA, Goncalves PR, Sakai JT, Mendes PFS, Varela ELP, Monteiro MC. Neuroprotective mechanisms of resveratrol in Alzheimer's disease: role of SIRT1. *Oxid Med Cell Longev.* 2018;2018:8152373.

Hu B, Dai F, Fan Z, Ma G, Tang Q, Zhang X. Nanotheranostics: congo red/rutin-MNPs with enhanced magnetic resonance imaging and H2O2-responsive therapy of Alzheimer's disease in APPswe/PS1dE9 transgenic mice. *Adv Mater.* 2015a;27:5499–5505.

Hu J, Lin T, Gao Y, Xu J, Jiang C, Wang G, Bu G, Xu H, Chen H, Zhang YW. The resveratrol trimer miyabenol C inhibits beta-secretase activity and beta-amyloid generation. *PloS One.* 2015b;10:e0115973.

Huang H, Shi H, Liu J, Min Y, Wang Y, Wang AZ, Wang J, Liu Y. Co-delivery of all-transretinoic acid enhances the anti-metastasis effect of albumin-bound paclitaxel nanoparticles. *Chem Commun.* 2017;53:212–215.

Ittner LM, Gotz J. Amyloid-β and tau—a toxic pas de deux in Alzheimer's disease. *Nat Rev Neurosci.* 2011;12:65–72.

Izquierdo V, Palomera-Avalos V, Lopez-Ruiz S, Canudas AM, Pallas M, Grinan-Ferre C. Maternal resveratrol supplementation prevents cognitive decline in senescent mice offspring. *Int J Mol Sci.* 2019;20:(In press).

Karuppagounder SS, Pinto JT, Xu H, Chen HL, Beal MF, Gibson GE. Dietary supplementation with resveratrol reduces plaque pathology in a transgenic model of Alzheimer's disease. *Neurochem Int.* 2009;54:111–118.

Kennedy DO, Wightman EL, Reay, JL, Lietz G, Okello EJ, Wilde A, Haskell CF. Effects of resveratrol on cerebral blood flow variables and cognitive performance in humans: a double-blind, placebo-controlled, crossover investigation. *Am J Clin Nutr.* 2010;91:1590–1597.

Kim D, Nguyen MD, Dobbin MM, Fischer A, Sananbenesi F, Rodgers JT, Delalle I, Baur JA, Sui G, Armour SM, Puigserver P, Sinclair DA, Tsai LH. SIRT1 deacetylase protects against neurodegeneration in models for Alzheimer's disease and amyotrophic lateral sclerosis. *EMBO J.* 2007;26:3169–3179.

Kobe T, Witte AV, Schnelle A, Tesky VA, Pantel J, Schuchardt JP, Hahn A, Bohlken J, Grittner U, Floel A. Impact of resveratrol on glucose control, hippocampal structure and connectivity, and memory performance in patients with mild cognitive impairment. *Front Neurosci.* 2017;11:105.

Kolarova M, Garcia-Sierra F, Bartos A, Ricny J, Ripova D. Structure and pathology of tau protein in Alzheimer disease. *Int J Alzheimers Dis*. 2012;2012:731526.

Kong D, Yan Y, He XY, Yang H, Liang B, Wang J, He Y, Ding Y, Yu H. Effects of Resveratrol on the mechanisms of antioxidants and estrogen in Alzheimer's disease. *Biomed Res Int*. 2019;2019:8983752.

Kores K, Lesnik S, Bren U, Janezic D, Konc J. Discovery of novel potential human targets of resveratrol by inverse molecular docking. *J Chem Inf Model*. 2019;59:2467–2478.

Kulkarni SS, Canto C. The molecular targets of resveratrol. *Biochim Biophys Acta*. 2015;1852:1114–1123.

Kwon HJ, Cha MY, Kim D, Kim DK, Soh M, Shin K, Hyeon T, Mook-Jung I. Mitochondria targeting ceria nanoparticles as antioxidants for Alzheimer's disease. *ACS Nano*. 2016;10:2860–2870.

Lagouge M, Argmann C, Gerhart-Hines Z, Meziane H, Lerin C, Daussin FN, Milne J, Lambert P, Elliott P, Geny B, Laakso M, Puigserver P, Auwerx J. Resveratrol improves mitochondrial function and protects against metabolic disease by activating SIRT1 and PGC-1α. *Cell*. 2006;127:1109–1122.

Lee J, Torosyan N, Silverman DH. Examining the impact of grape consumption on brain metabolism and cognitive function in patients with mild decline in cognition: a double-blinded placebo controlled pilot study. *Exp Gerontol*. 2017;87(Part A):121–128.

Lejri I, Agapouda A, Grimm A, Eckert A. Mitochondria- and oxidative stress-targeting substances in cognitive decline-related disorders: from molecular mechanisms to clinical evidence. *Oxid Med Cell Longev*. 2019;2019:9695412.

Li C, Xu X, Wang XJ, Pan Y. Imine resveratrol analogues: molecular design, Nrf2 activation and SAR analysis. *PloS One*. 2014;9:e101455.

Ma T, Tan MS, Yu JT, Tan L. Resveratrol as a therapeutic agent for Alzheimer's disease. *BioMed Res Int*. 2014;2014:350516.

Moussa C, Hebron M, Huang X, Ahn J, Rissman RA, Aisen PS, Turner RS. Resveratrol regulates neuroinflammation and induces adaptive immunity in Alzheimer's disease. *J Neuroinflamm*. 2017;14:1.

Murias M, Handler N, Erker T, Pleban K, Ecker G, Saiko P, Szekeres T, Jager W. Resveratrol analogues as selective cyclooxygenase-2 inhibitors: synthesis and structure–activity relationship. *Bioorg Med Chem*. 2004;12:5571–5578.

National Institutes of Health. *CTg, BDPP Treatment for Mild Cognitive Impairment (MCI) and Prediabetes (BDPP)*, June 2016. https://clinicaltrials.gov/ct2/show/NCT02502253.

Obulesu M. Chapter 4: natural compounds in the treatment of Parkinson's disease. In *Parkinson's Disease Therapeutics: Emphasis on Nanotechnological Advances*, 1st Edition. Elsevier, 2019 (In Press).

Ovesna Z, Horvathova-Kozics K. Structure-activity relationship of trans-resveratrol and its analogues. *Neoplasma*. 2005;52:450–455.

Pace-Asciak CR, Rounova O, Hahn SE, Diamandis EP, Goldberg DM. Wines and grape juices as modulators of platelet aggregation in healthy human subjects. *Clin Chim Acta*. 1996;246:163–182.

Palomera-Avalos V, Grinan-Ferre C, Izquierdo V, Camins A, Sanfeliu C, Canudas AM, Pallas M. Resveratrol modulates response against acute inflammatory stimuli in aged mouse brain. *Exp Gerontol*. 2018;102:3–11.

Palomera-Avalos V, Grinan-Ferre C, Izquierdo V, Camins A, Sanfeliu C, Pallas M. Metabolic stress induces cognitive disturbances and inflammation in aged mice: protective role of resveratrol. *Rejuv Res*. 2017;20:202–217.

Park D, Jeong H, Lee MN, Koh A, Kwon O, Yang YR, Noh J, Suh PG, Park H, Ryu SH. Resveratrol induces autophagy by directly inhibiting mTOR through ATP competition. *Sci Rep*. 2016;6:21772.

Pervaiz S. Resveratrol: from grapevines to mammalian biology. *FASEB J*. 2003;17:1975–1985.

Phan HTT, Samarat K, Takamura Y, Azo-Oussou AF, Nakazono Y, Vestergaard MC. Polyphenols modulate Alzheimer's amyloid beta aggregation in a structure-dependent manner. *Nutrients*. 2019;11:(In press).

Pirola L, Frojdo S. Resveratrol: one molecule, many targets. *IUBMB Life*. 2008;60:323–332.

Porquet D, Grinan-Ferre C, Ferrer I, Camins A, Sanfeliu C, Del Valle J, Pallas M. Neuroprotective role of trans-resveratrol in a murine model of familial Alzheimer's disease. *J. Alzheimer's Dis*. 2014;42:1209–1220.

Price NL, Gomes AP, Ling AJY, Duarte FV, Martin-Montalvo A, North BJ, Agarwal B, et al. SIRT1 Is Required for AMPK Activation and the Beneficial Effects of Resveratrol on Mitochondrial Function. *Cell Metab*. 2012 May 2;15(5):675–690.

Rahman I. Dietary polyphenols mediated regulation of oxidative stress and chromatin remodeling in inflammation. *Nutr Rev*. 2008;66 Supplement 1:S42–S45.

Raine CS. Inflammation in Alzheimer's disease: a view from the periphery. *Neurobiol Aging*. 2000;21:437–440.

Rayalam S, Della-Fera MA, Baile CA. Synergism between resveratrol and other phytochemicals: implications for obesity and osteoporosis. *Mol Nutr Food Res*. 2011;55:1177–1185.

Renaud S, de Lorgeril M. Wine, alcohol, platelets, and the French paradox for coronary heart disease. *Lancet.* 1992;339(8808):1523–1526.

Richard T, Pawlus AD, Iglesias ML, Pedrot E, Waffo-Teguo P, Merillon JM, Monti JP. Neuroprotective properties of resveratrol and derivatives. *Ann N Y Acad Sci.* 2011;1215:103–108.

Saqib U, Kelley TT, Panguluri SK, Liu D, Savai R, Baig MS, Schurer SC. Polypharmacology or promiscuity? Structural interactions of resveratrol with its bandwagon of targets. *Front Pharmacol.* 2018;9:1201.

Savio M, Ferraro D, Maccario C, Vaccarone R, Jensen LD, Corana F, Mannucci B, Bianchi L, Cao Y, Stivala LA. Resveratrol analogue 4, 4'-dihydroxy-trans-stilbene potently inhibits cancer invasion and metastasis. *Sci Rep.* 2016;6:19973.

Sawda A, Moussa C, Turner RS. Resveratrol for Alzheimer's disease. *Ann N Y Acad Sci.* 2017;1403:142–149.

Scarmeas N, Luchsinger JA, Schupf N, Brickman AM, Cosentino S, Tang MX, Stern Y. Physical activity, diet, and risk of Alzheimer disease. *JAMA.* 2009;302:627–637.

Siemann EH, Creasy LL. Concentration of the phytoalexin resveratrol in wine. *Am J Enol Viticult.* 1992;43:49–52.

Singh AP, Singh R, Verma SS, Rai V, Kaschula CH, Maiti P, Gupta SC. Health benefits of resveratrol: evidence from clinical studies. *Med Res Rev.* 2019:(In press).

Soares DG, Andreazza AC, Salvador M. Sequestering ability of butylated hydroxytoluene, propyl gallate, resveratrol, and vitamins C and E against ABTS, DPPH, and hydroxyl free radicals in chemical and biological systems. *J Agric Food Chem.* 2003;51:1077–1080.

Sun AY, Wang Q, Simonyi A, Sun GY. Resveratrol as a therapeutic agent for neurodegenerative diseases. *Mol Neurobiol.* 2010;41:375–383.

Sun J, Wei C, Liu Y, Xie W, Xu M, Zhou H, Liu J. Progressive release of mesoporous nano-selenium delivery system for the multi-channel synergistic treatment of Alzheimer's disease. *Biomaterials.* 2019;197:417–431.

Tou JC. Evaluating resveratrol as a therapeutic bone agent: preclinical evidence from rat models of osteoporosis. *Ann N Y Acad Sci.* 2015;1348:75–85.

Turner RS, Thomas RG, Craft S, van Dyck CH, Mintzer J, Reynolds BA, Brewer JB, Rissman RA, Raman R, Aisen PS, Alzheimer's Disease Cooperative Study. A randomized, double-blind, placebo-controlled trial of resveratrol for Alzheimer disease. *Neurology.* 2015;85:1383–1391.

Velander P, Wu L, Henderson F, Zhang S, Bevan DR, Xu B. Natural product-based amyloid inhibitors. *Biochem Pharmacol.* 2017;139:40–55.

Venkatesan B, Valente AJ, Reddy VS, Siwik DA, Chandrasekar B. Resveratrol blocks interleukin-18-EMMPRIN cross-regulation and smooth muscle cell migration. *Am J Physiol Heart Circ Physiol.* 2009;297:H874–H886.

Wang J, Ho L, Zhao Z, Seror I, Humala N, Dickstein DL, Thiyagarajan M, Percival SS, Talcott ST, Pasinetti GM. Moderate consumption of Cabernet Sauvignon attenuates Aβ neuropathology in a mouse model of Alzheimer's disease. *FASEB J.* 2006;20:2313–2320.

Wang J, Shi A, Agyei D, Wang Q. Formulation of water-in-oil-in-water (W/O/W) emulsions containing trans-resveratrol. *RSC Adv.* 2017;7:35917–35927.

Wei Z. The role of Alzheimer's disease and estrogen. Foreign Med Mol Biol Div. 2000;22:189–192.

Wightman EL, Reay JL, Haskell CF, Williamson G, Dew TP, Kennedy DO. Effects of resveratrol alone or in combination with piperine on cerebral blood flow parameters and cognitive performance in human subjects: a randomised, double-blind, placebo-controlled, cross-over investigation. *Brit J Nutr.* 2014;112:203–213.

Witte AV, Kerti L, Margulies DS, Floel A. Effects of resveratrol on memory performance, hippocampal functional connectivity, and glucose metabolism in healthy older adults. *J Neurosci.* 2014;34:7862–7870.

Xia D, Sui R, Zhang Z. Administration of resveratrol improved Parkinson's disease-like phenotype by suppressing apoptosis of neurons via modulating the MALAT1/miR-129/SNCA signaling pathway. *J Cell Biochem.* 2019;120:4942–4951.

Xie JC, Ma XY, Liu XH, Yu J, Zhao YC, Tan Y, Liu XY, Zhao YX. Hypoxia increases amyloid-beta level in exosomes by enhancing the interaction between CD147 and Hook1. *Am J Transl Res.* 2018;10:150–163.

Xie Y, Niu M, Ji C, Huang TY, Zhang C, Tian Y, Shi Z, et al. SNX8 Enhances Non-amyloidogenic APP Trafficking and Attenuates Aβ Accumulation and Memory Deficits in an AD Mouse. *Front. Cell. Neurosci.* 2019;13:410.

Yang T, Jiang M, Jia Y. The neuroprotective effect of estrogen in Alzheimer's disease. *J Dalian Med Univ.* 2012;34:1283–1284.

Yang Y, Liu H, Shi A, Liu L, Hu H, Wang Q. In vitro bioavailability of resveratrol encapsulated in liposomes: influence of chitosan coating and liposome compositions. *J Control Rel.* 2017;259:e172–e173.

Zhang J, Zhou X, Yu Q, Yang L, Sun D, Zhou Y, Liu J. Epigallocatechin-3-gallate (EGCG)-stabilized selenium nanoparticles coated with Tet-1 peptide to reduce amyloid-β aggregation and cytotoxicity. *ACS Appl Mater Interfaces*. 2014;6:8475–8487.

Zheng DW, Chen JL, Zhu JY, Rong L, Li B, Lei Q, Fan JX, Zou MZ, Li C, Cheng SX, Xu Z, Zhang XZ. Highly integrated nano-platform for breaking the barrier between chemotherapy and immunotherapy. *Nano Lett*. 2016;16:4341–4347.

Zhou P, Liu X, Li F, Wang Y. Resveratrol pretreatment attenuates traumatic brain injury in rats by suppressing NLRP3 inflammasome activation via SIRT1. *Mol Med Rep*. 2018;17:3212–3217.

Zhou X, Sun J, Yin T, Le F, Yang L, Liu Y, Liu J. Enantiomers of cysteine modified SeNPs (d/lSeNPs) as inhibitors of metal-induced Aβ aggregation in Alzheimer's disease. *J Mater Chem B*. 2015;3:7764–7774.

9 Pre-Clinical *In-Vivo* and *In-Vitro* Methods For Evaluation of Anti-Alzheimer's Drugs

Shilpa A. Deshpande and Niraj S. Vyawahare

CONTENTS

ABBREVIATIONS

Aβ β-amyloid
AChE Acetylcholineserase
AD Alzheimer's Disease
APP Amyloid Precursor Protein
ATC Acetylthiocholine

CA	Carnosic Acid
CS	Conditioned Stimulus
CSF	Cerebrospinal Fluid
DMEM	Dulbecco's Modified Eagle's Medium
DOPAC	Di- Hydroxyphenylacetic Acid
DTNB	5,5'-Dithiobis-2-nitrobenzoic Acid
ELISA	Enzyme-linked Immunosorbent Assay
GABA	Gamma-aminobutyric Acid
5-HIAA	5-Hydroxyindolacetic Acid
HVA	Homovanilic Acid
ICV	Intracerebroventricular
ITI	Inter-trial Interval
MAP-tau	Microtubule-associated Protein Tau
MWM	Morris Water Maze
NFT	Neurofibrillary Tangles
NGF	Nerve Growth Factor
NORT	Novel Object Recognition Test
NTP	Neural Thread Protein
PCR	Polymerase Chain Reaction
PDAPP	Platelet-derived Growth Factor-β Promoter
RAM	Radial Arm Maze
TNF	Tumor Necrosis Factor

9.1 INTRODUCTION

Alzheimer's disease (AD) is characterized by gradual deterioration of cognitive function, progressive impairment of daily activities, and neuropsychiatric symptoms. The hallmarks of the disease are accumulation of beta-amyloid (Aβ) protein, forming senile plaques in specific brain areas and tau protein hyperphosphorylation, promoting the formation and deposition of neurofibrillary tangles (NFT). Neural thread protein (NTP), which is a membrane-spanning phosphoprotein with a predicted 375-amino acid sequence, is overexpressed in AD and responsible for some of the important cell-death events associated with AD neurodegeneration. This leads to subsequent neuronal and synaptic loss, and memory loss, and the damage is irreversible and widespread at the time of clinical diagnosis (Laurijssens et al., 2013).

The experimental *in-vivo* models used to evaluate the drugs used for the treatment of AD are based on induction of AD-like conditions in animals or on genetic modification to produce transgenic animals mimicking AD-like symptoms. The drug effect can be studied using behavioral models or estimation of AD biomarkers in body fluids (Casadesus et al., 2010). The *in-vitro* techniques are based on cell line cultures of brain cells of AD patients or animals (Figure 9.1).

9.2 *IN-VIVO* MODELS FOR AD

The ideal animal model of any disease should be an imitation of the human disease, representing all the important features like cause, pathological changes, and symptoms, with a replication of the complexities of human behavior in rodents. Most of the experimental models of AD have the major goal to mimic the human aspect of disease by simulating the neuropathological changes of AD, resulting in the impairment of cognitive function (Cavanaugh et al., 2014). These neural and memory-related symptoms can be mimicked in animals and can then be evaluated using various behavioral models and biochemical assays.

These models are based on the amyloid, cholinergic, and tau hypotheses of AD (Ali, 2016).

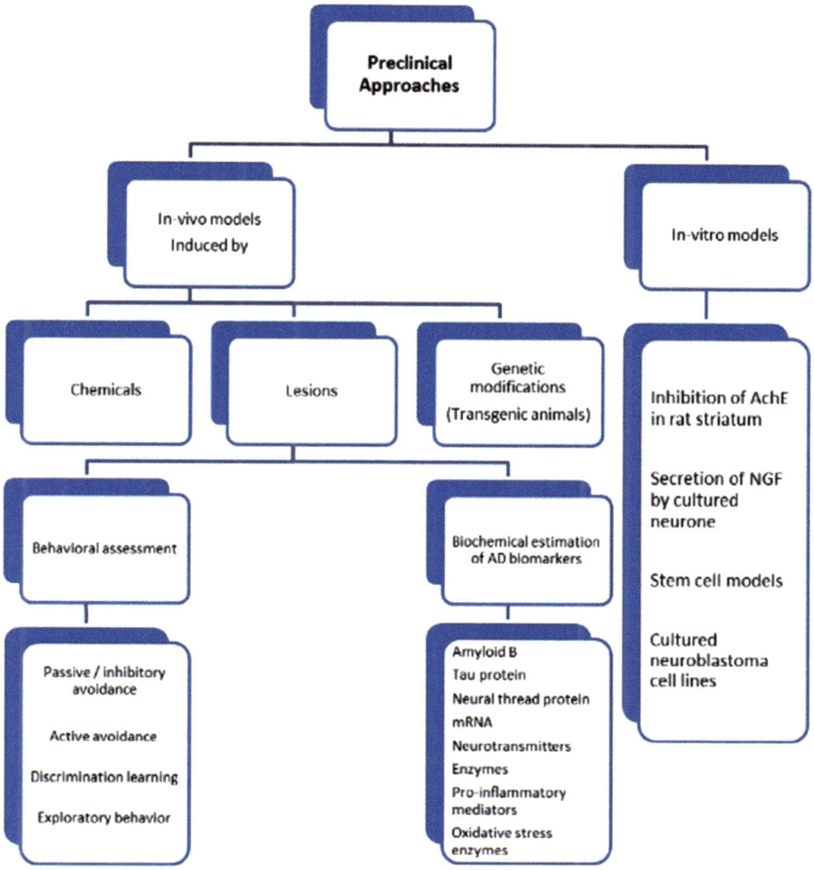

FIGURE 9.1 Concise pre-clinical approaches for evaluation of Anti-Alzheimer's drug.

The amyloid hypothesis: It states that the accumulation of senile plaques and NFTs causes neuronal atrophy and progressive synaptic failure, which initially appears in the medial temporal lobe, progressing to the limbic system, and subsequently to major areas of the neocortex, severely damaging the brain (Hardy and Allsop, 1991)

The tau hypothesis: It states that AD is characterized by the presence of pathological inclusions, such as Aβ plaques and NFTs composed of hyper-phosphorylated tau in the brain, leading to a gradual decline in cognitive function. "Tau tangles" or "neurofibrillary tangles" are formed from paired helical filaments of tau protein sub-units inside the neuron and result in neurodegeneration (Maccioni et al., 2010; Wischik et al., 2014).

The amyloid cascade hypothesis: It predicts that tau hyperphosphorylation occurs as a downstream consequence of Aβ accumulation.

The cholinergic hypothesis: It states that loss of cholinergic function in the AD brain is the reason for the significant decline in cognitive functions

The disruption of multiple neurotransmitter systems in AD is responsible for the pathophysiology of cognitive and behavioral disturbances associated with the disease. The majority of animal models are based on the cholinergic hypothesis of AD. Degeneration of cholinergic neurons in the nucleus basalis, situated in the basal forebrain and primarily projecting into the neocortex, occurs early in the course of the disease, resulting in cognitive impairment (Farooqui, 2016)

In-vivo models include induction of the pathological changes, characteristic features, and symptoms of AD, which can be achieved (Dam and De Deyn, 2011) with the help of:

1. Chemicals
2. Lesions
3. Genetic modification in animals

9.2.1 Chemically Induced AD-Like Conditions

The chemical or neurotoxin can be specifically introduced to a particular brain region using a small injection cannula. In animal research, a sturdy, large-bore guiding cannula is surgically implanted, using a stereotaxic procedure. After the animal has recovered, small injection cannulae can be inserted through the guide to deliver the agent to the target structure. The details of chemicals used to induce dementia, i.e memory impairment, such as their doses, route of administration, mode of action, type of memory loss, and experimental models used are shown in Table 9.1.

9.2.2 Brain Lesions

Brain lesions can be induced by physical destruction of specific brain areas, like the cholinergic nucleus basalis magnocellularis or the hippocampal, striatal, and cortical brain regions, or the lateral internal medullary lamina region of the thalamus in rats, which are involved in cognition. Some disadvantages of the lesion models may include the non-specificity of the lesion, and their failure to capture disease progression. The brain lesions can be produced by surgical removal of the targeted tissue, aspiration or suction of brain tissue through a glass pipette, or by introduction of a neurotoxin with the help of stereotaxic apparatus, whereas temporary lesions can be introduced using a cryoprobe.

9.2.3 Transgenic Rodent Models (LaFerla and Green, 2012; Wu et al., 2015)

As AD-associated genes are discovered, a number of transgenic animal models have been produced by introducing mutant genes into the existing genetic makeup or modifying genes of interest, using gene targeting technology, to mimic some features of human AD. Mice are the most commonly used species for transgenic modeling due to their ease of manipulation and their accessibility.

These models help to interpret the mechanistic importance of tau hyperphosphorylation and Aβ deposits, as well the relationship between each other, other pathological AD-related events, and memory loss.

Promoter sequences are connected to human genes to promote the pathological changes at early stages of development, which increases the chances of developing AD in the lifetime of the model animal.

Amyloid precursor protein (APP)-overexpressing transgenic animals may not develop NFTs, in spite of increased tau hyperphosphorylation. This could be because (1) human Aβ accumulation is not sufficient to cause NFT formation; (2) rodent tau has a different structure and sequence that may not be prone to aggregate formation; (3) the lifespan of mice is not long enough to allow for enough hyperphosphorylation/aggregation, as these pathologies develop over decades in humans. So Aβ accumulation in APP-overexpressing mice does not lead to NFT formation but these mice exhibit robust cognitive decline and also undergo more distinct alterations in tau that resemble the precursors to NFTs in the human brain. The details of transgenic animals with the mutant gene inserted and pathological features are shown in Table 9.2.

TABLE 9.1
Chemicals Used To Induce Dementia

Chemical	Dose in Animals	Type of Memory Loss Induced	Experimental Models Used	Mechanism of Action
Scopolamine (anticholinergic drug)	0.03 mg/ kg; i.p.	Spatial memory deficits, visual recognition and perception memory	• Estimation of neurotransmitters, AChE • Morris water maze task	• Non-selectively blocks the binding sites of ACh muscarinic receptors (M1 and M5) in the cerebral cortex • Causes disproportionate release of ACh, which destroys the hippocampus nerves
Colchicine	3–7.5 µg in 10 µl; intracerebroventricular (ICV)	Spatial memory impairment	• Estimation of oxidative stress enzymes, neurotransmitters, AChE • Morris water maze task	• Depolymerization and inhibition of microtubules • Cholinergic neurodegeneration and oxidative stress • Neurofibrillary degeneration • Hippocampal lesions • Increases cyclooxygenase (COX), glutamate/GABA ratio
Streptozotocin	3 mg/kg (sub-diabetogenic dose); ICV, twice at an interval of 48 h		Evaluation of oxidative stress enzymes (malondialdehyde assay)	• Appearance of synaptic plasticity in other cerebral structures and in the hippocampus • Neuronal damage by oxidative stress *via* the generation of reactive oxygen species (ROS) and reactive nitrogen species • Decreased activity of choline acetyltransferase (ChAT) in the hippocampus and augmented activity of acetylcholinesterase (AChE)
Amyloid-β 42	100 µM, 2.5 µl/mouse, ICV	Spatial learning and memory as well as hippocampal long-term potentiation	Morris water maze and novel object recognition tests	• Inhibition of ChAT to induce dysfunction of cholinergic neurons • Interfering with cAMP response element-binding (CREB) protein and calcium/calmodulin-dependent protein kinase II (CaMK-II) signaling pathways • Augments hyperphosphorylation of tau and stimulates the development of neurofibrillary tangles

(Continued)

TABLE 9.1 (CONTINUED)
Chemicals Used To Induce Dementia

Chemical	Dose in Animals	Type of Memory Loss Induced	Experimental Models Used	Mechanism of Action
Glucocorticoids (GCs)	40 mg/kg; i.p. for 21 d	Long-term memory impairment, Spatial memory deficit	Inhibitory avoidance task, Morris water maze task	Site-preferential downregulation of hippocampal GC receptors, involution of the dendritic processes of hippocampal neurons, inhibition of long-term potentiation
Diazepam	2 mg/kg; i.p. 20 min prior to test	Anterograde amnesia, spatial memory deficits	Morris water maze task and modified elevated plus-maze task	Suppression of LTP (Long Term Potentiation), reinforcement of GABAergic transmission
Lipopolysaccharide		Spatial memory deficits	Radial arm-maze task, Y-maze task	Oxidative and proinflammatory stress
Homocysteine	0.6 µmol/d, ICV for 7 days	Impairment of short- and long-term memories	Morris water maze task	Accumulation of amyloid and tau protein, activation of NMDA (N-methyl D-aspartate) receptors
High fat	-	Hippocampus-dependent learning deficits	Two-way active avoidance	Increases the brain cholesterol concentration by positive feedback association between cerebral and serum cholesterol levels. Increased cholesterol levels in the brain promote the generation and deposition of Aβ peptides, inducing inflammatory responses, as well as oxidative and nitrosative stress and cognitive decline

i.p. : Intraperitoneal; ICV: Intracerebroventricular

More, S. V., Kumar, H., Cho, D. Y., et al. 2016. Toxin-Induced Experimental Models of Learning and Memory Impairment. *Int J Mol Sci* 17:1447–1481.

TABLE 9.2
Transgenic Animal Models for AD

Model	Mutant Gene	Pathological Features
APP transgenic mice	Mutant human *APP* gene controlled by platelet-derived growth factor-β promoter (PDAPP)	Extensive extracellular Aβ deposits, synaptic loss and astrocytosis, with plaque formation at 6–9 months of age
Tau transgenic mice	Six tau isoform genes	Age- and gene-dependent development of NFTs in brain and spinal cord at 6 months; mild astrogliosis; synaptic loss; behavioral and motor deficit
APP and tau double transgenic mice	Human *APP* and *Tau* genes	Astrocytic tau pathology; mild blood–brain barrier (BBB) disruption; focal neuron damage, increase in NFT formation accompanied by enhanced Aβ deposits in the olfactory bulb and amygdala
Triple transgenic mice	Human *APP* and *Tau* genes with promoter sequence	Microglial activation and the upregulation of inflammatory markers were observed at 3 months of age, extracellular Aβ deposits from 6 months of age and a tau-related pathology at 10–12 months of age,

Li, X., Bao, X., and Wang, R. 2016. Experimental Models of Alzheimer's Disease for Deciphering the Pathogenesis and Therapeutic Screening (Review). *Int J Mol Med* 37:271–283.

9.2.4 Procedures for Behavioral Assessment of Dementia (Sivaraman et al., 2016; Lee et al., 2017)

9.2.4.1 Passive/Inhibitory Avoidance

In "passive avoidance" experiments, the animal learns that a particular response leads to punishment and passively avoids that noxious event by suppressing a particular behavior.

9.2.4.1.1 Step-Down Model

Principle: This is based on the principle that an animal in an open field spends most of the time close to the walls and in the corners. When placed on an elevated platform in the center of a rectangular compartment, it steps down almost immediately to the floor to explore the enclosure and to approach the wall. But if a punishment is given after descending (e.g. electric shock), the step-down latency may be reduced in the following trial as a result of learning.

Procedure: Mice or rats of either sex are divided into the control, standard, and treatment groups. The model consists of a rectangular box (50 cm × 50 cm) with an electrifiable grid floor and a 35 cm × 35 cm square platform on it. The foot shock can be delivered to the grid floor through a shock device. A typical paradigm consists of three phases: (1) familiarization – the animal is placed on the platform and the latency to descend is measured; it is returned to the home cage after 10 s of exploration; (2) learning – in the next trial, immediately after the animal has descended from the platform, an unavoidable foot shock of 50 Hz, 1.5 mA is applied for 1 s and the animal is returned to the home cage; (3) retention test – 24 h after the learning trial is performed, the animal is again placed on the platform and the step-down latency is measured; the test is finished when the animal steps down or after a cut-off time of 60 s if the animal remains on the platform.

Assessment: The time of descent during the learning phase and the time during the retention test are measured. A prolongation of the step-down latency is defined as learning.

9.2.4.1.2 Two-Compartment Model

Principle: A rodent in an open field has a tendency to enter any recesses in the walls and to hide there. If it is placed in a large box, connected with a small dark compartment through a narrow opening, it can rapidly find the narrow entrance into the small chamber, enter it and spend most of its time there. The times spent in the large and small compartments are measured. The latency of the first entrance into the dark chamber and the number of crossings from one compartment into the other can be measured as supplementary criteria.

Procedure: Mice or rats of either sex are divided into the control, standard, and treatment groups. The model consists of a rectangular box with a 50 cm × 50 cm grid floor and 35-cm high walls and a small 15 cm × 15 cm box with dark walls, electrifiable grid floor and removable ceiling. In the center of the common wall is a 6 cm × 6 cm opening connecting both the compartments. The opening can be closed by a transparent sliding door. The large compartment is illuminated with a 100 W bulb placed 150 cm above the center. Each animal is individually placed in the large bright chamber for training. Normally, after a brief orientation period, the animal enters the smaller, darker chamber. Once inside the second chamber, the door is closed which prevents the mouse from escaping, and a foot shock of 1 mA, is applied through the grid floor for 1 s. The animal is then returned to the home cage. The animal is again tested after 24 h by placing it again in the bright chamber. The time spent by the animal in the large and the small compartments, and the latency in entering the small darker chamber within a 5-min test session is measured. The percentage latency is calculated.

Assessment: Untreated control animals show a latency of about 250 s, whereas learning and memory loss reduce the latency to 50 s. The treatment is given 90 min before training. A prolonged latency indicates that the animal remembers that it has been punished and, therefore, avoids the darker chamber.

9.2.4.2 Active Avoidance

Active avoidance is a task which is motivated by fear of a noxious stimulus. In this task, the animal has to learn to anticipate the occurrence of an aversive event (shock) after the presentation of a specific stimulus (sound/light), to escape from the aversive event by moving to a different compartment.

9.2.4.2.1 Runway Avoidance

Principle: When the aversive stimulus is applied, the animal traverse across to the safe area to avoid the stimulus in speculated time.

Procedure: Mice or rats of either sex are divided into the control, standard, and treatment groups. The same box as used in the two-compartment model can be used in this experiment. The apparatus is provided with an overhead light source for uniform illumination, and an acoustic conditioned stimulus (CS; 80 dB, 2000 Hz) with a loudspeaker, mounted 50 cm above the start box. The foot shock is employed by the same source as in the step-down avoidance test. The animal is allowed to explore the whole area for 5 min. The connecting door is then closed, and the animal is placed into the larger, illuminated area. After 10 s, the acoustic CS is applied, the connecting door is simultaneously opened, and foot shock is turned on after 5 s. The CS is continued until the animal run away to reach the safe area. It is left there for an inter-trial interval (ITI) of 50–70 s and returned to the same area again. The training is continued on the same day until the animal avoids the stimulus nine times in ten consecutive trials. On the next day, the procedure is repeated until the same learning criterion is reached. The time needed to reach the safe area is measured.

Assessment: The time taken by the animal to reach the safe area on both days and the number of errors (not reaching the safe area) are measured.

9.2.4.2.2 Shuttle Box Avoidance

Principle: The principle is similar as runway paradigm, but two-way shuttle box avoidance is a more difficult task as it involves variable aversive stimuli and increased emotional factor. Since the animal is not handled between trials, the shuttle box can be easily automated, using a video tracking system.

Procedure: As shown in Figure 9.2, the apparatus consists of a rectangular box 50 cm × 15 cm, with 40-cm high metal walls, and an electrifiable grid floor. The box is divided by a wall with a manually operated connecting door (10 cm × 10 cm) into two 25 cm × 15 cm compartments, each illuminated by a 20 W bulb. A fixed resistance shock source is used. A computerized instrument

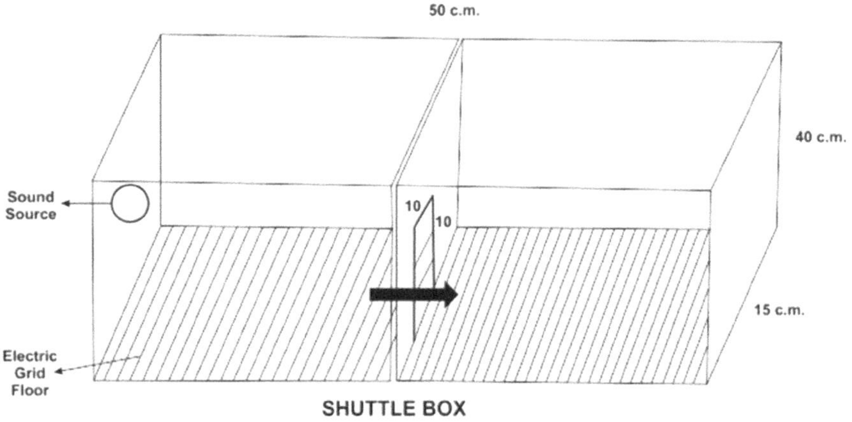

FIGURE 9.2 Shuttle box model.

facilitates the automatic delivery of the CS. The apparatus is placed in a dimly lit room with a masking noise background of 60 dB. The animal is allowed to explore the apparatus for 5 min with the connecting door open and the compartment lights switched off. The door is then closed. After 20 s, the light is switched on in the compartment containing the animal, and the door is opened. A CS, in the form of sound, is presented and floor shock is applied after 5 s and continued until the animal escapes to the dark side of the compartment; the connecting door is then closed, and the shock is discontinued. After a variable inter-trial interval (ITI; 30–90 s), the light is switched on in the previously dark compartment, the door is opened, and the animal is required to cross to the other side. The training is continued until the animal reaches the criterion of nine avoidances in ten consecutive trials. Retention is tested at different intervals after the original training by retraining the animal to the same criteria again.

Assessment: The time taken by the animal to reach the safe area on both days and the number of errors (not reaching the safe area) are measured. If the animal crosses to the safe side of the box during the sound (i.e. the avoidance CS), the shock is withdrawn and it is considered as a reward.

The higher the avoidance responses or the lower the number of mistakes in the test session indicates greater learning and memory retention i.e. the animal has learned the task correctly; the difference in the avoidance responses between the training and the test sessions indicates a measure of memory retention.

9.2.4.3 Discrimination Learning

In the above experiments, the animals have only one CS. There are certain procedures that illustrate the special techniques involving discrimination among different stimulus modalities. The experiments are based on spatial or visual discrimination and can be simultaneous or successive discrimination paradigms.

9.2.4.3.1 Morris Water Maze (MWM)

Principle: In the Morris water maze, a platform is submerged in a large, circular pool of water that remains in the same location in the pool for days. The animal's task is to find the platform by learning the spatial relationships between the platform's location and the other maze landmarks in the test environment. This is a reference memory task. Working memory can be tested with the platform in a different location on each day. The animal learns the location of the hidden platform in one trial, shown by a decreased latency to locate the platform on a second trial.

Procedure: The experimental apparatus consisted of a circular water tank of diameter 100 cm and height 35 cm, containing water at 28°C up to 15 cm in depth and made opaque by adding titanium dioxide or milk. Four points, equally distributed around the perimeter of the tank, serve as starting locations. The tank is divided into four equal quadrants and a small platform of diameter 4.5 cm and height 14.5 cm is placed 1-cm below the water surface at the midpoint of any one quadrant, as shown in Figure 9.3. The platform remains in the same position during the training days. The rat is released into the water and allowed to find the platform for 60–90 s. Each animal can undergo 2–4 trials per day for 4–5 d until they learn to escape onto the platform. A task is developed where animals learn to swim in the water and try to escape the fear stimulus by finding the hidden platform. After several trials, the test is conducted after the animal is subjected to chemically induced amnesia. In each training trial, the time required to escape to the platform, the number of annulus crossings (crossing of a virtual zone surrounding the platform) as well as the time the animal spent in the training quadrant are recorded, preferably with the aid of a video tracking system.

The probe trial is performed 24 h after the last trial, when the platform is removed. Where the animal spends its time is a measure of spatial bias. If the animal has learned the platform's location, it shows a preference for the quadrant in which the platform was located.

Assessment: Learning is said to be developed if escape latency is reduced and length of the path to find the platform is decreased. The platform can be located from outside the tank by providing some configurational cues.

9.2.4.3.2 Radial Arm Maze (RAM)

Principle: RAM is based on exploratory as well as spatial discrimination tasks for rodents, that have been extensively used to study the role of the hippocampus in learning and memory. The clues, like food pellets, are kept in the arms of the maze, and the animal efficiently locates the tempted/attracted arms by using spatial information provided by the clues in the maze. This is useful in studying spatial reference and working memory processes in the animals. In reference memory procedures, information is useful for many sessions/days and may usually be needed during the entire experiment. Working memory information presented in the maze is useful for only one session but not for subsequent ones; the animal has to remember the information during a delay interval (of between minutes to hours). Correct choices in the radial arm maze are rewarded by food. The RAM requires training for the assessment of learning and, before that, food is restricted to induce motivation, along with exposure to the rewards to make the animals familiar with them before being placed in the maze. Because the test measures trial-dependent memory, it is an assessment of working memory and, more specifically, spatial working memory.

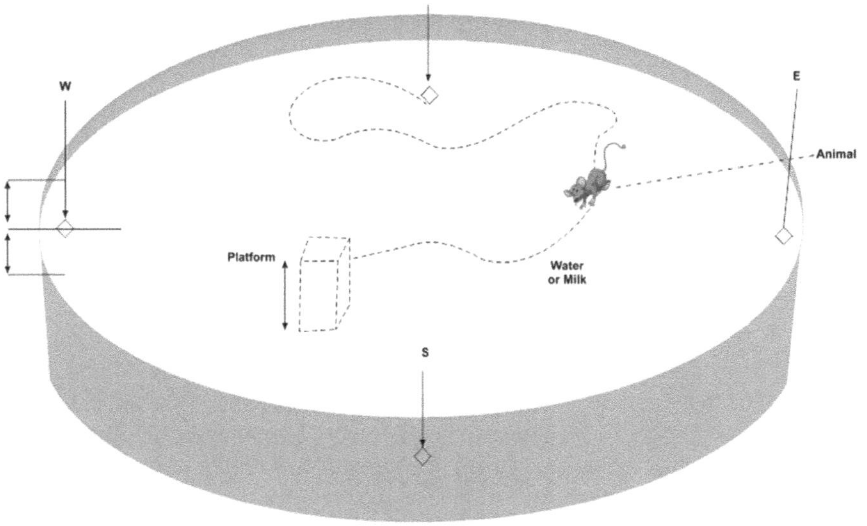

FIGURE 9.3 Morris water maze model.

Procedure: The model consists of a wooden elevated eight-arm radial maze with the arms (56 cm long and 5 cm wide) extending from a central platform (26 cm in diameter), as shown in Figure 9.4. Each arm has 2-cm high rails along the length of the arm. The maze is well illuminated and food pellets as a reward/clue are placed at the end of the arms. During the test, animals are trained on a daily basis in the maze to collect the food pellets. Training involves placing food pellet baits throughout the maze to encourage searching. Once this is learned, test trials begin by placing an animal in the center and allowing it to explore, with a single reward at the end of each arm. The session is terminated after eight choices and the animal has to obtain the maximum number of rewards with a minimum number of errors (entries to non-tempted arms).

Assessment: A single food pellet bait is placed at the end of each arm and the animal is placed on the central platform. The rat visits each arm to eat the pellet. It successfully completes the maze by going down each arm only once. It must use short-term memory along with spatial cues to remember the arms it has already visited. If it visits an arm twice, this is counted as an error. The performance of the animal on the maze is considered a test of short-term memory.

9.2.4.3.3 Y-Maze Task Consecutive Entries into Three Distinct Arms (e.g., ACB) in Overlapping Triplet Sets

Principle: The Y-maze task is used to measure spatial working through the spontaneous alternation of behavior.

Procedure: The maze is made of black painted wood. Each arm is 40 cm long, 3.5 cm high and 10 cm wide and joins at an equal angle as seen in Figure 9.5. A training session consists of free movement of the animal for 15 min through the maze by placing it at the end of one arm. Animals have a tendency to explore the maze systematically, entering each arm in turn. The animal is said to show alternation when it enters into three distinct arms consecutively in overlapping triplet sets. The ability to alternate requires that the animal know which arm they have already visited. The observations are for 5 min. The series of arm entries, including possible alternation, are recorded visually.

Assessment: The percentage of alternation is calculated as the ratio of actual alternations, defined as the total number of arm entries minus two and multiplied by 100. One arm of the Y-maze is blocked off and the animal is allowed to explore the other two arms for about 15 minutes. Then the animal is placed in the start arm and the blocked arm is uncovered. The animal's preference for

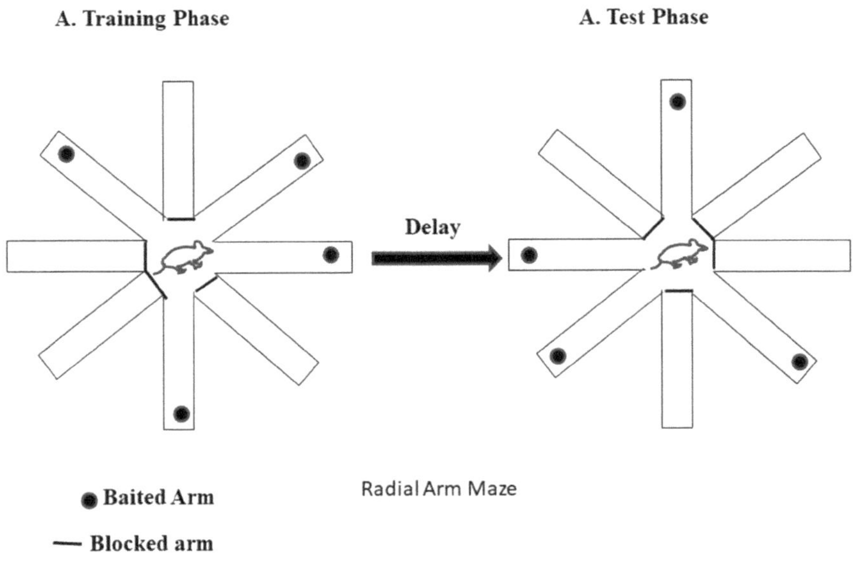

FIGURE 9.4 Radial arm maze.

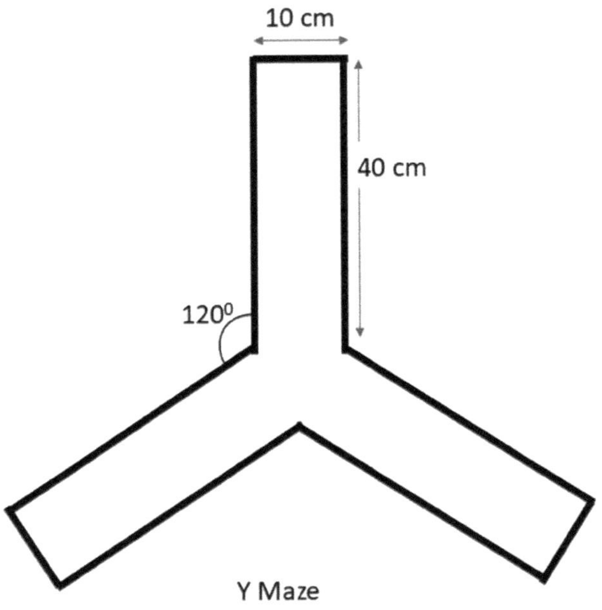

FIGURE 9.5 Y-maze.

the new arm or the known one is assessed. The test phase can be delayed from the familiarization phase to test the animal's memory.

9.2.4.4 Exploratory Behavior

This test is based on the natural tendency of rodents to explore novel environments/objects in order to open up new options for nutrition, reproduction, and lodging resources. The rate of exploration in an unfamiliar environment is restricted due to the inborn tendency to avoid dangers. Spatial habituation learning is defined as a decreased exploration in a novel environment after repeated exposure to the same environment because of memory or recognition of the specific physical characteristics of the environment. The test can be used to examine short-term spatial memory (within-trial reductions in exploratory activity) and/or long-term spatial memory (between-trial reductions in exploratory activity after a retention interval of 24, 48 or 96 h after the initial exposure).

9.2.4.4.1 The Open-Field Test

Principle: Rearings are instinctive exploratory postures of small rodents; the newer the environment, the higher the number of rearings. Exploration is also expressed as "crossings". The "test" session is performed after 24 h for long-term memory, less than 6 h for short-term memory, and up to 3 min for working memory by putting the same animal in the same arena under the same environmental conditions and measuring the same variables again. Normal memory retention is indicated by a reduction in the number of rearings and/or crossings between the training and the test sessions.

Procedure: The open-field apparatus shown in Figure 9.6 is a rectangular chamber (60 cm × 60 cm × 40 cm for rats and 26 cm × 26 cm × 40 cm for mice) made of painted wood or grey PVC. A red or green light bulb of 25 W is placed either directly above or beneath the maze to provide a uniform illumination at the center. A masking noise of 60 dB is provided by a noise generator. Prior to each trial, the apparatus is cleaned out with water, containing 0.1% acetic acid, to clean away the excreta. The rodent is placed in the center or in a corner of the open-field for 5–10 minute sessions. The animals are re-exposed to the open field 24 h and 96 h after the initial trial.

Assessment: The exploratory behaviors are recorded as: (1) the number of rearings and the duration of a single rearing (an animal stands on its hind legs with its forelegs in the air or against

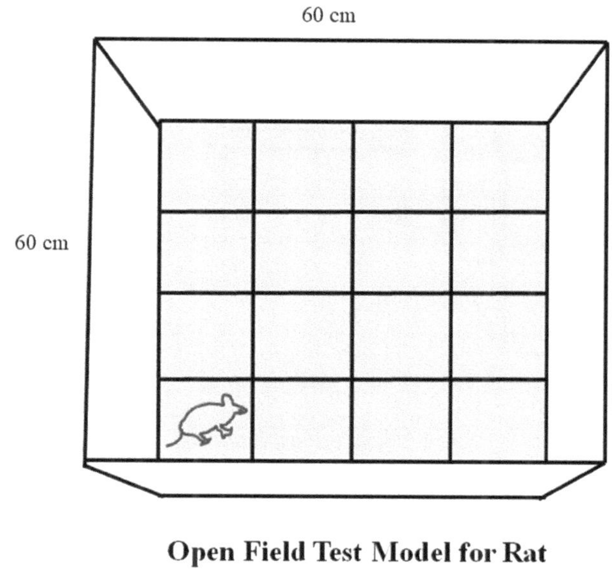

FIGURE 9.6 Open-field apparatus.

the wall; (2) locomotor activity or crossings: the distance (cm) which the animal moved. Decrease in the exploratory behavior during re-exposure indicates learning. The difference between training and test sessions, in the number of rearings (or of crossings), is the measure (or score) for retention of the habituation.

9.2.4.4.2 Exploratory Hole Board Test

Principle: The test arena has uniformly positioned holes in the floor with several of them, in an irregular pattern, are baited with a food pellet in every trial, leaving other holes always empty. Over the course of 5 d of training with six trials per d, the animals are tested for searching for the pellets in the same holes.

Procedure: The hole board apparatus shown in Figure 9.7 is used to predict the locomotor activity and memory of the animals; they are explored twice, with a 24-h interval, to a 40 cm × 40 cm × 60 cm

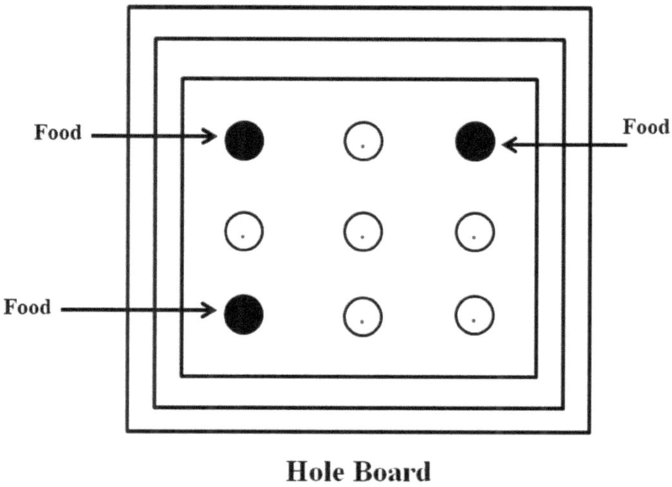

FIGURE 9.7 Exploratory hole board test model.

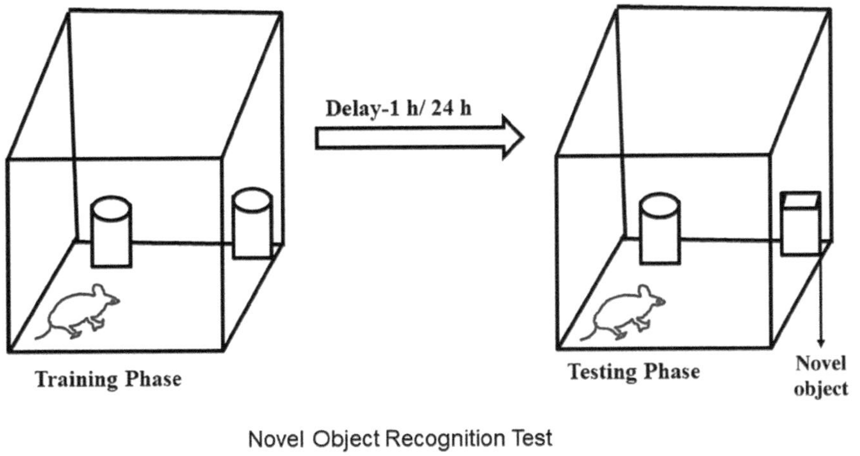

FIGURE 9.8 Novel object recognition test model.

open field, the brown linoleum floor of which was divided into 9 or 16 equal squares with holes separated by white lines.

The procedure is appetitive and therefore requires food restriction and reduction in free-feeding body weight to 80–85% of the normal weight. After 1 h of administration of the test drug, the animal is placed in the rear left square and left to explore it freely for 5 min.

Assessment: During the time of exploration, the number of line crossings, head dippings, and rearings are counted.

9.2.4.4.3 Novel Object Recognition Test

Principle: This test is based on the animal's spontaneous tendency to spend more time in exploring for a novel object than for a familiar one. It is used to evaluate the recognition memory.

Procedure: The apparatus consists of a wooden box (70 cm × 60 cm × 30 cm) with a grid floor that can be easily cleaned after each trial, which is shown in Figure 9.8. The two different-shaped objects are placed at diagonally opposite corners of the box for discrimination (pyramid of 8-cm side and cylinder of 8-cm height). On day 0, animals are allowed to explore the box without any object for 2 min. On the first trial (T1), two identical objects are placed in two opposite corners of the box and animals are allowed to explore the objects for 20 s. Exploration means directing the nose to a distance of less than 2 cm from an object and/or touching the object with the nose. At 90 min after T1, the second trial (T2) is initiated, with one of the objects replaced by a new different object present in T1, and the animal is left in the box for 5 min.

Assessment: The time spent for exploring the New (N) and Familiar (F) objects are recorded separately. Care is taken to avoid place preferences and olfactory stimuli by randomly changing the position of the two objects during T2 and cleaning them carefully.

9.2.5 Biochemical Estimation in Body Fluids Such As Cerebrospinal Fluid (CSF), Blood, and Urine

9.2.5.1 Estimation of AD Biomarkers (Sharma and Singh, 2016)

An ideal diagnostic marker should enable predictive testing, monitoring of disease progression, and determination of the effects of a treatment, using novel therapeutic compounds. A diagnostic marker of AD should reflect a central pathogenic process of the disorder, like degeneration of neurons and synapses, or the development of typical lesions as neuritic plaques and neurofibrillary tangles (NFT). Markers should be validated in neuropathologically confirmed AD cases and should have a sensitivity of at least 80% for detecting AD and a specificity of at least 80% for distinguishing it from other dementias. Moreover, the biological marker should be present in body fluids that are easily accessible, cheap, less invasive and easy to collect, like urine, blood or CSF. The main advantages of using blood serum for diagnosis are that it is easily obtainable, whereas analyzing blood cells (e.g. peripheral blood mononuclear cells, lymphocytes, monocytes, or platelets) can be more specifically related to AD pathologies. Extensively evaluated markers that can be helpful for diagnosing sporadic AD are amyloid-β protein (Aβ), microtubule-associated protein tau (MAP-tau), neural thread protein, and mRNA expression.

1. **Amyloid-β (Aβ40 and Aβ42):** Aβ is generated continuously as a soluble protein resulting from the normal constitutive amyloid precursor protein (APP) metabolism and is secreted into the extracellular space, allowing its detection in the CSF and plasma (Sobów et al., 2004).
2. **Tau protein (total and phosphorylated):** Both MAP-tau and phosphorylated MAP-tau can be detected in the CSF. CSF MAP-tau concentration has been suggested to reflect: (i) neuronal and axonal degeneration or damage, (ii) formation of NFT. Contrary to total MAP-tau, phosphorylated (P)-MAP-tau is not merely a marker of neuronal damage (P-MAP-tau does not change after acute stroke), but rather is a reflection of hyperphosphorylation of tau and possibly formation of NFTs. The sensitivity and specificity of CSF total MAP-tau and Aβ42 simultaneous measurements and P-MAP-tau/total MAP-tau ratio are high enough for discriminating between AD and normal aging when combined with the assessment of cognitive functions (Sobów et al., 2004).
3. **Neural thread protein (NTP):** NTP is selectively elevated in urine in AD patients and can be detected by a competitive ELISA assay. NTP in a urine sample competes with an alkaline phosphatase (AP)-labeled immunoglobulin G (IgG) for binding. The free labeled IgG shows high absorbance, whereas absorbance is decreased in the presence of NTP. It competes with AP for binding with IgG and the decrease in absorbance is proportional to the amount of NTP present. The sample concentration of NTP is read from the standard concentration curve (Levy et al., 2007).
4. **mRNA:** Downregulation of mRNAs 29b and 15a, which regulate transcription factor Sp1 responsible for expression of APP and tau, along with other target genes, can be detected in CSF by polymerase chain reaction (PCR), northern blot, or microarray techniques.

9.2.5.2 Estimation of Brain Neurotransmitters and Enzymes (Rahman and Eswaraiah, 2013; Strac et al., 2015; Sivaraman et al., 2016; Si and Song, 2018)

Specific degeneration of cholinergic neurons, downregulation of choline acetyltransferase, the enzyme responsible for the synthesis of acetylcholine (ACh), and elevation of acetylcholineserase (AChE) enzyme, as well as reduced choline uptake and ACh release, result in severe deficits of cholinergic function observed in AD. The concentrations of the monoamine metabolites homovanilic acid (HVA), di- hydroxyphenylacetic acid (DOPAC), and 5-hydroxyindolacetic acid (5-HIAA), as well as the monoamine synthesis cofactor biopterin, are found to be significantly decreased in AD. Glutamate plays an especially important role in neuronal plasticity underlying learning and memory, and is found to be significantly elevated in the CSF of AD subjects. Reduced levels of the major inhibitory neurotransmitter gamma-aminobutyric acid (GABA) in CSF were also observed in patients with AD.

9.2.5.2.1 Acetylcholineserase (AChE) Enzyme Determination

AChE enzyme activity is estimated by the Ellman method.

Principle: Acetylcholinesterase activity is measured by using an artificial substrate, acetylthiocholine (ATC). It is cleaved by AChE to release thiocholine, which is allowed to react with the -SH reagent, DTNB (5,5'-dithiobis-2-nitrobenzoic acid). DTNB is reduced to thionitrobenzoic acid, a yellow-colored anion which gives an absorption maximum at 412 nm.

Reagents:

1. 0.1 M phosphate buffer is prepared by adding Solution A (5.22 g of K_2HPO_4 and 4.68 g of NaH_2PO_4 dissolved in 150 ml of distilled water) and Solution B (6.2 g NaOH dissolved in 150 ml of distilled water) and the pH is adjusted to the desired level (pH 8.0 or 7.0).
2. DTNB reagent is prepared by dissolving 39.6 mg of DTNB with 15 mg $NaHCO_3$ in 10 ml of 0.1 M phosphate buffer, and the pH is adjusted to 7.0.
3. Acetylthiocholine (ATC) solution (0.075 M) is prepared by dissolving 21.67 mg of acetyl-thiocholine in 1 ml of distilled water.

Procedure: The treated animals are decapitated, and the brains are removed quickly and placed in ice-cold saline. Frontal cortex, hippocampus, and septum are quickly dissected out in a Petri plate chilled on crushed ice. The tissues are weighed and homogenized with tissue a homogenizer in 0.1 M phosphate buffer (pH 8). An aliquot (0.4 ml) of the homogenate is added to a cuvette containing 2.6 ml phosphate buffer (0.1 M, pH 8) and 100 µl of DTNB reagent. The contents of the cuvette are mixed thoroughly, and the basal absorbance is measured at 412 nm in a spectrophotometer. An aliquot (20 µl) of substrate, i.e., acetylthiocholine is added, and the change in the absorbance per minute is determined.

Calculations:
The enzyme activity is calculated using the following equation:

$$\text{Acetylcholinesterase activity}\left(\text{M/ml}\right) = \frac{\text{A/min} \times V_t}{\varepsilon \times b \times V_s}$$

where

A/min= Change in absorbance per min
$\varepsilon = 1.361 \times 10^4\ M^{-1}\ cm^{-1}$
b = path length (1-cm)
V_t = total volume (3.1 ml)
V_s = sample volume (0.4 ml)

The final reading of enzyme activity is expressed as µ moles/minute/mg tissue.

$$\mu\,\text{moles/minute/mg protein} = \frac{\mu\,\text{moles /ml sample}}{\text{mg protein/ml sample dilution}}$$

9.2.5.2.2 Estimation of Monoamine Oxidase (MAO) A and B

The MAO-A and B activities are estimated by the method of Tipton and Dawson (1968).

Principle: MAO reacts with *p*-tyramine, a substrate for both MAO-A and MAO-B, resulting in the formation of H_2O_2, which is determined by a fluorometric method (λ_{ex} = 530 nm, λ_{em} = 585 nm).

Reagents:
Sucrose (0.25 M), Tris buffer (0.1 M), EDTA (0.02 M), sodium phosphate buffer (100 mM, pH 7.4), i.e. assay buffer, pH 7.4, pargyline (20 mM) (MAO-B inhibitor), Clorgyline (20 mM) (MAO-A inhibitor), 3% Hydrogen peroxide, *p*-tyramine, Horseradish Peroxidase (HRP) enzyme, Vanillic acid as dye reagent

Procedure: The brain mitochondrial fraction is rinsed in 0.25 M sucrose, 0.1 M Tris, and 0.02 M EDTA (pH 7.41) to remove blood, and homogenized for 45 s with 400 ml of the same buffer.

The homogenate is subjected to differential centrifugation with the same buffer. The precipitate is washed twice more with 100 ml of the sucrose–Tris–EDTA buffer and resuspended in 50 ml of the same buffer. The protein concentration was adjusted to 1 mg/ml.

The MAO inhibitor solution is prepared by adding 5 µl of 20 mM inhibitor to 10 ml water to generate a 10 µM solution. An aliquot (45 µl) of the sample homogenate and 5 µl water are mixed with 5 µl of inhibitor solution and It is incubated at room temperature for 10 min. One aliquot of 1 µL each of *p*-tyramine, HRP, and dye reagent, and 50 µl of assay buffer are added. The solution is incubated at room temperature for 20 min in the dark. The fluorescence (FLU) of the samples and standards were measured at $\lambda_{ex} = 530$, $\lambda_{em} = 585$ nm.

The MAO enzyme activity in the sample is calculated as:

$$\text{MAO Activity}(\text{units/L}) = \frac{\text{FLU}_{\text{sample}} - \text{FLU}_{\text{control}}}{\text{Slope} \times \text{t}}$$

where

$\text{FLU}_{\text{sample}}$ = Absorbance measured in unknown sample
$\text{FLU}_{\text{control}}$ = Absorbance measured in sample control
(i.e. sample in presence of inhibitor)
Slope = determined from calibration curve (μM^{-1})
t = incubation time (i.e. 20 minutes)

9.2.5.2.3 Estimation of Dopamine, Adrenaline, and Serotonin

Reagents:

1. HCl–butanol solution (0.85 ml of 37% hydrochloric acid in 1 l n-butanol)
2. Heptane
3. 0.1 M HCl (0.85 ml concentrated HCl, made up to 100 ml with H_2O)

Preparation of tissue extracts:

After dissecting the brain, the sub cortical region including the striatum is separated. The tissue is weighed and is homogenized in 5 ml HCl–butanol for about 1 minute and then centrifuged at 2000 rpm for 10 minutes. The supernatant phase is taken in centrifuge tube containing 2.5 ml heptane and 0.31 ml HCl of 0.1 M. After 10 minutes of vigorous shaking, the tube is centrifuged under the same conditions and the overlaying organic phase is discarded. The aqueous phase is used for estimation of dopamine, adrenaline, and serotonin. All steps should be carried out at 0°C.

9.2.5.2.4 Estimation of Noradrenaline and Dopamine

Reagents:

1. 0.4 M HCl
2. Sodium acetate buffer (pH 6.9)
3. 5 M NaOH
4. 0.1 M iodine solution (in ethanol)
5. Na_2SO_3 solution
6. 10 M acetic acid

Procedure:

Aliquots of 0.05 ml 0.4 M HCl and 0.1 ml of EDTA/sodium acetate buffer (pH 6.9) are added to 0.2 ml of the aqueous phase, followed by 0.1 ml of 0.1 M iodine solution (in ethanol) for oxidation. The reaction is stopped after 2 min by addition of 0.1 ml Na_2SO_3 solution, and 0.1 ml acetic acid is added after a further 1.5 min. The solution is then heated to 100°C for 6 min. Excitation and emission spectra are recorded from the spectrofluorometer when the sample reaches room temperature. The readings are taken at 330 (excitation) and 375 nm (emission) for dopamine and at 395 and 485 nm for noradrenaline.

9.2.5.2.5 *Estimation of Serotonin*

Reagents:

1. *O*-phthaldialdehyde (OPT) reagent (20 mg in 100 ml concentrated HCl)

Procedure:

An aliquot (0.25 ml) of OPT reagent is added to 0.2 ml aqueous extract. The fluorophore is developed by heating to 100°C for 10 min. After the samples reaches equilibrium with the room temperature after cooling, readings are taken at 360 (excitation) and 470 nm (emission) in a spectrofluorometer. An aliquot of 0.25 ml concentrated HCI without OPT is used as the blank. Serotonin (500 µg/ml) in distilled water: HCl-butanol in a 1:2 ratio is used as the internal standard.

9.2.5.2.6 *Estimation of Glutamate*

Reagents:

1. butanol: acetic acid: water: 12: 3: 5
2. 0.25% ninhydrin reagent
3. 0.005% copper sulphate solution
4. standard glutamate solution

Procedure:

An aliquot (1.0 ml) of the supernatant from the brain homogenate is evaporated to dryness at 70°C in an oven and the residue is reconstituted in 100 ml of distilled water. A standard solution of glutamate at a concentration of 2 mM and the samples are spotted on chromatography paper using a micropipette. The paper is placed in a tank containing butanol: acetic acid: water (12: 3: 5 v/v) as the mobile phase. After chromatography is completed, the paper is removed, dried, and sprayed with ninhydrin reagent and placed in an oven at 100°C for 4 minutes. The portions which contain glutamate corresponding with the standard are cut and eluted with 0.005% $CuSO_4$ in 75% ethanol. Optical density (OD) is read against the blank at 515 nm in a spectrophotometer.

Calculation:

Glutamate concentration is calculated by using the following equation:

$$A = \frac{\text{Unknown OD} \times \text{Standard in mg}\,(3\,\mu g) \times 1000}{\text{Standard OD} \times \text{Volume spotted}\,(10\,\mu l) \times W}$$

where

A = amino acid content in umoles/g wet weight tissue
1000 = conversion factor for g wet weight tissue
W = weight of the tissue in g

9.2.5.3 Estimation of Pro-Inflammatory Mediators and Oxidative Stress Enzymes

The inflammatory biomarkers play a crucial role in neurodegeneration during progression of AD. Chemokines, cytokines, tumor necrosis factor (TNF)-α, interleukin β (IL- β), lipid peroxidase and malondialdehyde overexpression are the key players in AD.

9.2.6 *In-Vitro* Techniques

In-vitro techniques provide accurate and reproducible control of the living environment and help in reduction of the use of animals. Such techniques provide a prompt and direct manner with which to reveal the pathological changes occurring in AD and also to study the responses of nerve cells to treatments at the molecular and cellular levels.

9.2.6.1 Inhibition of AChE in the Rat Striatum

The purpose of this assay is to estimate inhibition of acetylcholinesterase (AChE) activity in isolated brain cells. Inhibitors of this enzyme may be useful for the treatment of AD.

Male Wistar rats are decapitated and the brains are rapidly removed. They are weighed and homogenized in 0.05 M NaH_2PO_4 (pH 7.2). A 25-μl aliquot of this suspension is added to 1 ml of the various concentrations of the test drug and incubated for 10 min at 37°C. Reagents (PO_4 buffer/DTNB/enzyme and Acetylthiocholine as substrate are added to the blank and sample cuvettes. Half-maximal inhibitory concentration (IC_{50}) values are calculated by log-probit analysis.

9.2.6.2 Secretion of NGF By Cultured Neurons

Nerve growth factor (NGF) is essential for the development and maintenance of peripheral and sensory neurons, and it prevents neuronal death after brain injury especially in the basal forebrain nuclei involved in memory processes. Increases in NGF secretion by any drug may prove beneficial in treating primary degenerative dementia. Cultured brain cells can be used for investigation of synthesis and secretion of NGF or for testing neuroprotective drugs.

Whole brains of 8-day-old mice are removed and are washed with phosphate-buffered saline, then treated with 0.25% trypsin at 37°C for 30 min. The excess trypsin is removed by centrifugation for 5 min. The brain cells are cultured in a culture bottle containing Dulbecco's modified Eagle's medium (DMEM) (10% fetal calf serum (FCS), 50 milliunits/ml penicillin, and 50 mg/ml of streptomycin) at 37°C in a humid atmosphere of 5% CO_2 for 1–2 weeks, changing the medium every 3 d. After complete confluence is achieved, the cells in each bottle are dissociated by trypsin treatment and recultured in new bottles. This procedure is repeated thrice to obtain a morphologically uniform cell culture. NGF concentration in the culture medium is determined by a two-site enzyme immunoassay. Time-response curves of release of NGF into the medium are established after addition of the test drug and compared with controls. Dose-response curves can be prepared after addition of various amounts of the test drug.

9.2.6.3 Stem Cell Models

AD-specific pluripotent stem cell lines have been generated from patients with AD, providing an effective approach for disease modeling and drug discovery.

9.2.6.4 Cultured Neuroblastoma Cell Lines

Human neuroblastoma cell lines are also used as a model to simulate AD pathophysiological features. The APP-processing pathway, expressing components of the amyloidogenic cascade observed in AD, can be mimicked in human neuroblastoma cells. Carnosic acid (CA) is used to treat human neuroblastoma cells to cause intracellular Aβ aggregation. Neuroblastoma cells exposed to aluminum chloride can induce Aβ toxicity. Thus, human neuroblastoma cell lines can be modified to induce certain aspects of AD pathophysiology to explore the underlying mechanisms and to develop potential new therapies.

9.3 SUMMARY

This chapter includes the experimental techniques for studying the pathophysiology of AD and for evaluating any new therapeutic agent for its treatment before actual clinical use. These preclinical studies involve *in-vivo* and *in-vitro* methods, such as induction of AD or its symptoms in experimental animals, use of transgenic Alzheimer's animals, or cell culture techniques. In this way, new pharmacologically active anti-Alzheimer's drugs can undergo clinical trials and may prove beneficial for society.

ACKNOWLEDGMENT

The authors are thankful to Mr. Prashant Amale, Assistant Professor, and Mr. Salil Pophali of Priyadarshini J. L. College of Pharmacy, Nagpur for their help.

REFERENCES

Ali, A. A. 2016. Alzheimer's Disease: Pathophysiology, Hypotheses and Treatment Strategies. *Acta Psychopathol* 2:23.

Casadesus, G., Arendash, G., Laferla, F. et al. 2010. Animal Models of Alzheimer's Disease. *Int J Alzhs Dis.* Article ID 606357, 2 pages. doi:10.4061/2010/606357.

Cavanaugh, S. E., Pippin, J. J., and Barnard, N. D. 2014. Animal Models of Alzheimer Disease: Historical Pitfalls and a Path Forward. *ALTEX* 31:279–302.

Dam, D. V. and De Deyn, P. P. 2011. Animal Models in the Drug Discovery Pipeline for Alzheimer's Disease. *Brit J Pharmacol* 164:1285–1300.

Farooqui, A. A. 2016. Potential Animal Models of Alzheimer Disease and Their Importance in Investigating the Pathogenesis of Alzheimer Disease. In *Therapeutic Potentials of Curcumin for Alzheimer Disease* 77. Springer International Publishing: Switzerland.

Hardy, J. and Allsop, D. 1991. Amyloid Deposition as the Central Event in the Aetiology of Alzheimer's Disease. *Trends Pharmacol Sci* 12:383–388.

LaFerla, F. M. and Green, K. N. 2012. Animal Models of Alzheimer Disease. *Cold Spring Harb Perspect Med* 1:2.

Laurijssens, B., Aujard, F., and Rahman, A. 2013. Animal Models of Alzheimer's Disease and Drug Development. *Drug Discov Today Technol* 10:e319–e327.

Lee, G. Y., Lee, C., Park, G. H., et al. 2017. Amelioration of Scopolamine-Induced Learning and Memory Impairment by α-Pinene in C57BL/6 Mice. *Evid Based Complement Alternat Med* 2017:4926815.

Levy, S., McConville, M., Lazaro, G. A., et al. 2007. Competitive ELISA Studies of Neural Thread Protein in Urine in Alzheimer's Disease. *J Clin Lab Anal* 21:24–33.

Li, X., Bao, X., and Wang, R. 2016. Experimental Models of Alzheimer's Disease for Deciphering the Pathogenesis and Therapeutic Screening (Review). *Int J Mol Med* 37:271–283.

Maccioni, R. B., Farías, G., Morales, I., et al. 2010. The Revitalized Tau Hypothesis on Alzheimer's Disease. *Arch Med Res* 41:226–231.

More, S. V., Kumar, H., Cho, D. Y., et al. 2016. Toxin-Induced Experimental Models of Learning and Memory Impairment. *Int J Mol Sci* 17:1447–1481.

Rahman, H. and Eswaraiah, M. C. 2013. Simple Spectroscopic Methods for Estimating Brain Neurotransmitters, Antioxidant Enzymes of Laboratory Animals like Mice: A Review. *PharmaTutor*, https://www.pharmatutor.org/articles/simple-spectroscopic-method-estimating-brain-neurotransmitter-antioxidnat-enzymes-lab-animals

Sharma, N. and Singh, A. N. 2016. Exploring Biomarkers for Alzheimer's Disease. *J Clin Diagn Res* 10:KE01–KE06.

Si, B. and Song, E. 2018. Recent Advances in the Detection of Neurotransmitters. *Chemosensors* 6:1–24.

Sivaraman, D., Panneerselvam, P., and Muralidharan, P. 2016. Memory and Brain Neurotransmitter Restoring Potential of Hydroalcoholic Extract of Ipomoea Aquatica Forsk on Amyloid Beta Aβ (25–35) Induced Cognitive Deficits in Alzheimer's Mice. *Int J Pharmacol* 12(2):52–65.

Sobów, T., Flirski, M., and Liberski, P. P. 2004. Amyloid-Beta and Tau Proteins as Biochemical Markers of Alzheimer's Disease. *Acta Neurobiol Exp* 64:53–70.

Strac, D. S., Muck-Seler, D., and Pivac, N. 2015. Neurotransmitter Measures in the Cerebrospinal Fluid of Patients with Alzheimer's Disease: A Review. *Psychiatr Danub* 27:14–24.

Wischik, C. M., Harrington, C. R., and Storey, J. 2014. Tau-Aggregation Inhibitor for Alzheimer's Disease. *Biochem Pharmacol* 88:529–539.

Wu, X., Li, J., Zhou, W., et al. 2015. Animal Models for Alzheimer's Disease: A Focused Review of Transgenic Rodent Models and Behavioral Assessment Methods. *ADMET and DMPK* 3:242–253.

10 Antioxidant Phytochemicals and Alzheimer's Disease

Current Understanding and Future Scope

Saikat Sen, Raja Chakraborty, and Atanu Bhattacharjee

CONTENTS

ABBREVIATIONS

ACh	Acetylcholine
AChE	Acetylcholinesterase
AD	Alzheimer's Disease
APP	Amyloid-β
APP	Amyloid Precursor Protein
BACE	β-secretases
BDNF	Brain-derived Neurotrophic Factor
cAMP	Cyclic Adenosine Monophosphate
CAT	Catalase
COX	Cyclooxygenase
EGCG	Epigallocatechin-3-gallate

GPx	Glutathione Peroxidase
GR	Glutathione Reductase
GSH	Reduced Glutathione
GSK-3	Glycogen Synthase Kinase 3
H_2O_2	Hydrogen Peroxide
hMAPτ	Microtubule-associated Protein Tau
HO-1	Heme Oxygenase-1
IL	Interleukin
iNOS	Inducible Nitric Oxide Synthase
JNK	c-Jun N-terminal Kinases
MAPK	Mitogen-activated Protein Kinase
MDA	Malondialdehyde
NFTs	Neurofibrillary Tangles
NF-κB	Nuclear Factor Kappa-light-chain-enhancer of Activated B cells
Nrf2	Nuclear Erythroid-2 Related Factor
PGE	Prostaglandin E
RNS	Reactive Nitrogen Species
ROS	Reactive Oxygen Species
SCN	Suprachiasmatic Nucleus
SOD	Superoxide Dismutase
TNF	Tumor Necrosis Factor

10.1 REDOX HOMEOSTASIS, OXIDATIVE STRESS, AND ANTIOXIDANTS

Reactive oxygen species (ROS) and reactive nitrogen species (RNS) include reactive free radicals and non-radicals that are the by-products of cellular redox processes. In the normal physiological state, the production and accumulation of ROS are tightly controlled by endogenous antioxidant defense mechanisms, that consist of enzymatic and non-enzymatic antioxidants. The "steady-state" level of ROS is maintained by the equilibrium between their production rate and their removal rate by the antioxidant system. The redox state of a cell and its alternation controls cellular function. ROS-mediated actions and protection of the cell from ROS-mediated damage, to maintain the "redox balance", is known as "redox homeostasis" (Sen and Chakraborty, 2011).

Free radicals are produced continuously from both endogenous and exogenous sources. ROS are produced in the body during the immune response, metabolic processes, inflammation, respiratory processes, and stress, whereas the major exogenous sources of ROS include pollution, radiation, drugs, toxin, junk foods, smoking, etc. (Sen and Chakraborty, 2011; Sen et al., 2010). Different free radicals include superoxide ($O_2^{\bullet -}$), hydroxyl (•OH), peroxyl (ROO•), alkoxyl (RO•), nitric oxide (NO•), lipid peroxyl (LOO•), and nitrogen dioxide ($NO_2^{\bullet}$) radicals. Examples of non-radical reactive species are peroxide (H_2O_2), singlet oxygen ($^1O_2$), ozone (O_3), dinitrogen trioxide (N_2O_3), hypochlorous acid (HOCl), nitrous acid (HNO_2), peroxynitrite (ONOO–), and lipid peroxide (LOOH). In low to moderate levels, ROS/RNS are beneficial for the body as they play an important role by enhancing immunity (killing microorganisms by phagocytosis), destroying cancer cells, detoxifying xenobiotics, generating ATP, promoting cell growth, inducing mitogenic responses, and promoting cellular signaling (Sen and Chakraborty, 2011).

Increased production of ROS and/or reduced levels of endogenous antioxidant defense results in oxidative stress. Oxidative stress is responsible for damage to cells, including lipids and membranes, proteins, and DNA, and disruption of cell function and signaling. Oxidative stress has been described as a key mechanism underlying the pathophysiology of various diseases, such as cancer, neurodegenerative diseases, cardiovascular diseases, neurological disorders, diabetes, and aging, etc. (Sen and Chakraborty, 2011). Antioxidants are any materials that delay or inhibit oxidative stress damage. An antioxidant molecule reacts with free radicals and scavenges them by donating one of their electrons, and thus stopping the free radical-induced carbon-stealing reaction.

Antioxidants avert damage to cells and tissues as they act as ROS scavengers. The human body is well equipped with an endogenous antioxidant system that plays a key role in maintaining redox homeostasis, whereas exogenous antioxidants, such as various phytomolecules, also achieve health-promoting effect by scavenging ROS (Sen and Chakraborty, 2011; Sen et al., 2010). Table 10.1 and Table 10.2 list details of various endogenous and exogenous antioxidants.

10.2 ALZHEIMER'S DISEASE

Dementia is associated with progressive weakening of the intellectual ability or functionS like memory, decision making, language, attention, reasoning, etc. Dementia can be categorized as reversible or irreversible. Alzheimer's disease (AD) is considered to be the most common cause of (irreversible) dementia, accounting for most cases of dementia. Other forms of primary dementia are vascular dementia, dementia linked with Parkinson's disease, frontotemporal dementia, and dementia with Lewy bodies (Korolev, 2014). In 2018, it was estimated that about 50 million people were living with dementia worldwide, and the number will reach 152 million by 2050. The total worldwide cost of dementia was estimated to be US$1 trillion in 2018, a figure which is predicted to double by 2050 (Patterson, 2018).

TABLE 10.1
Different Endogenous Antioxidants and Their Action

Major Endogenous Antioxidant	Details
Superoxide dismutase (SOD)	• SOD is a protein containing zinc/copper, or manganese, iron, or nickel. • Acts as the first-line defense system against ROS. • Scavenges superoxide radicals. • SOD catalyzes the neutralization of $O_2^{\bullet-}$ to H_2O_2 and O_2. • Humans have three types of SOD: SOD-1,which is located in the cytoplasm, SOD-2 located in the mitochondria, and SOD-3 present in extracellular spaces.
Glutathione peroxidase (GPx)	• GPx exists in two forms, i.e. selenium-dependent and selenium-independent. • They have different subunits with different active sites. • They catalyze the reduction of H_2O_2/ROOH to H_2O or alcohol; this process requires reduced glutathione (GSH), which is converted to GSSG (oxidized glutathione). • GPx has four isoforms: GPx1 is cytosolic and mitochondrial, GPx2 is cytosolic, GPx3 is extracellular, and GPx4 is a phospholipid peroxidase. • Kidneys and liver contain highest GPx activities. • GPx enzymes act as the first line of defense against oxidative stress.
Reduced glutathione (GSH)	• In the nucleus, GSH maintains the redox state and causes DNA repair and expression. • It is the major nonprotein intracellular thiol compound, biosynthesized from cysteine, glutamate, and glycine. • GSH is important for detoxifying free radicals and also xenobiotics. • It is capable of neutralizing hydroxyl radicals and singlet oxygen. • It also helps the catalytic detoxification of hydrogen peroxide and lipid peroxides by GPx.
Glutathione reductase (GR)	• GR is a flavoprotein enzyme and is important for cellular antioxidant defense and is also necessary for the conversion of GSH. • The Oxidized glutathione (GSSG) is reduced back to GSH by the presence of GR. It uses NADPH as the electron donor.
Catalase (CAT)	• It catalyzes the conversion of H_2O_2 to H_2O and O_2. • It is mainly located in peroxisomes.
CoQ10	• It is mainly involved in the inhibition of lipid peroxidation and reduces oxidative stress in mitochondria • It also recycles vitamin E.

TABLE 10.2
Different Exogenous Antioxidants and Their Actions

Exogenous Antioxidant	Antioxidant Mechanism
Flavonoids 1. Anthocyanidins e.g. cyanidin, delphinidin 2. Flavonols e.g. kaempferol, quercetin 3. Isoflavonoids e.g. daidzein, genistein 4. Flavones e.g. apigenin, luteolin 5. Flavanones e.g. naringenin, hesperetin 6. Flavanols e.g. epicatechin, catechin, 7. Condensed tannins 8. Hydroxybenzoic acid e.g. gallic acid, protocatechuic acid 9. Hydroxycinnamic acids e.g. caffeic acid, chlorogenic acid, coumaric acid, ferulic acid	• Flavonoids scavenge hydroxyl radicals, lipid peroxy radicals, and superoxide anions.
Vitamin E	• Scavenges superoxide, hydroxyl radicals • Involved in upregulation of antioxidant enzymes and breaks chain reactions of lipid peroxidation
Bilirubin	• It has the efficiency to neutralize peroxyl radicals and protects human cells from peroxyl radical-induced oxidation of albumin-bound linoleic acid
Vitamin C	• It is involved in neutralization of superoxide, hydroxyl radicals; protects stimulated neutrophils from oxidants and regenerates vitamin E
Carotenoids 1. α-carotene 2. β-carotene 3. γ-carotene 4. crocin 5. β-cryptoxanthin 6. Lycopene 7. lutein 8. Zeaxanthin 9. bixin 10. Astaxanthin 11. Capsorubin 12. Canthaxanthin	• Antioxidant activity of carotenoids is due to the capacity to quench singlet oxygen • Vitamin A can be biosynthesized from α- and β-carotene and β-cryptoxanthin, and is involved in its related role of disease prevention

AD is a multifactorial, progressive, neurodegenerative disease that involves major disruption of brain function and structure. No single cause is associated with AD, although a number of non-modifiable and modifiable risk factors are linked with disease development and progression. The risk of AD is increased by age, particularly in old-aged people. Progressive loss of or damage to cortical neurons (particularly pyramidal cells), synaptic dysfunction (in the early stage of AD), and problems with communication within neural circuits are some characteristics of AD. Neurodegeneration in AD starts in the medial temporal lobe, particularly in the entorhinal cortex and hippocampus, and then it spreads throughout the temporal linked cortex and to the parietal areas. In advanced stages, degeneration can be seen in the frontal cortex, and, ultimately, in most of the remaining neocortex area (Korolev et al., 2014).

10.3 PATHOGENESIS OF AD

Extracellular accumulation of amyloid plaques and intracellular deposition of neurofibrillary tangles (NFTs) in the brain of patient with AD are considered to be hallmarks of AD. Activation of the inflammatory response, along with the innate immune reaction, excessive deposition of iron, and damage to mitochondria are also linked with the pathogenesis of AD (Wojsiat et al., 2018).

Amyloid-β (Aβ) is usually a secreted and soluble protein, that exists in several isoforms. Aβ is the key element of neuritic/amyloid peptide plaques generated by the improper cleavage of amyloid precursor protein (APP). Isoform Aβ42 is insoluble in nature and is generated by unusual APP processing, that accumulates in the form of aggregates, which enclose the amyloid protein in the form of oligomers, fibrils, or protofibrils (Sajjad et al., 2018). The proteolytic process happens near or within the APP transmembrane domain. β-secretases (β-site APP cleaving enzymes; BACEs) and γ-secretases are the key proteases responsible for the formation of Aβ. In the first step, β-secretase cleaves APP to form the N terminus of Aβ that results in the formation of the C-terminal fragment known as C99. In the next step, γ-secretase cleaves C99 to produce the mature Aβ peptide. The third protease, α-secretase, cleaves APP within the Aβ domain, thus preventing Aβ formation (Sajjad et al., 2018; Vassar et al., 2009).

NFTs are produced due to abnormal hyperphosphorylated tau (p-τ) proteins. The tau protein is a member of a family of microtubule-linked proteins, which are available in the cytosol and in neuronal axons. Hyperphosphorylation of tau protein increases its capacity to accumulate into tangles of paired helical filaments, gathering in the form of aggregates and leading to the loss of axonal/dendritic transport, and the disassembly of microtubules. APP dysfunction, following tau pathology, within the entorhinal cortex and hippocampus, is linked to AD (Sajjad et al., 2018). Scientific evidence indicates that alteration in τ protein and Aβ oligomers are the key factors that account for neuronal dysfunction in the pathogenesis of AD (Sanabria-Castro et al., 2017).

Acetylcholine (ACh) is a key neurotransmitter in the brain, with action occurring throughout the cortex, basal ganglia, and basal forebrain. Association of AD with the cholinergic system was one of the earliest mechanisms analyzed in relation to AD pathogenesis. Pathological observation of AD brains showed that the cholinergic lesion, considered an early asymptomatic or prodromal phase of AD, is largely presynaptic rather than postsynaptic. Loss of cholinergic neurons or degeneration of cholinergic neurons is associated with the pathogenesis of AD. Nicotinic and muscarinic receptors in the cerebral cortex undergo changes as part of the cholinergic lesion. A number of studies have shown that nicotinic receptors in the cerebral cortex are lost during AD. Evidence also found the postsynaptic M1 receptors of the cerebral cortex are dysfunctional. The cholinergic hypothesis of AD focuses on the gradual loss of limbic and neocortical cholinergic innervation. In the basal forebrain, neurofibrillary degeneration is considered to be the main cause of the dysfunction and death of forebrain cholinergic neurons (Hampel et al., 2018).

Association between increased production of free radicals, depletion of endogenous antioxidants, and the resulting oxidative stress damage are other key causes of AD, which will be discussed in detail in the next section.

10.4 ASSOCIATION OF OXIDATIVE STRESS AND AD

Oxidative stress is considered to be a major cause of AD, although the exact nature of the relationship is still uncertain and needs to be investigated further. ROS have been found to modulate the generation/secretion of Aβ, with overproduction of Aβ, related to APP overexpression, also being associated with increased generation of ROS (Wojsiat et al., 2018). Free radical-induced oxidative stress also increases the aggregation of Aβ and increases tau protein hyperphosphorylation and polymerization. Depletion of antioxidant enzymes increases the risk of AD through increased Aβ oligomerization and aggravated memory dysfunction. It has been hypothesized that α-secretase activity/expression is decreased by oxidative stress, while β- and γ-secretase activities are increased by oxidative stress (Kim et al., 2015). The excessive generation and accumulation of ROS can lead to oxidative stress in the brain of patients with AD, that may induce mitochondrial dysfunction. On the other hand, loss of functional and structural integrity of mitochondria also induces ROS production. A number of studies showed that Aβ-induced oxidative imbalance may raise the concentration of byproducts associated with lipid peroxidation (e.g. 4-hydroxynonal, malondialdehyde [MDA]), oxidation of DNA and RNA (e.g. 8-hydroxyldeoxyguanosine and 8-hydroxylguanosine), and protein oxidation (e.g. carbonyl groups) (Wojsiat et al., 2018; Kim et al., 2015).

Oxidative stress and dysfunctional glucose metabolism are interlinked, and play a key role in AD. The brain utilizes glucose for energy, but, during AD, the metabolism of glucose is radically reduced, due possibly to oxidative injury to enzymes that play a key role in glycolysis, the TCA cycle, and ATP biosynthesis. Other proteins (e.g. BVRA – biliverdin reductase A, UCHL1 – ubiquitin carboxyterminal hydrolase L1, and the proteasome) are also susceptible to oxidative damage. Reduced generation of ATP causes a number of changes in brain function, e.g. damage to membrane potentials and increases in Ca^{2+} levels (intracellular), which reduces cell function and survival. Aβ42 also promotes oxidative stress, that leads to lipid peroxidation and impairs glucose metabolism. These changes lower the activity of the brain and cause synaptic dysfunction and neuronal death. Presynaptic membranes are also susceptible to oxidative damage, that causes reduced learning and memory, and ultimately dementia (Butterfield and Halliwell, 2019).

The loss of synapses in the brains of AD patients is associated with the cognitive impairment believed to be an early mechanism of AD that leads to neuronal loss. Evidence showed that increased levels of ROS are linked with the destruction/reduction of mitochondrial function, distortion of metal homeostasis, and a decreased level of antioxidant defense that negatively impacts upon synaptic activity and neurotransmission. Increased levels of ROS also destroy nuclear and mitochondrial DNA, proteins, lipids, and cellular architecture, alter calcium and energy homeostasis, and induce trafficking of receptors and endocytosis. Such effects again increase production and accumulation of the p-τ proteins (Tonnies and Trushina, 2017).

It has also been shown that expression of the nicotinic and muscarinic receptors can be influenced by high levels of free radicals. Cholinergic receptors are located on the phospholipid-based cell membranes. The brain is more susceptible to the induction of free radicals as it requires more oxygen and energy than other parts of the body, and it is also enriched in oxy-radical-susceptible polyunsaturated fatty acids. Lipids that surround the receptor are vulnerable to attack by free radicals. The relationship between oxidative stress and the loss/destruction of the nicotinic receptor from the temporal cortex area was investigated and the report described a significant relationship between increased lipid peroxidation and a reduced number of nicotinic receptors. Another study reported that Aβ-induced lipid peroxidation may induce a scarcity of nicotinic receptors. Reports also indicated that COS-7 cells transfected with muscarinic receptors (M1, M2, M4) exhibited greater oxidative stress sensitivity than cells without the receptors (Guan, 2008)

10.5 ANTIOXIDANT PHYTOCHEMICALS/EXTRACTS AND AD

10.5.1 Possible Role of Antioxidants in AD

The human antioxidant defense is important for good health and protection from diseases. The endogenous antioxidant defense system helps us to avert various diseases *via* different mechanisms. Antioxidants act against the harmful effects of ROS and maintain the optimum level of ROS in body (Sajjad et al., 2019). Exogenous antioxidants supplied by plants in the diet or as supplements can help to scavenge excess ROS, and act in synergy with endogenous antioxidants. Free radical-induced oxidative stress is considered to be one of the mechanisms underlying the pathogenesis of AD. Several types of research have shown that antioxidant phytochemicals attenuate Aβ-induced apoptosis, reduce Aβ production and aggregation, inhibit tau aggregation, inhibit oxidative stress-induced DNA/RNA/lipid/protein modification, and reduce lipid peroxidation, etc. (Feng and Wang, 2012). Considering the above observations, it may be predicted that using antioxidant phytoextracts/phytomolecules could be one of the key approaches in the future to prevent or reduce oxidative damage in the brain, and that could, at least in part, help in the prevention/management of AD.

10.5.2 Plants Active against AD

A number of plants have been investigated in different *in-vitro* and *in-vivo* studies to determine their effectiveness as a future source of antioxidant drugs in the management of AD. These plants have also been investigated for their antioxidant properties and have shown potent free radical scavenging effects. In Table 10.3, a number of plants are listed that have been investigated in preclinical trials.

Mathew and Subramanian (2014) investigated a number of Indian traditional medicinal plants, namely *Acorus calamus, Bacopa monnieri, Cedrus deodera, Celastrus paniculatus, Centella asiatica, Convolvulus pluricaulis, Coriandrum sativum, Emblica officinalis, Evolvulus alsinoides, Glycyrrhiza glabra, Nardostachys jatamansi, Nelumbo nucifera, Punica granatum, Rauwolfia serpentina, Saussurea lappa, Terminalia chebula, Tinospora cordifolia, Trigonella foenum-graecum, Valeriana wallichii,* and *Withania somnifera* for their *in-vitro* antioxidant and AChE inhibitory activities. Among the plant extracts, *E. officinalis, N. jatamansi, N. nucifera, P. granatum and R. serpentina* exhibited strong AChE inhibitory activity.

Adewusi et al. (2010) documented different plants with cholinesterase inhibitory activity: *Tribulus terrestris* (whole plant), *Zygophyllum fabago* (whole plant), *Symplocos chinensis* (whole plant), *Meliosma oldhamii* (whole plant), *Pyrola japonica* (whole plant), *Teucrium polium* (aerial parts), *Salvia syriaca* (whole plant), *Salvia sclarea* (whole plant), *Salvia multicaulis* (whole plant), *Salvia migrostegia* (whole plant), *Salvia aucheri* (whole plant), *Origanum syriacum* (aerial parts), *Origanum ehrenbergii* (aerial parts), *Fumaria vaillantii* (whole plant), *Fumaria petteri* (whole plant), *Fumaria kralikii* (whole plant), *Fumaria asepala* (whole plant), *Vicia faba* (whole plant), *Capsella bursa-pastoris* (whole plant), *Tabernaemontana divaricata* (whole plant), *Rhododendron schlippenbachii* (whole plant), *Rhododendron ponticum* (whole plant), *Chamaecyparis pisifera* (whole plant), *Robinia pseudoacacia* (whole plant), and *Terminalia chebula* (fruit), etc. exerted both AChE and butyrylcholinesterase (BChE) inhibitory activities. Plants which exhibited only AChE inhibitory include *Alpinia galangal* (rhizomes), *Lantana camara* (aerial parts), *N. jatamansi* (rhizomes), *C. asiatica* (whole plant), *Myricaria elegans* (aerial parts), *W. somnifera* (root), *B. monnieri* (whole plant), *Mimusops elengi* (flower), *Salix mucronata* (bark), *Ruta graveolens* (whole plant), *Aegle marmelos* (fruit pulp), *Rubia cordifolia* (stem), *Paederia linearis* (whole plant), *Sanguisorba minor* (aerial parts), *Cymbopogon schoenanthus* (whole plant), *Plumbago indica* (root), *Piper nigrum* (seed), *Piper interruptum* (stem), *Corydalis solida* (whole plant, tuber), *Corydalis intermedia* (whole plant), *Corydalis cava* (whole plant, tuber), *Ptychopetalum olacoides* (root), *Boerhavia diffusa* (whole plant), *Nelumbo nucifera* (stamen), *Embelia ribes* (fruit, root, seeds), *Musa sapientum* (fruit), *Moringa oleifera* (bark), *Ficus religiosa* (bark), *Streblus asper* (seed), *Acacia sieberiana* (root), *Acacia nilotica* (leaf, bark), *T. cordifolia* (stem), *Tiliacora triandra* (root), *Stephania suberosa* (root), *Trichilia dregeana* (bark), *Azadirachta indica* (bark), and *Malva sylvestris* (aerial parts).

Dastmalchi et al. (2007) reviewed potential source of drugs from herbal medicinal plants for treatment of AD. Preclinical studies have shown the potential of different medicinal plants, namely *A. calamus, Angelica archangelica, B. monnieri, Biota orientalis, C. paniculatus, C. asiatica, Clitoria ternatea, Codonopsis pilosula, C. pluricaulis, Coptis chinensis, Crocus sativus, Curcuma longa, Evodia rutaecarpa, Ginkgo biloba, Hypericum perforatum, Magnolia officinalis, Melissa officinalis, Piper methysticum, Polygala tenuifolia, Rheum* spp., *Salvia lavandulaefolia, Salvia miltiorrhizia, Salvia officinalis, Terminalia chebula,* and *W. somnifera* as future sources of candidate drugs against AD.

10.5.3 Phytoconstituents and AD

10.5.3.1 Curcumin

Curcumin is the main constituent of *Curcuma longa* and has shown diverse pharmacological activities. *In-vitro, in-vivo,* and epidemiological studies have shown the possible effectiveness of

TABLE 10.3
Different Plants and Their Effect Investigated for Future Sources of Drugs in Management of AD

Plant Name	Observation From Preclinical Trials
Melissa officinalis	Ethanol extract of leaves reduced AChE enzyme activity in rat hippocampus after intraperitoneal injection. Oral administration of ethanol extract improved spatial memory and reduced amyloid plaques in hippocampus. The extract also improved the underlying behavioral and cognitive reaction of rats treated with scopolamine. *M. officinalis* showed AChE and BChE inhibitory activity and also reduced BACE mRNA expression in brain. Anti-inflammatory and strong antioxidant activity exerted by the plant extract may also contribute to its activity against AD (Mahboubi, 2019).
Salvia species	*Salvia* species exerted Aβ peptide effect, cholinergic, neurotrophic, anxiolytic, anti-inflammatory, and antioxidant effects. *S. miltiorrhiza* displayed a protective effect against neurotoxicity in mice induced by Aβ that may link with its effect i.e. inhibition of TNF-α, IL-6 and AChE activity. *S. sahendica* WAS found to attenuate memory deficits, modulate cAMP response, and reduce apoptosis in Aβ-injected experimental animals. *S. officinalis* extracts reduced AChE and BChE activity. *S. sahendica* in mice ameliorated AChE activity and cognitive ability positively. Tanshinones isolated from *S. miltiorrhiza* inhibited AChE and BChE activities. *S. miltiorrhiza* mitigated Aβ-induced reductions in brain-derived neurotrophic factor in mice (Lopresti, 2017).
Ginkgo biloba	This plant is known for its diverse biological activities. Different *in-vitro*, preclinical, and clinical studies have confirmed the effectiveness of *G. biloba* in age-related disorders. *G. biloba* exhibits strong free radical scavenging and antioxidant activity. Extract of *G. biloba* possesses antiapoptosis and anti-inflammatory activity. The extract was found to be effective against dysfunction of mitochondria, amyloidogenesis, aggregation of Aβ, modulation of phosphorylation of tau protein, etc (Shi et al., 2010).
Kigelia africana	Methanol extract of *K. africana* leaves and its flavonoid-rich fraction found to be effective against $AlCl_3$-induced AD in the experimental animal. Treatment with the fraction effectively reversed neurological deficits in different experimental models. Fraction effectively reduced oxidative stress and also decreased cholinesterase activities (Falode et al., 2017).
Elatostema papillosum	80% methanol extract of *E. papillosum* leaves exhibited strong AChE and BChE inhibitory activity. The extract also potentially showed free radical scavenging activity (Reza et al., 2018).
Panax ginseng	Extract of ginseng were found to be effective against AD in preclinical studies. Ginseng was found to inhibit Aβ-induced neurotoxicity and attenuated the accumulation of Aβ in brains of experimental animals. Ginseng extract also improved memory function in experimental models. Extract of white ginseng was found to normalize synaptophysin and choline acetyltransferase activity in Aβ oligomer-injected mice. Two major components of ginseng, i.e. ginsenosides and gintonin, also showed AD-related neuroprotective activities. Ginsenosides reduced formation of Aβ formation through inhibition of β- and δ-secretase activities or through activation of the nonamyloidogenic pathway. Phytochemicals also inhibited AChE activity, reduced neurotoxicity and neuroinflammation, and exerted antioxidant activity (Kim et al., 2018).
Convolvulus pluricaulis	Effect of *C. pluricaulis* aqueous extract against human microtubule-associated protein tau *(hMAPτ)* induced neurotoxicity in AD *Drosophila* model. Supplementation of *C. pluricaulis* reduced hMAPτ-induced early death and enhanced the lifespan and reduced the τ protein level in tauopathic *Drosophila*. Extract also increased antioxidant enzyme and ameliorated oxidative stress; it also restored the reduced AChE activity in the fly model (Anupama et al., 2019).
Pinus halepensis	An essential oil obtained from *Pinus halepensis* was tested for neuroprotective and nootropic activity in acute Aβ1-42-induced toxicity in rat. The oil enhanced cognitive ability and memory, reduced the elevated AChE effect, and enhanced hippocampal SOD, CAT, GPX and GSH levels while reducing MDA level (Postu et al., 2019).
Cajanus cajan	Hydroalcoholic extract of *C. cajan* leaves conferred protective effect against memory impairment when tested on sleep-deprived experimental rats. Extract also exerted AChE inhibitory activity and enhanced level of endogenous antioxidants significantly (Ahmad et al., 2019).

(Continued)

TABLE 10.3 (CONTINUED)
Different Plants and Their Effect Investigated for Future Sources of Drugs in Management of AD

Plant Name	Observation From Preclinical Trials
Withania somnifera	Ashwagandha (*W. somnifera*) root is one of the popular Ayurvedic medicines for enhancing memory and for treating general debility, insomnia, etc. The plant causes neurite outgrowth, enhances memory, exerts neuroprotective effects, and causes clearance of Aβ. It also inhibits NF-κB activation, blocks the production of Aβ, decreases apoptotic cell death, restores synaptic function, increases antioxidant activity through Nrf2 migration to the nucleus, and enhances antioxidant enzyme activities (Kuboyama et al., 2014; Farooqui et al., 2018).
Rosmarinus officinalis	Extract of *R. officinalis* leaves was found to improve cognitive responses of rats. Extract also inhibited AChE and BChE activities and their mRNA expression levels in the brain (Ozarowski et al., 2013).
Bacopa monnieri	It is used in Ayurvedic medicine and has been investigated widely to confirm its therapeutic potential. The plant showed excellent free radical scavenging, antioxidant, and iron-chelating properties. The plant also exerted positive effects on the cholinergic system. *B. monnieri* was also found to attenuate sodium nitrite and scopolamine-induced amnesia, and also increased cerebral blood flow. An extract of the plant enhanced the expression of BDNF and the activity-regulated cytoskeleton-associated protein Arc in scopolamine-treated mice. Treatment with the extract averted Aβ protein-induced cell death and the associated increase in AChE activity. A clinical trial also confirmed the positive effect of *B. monnieri* extract (Chaudhari et al., 2017).

curcumin and its derivatives against AD. Curcumin or its derivatives were found to reduce the level of certain Aβ isoforms in primary neuronal cells of mouse, positively alter the immature-to-mature APP turnover, inhibit β-sheet aggregation, decrease APP and BACE1 overexpression, exert anti-Aβ aggregation potential, and γ-secretase inhibitory effect. In addition, curcumin is a strong antioxidant compound and also exerts anti-inflammatory activity by reducing COX (cyclooxygenase), TNF-α (tumor necrosis factor alpha), NFκB, and MAPK (mitogen-activated protein kinas), and levels of other inflammatory or pro-inflammatory cytokines like IL-1, IL-2, IL-6, IL-8, and IL-12. Preclinical evaluation also confirmed the neuroprotective effect of curcumin. Results obtained from different animal studies have shown that curcumin is effective at reducing levels of insoluble amyloid and Aβ plaque, exhibits antioxidant activity by increasing concentrations of endogenous antioxidants, reduces inflammatory or pro-inflammatory cytokines, suppresses JNK and tau phosphorylation, prevents the aggregation of Aβ, and increases the memory of experimental animals, etc. Epidemiological studies in India have also concluded that regular consumption of curcumin was associated with reduced prevalence of AD (Das and Devi, 2019).

10.5.3.2 Rosmarinic Acid

Rosmarinic acid showed anti-AChE activity and thus increased acetylcholine content. It also exhibited strong BChE stimulatory effect in the hippocampus. In a preclinical study, rosmarinic acid improved behavioral and cognitive responses in rats treated with scopolamine. Rosmarinic acid is a strong antioxidant molecule found in a range of plant species. In *in-vitro* experiments, rosmarinic acid inhibited Aβ-related ROS accumulation and the formation of Aβ fibrils, and also destabilized the fibrils of Aβ. Rosmarinic acid inhibited the production of pro-inflammatory cytokines, shielded the cells from toxicity induced by Aβ-induced toxicity, and inhibited phosphorylated-p38 mitogen-activated protein kinases and lipid peroxidation. It also inhibited the hyperphosphorylation of tau proteins and Aβ-induced apoptosis and DNA fragmentation (Mahboubi, 2019).

10.5.3.3 Huperzine A

Huperzine A, a major constituent of the toothed clubmoss *Huperzia serrata*, exhibited strong AChE inhibitory activity. Huperzine A is also found to decrease Aβ production and to preserve cells from

Aβ-induced damage. Clinical use of huperzine A to recover cognition and memory in patients with AD/dementia is recognized in China. It is also available in US as a memory- enhancing supplement (Damar et al., 2017). A number of clinical trials were conducted to test the effectiveness of huperzine A in treatment of patients with AD, where it was found to be effective and to improve cognitive ability, daily living activity, and global clinical assessment (Yang et al., 2013). Huperzine A possesses strong antioxidant and anti-inflammatory properties and demonstrated. amelioration of cognitive dysfunction and neuroinflammation through its antioxidant activity and inhibition of the NLRP3/caspase-1 inflammasome pathway (Mohseni-Moghaddam et al., 2019).

10.5.3.4 Pentylcurcumene

Pentylcurcumene, a terpene isolated from a *Geophila repens* hydroalcohol extract, has shown AChE and BChE inhibitory activities. A docking study also confirmed the binding capacity of the isolated compound with these two target enzymes. Pentylcurcumene also showed strong antioxidant activity (Dash et al., 2019).

10.5.3.5 Vitamin E

Vitamin E is an antioxidant, which is considered to be a neuroprotector. It exhibited anti-inflammatory properties, thought to be important for brain health. The α-tocopherol form is considered to be a potent antioxidant in the brain. *In-vitro* and preclinical studies indicated the effectiveness of vitamin E in treatment of AD. Several research studies were also carried out to correlate the level of vitamin E and AD incidence. A clinical trial with vitamin E supplementation was one of the most-popular areas of research in patients with AD or dementia in the past few decades Vitamin E has shown positive effects on cognition and in the treatment of dementia, but the results were not consistent and the findings were unreliable. Therefore, further studies are required to establish the effectiveness of vitamin E (Gugliandolo et al., 2017; Lloret et al., 2019).

10.5.3.6 Resveratrol

Resveratrol is a strong antioxidant and has shown its effectiveness in treatment/management of various disorders, including neurological disorders. It was believed that resveratrol is beneficial in neurological disorders as it has shown strong antioxidant and anti-inflammatory activity, overcoming two key pathological conditions which are known to induce CNS damage. Resveratrol is considered a potent SIRT1 activator that may contribute to mimicking caloric restriction in a way that averts diseases related to ageing. Preclinical studies showed that resveratrol was useful at improving age-dependent decline of cognitive ability and AD-like pathologies. It also causes vasodilation through the activation of nitric oxide (NO), which is helpful in improving post-ischemic cerebral perfusion in rats. Resveratrol effectively reduces pro-inflammatory and anti-inflammatory chemokines and cytokines. It has been reported that resveratrol can reduce levels of matrix metalloproteinase-9 (MMP-9) in CSF, enhance the cytokine interleukin-4 (IL-4), and decrease levels of Aβ40 and Aβ42, although few clinical studies on resveratrol have been reported (Berman et al., 2017; Sawda et al., 2018).

10.5.3.7 Luteolin

Luteolin is a well-known flavonoid which has been investigated widely for its beneficial effects on the CNS. Luteolin was found to enhance brain-derived neurotrophic factor (BDNF), synapsin I, and postsynaptic density protein 95 in the brains of obese mice, and to avert neuronal apoptosis. Luteolin also inhibits neuroinflammation by inhibiting the production of inflammatory markers. Luteolin reduces the activation of GSK-3, that also causes reduced levels of Aβ in the cerebral cortex of experimental animals. Luteolin also downregulates expression of BACE1 and NF-κB, the latter being key to a proinflammatory signaling pathway, followed by removal of Aβ peptides from the cerebral cortex and hippocampus. Luteolin reduces TNFα-induced inflammation through decreasing NF-κB and activator protein 1. Luteolin was found to inhibit activities of IL-6, IL-1β,

COX-2, TNFα, and interferon gamma and to decrease activity of cholinesterase in the cortex and the hippocampus area of obese mice. Luteolin exerted strong antioxidant activity that may also contribute to its neuroprotective effect in AD (Kwon, 2017).

10.5.3.8 Epigallocatechin-3-Gallate (EGCG)

EGCG is a flavanol that is abundantly available in tea and vegetables. EGCG is considered to be a very powerful antioxidant that actively scavenges ROS and also increases the activities of antioxidant enzymes. EGCG activates nuclear erythroid-2 related factor (Nrf2) and heme oxygenase-1 (HO-1), that would also contribute to its antioxidant property. EGCG is a highly anti-inflammatory compound and was found to reduce TNF-α, IL-1β, IL-6, IL-8, inducible nitric oxide synthase (iNOS), PGE, cyclooxygenase-2 (COX-2), NFκB, MAPK, and JNK. Administration of EGCG causes reduced levels of Aβ and repairs the mitochondrial respiratory status by decreasing generation of ROS in APP/PS1 mice. It is also found to reduce activities of the Aβ-synthesizing secretases (β- and γ-), while enhancing non-amyloidogenic α-secretase activity. EGCG also inhibits ERK/NFκB and JNK/cleaved-caspase3. A clinical trial with EGCG is in progress to assess the effectiveness of the molecule in patients with AD (Libro et al., 2016).

10.5.3.9 Withanolide

Different phytochemicals from Ashwagandha (*Withania somnifera*) roots have been considered to be potential leads for future drug molecules active against AD and dementia. An *in-vitro* study reported that withanolide A, withanoside IV, and withanoside VI caused neurite outgrowth when tested on rat cortical neurons and human neuroblastoma SH-SY5Y cells. Phytomolecules also caused axonal regeneration and synaptic reconstruction activity, and improved memory. Withaferin A may cause translocation of Nrf2 to the nucleus and is considered a key molecule for management of AD and dementia, as it can repair damaged neuronal networks (Kuboyama et al., 2014; Farooqui et al., 2018).

Flavonoids are well-known antioxidant molecules that are widely available in plants and which have demonstrated numerous beneficial effects on cognition and behavior. Flavonoids reduce oxidative stress and free radical-induced damage, enhance endogenous antioxidant levels, reduce neuroinflammation, increase neurogenesis and communication between cells (e.g. the cholinergic system), decrease the amyloid level, cause production of neurotrophins (e.g. BDNF), inhibit apoptosis and increase neuronal survival, causing induction of long-term potentiation. Flavonoids act through the extracellular signal-regulated kinases (ERK), cyclic adenosine monophosphate response element binding protein (CREB), brain-derived neurotrophic factor (BDNF), and phosphatidylinositol-3-kinase (PI3K), protein kinase B (AKT) pathways and enhance neuronal survival and proliferation. Plants rich in flavonoids showed effectiveness against AD or other forms of dementia during *in-vitro* or *in-vivo* studies. Flavonoids like quercetin, naringenin, hesperitin, acacetin, liquiritigenin, puerarin, swertisin, phloretin, etc have shown strong antioxidant activity and effectiveness as future drug candidates for the treatment of AD (Bakoyiannis et al., 2019) (Figure 10.1).

Research is being carried out to identify the most effective natural phytochemicals for the prevention and management of AD and other forms of dementia. Many phytochemicals, such as isothiocyanates (sulforaphane, moringin), phytocannabinoids (cannabidiol), physostigmine, phenolic compounds (such as nobiletin, quercetin, sinecatechins), terpenoids of *Ginkgo biloba*, such as limonoids), S-allyl cysteine, omega-3 fatty acids (e.g. α-linolenic acid, eicosapentaenoic acid, docosahexaenoic acid), alkaloids like rivastigmine, berberine, caffeine, galantamine, morphine, nicotine, and plumbagin have been investigated to evaluate their potency in treatment for prevention of AD, and preclinical results have been satisfactory (Libro et al., 2016; D'Onofrio et al., 2017; Velmurugan et al., 2018; Nakhate et al., 2018; Hartman and Ross, 2018; Williams et al., 2011). Phytochemicals like arecoline, asiaticosides, bacosides, biphenolic lignans, crocin, hyperforine, pilocarpine, srotoberberine alkaloids, stilbenes, tanshinones, terpenoid indole alkaloids, terpenoid

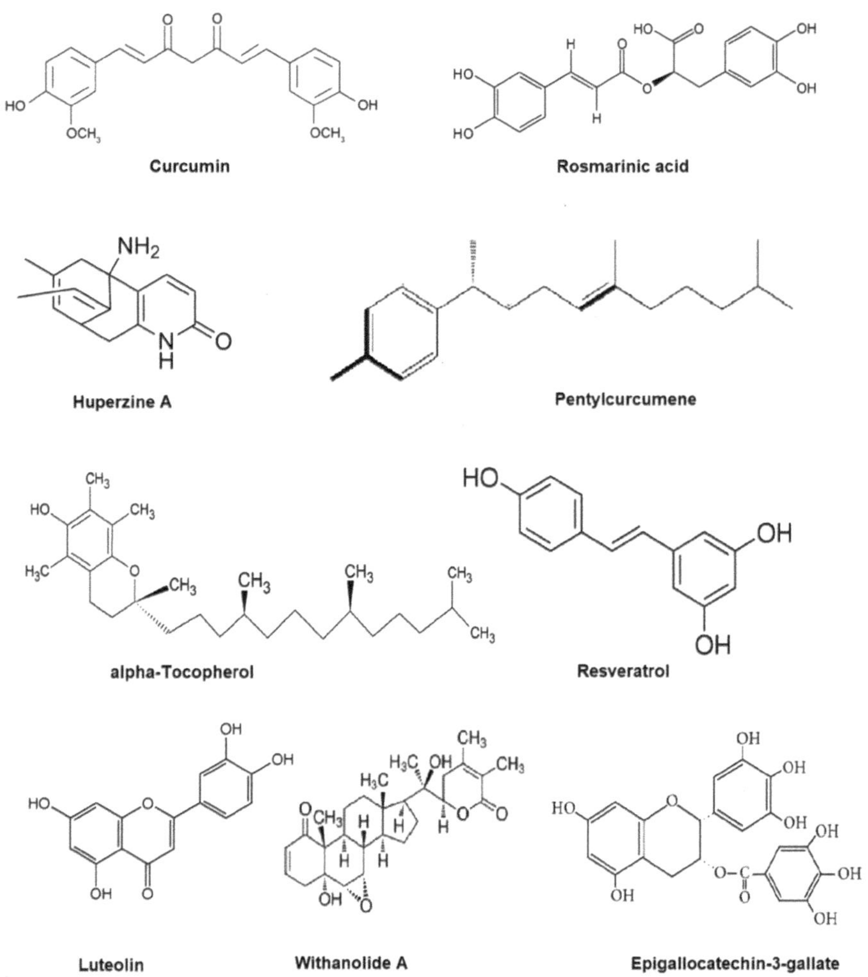

FIGURE 10.1 Chemical structures of different phytomolecules tested for their potential against AD.

trilactones, withanolides, and zeatin have also been investigated in preclinical trials for their potency as future drug molecules against AD (Dastmalchi et al., 2007).

It has clearly been shown that specific phytoextracts/phytomolecules are effective against AD, acting by various mechanisms, such as inhibition of oxidative stress, enhanced endogenous antioxidant levels, inhibition of lipid peroxidation, inhibition of beta- & gamma-secretases, Aβ production and aggregation, inhibited production of anti-inflammatory mediators, inhibition of modification of DNA/RNA, proteins, and lipids, induced BDNF secretion, and enhanced cholinergic activity, inhibited AChE and BChE activity, induced neurite outgrowth, inhibited formation of neurofibrillary tangles and tau proteins, achieved prevention of tau hyperphosphorylation, inhibition of tau aggregation, and stimulation of nicotinic and muscarinic receptors, etc. (Figure 10.2). Antioxidant activity of phytochemicals is considered to be one of the key mechanisms by which they act. In Figure 10.3, the pathogenesis of AD and the possible role of antioxidant phytochemicals/ phytoextracts is described.

10.6 FOOD SUPPLEMENTS AND CLINICAL TRIALS

A diet containing plant and animal sources rich in antioxidant molecules may reduce the risk of different diseases, including neurodegenerative diseases. Aging, inflammation, deposition of amyloid,

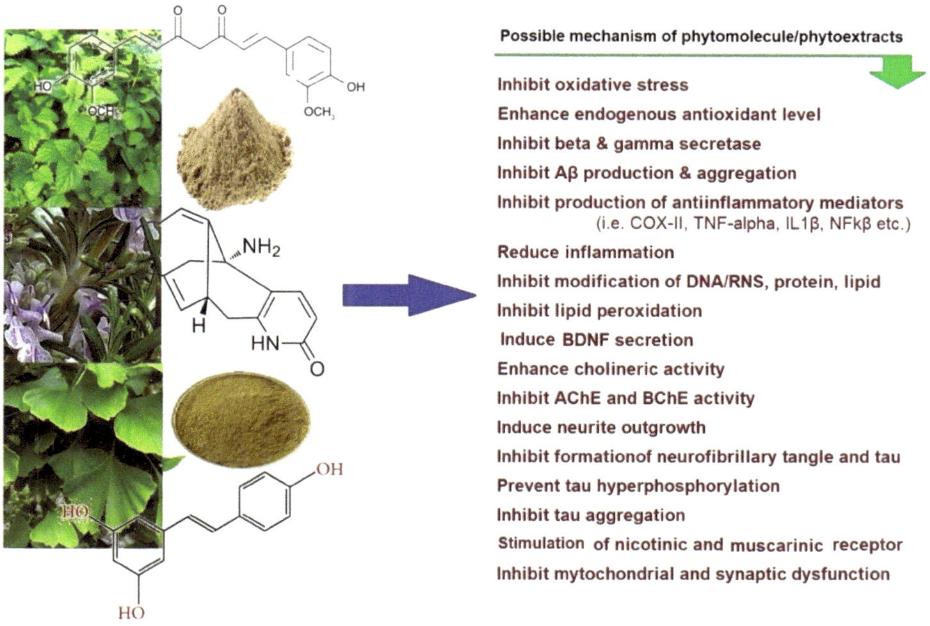

FIGURE 10.2 Different anti-AD mechanisms of phytochemicals/phytoextracts.

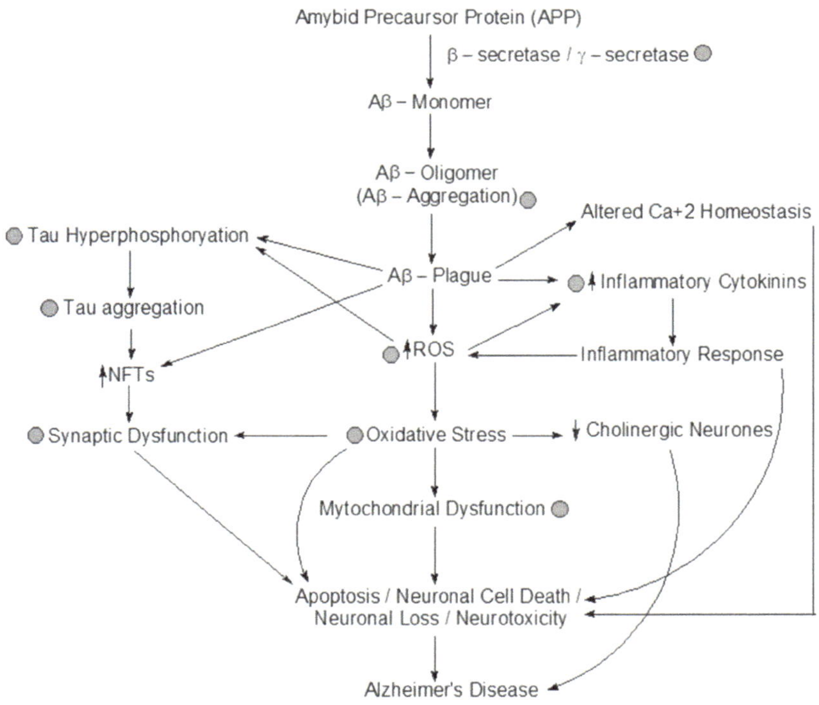

FIGURE 10.3 General causes and pathophysiology of AD. '○' is the area where antioxidant phytochemicals can innervate.

loss of synapse, neurofibrillary degeneration, oxidative stress, metabolic compromise, reduced/loss of vascular integrity, and injury/loss of neurons are some of the key pathological conditions associated with AD. Antioxidants (e.g. flavonoids & other phenolics), trace minerals, vitamins, metabolic substrates and modulators, and omega-3 fatty acids play important roles in maintaining normal brain health and slowing down/preventing the progression of AD. More, larger, and better clinical trials are essential to test the veracity of these claims of beneficial effects of such compounds in relation to AD (Swaminathan and Jicha, 2014). A diet supplemented with foods high in oxygen radical absorbance capacity (e.g. apple, spirulina) was found to reverse age-related reduction in the function of cerebellar β-adrenergic receptors and to reduce proinflammatory cytokine levels in aged rats. Levels of malondialdehyde (MDA) decreased after supplementation with apple and spirulina (Gemma et al., 2002). Dai et al. (2006) evaluated the effect of fruit and vegetable juices on human volunteers under the *Kame* project. It was observed that fruit and vegetable juices were effective in delaying the beginning of AD, particularly in people who are at high risk of developing the disease. A number of studies indicated that vitamin E, vitamin C, and flavonoids from food are effective in management/prevention of AD. Although the data were not sufficient to draw a conclusion, it was believed that a balanced increase in the intake of fruits, grains, and vegetables could be helpful in maintaining redox balance and modulating inflammatory processes, both of which can be helpful in decreasing the risk of developing neurodegenerative diseases like AD (Guest and Grant, 2012). Another study evaluated the effect of antioxidant supplements (vitamin E, vitamin C, lipoic acid, and coenzyme Q3) and found that the introduction of antioxidants did not alter CSF biomarkers related to amyloid or tau pathology, though the supplements did reduce oxidative stress in the brain (Galasko et al., 2012).

The effect of a standardized ethanol extract of *Melissa officinalis* was evaluated on patients with mild to moderate AD. Results concluded that the *M. officinalis* extract inhibited the progress of severe symptoms and reduce agitation of the patients. Another study showed that topical administration of the essential oil of *M. officinalis* (major components being citronellol, caryophyllene, neral, geraniol, geranyl acetate, and citronellal) reduced agitation in geriatric patients with severe dementia. A clinical trial on healthy individuals indicated that *M. officinalis* extract may improve the memory when administrated up to a certain dosage (Mahboubi, 2019).

A systematic review summarized the clinical potential of *Salvia officinalis* and *Salvia lavandulaefolia* against AD. The effect of these plants was investigated on both healthy individuals and on patients with AD. Studies on the healthy individuals found that plant was useful in improving memory, mood, and cognitive performance. Plants also proved useful for managing mild-to-moderate AD, improving attention and decreasing neuropsychiatric symptoms in patients with AD, although the systematic review also concluded that better-designed studies were required in this area (Miroddi et al., 2014). *Ginkgo biloba* extracts were also investigated in clinical trials. High doses of ginkgo (240 mg) elicited beneficial effects, in terms of improving cognitive ability and associated psychopathological symptoms (Janßen et al., 2010).

10.7 GENERAL CONSIDERATIONS, CONFUSION, AND FUTURE DIRECTIONS

Effects of a number of molecules/extracts with antioxidant properties, such as vitamin E, epigallocatechine gallate, resveratrol, curcumin, lipoic acid, and *Ginkgo biloba* extract, have been studied through clinical trials. But clinical trials of the roles of antioxidants in AD treatment have come to conflicting conclusions. A number of limitations of those studies, such as improper study design itself, lack of established efficacy on oxidative stress biomarkers, less/no nutritional information, lack of properly established neuropsychological parameters and lifestyle endpoints, and disease severity, etc. suggest that variation in these factors could be responsible for such conflicting conclusions (Mecocci and Polidori, 2012). Usually, it was believed that antioxidant molecules can cause only beneficial effects. However, when the effect of antioxidant supplements was investigated through different epidemiological/clinical trials for the treatment of various diseases, it was found that antioxidant supplementation may also increase the risk of particular diseases or may produce a null effect. Therefore, a well-balanced antioxidant-rich diet (with plenty of fruits and vegetables) are better options than supplements to meet the need of body (Sen and Chakraborty, 2015).

The current understanding from various clinical and preclinical research justifies the use of antioxidant molecules or foods rich in antioxidant molecules in the management of different degenerating disorder including AD. Sufficient research has confirmed the role of free radical-induced oxidative stress in the pathogenesis of AD, so that the role of antioxidant substances in the prevention/treatment of AD could be a future strategy for preventing several pathways of AD progression, such as inhibition of tau aggregation, Aβ aggregation, prevention of oxidative stress-induced cell damage, promotion of the cholinergic system, etc. Due to the lack of well-designed and long-term clinical trials, the beneficial effects of antioxidant molecules have not yet been confirmed. Although food rich in antioxidants has shown its potency against oxidative stress-related neurodegenerative disorders, current research continues to establish different antioxidant molecules as future drugs for the management of AD.

REFERENCES

Adewusi, E. A., Moodley, N., and Steenkamp, V. 2010. Medicinal plants with cholinesterase inhibitory activity: a review. *Afr J Biotechnol* 9(49): 8257–8276.

Ahmad, L., Mujahid, M., Mishra, A., and Rahman, M. A. 2019. Protective role of hydroalcoholic extract of *Cajanus cajan* Linn leaves against memory impairment in sleep deprived experimental rats. *J-AIM* (Article in Press). doi:10.1016/j.jaim.2018.08.003.

Anupama, K. P., Shilpa, O., Antony, A., Siddanna, T. K., and Gurushankara, H. P. 2019. *Convolvulus pluricaulis* (Shankhapushpi) ameliorates human microtubule-associated protein tau (hMAPτ) induced neurotoxicity in Alzheimer's disease Drosophila model. *J Chem Neuroanat* 95: 115–122.

Bakoyiannis, I., Daskalopoulou, A., Pergialiotis, V., and Perrea, D. 2019. Phytochemicals and cognitive health: are flavonoids doing the trick? *Biomed Pharmacother* 109: 1488–1497.

Berman, A. Y., Motechin, R. A., Wiesenfeld, M. Y., and Holz, M. K. 2017. The therapeutic potential of resveratrol: a review of clinical trials. *NPJ Precision Oncol* 35: 1–9.

Butterfield, D. A., and Halliwell, B. 2019. Oxidative stress, dysfunctional glucose metabolism and Alzheimer disease. *Nat Rev Neurosci* 20: 148–160.

Chaudhari, K. S., Tiwari, N. R., Tiwari, R. R., and Sharma, R. S. 2017. Neurocognitive effect of nootropic drug brahmi (Bacopa monnieri) in Alzheimer's disease. *Ann Neurosci* 24: 111–122.

Dai, Q., Borenstein, A. R., Wu, Y., Jackson, J. C., and Larson, E. B. 2006. Fruit and vegetable juices and Alzheimer's disease: the Kame project. *Am J Med* 119(9): 751–759.

Damar, U., Gersner, R., Johnstone, J. T., Schachter, S., and Rotenberg, A. 2017. Huperzine A: a promising anticonvulsant, disease modifying, and memory enhancing treatment option in Alzheimer's disease. *Med Hypotheses* 99: 57–62.

Das, M., and Devi, K. P. 2019. Potential role of curcumin and its derivatives against Alzheimer disease. In *Curcumin for Neurological and Psychiatric Disorders*, ed. T. Farooqui, and A. A. Farooqui, 211–230. Academic Press.

Dash, U. C., Kanhar, S., Dixit, A., Dandapat, J., and Sahoo, A. K. 2019. Isolation, identification, and quantification of Pentylcurcumene from *Geophila repens*: a new class of cholinesterase inhibitor for Alzheimer's disease. *Bioorg Chem* 88: 102947. doi:10.1016/j.bioorg.2019.102947.

Dastmalchi, K., Dorman, H. J. D., Vuorela, H., and Hiltunen, R. 2007. Plants as potential sources for drug development against Alzheimer's disease. *IJBPS* 1(2): 83–104.

Falode, J. A., Akinmoladun, A. C., Olaleye, M. T., and Akindahunsi, A. A. 2017. Sausage tree *(Kigelia africana)* flavonoid extract is neuroprotective in $AlCl_3$-induced experimental Alzheimer's disease. *Pathophysiology* 24(4): 251–259.

Farooqui, A. A., Farooqui, T., Madan, A., Ong, J. H., and Ong, W. 2018. Ayurvedic medicine for the treatment of dementia: mechanistic aspects. *Evid Based Complement Alternat Med* 2481076: 1–11. doi:10.1155/2018/2481076.

Feng, Y., and Wang, X. 2012. Antioxidant therapies for Alzheimer's disease. *Oxid Med Cell Longev* 472932: 1–17. doi:10.1155/2012/472932.

Gemma, C., Mesches, M. H., Sepesi, B., Choo, K., Holmes, D. B., and Bickford, P. C. 2002. Diets enriched in foods with high antioxidant activity reverse age-induced decreases in cerebellar-adrenergic function and increases in proinflammatory cytokines. *J Neurosci* 22(14): 6114–6120.

Guan, Z. 2008. Cross-talk between oxidative stress and modifications of cholinergic and glutaminergic receptors in the pathogenesis of Alzheimer's disease. *Acta Pharmacol Sin* 29(7): 773–780.

Guest, J. A., and Grant, R. S. 2012. Effects of dietary derived antioxidants on the central nervous system. *Int J Nutr Pharmacol Neurol Dis* 2(3): 185–197.

Gugliandolo, A., Bramanti, P., and Mazzon, E. 2017. Role of vitamin E in the treatment of Alzheimer's disease: evidence from animal models. *Int J Mol Sci* 18: 2504.

Hampel, H., Mesulam, M. M., Cuello, A. C., et al. 2018. The cholinergic system in the pathophysiology and treatment of Alzheimer's disease. *Brain* 2018: 1–17. doi:10.1093/brain/awy132.

Hartman, R. E., and Ross, D. M. 2018. Effects and mechanisms of actions of phytochemicals on Alzheimer's disease neuropathology. Front Biosci (Elite Ed) 10: 300–333.

Janßen, I. M., Sturtz, S., Skipka, G., Zentner, A., Garrido, M. V., and Busse, R. 2010. *Ginkgo biloba* in Alzheimer's disease: a systematic review. *Wien Med Wochenschr* 160/21–22: 539–546.

Kim, G. H., Kim, J. E., Rhie, S. J., and Yoon, S. 2015. The role of oxidative stress in neurodegenerative diseases. *Exp Neurobiol* 24(4): 325–340.

Kim, H. J., Jung, S. W., Kim, S. Y., et al. 2018. *Panax ginseng* as an adjuvant treatment for Alzheimer's disease. *J Ginseng Res* 42: 401–411.

Korolev, I. O. 2014. Alzheimer's disease: a clinical and basic science review. *Med Student Res J* 4: 24–33.

Kuboyama, T., Tohda, C., and Komatsu, K. 2014. Effects of Ashwagandha (roots of *Withania somnifera*) on neurodegenerative diseases. *Biol Pharm Bull* 37(6): 892–897.

Kwon, Y. 2017. Luteolin as a potential preventive and therapeutic candidate for Alzheimer's disease. *Exp Gerontol* 95: 39–43.

Libro, R., Giacoppo, S., Rajan, T. S., Bramanti, P., and Mazzon, E. 2016. Natural phytochemicals in the treatment and prevention of dementia: an overview. *Molecules* 21: 518. doi:10.3390/molecules21040518.

Lloret, A., Esteve, D., Monllor, P., Cervera-Ferri, A., and Lloret, A. 2019. The effectiveness of vitamin E treatment in Alzheimer's disease. *Int J Mol Sci* 20: 879. doi:10.3390/ijms20040879.

Lopresti, A. L. 2017. Salvia (Sage): a review of its potential cognitive-enhancing and protective effects. *Drugs R D* 17: 53–64.

Mahboubi, M. 2019. *Melissa officinalis* and rosmarinic acid in management of memory functions and Alzheimer disease. *Asian Pac J Trop Biomed* 9(2): 47–52.

Mathew, M., and Subramanian, S. 2014. *In vitro* screening for anti-cholinesterase and antioxidant activity of methanolic extracts of ayurvedic medicinal plants used for cognitive disorders. *PLoS One* 9(1): e86804. doi:10.1371/journal.pone.0086804.

Mecocci, P., and Polidori, M. C. 2012. Antioxidant clinical trials in mild cognitive impairment and Alzheimer's disease. *Biochim Biophys Acta* 1822: 631–638.

Miroddi, M., Navarra, M., Quattropani, M. C., Calapai, F., Gangemi, S., and Calapai, G. 2014. Systematic review of clinical trials assessing pharmacological properties of *Salvia* species on memory, cognitive impairment and Alzheimer's disease. *CNS Neurosci Ther* 20(6): 485–495.

Moghaddam, P. M., Sadr, S. S., Roghani, M., et al. 2019. Huperzine A ameliorates cognitive dysfunction and neuroinflammation in kainic acid-induced epileptic rats by antioxidant activity and NLRP3/caspase-1 pathway inhibition. *Clin Exp Pharmacol Physiol* (Online Published). doi:10.1111/1440-1681.13064.

Nakhate, K. T., Bharne, A. P., Verma, V. S., Aru, D. N., and Kokare, D. M. 2018. *Plumbagin ameliorates* memory dysfunction in streptozotocin induced Alzheimer's disease via activation of Nrf2/ARE pathway and inhibition of β-secretase. *Biomed Pharmacother* 101: 379–390.

Onofrio, G., Sancarlo, D., Ruan, Q., et al. 2017. Phytochemicals in the treatment of Alzheimer's disease: a systematic review. *Curr Drug Target* 18: 1487–1498.

Ozarowski, M., Mikolajczak, P. L., Bogacz, A., et al. 2013. *Rosmarinus officinalis* L. leaf extract improves memory impairment and affects acetylcholinesterase and butyrylcholinesterase activities in rat brain. *Fitoterapia* 91: 261–271.

Patterson, C. 2018. *World Alzheimer Report –2018. The State of the Art of Dementia Research: New Frontiers.* Published by Alzheimer's Disease International (ADI), London, September 2018.

Postu, P. A., Sadiki, F. Z., Idrissi, M. E., et al. 2019. *Pinus halepensis* essential oil attenuates the toxic Alzheimer's amyloid beta (1–42)-induced memory impairment and oxidative stress in the rat hippocampus. *Biomed Pharmacother* 112: 108673. doi:10.1016/j.biopha.2019.108673.

Reza, A. S. M. A., Hossain, M. S., Akhter, S., et al. 2018. *In vitro* antioxidant and cholinesterase inhibitory activities of *Elatostema papillosum* leaves and correlation with their phytochemical profiles: a study relevant to the treatment of Alzheimer's disease. *BMC Complement Altern Med* 18: 123. doi:10.1186/s12906-018-2182-0.

Sajjad, N., Wani, A., Hassan, S., et al. 2019. Interplay of antioxidants in Alzheimer's disease. *J Transl Sci* 5: 1–11.

Sajjad, R., Arif, R., Shah, A. A., Manzoor, I., and Mustafa, G. 2018. Pathogenesis of Alzheimer's disease: role of amyloid-β and hyperphosphorylated tau protein. *Indian J Pharm Sci* 80(4): 581–591.

Sanabria-Castro, A., Alvarado-Echeverría, I., and Monge-Bonilla, C. 2017. Molecular pathogenesis of Alzheimer's disease: an update. *Ann Neurosci* 24: 46–54.

Sawda, C., Moussa, C., and Turner, R. S. 2018. Resveratrol for Alzheimer's disease. *Ann N Y Acad Sci* 1403(1): 142–149.

Sen, S., and Chakraborty, R. 2011. The role of antioxidants in human health. In *Oxidative Stress: Diagnostics, Prevention, and Therapy*, ed. A. Silvana, and M. Hepel, 1–37. Washington, DC: American Chemical Society.

Sen, S., and Chakraborty, R. 2015. Antioxidant supplements: friend or foe? In *Free Radicals in Human Disease and Health*, ed. V. Rani, and U. C. C. S. Yadav, 293–322. New Delhi: Springer Publication.

Sen, S., Chakraborty, R., Sridhar, C., Reddy, Y. S. R., and De, B. 2010. Free radicals, antioxidants, diseases and phytomedicines: current status and future prospect. *Int J Pharma Sci Rev Res* 3: 91–100.

Shi, C., Liu, J., Wu, F., and Yew, D. T. 2010. *Ginkgo biloba* extract in Alzheimer's disease: from action mechanisms to medical practice. *Int J Mol Sci* 11: 107–123.

Swaminathan, A., and Jicha, G. A. 2014. Nutrition and prevention of Alzheimer's dementia. *Front Aging Neurosci* 6: 282. doi:10.3389/fnagi.2014.00282.

Tonnies, E., and Trushina, E. 2017. Oxidative stress, synaptic dysfunction, and Alzheimer's disease. *J Alzheimers Dis* 57: 1105–1121.

Vassar, R., Kovacs, D. M., Yan, R., and Wong, P. C. 2009. The *β*-secretase enzyme BACE in health and Alzheimer's disease: regulation, cell biology, function, and therapeutic potential. *J Neurosci* 29(41): 12787–12794.

Velmurugan, B. K., Rathinasamy, B., Lohanathan, B. P., Thiyagarajan, V., and Weng, C. 2018. Neuroprotective role of phytochemicals. *Molecules* 23: 2485. doi:10.3390/molecules23102485.

Williams, P., Sorribas, A., and Howes, M. R. 2011. Natural products as a source of Alzheimer's drug leads. *Nat Prod Rep* 28: 48. http://pubs.rsc.org|doi:10.1039/C0NP00027B.

Wojsiat, J., Zoltowska, K. M., Laskowska-Kaszub, K., and Wojda, U. 2018. Oxidant/antioxidant imbalance in Alzheimer's disease: therapeutic and diagnostic prospects. *Oxid Med Cell Longev* 6435861: 1–16. doi:10.1155/2018/6435861.

Yang, G., Wang, Y., Tian, J., and Liu, J. 2013. Huperzine A for Alzheimer's disease: a systematic review and meta-analysis of randomized clinical trials. *PLoS One* 8(9): e74916. doi:10.1371/journal.pone.0074916.

11 Neuroprotective Role of Curcumin in Alzheimer's Disease

Magisetty Obulesu and B. Mahendran

CONTENTS

ABBREVIATIONS

AD	Alzheimer's Disease
ADP/ATP	Adenosine Diphosphate/Adenosine Triphosphate
ApoE	Apolipoprotein E
APP/PS1	Amyloid precursor Protein/Presenilin1
Aβ	Amyloid Beta
BACE1	Beta Amyloid Cleaving Enzyme-1
BBB	Blood–brain Barrier
CNS	Central Nervous System
COX-2	Cyclooxygenase-2
DDS	Drug Delivery Systems
GSH	Glutathione
HD	Huntington's Disease
IL-10	Interleukin-10
IL-1β	Interleukin-1β
IL-4	Interleukin-4
iNOS	inducible Nitric Oxide Synthase
JAK	Janus Kinases
LPS	Lipopolysaccharide
MDA	Malondialdehyde
NDs	Neurodegenerative Diseases
NF-κβ	Nuclear factor κ Beta
NLCs	Nanolipid Capsules

NPs	Nanoparticles
PD	Parkinson's Disease
PSD95	Post-synaptic Density Protein 95
RES	Reticuloendothelial System
ROS	Reactive oxygen Species
SLNs	Solid Lipid Nanoparticles
SOCS-1	Suppressors of Cytokine Signaling
SOD	Superoxide Dismutase
STAT3	Signal Transducer and Activator of Transcription
TNF-α	Tumor Necrosis Factor-α

11.1 INTRODUCTION

The most critical diseases of the central nervous system (CNS) are neurodegenerative diseases (NDs), leading to neuronal death (Yavarpour et al., 2019). The vital mechanisms involved in these diseases include oxidative stress, protein aggregation, and neuroinflammation (Koo et al., 1999; Emerit et al., 2004; Amor et al., 2010; Yavarpour et al., 2019). Brain tissue is particularly susceptible to oxidative stress, due to its demand for increased amounts of oxygen and the presence of unsaturated fatty acids, that may induce structural and functional impairment in nerve cells (Sadegh Malvajerd et al., 2019).

11.1.1 Curcumin

Curcumin, the main curcuminoid isolated from turmeric, *Curcuma longa* L., has been extensively used as a dietary supplement, and it exerts many health benefits such as antioxidant, antitumor, anti-inflammatory, and neuroprotective effects (Lopez-Lazaro, 2008; Ishrat et al., 2009; Gazal et al., 2014; Zhang et al., 2015; Yu et al., 2018; Giacomeli et al., 2019). Curcumin has been used extensively in India and East Asian countries to enhance digestion, improve circulation, and inhibit inflammation (Kim et al., 2019a; Yavarpour-Bali et al., 2019). Curcumin has been extensively used as a dietary supplement, due to its robust antioxidant activity, particularly in Indian cuisine (Toda et al., 1985; Tharakan et al., 2010; Tsai et al., 2011; Canales-Aguirre et al., 2012; Massimino et al., 2017; Kim et al., 2019a). Its role as a potential antioxidant inhibits the production of free radicals (Kim et al., 2005; Sadegh Malvajerd et al., 2019) and also decreases lipid peroxidation considerably (Frautschy et al., 2001; Sadegh Malvajerd et al., 2019). Curcumin has also been known to ameliorate impairment of memory and cognition in Alzheimer's disease (AD) (Mishra and Palanivelu, 2008; Yu et al., 2013; McClure et al., 2015; Kim et al., 2019a).

Mounting evidence has also shown that curcumin exerts pharmacological functions, thus ameliorating cognitive functions, inhibiting cerebral edema (Zhu et al., 2014; Li et al., 2019), and increasing cell proliferation in embryonic cortical neural stem cells (Kim et al., 2008; Tiwari et al., 2014; Li et al., 2019). Downstream pro-inflammatory and nitrosative mediators, such as tumor necrosis factor-α (TNF-α), interleukin-1β (IL-1β), cyclooxygenase-2 (COX-2) and inducible nitric oxide synthase (iNOS), were also attenuated. Large numbers of polyphenols were tested for their efficacy against AD, of which curcumin showed substantial therapeutic efficacy (Goozee et al., 2015; Venigalla et al., 2016; Khalil et al., 2019). Curcumin treatment caused remarkable increases in learning and memory in amyloid precursor protein/presenilin1 (APP/PS1) mice by increasing the number of new neural stem cells and newborn neurons in the hippocampus, and decreasing the number of apoptotic neurons (Li et al., 2019).

11.1.2 Anti-Amyloidogenic Activity

Curcumin has also been known to exert anti-amyloidogenic activity (Sishodia et al., 2009; Kim et al., 2019b). It plays a crucial role in inhibiting amyloid-β (Aβ) oligomer and fibril formation, reducing neurotoxicity of Aβ, and inhibiting inflammation in the transgenic mouse brain (Liu et al., 2016; Sun et al., 2017; Sundaram et al., 2017; Li et al., 2019). Several other lines of evidence have also shown that curcumin curbs neuronal death in animal models of neurodegeneration (Kim et al., 2008; Feng et al., 2016; Maiti and Dunbar 2018a; Srivastava et al., 2018; Li et al., 2019). In contrast, a plethora of AD-targeted drugs, aimed at attenuation of Aβ plaques, such as γ-secretase inhibitors, BACE1 inhibitors, and amyloid vaccines, did not succeed in clinical trials (Karunaweera et al., 2015; Khalil et al., 2019).

The transcription factor nuclear factor κ beta (NF-κβ) plays an essential role in the pathophysiology of AD (Khalil et al., 2019). Its increased expression leads to the upregulation of Aβ-generating genes, proinflammatory cytokines, BACE1, and oxidative stress-related genes (Srinivasan and Lahiri, 2015; Shi et al., 2016; Khalil et al., 2019). NF-κβ is a redox-sensitive transcription factor (Kaur et al., 2015; Khalil et al., 2019), where mitochondrial impairment, NF-κβ, and iNOS pathways were observed to be greatly perturbed (Li et al., 2015; Khalil et al., 2019). A wealth of studies has shown that curcumin attenuates the NF-κβ signaling pathway (Manikandan et al., 2011; Huang et al., 2011; Huang et al., 2017; Akaishi and Abe, 2018; Yu et al., 2018; Giacomeli et al., 2019). Despite its low bioavailability, curcumin shows promising therapeutic efficacy against AD, with its potential to target NF-κβ (Khalil et al., 2019). Despite the remarkable activities of curcumin, however, the mechanism of its action remains elusive (Anand et al., 2007; Khalil et al., 2019a).

11.1.3 The Influence of Curcumin on Signaling

Curcumin stimulates the generation of the anti-inflammatory cytokines, IL-10 and IL-4 in murine BV2 microglial cells exposed to lipopolysaccharide (LPS) (Porro et al., 2019). In line with this, curcumin exposure also increases the expression of suppressors of cytokine signaling (SOCS-1), whereas phosphorylation of the Janus kinases (JAK) and the signal transducer and activator of transcription (STAT3) was decreased (Porro et al., 2019). Based on these findings, it can be concluded that curcumin can mediate neuroinflammatory reactions by exerting anti-inflammatory responses in microglia *via* changes in the JAK/STAT/SOCS pathway (Porro et al., 2019). Nevertheless, the mechanism by which curcumin inhibits the inflammatory responses activated by microglia is elusive (Porro et al., 2019). LPS stimulation substantially upregulated the expression of pro-inflammatory factors TNF-α and IL-1β, with a moderate increase in IL-10 levels. Nevertheless, remarkable reduction of TNF-α and IL-1β levels, and a marked increase in the levels of the anti-inflammatory cytokines IL-10 and IL-4 were observed in response to curcumin treatment (Porro et al., 2019). Curcumin stimulated increased production of IL-4, which is highly anti-inflammatory and offers microglia-mediated neuroprotection (Chao et al., 1993; Dooley et al., 2014; Porro et al., 2019).

11.2 THERACURMIN

Theracurmin was obtained by using the submicron colloidal dispersion technique, by which its bioavailability was increased to nearly 27 times that of curcumin (Sasaki et al., 2011; Kim et al., 2019a). Theracurmin, a more bioavailable form of curcumin, substantially improved recognition and spatial memories in 5xFAD mice (Kim et al., 2019b). Moreover, the antioxidant activity of Theracurmin, as evaluated by superoxide dismutase (SOD) activity and levels of reduced glutathione (GSH) and malondialdehyde (MDA), showed marked improvements (Kim et al., 2019a). Studies have shown that intake of Theracurmin on a daily basis for 18 months resulted in improved memory and attention in adults without dementia (Small et al., 2018; Kim et al., 2019a). Post-synaptic density protein 95 (PSD95), a vital structural protein with a significant role in memory, has been found to be present in low levels in 5xFAD mice, a strain which rapidly develops severe amyloid pathology (Meyer et al., 2014; Grinan-Ferre et al., 2018; Kim et al., 2019a). Theracurmin administration significantly increased the levels of PSD95 (Kim et al., 2019a).

11.3 CHALLENGES ASSOCIATED WITH CURCUMIN

Low bioavailability is a major issue for curcumin and impedes its success significantly (Khalil et al., 2019). A few factors contribute to its low bioavailability, including lipophilicity, instability in the alkaline intestinal environment, degeneration during transport, rapid metabolism, intracellular accumulation, and excretion (Wahlang et al., 2011; Khalil et al., 2019). A number of pharmaceutical technologies have been used to overcome the bioavailability issues of curcumin (Serafini et al., 2017; Khalil et al., 2019a).

11.4 THE ROLE OF CURCUMIN IN AD DIAGNOSIS

Recent studies have shown that difluoroboron complexes of fluorine-substituted curcumin derivatives bind strongly to amyloid plaques in APP/PS1 transgenic mouse brain sections (Kim et al., 2019b). A few radiolabeled forms of curcumin derivatives, such as 4'-*O*-^{18}F-fluoropropyl curcumin and other ^{18}F-labeled curcumins, showed low brain-spanning capability, despite their ability to bind to Aβ plaques (Ryu et al., 2006; Lee et al., 2011; Rokka et al., 2014; Kim et al., 2019b). Therefore, difluoroboron complexes of fluorine-substituted curcumin derivatives, with adequate lipophilicity, showed enhanced blood–brain barrier (BBB) ferrying efficacy, in turn, binding to the Aβ plaques (Kung et al., 2010; Kim et al., 2019b). Imaging the Aβ plaques, using curcumin, has long been in use (Cole et al., 2004; Garcia-Alloza et al., 2007; den Haan et al., 2018; Lichtenegger et al., 2019). In another study, fluorescence of curcumin was explored to detect amyloid plaques in brain slices, using the multimodal visible light optical coherence microscopy technique (Lichtenegger et al., 2019).

11.5 NANOTECHNOLOGY

Multiple approaches have been employed to date to increase the solubility and bioavailability of curcumin, include the use of adjuvants, such as quercetin, silibinin, or piperine, introduction of structural analogs of curcumin, chemical complex formation with curcumin and proteins, phospholipids or polysaccharides, and the formation of curcumin bioconjugates with turmeric oil or alanine (Naksuriya et al., 2014; Yallapu et al., 2015; Yavarpour et al., 2019). Despite the improvements in bioavailability and solubility of curcumin by these methods, they failed to stop its rapid metabolism.

To overcome these challenges, a number of nanobased delivery systems have been designed and extensively used by researchers for several decades (Mouhieddine et al., 2015; Yavarpour et al., 2019). These delivery systems became valuable tools which enhance the properties of several bioactive compounds such as curcumin, for a short period (Yavarpour et al., 2019).

Curcumin is highly unstable, due to the presence of hydroxyl groups in its structure. It is easily metabolized by liver and kidney enzymes, thus exhibiting low absorption and brain bioavailability (Leung and Kee, 2009; Ringman et al., 2012; Sadegh Malvajerd et al., 2019). In addition, its BBB-spanning is relatively inadequate (Tsai et al., 2011; Sadegh Malvajerd et al., 2019). A few studies have shown that encapsulation of curcumin in nanoparticles (NPs) profoundly improved its stability and inhibited its enzymatic and pH-based degradation, in turn improving its systemic circulation (Anand et al., 2007; Szymusiak et al., 2016; Maiti et al., 2018b; Yavarpour et al., 2019).

11.6 SOLID LIPID NANOPARTICLES AND LIPID CORE NANOCAPSULES

The use of nanoparticles has been extensively studied to circumvent the BBB problems exhibited by curcumin and to enhance drug delivery to the brain (Obulesu, 2019, 2020; Vergoni et al., 2009; Reddy and Labhasetwar, 2009; Sadegh Malvajerd et al., 2019). In line with this, solid lipid nanoparticles (SLNs) and nanolipid capsules (NLCs) have been extensively used to improve brain delivery, since their lipidic nature makes them readily localizable to brain tissue (Kaur et al., 2008;

Aboutaleb et al., 2014; Sadegh Malvajerd et al., 2019). Apolipoproteins have been used in SLNs and NLCs, since their transport through a plethora of apolipoprotein receptors on brain tissue is feasible (Michaelis et al., 2006; Emami et al., 2012; Dal Magro et al., 2017; Neves et al., 2017; Sadegh Malvajerd et al., 2019).

Usually, nanoencapsulation of drugs markedly improves their efficacy, reduces their toxicity, and facilitates the use of lower doses (Bernardi et al., 2012; Dimer et al., 2015; Giacomeli et al., 2019). NLC–curcumin showed robust neuroprotective efficacy against Aβ1-42-induced cognitive impairment, compared with free curcumin, in aged female mice (Giacomeli et al., 2019). Enhanced attention was paid to the development of nanotechnology-based delivery systems to improve various formulations and bioactive substance delivery systems (Serafini et al., 2017; Hussain et al., 2017; Giacomeli et al., 2019). Innovative NLCs comprised a dispersion of sorbitan monostearate as a core and poly(epsiloncaprolactone) as an outer layer, with polysorbate 80 micelles as stabilizers (Giacomeli et al., 2019). Using this delivery system, several drugs, such as indomethacin, curcumin, *trans*-resveratrol, and olanzapine, were successfully delivered to the brain (Bernardi et al., 2012; Hoppe et al., 2013; Dimer et al., 2015; Giacomeli et al., 2019). The enhanced efficacy of curcumin-loaded LNCs can be attributed to their increased brain biodistribution and potential to ferry curcumin across the BBB (Rodrigues et al., 2016; Giacomeli et al., 2019). The results of this study were also in accordance with those from other curcumin-loaded nanocapsules (Coradini et al., 2015; Marin et al., 2017; Velasques et al., 2018; Giacomeli et al., 2019).

The neuroprotective role of curcumin toward neurons, with its robust antioxidant and free radical removal activity, has been extensively studied (Sadegh Malvajerd et al., 2019). NLCs, designed recently to enhance BBB ferrying of curcumin, substantially improved the level of curcumin in the brain, thus increasing its therapeutic effect (Sadegh Malvajerd et al., 2019). The protective efficacy of curcumin-loaded NLCs was also confirmed in rats by decreased oxidative stress parameters (lipid peroxidation, reactive oxygen species (ROS) formation, and ADP/ATP ratio) in the hippocampal tissue, and amelioration of spatial memory (Sadegh Malvajerd et al., 2019). Interestingly, the nano sizes of the NPs and the presence of Tween 80 on the NLC surface allow them to evade the reticuloendothelial system (RES) (Goppert and Muller, 2005; Sadegh Malvajerd et al., 2019). Moreover, binding of circulating plasma apolipoprotein E (ApoE) on the surface of NPs can increase curcumin uptake into the brain by targeting low-density lipoprotein (LDL) receptors on BBB endothelial cells (Gulyaev et al., 1999; Olivier et al., 1999; Sadegh Malvajerd et al., 2019).

11.7 CONCLUSIONS AND FUTURE PERSPECTIVES

Curcumin has long been a vital culinary ingredient, in the form of turmeric, in Asian countries. It offers potential health benefits against numerous diseases which are specifically associated with inflammation, such as NDs. However, its low bioavailability and poor water solubility impede its success. To overcome these challenges, multiple nanotechnological methods have been used which profoundly improved the bioavailability and solubility of curcumin. Despite the voluminous data on curcumin's efficacy and the development of drug-delivery systems (DDS) for curcumin, there is an increasing need to develop more appropriate formulations to fully utilize the efficacy of this valuable phytochemical.

REFERENCES

Aboutaleb E, Atyabi F, Khoshayand MR, Vatanara AR, Ostad SN, Kobarfard F, Dinarvand R. Improved brain delivery of vincristine using dextran sulfate complex solid lipid nanoparticles: optimization and *in vivo* evaluation. *J Biomed Mater Res A*. 2014;102:2125–2136.

Akaishi T, Abe K. CNB-001, a synthetic pyrazole derivative of curcumin, suppresses lipopolysaccharide-induced nitric oxide production through the inhibition of NF-κB and p38 MAPK pathways in microglia. *Eur J Pharmacol*. 2018;819:190–197.

Amor S, Puentes F, Baker D, Van Der Valk PJI. Inflammation in neurodegenerative diseases. *Immunology*. 2010;129:154–169.

Anand P, Kunnumakkara AB, Newman RA, Aggarwal BB. Bioavailability of curcumin: problems and promises. *Mol Pharm*. 2007;4:807–818.

Bernardi A, Frozza RL, Meneghetti A, Hoppe JB, Battastini AM, Pohlmann AR, Guterres SS, Salbego CG. Indomethacin-loaded lipid-core nanocapsules reduce the damage triggered by Aβ1-42 in Alzheimer's disease models. *Int J Nanomed*. 2012;7:4927–4942.

Canales-Aguirre AA, Gomez-Pinedo UA, Luquin S, Ramirez-Herrera MA, Mendoza-Magana ML, Feria-Velasco A. Curcumin protects against the oxidative damage induced by the pesticide parathion in the hippocampus of the rat brain. *Nutr Neurosci*. 2012;15:62–69.

Chao CC, Molitor TW, Hu S. Neuroprotective role of IL-4 against activated microglia. *J Immunol*. 1993;151:1473–1481.

Cole GM, Morihara T, Lim GP, Yang F, Begum A, Frautschy SA. NSAID and antioxidant prevention of Alzheimer's disease: lessons from in vitro and animal models. *Ann N Y Acad Sci*. 2004;1035:68–84.

Coradini K, Friedrich RB, Fonseca FN, Vencato MS, Andrade DF, Oliveira CM, Battistel AP, Guterres SS, da Rocha MI, Pohlmann AR, Beck RC. A novel approach to arthritis treatment based on resveratrol and curcumin co-encapsulated in lipid-core nanocapsules: in vivo studies. *Eur J Pharm Sci*. 2015;78:163–170.

Dal Magro R, Ornaghi F, Cambianica I, Beretta S, Re F, Musicanti C, Rigolio R, Donzelli E, Canta A, Ballarini E. ApoE-modified solid lipid nanoparticles: a feasible strategy to cross the blood-brain barrier. *J Control Rel*. 2017;249:103–110.

Den Haan J, Tjado H, Morrema J, Rozemuller AJ, Bouwman FH, Hoozemans JJM. Different curcumin forms selectively bind fibrillary amyloid beta in post mortem Alzheimer's disease brains: implications for in-vivo diagnostics. *Acta Neuropathol Commun*. 2018;6:75.

Dimer FA, Pigatto MC, Boque CA, Pase CS, Roversi K, Pohlmann AR, Burger ME, Rates MK, Dalla Costa T, Guterres SS. Nanoencapsulation improves relative bioavailability and antipsychotic effect of olanzapine in rats. *J Biomed Nanotechnol*. 2015;11:1482–1493.

Dooley D, Vidal P, Hendrix S. Immunopharmacological intervention for successful neural stem cell therapy: new perspectives in CNS neurogenesis and repair. *Pharmacol Ther*. 2014;141:21–31.

Emami J, Rezazadeh M, Varshosaz J. Formulation of LDL targeted nanostructured lipid carriers loaded with paclitaxel: a detailed study of preparation, freeze drying condition, and *in vitro* cytotoxicity. *J Nanomater*. 2012;2012:3.

Emerit J, Edeas M, Bricaire F. Neurodegenerative diseases and oxidative stress. *Biomed Pharmacother*. 2004;58:39–46.

Feng HL, Dang HZ, Fan H, Chen XP, Rao YX, Ren Y, Yang JD, Shi J, Wang PW, Tian JZ. Curcumin ameliorates insulin signalling pathway in brain of Alzheimer's disease transgenic mice. *Int J Immunopathol Pharmacol*. 2016;29:734–741.

Frautschy S, Hu W, Kim P, Miller S, Chu T, Harris-White M, Cole G. Phenolic anti-inflammatory antioxidant reversal of Aβ-induced cognitive deficits and neuropathology. *Neurobiol Aging*. 2001;22:993–1005.

Garcia-Alloza M, Borrelli LA, Rozkalne A, Hyman BT, Bacskai BJ. Curcumin labels amyloid pathology in vivo, disrupts existing plaques, and partially restores distorted neurites in an Alzheimer mouse model. *J Neurochem*. 2007;102;1095–1104.

Gazal M, Valente MR, Acosta BA, Kaufmann FN, Braganhol E, Lencina CL, Stefanello FM, Ghisleni G, Kaster MP. Neuroprotective and antioxidant effects of curcumin in a ketamine-induced model of mania in rats. *Eur J Pharmacol*. 2014;724:132–139.

Giacomelia R, Izoton JC, Santos RB, Boeiraa SP, Jessea CR, Haasa SE. Neuroprotective effects of curcumin lipid-core nanocapsules in a model Alzheimer's disease induced by β-amyloid 1–42 peptide in aged female mice. *Brain Res*. 2019;1721:146325.

Goozee KG, Shah TM, Sohrabi HR, Rainey-Smith SR, Brown B, Verdile G, et al. Examining the potential clinical value of curcumin in the prevention and diagnosis of Alzheimer's disease. *Brit J Nutr*. 2015;115:449–465.

Goppert TM, Muller RH. Polysorbate-stabilized solid lipid nanoparticles as colloidal carriers for intravenous targeting of drugs to the brain: comparison of plasma protein adsorption patterns. *J Drug Deliv*. 2005;13:179–187.

Grinan-Ferre C, Izquierdo V, Otero E, Puigoriol-Illamola D, Corpas R, Sanfeliu C, Ortuno-Sahagun D, Pallas M. Environmental enrichment improves cognitive deficits, AD hallmarks and epigenetic alterations presented in 5xFAD mouse model. *Front Cell Neurosci*. 2018;12:224.

Gulyaev AE, Gelperina SE, Skidan IN, Antropov AS, Kivman GY, Kreuter J. Significant transport of doxorubicin into the brain with polysorbate 80-coated nanoparticles. *Pharm Res*. 1999;16:1564–1569.

Hoppe JB, Coradini K, Frozza RL, Oliveira CM, Meneghetti AB, Bernardi A, Pires ES, Beck RC, Salbego CG. Free and nanoencapsulated curcumin suppress β-amyloid-induced cognitive impairments in rats: involvement of BDNF and Akt/GSK-3b signaling pathway. *Neurobiol Learn Mem.* 2013;106:134–144.

Huang F, Yao Y, Wu J, Liu Q, Zhang J, Pu X, Zhang Q, Xia L. Curcumin inhibits gastric cancer-derived mesenchymal stem cells mediated angiogenesis by regulating NF-κB/VEGF signaling. *Am J Transl Res.* 2017;12:5538–5547.

Huang G, Yang Y, Xu Z, Zhou P, Gong W, Li Y, Fan J, He F. Downregulation of B lymphocyte stimulator expression by curcumin in B lymphocyte via suppressing nuclear translocation of NF-κB. *Eur J Pharmacol.* 2011;650:451–457.

Hussain Z, Thu HE, Amjad MW, Hussain F, Ahmed TA, Khan S. Exploring recent developments to improve antioxidant, anti-inflammatory and antimicrobial efficacy of curcumin: a review of new trends and future perspectives. *Mater Sci Eng C.* 2017;77:1316–1326.

Ishrat T, Hoda MN, Khan MB, Yousuf S, Ahmad M, Khan MM, Ahmad A, Islam F. Amelioration of cognitive deficits and neurodegeneration by curcumin in rat model of sporadic dementia of Alzheimer's type (SDAT). *Eur Neuropsychopharmacol.* 2009;19:636–647.

Karunaweera N, Raju R, Gyengesi E, Munch G. Plant polyphenols as inhibitors of NF-κB induced cytokine production—a potential anti-inflammatory treatment for Alzheimer's disease? *Front Mol Neurosci.* 2015;8:24.

Kaur IP, Bhandari R, Bhandari S, Kakkar V. Potential of solid lipid nanoparticles in brain targeting. *J Control Rel.* 2008;127:97–109.

Kaur U, Banerjee P, Bir A, Sinha M, Biswas A, Chakrabarti S. Reactive oxygen species, redox signaling and neuroinflammation in Alzheimer's disease: the NF-κB connection. *Curr Top Med Chem.* 2015;15:446–457.

Khalil MNA, Choucry MA, El Senousy AS, Hassan A, El-Marasy SA, El Awdan SA, Omar FA. Ambrosin, a potent NF-κβ inhibitor, ameliorates lipopolysaccharide induced memory impairment, comparison to curcumin. *PLoS One.* 2019;14:e0219378.

Kim GY, Kim KH, Lee SH, Yoon MS, Lee HJ, Moon DO, Lee CM, Ahn SC, Park YC, Park YM. Cur cumin inhibits immunostimulatory function of dendritic cells: MAPKs and translocation of NF-κB as potential targets. *J Immunol.* 2005;174:8116–8124.

Kim H, Im YH, Ahn J, Yang J, Choi JY, Lee KH, Kim BT, Choe YS. Synthesis and in vivo characterization of $_{18}$F-labeled difluoroboron-curcumin derivative for β-amyloid plaque imaging. *Sci Rep.* 2019a;9:6747.

Kim J, Kim J, Huang Z, Goo N, Bae HJ, Jeong Y, Park HJ, Cai M, Cho K, Jung SY, Bae SK, Ryu JH. Theracurmin ameliorates cognitive dysfunctions in 5XFAD mice by improving synaptic function and mitigating oxidative stress. Biomol Ther (Seoul). 2019b;27:327–335.

Kim SJ, Son TG, Park HR, Park M, Kim MS, Kim HS, Chung HY, Mattson MP, Lee J. Curcumin stimulates proliferation of embryonic neural progenitor cells and neurogenesis in the adult hippocampus. *J Biol Chem.* 2008;283:14497–14505.

Koo EH, Lansbury PT, Kelly JWJ. Amyloid diseases: abnormal protein aggregation in neurodegeneration. *Proc Natl Acad Sci.* 1999;96:9989–9990.

Kung HF, Choi SR, Qu W, Zhang W, Skovronsky D. 18F Stilbenes and styrylpyridines for PET imaging of Aβ plaques in Alzheimer's disease: a miniperspective. *J Med Chem.* 2010;53:933–941.

Lee I, Yang J, Lee JH, Choe YS. Synthesis and evaluation of 1-(4-[^{18}F]fluoroethyl)-7-(4′-methyl)curcumin with improved brain permeability for β-amyloid plaque imaging. *Bioorg Med Chem Lett.* 2011;21:5765–5769.

Leung MH, Kee TW. Effective stabilization of curcumin by association to plasma proteins: human serum albumin and fibrinogen. *Langmuir.* 2009;25:5773–5777.

Li J, Han Y, Li M, Nie C. Curcumin promotes proliferation of adult neural stem cells and the birth of neurons in Alzheimer's disease mice via notch signaling pathway. *Cell Reprogram.* 2019;21:152–161.

Li X, Long J, He T, Belshaw R, Scott J. Integrated genomic approaches identify major pathways and upstream regulators in late onset Alzheimer's disease. *Sci Rep.* 2015;5:12393.

Liu ZJ, Li ZH, Liu L, Tang WX, Wang Y, Dong MR, Xiao C. Curcumin attenuates beta-amyloid induced neuroinflammation via activation of peroxisome proliferator-activated receptor-gamma function in a rat model of Alzheimer's disease. *Front Pharmacol.* 2016;7:261.

Lopez-Lazaro M. Anticancer and carcinogenic properties of curcumin: considerations for its clinical development as a cancer chemopreventive and chemotherapeutic agent. *Mol Nutr Food Res.* 2008;52 Supplement 1:103–127.

Maiti P, Dunbar GJ. Use of curcumin, a natural polyphenol for targeting molecular pathways in treating age-related neurodegenerative diseases. *Int J Mol Sci.* 2018;19:1637.

Maiti P, Paladugu L, Dunbar GL. Solid lipid curcumin particles provide greater anti-amyloid, anti-inflammatory and neuroprotective effects than curcumin in the 5xFAD mouse model of Alzheimer's disease. *BMC Neurosci.* 2018b;19:7.

Manikandan R, Beulaja M, Thiagarajan R, Priyadarsini A, Saravanan R, Arumugam M. Ameliorative effects of curcumin against renal injuries mediated by inducible nitric oxide synthase and nuclear factor kappa B during gentamicin-induced toxicity in Wistar rats. *Eur J Pharmacol.* 2011;670:578–585.

Marin E, Briceno MI, Torres A, Caballero-George C. New curcumin-loaded chitosan nanocapsules: in vivo evaluation. *Planta Med.* 2017;83:877–883.

Massimino LC, Faria HAM, Yoshioka SA. Curcumin bioactive nanosizing: increase of bioavailability. *Ind Crops Prod.* 2017;109:493–497.

McClure R, Yanagisawa D, Stec D, Abdollahian D, Koktysh D, Xhillari D, Jaeger R, Stanwood G, Chekmenev E, Tooyama I. Inhalable curcumin: offering the potential for translation to imaging and treatment of Alzheimer's disease. *J Alzheimers Dis.* 2015;44:283–295.

Meyer D, Bonhoeffer T, Scheuss V. Balance and stability of synaptic structures during synaptic plasticity. *Neuron.* 2014;82:430–443.

Michaelis K, Hoffmann M, Dreis S, Herbert E, Alyautdin R, Michaelis M, Kreuter J, Langer K. Covalent linkage of apolipoprotein e to albumin nanoparticles strongly enhances drug transport into the brain. *J Pharmacol Exp Therap.* 2006;317:1246–1253.

Mishra S, Palanivelu K. The effect of curcumin (turmeric) on Alzheimer's disease: an overview. *Ann Indian Acad Neurol.* 2008;11:13–19.

Mouhieddine TH, Itani MM, Nokkari A, Ren C, Daoud G, Zeidan A, Mondello S, Kobeissy FH. Nanotheragnostic applications for ischemic and hemorrhagic strokes: improved delivery for a better prognosis. *Curr Neurol Neurosci Rep.* 2015;15:505.

Naksuriya O, Okonogi S, Schiffelers RM, Hennink WE. Curcumin nanoformulations: a review of pharmaceutical properties and preclinical studies and clinical data related to cancer treatment. *Biomaterials.* 2014;35:3365–3383.

Neves AR, Queiroz JF, Lima SAC, Reis S. Apo E-functionalization of solid lipid nanoparticles enhances brain drug delivery: uptake mechanism and transport pathways. *Bioconjug Chem.* 2017;28:995–1004.

Obulesu M. *Alzheimer's Disease Theranostics*, 1st Edition, Elsevier, 2019.

Obulesu M. *Parkinson's Disease Therapeutics: Emphasis on Nanotechnological Advances*, 1st Edition, Elsevier, 2020.

Olivier JC, Fenart L, Chauvet R, Pariat C, Cecchelli R, Couet W. Indirect evidence that drug brain targeting using polysorbate 80-coated polybutylcyanoacrylate nanoparticles is related to toxicity. *Pharm Res.* 1999;16:1836–1842.

Porro C, Cianciulli A, Trotta T, Lofrumento DD, Panaro MA. Curcumin regulates anti-inflammatory responses by JAK/STAT/SOCS signaling pathway in BV-2 microglial cells. Biology (Basel). 2019;8:(in press).

Reddy MK, Labhasetwar V. Nanoparticle-mediated delivery of superoxide dismutase to the brain: an effective strategy to reduce ischemia-reperfusion injury. *FASEB J.* 2009;23:1384–1395.

Ringman JM, Frautschy SA, Teng E, Begum AN, Bardens J, Beigi M, Gylys KH, Badmaev V, Heath DD, Apostolova LG. Oral curcumin for Alzheimer's disease: tolerability and efficacy in a 24-week randomized, double blind, placebo-controlled study. *Alzheimers Res Ther.* 2012;4:43.

Rodrigues SF, Fiel LA, Shimada AL, Pereira NR, Guterres SS, Pohlmann AR, Farsky SH. Lipid-core nanocapsules act as a drug shuttle through the blood brain barrier and reduce glioblastoma after intravenous or oral administration. *J Biomed Nanotechnol.* 2016;12:986–1000.

Rokka J, Snellman A, Zona C, La Ferla B, Nicotra F, Salmona M, Forloni G, Haaparanta-Solin M, Rinne JO, Solin O. Synthesis and evaluation of a ^{18}F-curcumin derivate for β-amyloid plaque imaging. *Bioorg Med Chem.* 2014;22:2753–2762.

Ryu EK, Choe YS, Lee KH, Choi Y, Kim BT. Curcumin and dehydrozingerone derivatives: synthesis, radiolabeling, and evaluation for β-amyloid plaque imaging. *J Med Chem.* 2006;49:6111–6119.

Sadegh Malvajerd S, Izadi Z, Azadi A, Kurd M, Derakhshankhah H, Sharif Zadeh M, Akbari Javar H, Hamidi M. Neuroprotective potential of curcumin-loaded nanostructured lipid carrier in an animal model of Alzheimer's disease: behavioral and biochemical evidence. *J Alzheimers Dis.* 2019;69:671–686.

Sasaki H, Sunagawa Y, Takahashi K, Imaizumi A, Fukuda H, Hashimoto T, Wada H, Katanasaka Y, Kakeya H, Fujita M, Hasegawa K, Morimoto T. Innovative preparation of curcumin for improved oral bioavailability. *Biol Pharm Bull.* 2011;34:660–665.

Serafini MM, Catanzaro M, Rosini M, Racchi M, Lanni C. Curcumin in Alzheimer's disease: can we think to new strategies and perspectives for this molecule? *Pharmacol Res.* 2017;124:146–155.

Shi ZM, Han YW, Han XH, Zhang K, Chang YN, Hu ZM, Qi HX, Ting C, Zhen Z, Hong W. Upstream regulators and downstream effectors of NF-κB in Alzheimer's disease. *J Neurol Sci.* 2016;366:127–134.

Sishodia S, Misra K, Aggarwal BB. Turmeric as cure-cumin: promises, problems, and solutions. In Surh YJ, Dong Z, Cadenas E, and Packer L (eds.), *Dietary Modulation of Cell Signaling Pathways*. CRC Press, 2009, 91–99.

Small GW, Siddarth P, Li Z, Miller KJ, Ercoli L, Emerson ND, Martinez J, Wong KP, Liu J, Merrill DA, Chen ST, Henning SM, Satyamurthy N, Huang SC, Heber D, and Barrio JR. Memory and brain amyloid and tau effects of a bioavailable form of curcumin in non-demented adults: a doubleblind, placebo-controlled 18-month trial. *Am J Geriatr Psychiatr.* 2018;26:266–277.

Srinivasan M, Lahiri DK. Significance of NF-κB as a pivotal therapeutic target in the neurodegenerative pathologies of Alzheimer's disease and multiple sclerosis. *Expert Opin Ther Tar.* 2015;19:471–487.

Srivastava P, Dhuriya YK, Kumar V, Srivastava A, Gupta R, Shukla RK, Yadav RS, Dwivedi HN, Pant AB, Khanna VK. PI3K/Akt/GSK3b induced CREB activation ameliorates arsenic mediated alterations in NMDA receptors and associated signaling in rat hippocampus: neuroprotective role of curcumin. *Neurotoxicology.* 2018;67:190–205.

Sun J, Zhang X, Wang C, Teng Z, Li Y. Curcumin decreases hyperphosphorylation if Tau by downregulating caveolin-1/GSK-3b in N2a/APP695swe cells and APP/PS1 double transgenic Alzheimer's disease mice. *Am J Chin Med.* 2017;45:1667–1682.

Sundaram JR, Poore CP, Sulaimee NHB, Pareek T, Cheong WF, Wenk MR, Pant HC, Frautschy SA, Low CM, Kesavapany S. Curcumin ameliorates neuroinflammation, neurodegeneration, and memory deficits in p25 transgenic mouse model that bears hallmarks of Alzheimer's disease. *J Alzheimers Dis.* 2017;60:1429–1442.

Szymusiak M, Hu X, Plata PAL, Ciupinski P, Wang ZJ, Liu YJ. Bioavailability of curcumin and curcumin glucuronide in the central nervous system of mice after oral delivery of nano-curcumin. *Int J Pharma.* 2016;511:415–423.

Tharakan B, Hunter FA, Smythe WR, Childs EW. Curcumin inhibits reactive oxygen species formation and vascular hyperpermeability following haemorrhagic shock. *Clin Exp Pharmacol Physiol.* 2010;37:939–944.

Tiwari SK, Agarwal S, Seth B, Yadav A, Nair S, Bhatnagar P, Karmakar M, Kumari M, Chauhan LK, Patel DK, Srivastava V, Singh D, Gupta SK, Tripathi A, Chaturvedi RK, Gupta KC. Curcumin-loaded nanoparticles potently induce adult neurogenesis and reverse cognitive deficits in Alzheimer's disease model via canonical Wnt/b-catenin pathway. *ACS Nano.* 2014;8:76–103.

Toda S, Miyase T, Arichi H, Tanizawa H, Takino Y. Natural antioxidants. III. Antioxidative components isolated from rhizome of Curcuma longa L. Chem Pharm Bull (Tokyo). 1985;33:1725–1728.

Tsai YM, Chien CF, Lin LC, Tsai TH. Curcumin and its nano-formulation: the kinetics of tissue distribution and blood–brain barrier penetration. *Int J Pharm.* 2011;416:331–338.

Velasques KP, Maciel TR, de Castro Dal Forno AH, Teixeira FEG, da Fonseca AL, Varotti FP, Fajardo AR, Avila DS, Haas SE. Co-nanoencapsulation of antimalarial drugs increases their in vitro efficacy against Plasmodium falciparum and decreases their toxicity to Caenorhabditis elegans. *Eur J Pharm Sci.* 2018;118:1–12.

Venigalla M, Sonego S, Gyengesi E, Sharman MJ, Munch G. Novel promising therapeutics against chronic neuroinflammation and neurodegeneration in Alzheimer's disease. *Neurochem Int.* 2016;95:63–74.

Vergoni AV, Tosi G, Tacchi R, Vandelli MA, Bertolini A, Costantino L. Nanoparticles as drug delivery agents specific for CNS: *in vivo* biodistribution. *Nanomedicine.* 2009;5:369–377.

Wahlang B, Pawar YB, Bansal AK. Identification of permeability-related hurdles in oral delivery of curcumin using the Caco-2 cell model. *Eur J Pharma Biopharma.* 2011;77:275–282.

Yallapu MM, Nagesh PKB, Jaggi M, Chauhan SC. Therapeutic applications of curcumin nanoformulations. *Aaps J.* 2015;17:1341–1356.

Yavarpour-Bali H, Ghasemi-Kasman M, Pirzadeh M. Curcumin-loaded nanoparticles: a novel therapeutic strategy in treatment of central nervous system disorders. *Int J Nanomedicine.* 2019;14:4449–4460.

Yu SY, Zhang M, Luo J, Zhang L, Shao Y, Li G. Curcumin ameliorates memory deficits via neuronal nitric oxide synthase in aged mice. *Prog Neuropsychopharmacol Biol Psychiatr.* 2013;45:47–53.

Yu Y, Shen Q, Lai Y, Park SY, Ou X, Lin D, Jin M and Zhang W. Anti-inflammatory Effects of Curcumin in Microglial Cells. *Front. Pharmacol.* 2018;9:386.

Zhang L, Fang Y, Xu Y, Lian Y, Xie N, Wu T, Zhang H, Sun L, Zhang R, Wang Z. Curcumin improves amyloid β-peptide (1–42) induced spatial memory deficits through BDNF-ERK signaling pathway. *PLoS One.* 2015;10:1–17.

Zhu HT, Bian C, Yuan JC, Chu WH, Xiang X, Chen F, Wang CS, Feng H, Lin JK. Curcumin attenuates acute inflammatory injury by inhibiting the TLR4/MyD88/NF-kappaB signaling pathway in experimental traumatic brain injury. *J Neuroinflamm.* 2014;11:59.

12 Epigenetic Alterations in Alzheimer's Disease and Its Therapeutic and Dietary Interventions

P. M. Aswathy, C. M. Shafeeque, and Moinak Banerjee

CONTENTS

ABBREVIATIONS

5,10-MTHF	5,10-Methylenetetrahydrofolate
5hmC	5-hydroxymethyl Cytosine
5mC	5-methyl Cytosine
ABCA1	ATP-binding Cassette Transporter Subfamily A Number 1
AD	Alzheimer's Disease
ANK1	Ankyrin 1
APOE	Apolipoprotein E
APOJ	Apolipoprotein J
APP	Amyloid Precursor Protein

Aβ	Amyloid-beta
BACE	Beta-secretase (beta-site APP Cleaving Enzyme 1)
BDNF	Brain-derived Neurotropic Factor
BIN1	Bridging Integrator 1
CA3	Cornu Ammonis 3
CBS	Cystathionine β-synthase
CDK5R1	Cyclin-dependent Kinase 5 Regulatory Subunit 1
CLU	Clusterin
COX-2	Cyclooxygenase-2
CREB	Cyclic AMP-responsive Element-binding Protein
DG	Dentate Gyrus
DHA	Docosahexaenoic Acid
DhMRs	Differentially Hydroxymethylated Regions
DNMT	DNA Methyltransferase
DUSP22	Dual-specificity Phosphatase 22
EPA	Eicosapentaenoic Acid
ERK1	Extracellular Signal-regulated Kinase 1
FOXO3a	Forkhead Box Protein O3
GCF	GC-rich Sequence DNA-binding Factor
GSH	Glutathione
GSK3	Glycogen Synthase Kinase 3
HAT	Histone Acetyltransferases
HDAC	Histone Deacetylases
HDACi	Histone Deacetylase inhibitors
HDMTs	Histone Demethylases
HMTs	Histone Methyltransferases
HP1	Heterochromatin Protein 1
IRS-1	Insulin Receptor Substrate 1
LOAD	Late-onset AD
LRPAP1	Low-density Lipoprotein-related Protein-associated Protein 1
MAT	Methionine Adenosyltransferase
MCI	Mild Cognitive Impairment
MFG	Middle Frontal Gyrus
miRNAs	MicroRNAs
mtDNA	Mitochondrial DNA
MTG	Middle Temporal Gyrus
MTHFR	Methylene Tetrahydrofolate Reductase
MTR	Methionine Synthase
MTRR	Methionine Synthase Reductase
ncRNAs	Non-coding RNAs
NEP	Neprilysin
NMDA	N-methyl-D-aspartate
OPRD1	Opioid Receptor Delta 1
PIK3R2	Phosphoinositide-3-kinase Regulatory Subunit 2
PKA	Protein Kinase A
PS	Presenilin
PTBP1	Polypyrimidine Tract Binding Protein 1
PTEN	Phosphatase and Tensin Homolog
RFC1	Reduced Folate Carrier
ROCK1	Rho-associated Coiled Coil Containing Protein Kinase 1
SAH	S-adenosylhomocysteine

SAM	S-adenosylmethionine
SHMT1	Serine Hydroxymethyltransferase 1
shRNA	Short Hairpin RNA
siRNA	Short Interfering RNA
SIRTs	Sirtuins
SNPs	Single Nucleotide Polymorphisms
SORL1	Sortilin Related Receptor 1
SYP	Synaptophysin
TC	Transcobalamin
THF	Tetrahydrofolate
THF	Tetrahydrofolate
TMEM59	Transmembrane Protein 59
TREM2	Triggering Receptor Expressed in Myeloid Cells 2

12.1 INTRODUCTION

Alzheimer's disease (AD) is the most common cause of dementia in the elderly. According to 'The World Alzheimer Report 2018', approximately 50 million people are living with dementia worldwide, out of which 35 million cases are classified as AD. In India, 4.1 million people suffer from dementia, among which 2.9 million cases are diagnosed as suffering from AD (GBD 2016 Dementia Collaborators) and this number is set to triple by 2050. Neuropathological analysis revealed selective degeneration of brain regions that control the memory, such as the hippocampus, with extracellular accumulation of β-amyloid (Aβ) plaques and intracellular accumulation of neurofibrillary tangles as two hallmarks of AD, leading to neuronal death and impairment of cognitive abilities.

To date, the major risk factor for developing AD is age, independent of any genetic background. Familial cases account for ~10% of total AD cases, caused by fully penetrant mutations in three genes, namely those encoding the amyloid precursor protein (APP), presenilin 1 (PS-1) and presenilin 2 (PS-2). More than 90% of AD cases are sporadic, likely to result from complex interactions of genetic and environmental factors. The most widely distributed genetic risk factor associated with sporadic AD is the possession of the ε4 allele of the apolipoprotein E gene (*APOEε4*). The onset of the disease normally occurs only after 50 years of age even in familial cases. This implies that even in genetically predisposed individuals cumulative events act together with the interplay of genes and the environment during the aging process to result in AD. Increasing evidence supports a major role for epigenetic modifications in AD pathogenesis. In recent times, several studies have emerged that identify a role for epigenetic mechanisms in neuronal function and cognition. Reversing these epigenetic events would be simpler than for the genetic events.

12.1.1 What Is Epigenetics?

Epigenetics refers to any process that alters gene activity without changing the primary DNA sequence, and these modifications can be transmitted to daughter cells. The three most relevant epigenetic modifications are DNA methylation, histone modification, and gene regulation by non-coding RNAs. Together, histone modifications (acetylation, methylation, phosphorylation, ubiquitination) and DNA methylation constitute a higher-order epigenetic modification, defined as chromatin remodeling (Figure 12.1). Alteration of chromatin structure will affect gene transcription and gene expression, resulting in long-term phenotypic changes (Jaenisch and Bird 2003).

12.1.2 DNA Methylation

One of the best-studied epigenetic modifications is DNA methylation, which refers to the binding of a methyl group ($-CH_3$) to the carbon in position 5 of a cytosine moiety, resulting in the formation

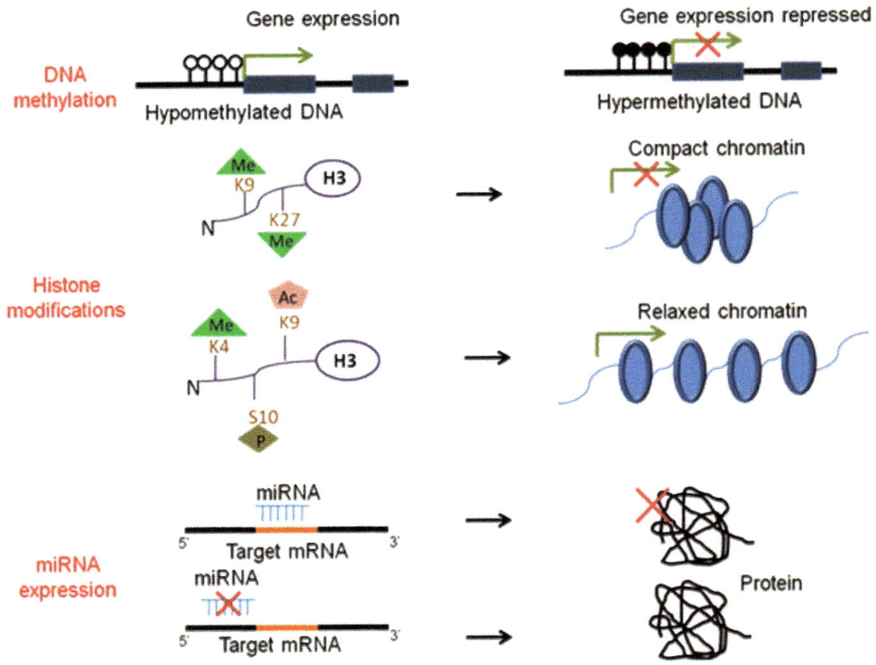

FIGURE 12.1 Modes of epigenetic modulation by DNA methylation, histone modification, and microRNA expression.

of 5-methylcytosine (5mC). The classic functions of DNA methylation are genomic imprinting, X-chromosome inactivation in mammalian females, and gene silencing. This reaction occurs mostly at so-called CpG islands and is catalyzed by enzymes known as DNA methyltransferases (DNMTs). DNMTs are of four types, namely DNMT1, DNMT2, DNMT3a, and DNMT3b. DNA methylation appears to be frequently involved in the processes associated with both healthy and diseased aging, particularly in neurological and neurodegenerative diseases. Finally, the 5mC can be converted into 5-hydroxymethyl cytosine (5hmC), which is abundant in the brain (Tognini et al. 2015). The appropriate balance between methylated and demethylated states defines the state of health and disease.

12.1.3 One-Carbon Metabolism (Folate Pathway)

Folate is an important component in the functions of one-carbon metabolism, where it acts as a methyl donor required for the production of S-adenosylmethionine (SAM), which is the major DNA methylating agent. Through a sequence of reactions, dietary folate donates a methyl group to homocysteine, forming methionine, and then SAM, which is a global methyl donor for numerous methylation reactions, including DNA methylation. After demethylation, SAM is converted into S-adenosylhomocysteine (SAH) which is then converted back to homocysteine, thereby closing the cycle.

In the one-carbon metabolism pathway, serine hydroxymethyltransferase 1 (SHMT1) is an enzyme that is involved in the reversible conversion of serine and tetrahydrofolate (THF) to glycine and 5,10-methylenetetrahydrofolate (5,10-MTHF). Methylene tetrahydrofolate reductase (MTHFR) is another enzyme in the pathway that irreversibly reduces 5,10-MTHF to 5-MTHF. 5-MTHF is the most stable and abundant form of the folate metabolites, and is the methyl donor for the pathway. Subsequently, methionine synthase (MTR) transfers a methyl group from 5-MTHF to homocysteine, forming methionine and tetrahydrofolate (THF), with the help of methionine synthase reductase (MTRR). Methionine is then converted back to SAM in a reaction catalyzed by methionine

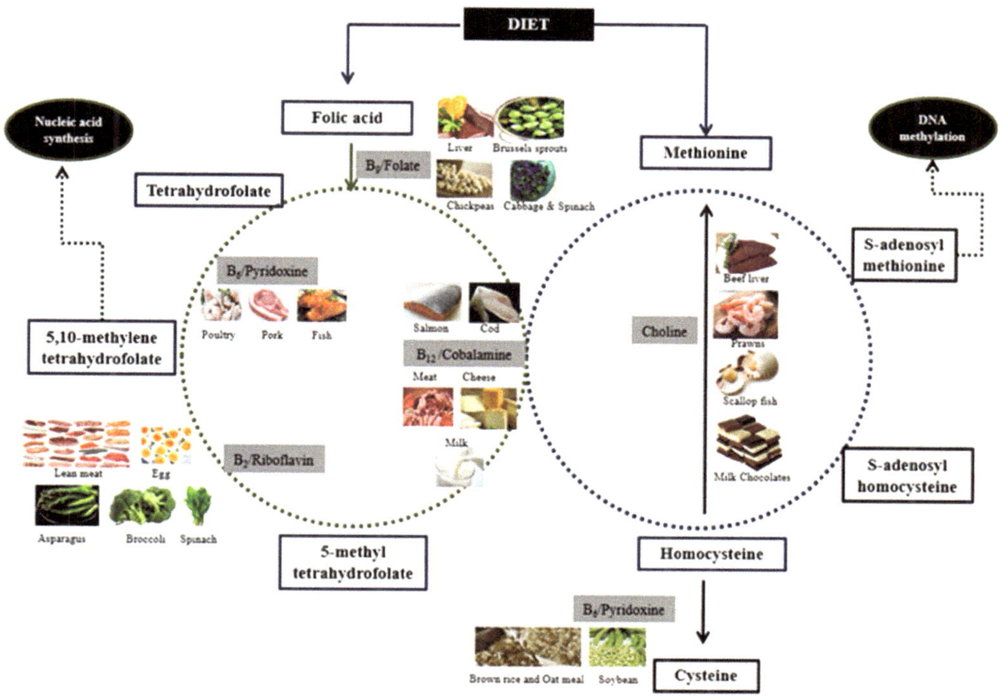

FIGURE 12.2 Overview of the folate pathway and its intervention by nutritional supplements.

adenosyltransferase (MAT). Most of the SAM generated is used in transmethylation reactions, whereby SAM is converted to SAH by transferring the methyl group to diverse biological acceptors, including proteins and DNA. Vitamins B_2 (riboflavin), B_6 (pyridoxine), and B_{12} (cobalamin) are the cofactors of MTHFR, SHMT1, and MTRR, respectively, that are required for the maintenance of MTR in its active state (Figure 12.2).

12.1.4 Histone Modifications

Nucleosomes are the fundamental units of chromatin, and each nucleosome is composed of 147 DNA base pairs, wrapped tightly around an octamer of histone proteins, which consists of two copies of each of the four core histones, H2A, H2B, H3, and H4. The linker histone, H1, binds to the DNA between the nucleosomal core particles, and is essential to stabilize higher-order chromatin structures. Each histone protein consists of a central globular domain and an N-terminal tail that contains multiple sites for various post-translational modifications (Bowman and Poirier 2015), such as acetylation, methylation, phosphorylation, ADP-ribosylation, ubiquitylation, sumoylation, crotonylation, propionylation, deimination, and *O*-GlcNAcylation (Sanchez-Mut and Gräff 2015). These modifications can occur on different amino acids; lysines can be acetylated, methylated, ubiquitylated, or sumoylated, arginines can be deiminated, methylated, or ADP-ribosylated, histidine residues can be methylated, and serine or threonine residues can be phosphorylated or *O*-GlcNAcylated, whereas glutamate residues can be ADP-ribosylated, tyrosines can be phosphorylated, and prolines can be isomerized (Hanes 2015; Xu et al. 2014; Bowman and Poirier 2015).

Each of these post-translational modification is catalyzed by a specific set of enzymes and has different effects on gene expression (Strahl and Allis 2000). Histone acetylation is a reversible process, and the enzymes involved are histone acetyltransferases (HATs) and histone deacetylases (HDACs). Generally, acetylation of histones occurs on the ε amino group of lysine residues in the N-terminal region of histone tails, which effectively neutralizes the positive charge. This reduces the electrostatic interactions between the positively charged histones and the negatively charged DNA backbone, thereby increasing gene expression and also mediating the chromatin remodeling, to allow an open chromatin structure. HDACs are generally divided into four subclasses: Class I (HDAC 1, 2, and 8), Class II (HDAC 4, 5, 6, 7, 9, and 10), Class III, also known as sirtuins (SIRTs 1, 2, 3, 4, 5, 6, and 7), and Class IV (HDAC 11) (Dokmanovic et al. 2007). The SIRT family of enzymes requires NAD^+ for their activity, whereas the other classes of HDACs are zinc dependent. The expression patterns of HDACs are region or cell specific, with HDAC2 being specifically expressed in most brain regions and being predominantly active in differentiated neurons (Guan et al. 2009). Currently, the use of HDAC inhibitors are the most common method of manipulating the epigenome pharmacologically.

Histone methylation is also dynamic and is carried out by the opposing actions of histone methyltransferases (HMTs) and histone demethylases (HDMTs). Methylation occurs on lysine (mono-, di- or tri-methylated) or arginine residues and does not seem to alter the charge of the altered residues but confers unique structural alterations. Similarly, histone phosphorylation is mediated by the opposing activities of protein kinases and phosphatases. Histone phosphorylation regulates multiple processes, such as DNA damage response, gene expression, chromatin condensation etc.

12.1.5 Non-Coding RNAs

The majority of the eukaryotic genome is transcribed into non-coding RNAs (ncRNAs), and only ~2% is translated. Non-coding RNAs are mainly classified into two types, based on their size, namely small RNAs (sRNAs) (<200 nucleotides) and long non-coding RNAs (lncRNAs) (>200 nucleotides). ncRNAs play crucial roles in the regulation of most epigenetic mechanisms. The small ncRNAs are involved in silencing of transposable elements (Lisch 2012), miRNAs are involved in gene expression control, lncRNAs in X-chromosome inactivation and DNA imprinting (Jeon et al. 2012), and so on. Moreover, these ncRNAs can also regulate DNA methylation and histone modifications. Thus, ncRNAs are directly and/or indirectly implicated in epigenetic mechanisms.

12.2 EPIGENETIC REGULATION OF AGING

Aging is a multifactorial, physiological condition, resulting from the accumulation of damage at the molecular level over a lifetime, and it depends on genetic, epigenetic, environmental, and stochastic factors. Aberrant epigenetic alterations, such as DNA methylation and histone modifications, have been reported during the aging process (reviewed in Mastroeni et al. 2011). Genomic methylation, which influences gene expression and chromatin organization, has been shown to exhibit a genome-wide tendency toward DNA hypomethylation with age in different vertebrate species, including humans. In line with this finding, the activity of DNMT1, an enzyme responsible for maintaining DNA methylation, has also been found to decrease with aging (Lopatina et al. 2002).

12.3 EPIGENETICS IN THE PATHOPHYSIOLOGY OF ALZHEIMER'S DISEASE

The best-known risk factor for AD is aging. Neurodegeneration in AD is associated with selective degeneration of temporal and parietal lobes, including the hippocampus and entorhinal cortex and selected regions within the frontal cortex and the cingulate gyrus. These regions are characterized by intraneuronal aggregates of hyperphosphorylated tau proteins in the form of neurofibrillary tangles and accumulation of extracellular aggregates of amyloid-beta (Aβ) peptides, termed amyloid plaques.

Aβ is the primary component of senile plaques in the degenerating brain regions of AD patients. Pathogenic mutations within the genes encoding APP, PS-1, and PS-2 have been identified in familial AD. These genes contain manipulable methylated CpG sites (Fuso et al. 2005). APP is a single-pass *trans*-membrane protein expressed at high levels in the brain and metabolized in a rapid and highly complex fashion by sequential cleavages by proteases, such as β-secretase and γ-secretase. Identification of familial AD cases harboring pathogenic mutations in genes encoding *APP*, beta-secretase (*BACE*) and *PSEN1* suggested that proteolysis of APP is a crucial step in the development of AD. Cleavage of APP by γ-secretase results in the production of Aβ40 or Aβ42. Aβ42 has been suggested to be neurotoxic in nature. Aβ42 can be cleaved by proteases such as the insulin-degrading enzyme (Kurochkin and Goto 1994), neprilysin (NEP) (Iwata et al. 2000), BACE1 (Huse et al. 2002), and cathepsin B (only Aβ1–42) (Mueller-Steiner et al. 2006). What are the possible modifiable mechanisms that are known to prevent or aggravate these neurotoxic events?

12.3.1 DNA Methylation Patterns in Disease-Associated Genes in AD

The studies addressing DNA methylation status in AD began in 1995 when West et al. reported an AD-specific hypomethylation of the *APP* promoter in a single patient (West et al. 1995). Subsequently, evidence for epigenetic changes in AD pathogenesis has been extensively investigated, using various human tissue samples, animal models, and cell culture models. Most of these studies identified aberrant DNA methylation patterns in patients with AD. The promoter region of the *APP* gene was found to be frequently methylated in AD patients and was suggested to have a significant role in the development of Aβ deposition in the aged brain (Tohgi et al. 1999). However, studies using larger sample sizes could not replicate these findings (Barrachina and Ferrer 2009). DNA methylation has been shown to be involved in APP processing and Aβ formation through the regulation of *PSEN1* expression. Administration of SAM silences the *APP* gene, thereby preventing Aβ production. AD is characterized by high levels of homocysteine and low levels of folate and vitamin B_{12}. Studies in mice and neuroblastoma cell lines demonstrate that *PSEN1* gene expression is regulated by promoter DNA methylation, depending on vitamin B (folate, B12 and B6) availability (Fuso et al. 2011, 2005). However, few studies failed to demonstrate an alteration in methylation levels at *APP*, *PSEN1* or *PSEN2* in peripheral blood DNA or post-mortem brain samples of AD (Barrachina and Ferrer 2009; Brohede et al. 2010). Methylation at the promoter region of the gene encoding Transmembrane Protein 59 (*TMEM59*) has been functionally associated with expression levels of *TMEM59*, which is implicated in APP post-translational processing, supporting a role for epigenetic change in late-onset AD (LOAD) pathology.

Aβ itself has been shown to trigger the epigenetic changes. In a murine cerebral endothelial cell model, Aβ induced global DNA hypomethylation and reduced NEP expression, resulting in an increase in Aβ accumulation and deposition (Chen et al. 2009). The tau protein is the major component of the neurofibrillary tangles present in AD. The *Tau* gene contains differentially methylated binding sites for transcription factors, and it is subjected to complex epigenetic regulations. The binding sites for *Sp1*, a transcriptional activator, within the *Tau* gene promoter was shown to be significantly hypermethylated with age, whereas the binding sites for the GC-rich sequence DNA-binding factor (GCF), a repressor of GC-rich promoters, was shown to be significantly hypomethylated with age, suggesting that transcriptional activity of the *Tau* gene decreased with age in the human cerebral cortex (Tohgi et al. 1999). However no significant differences in promoter methylation of the *Tau* gene have been observed in the frontal cortex or hippocampus of post-mortem AD samples (Barrachina and Ferrer 2009).

DNA methylation profiles of hippocampal tissues from control and AD patients have identified the presence of promoter hypermethylation of the gene *Dual-Specificity Phosphatase 22* (*DUSP22*), that inhibits protein kinase A (PKA) activity and, thereby determines tau phosphorylation status and cyclic AMP-responsive element-binding protein (CREB) signaling in AD (Sanchez-Mut et al. 2014). The methylation status of *DUSP22* correlated positively with the Braak stages of the patient (Sanchez-Mut et al. 2014). Decreased expression of another phosphatase, DUSP6, that regulates tau production, through hypermethylation, was recently shown in AD brains (Watson et al. 2016). The Bridging Integrator1 (BIN1), which mediates AD risk by modulating tau pathology (Chapuis et al. 2013), was shown to be aberrantly hypermethylated in AD, resulting in Aβ load (De Jager et al. 2014; Yu et al. 2015).

One of the best-known genetic risk factors for developing AD is the possession of an *APOE* ε4 allele. The *APOE* gene promoter has a lower CpG content and so exhibits low levels of DNA methylation. However, the sequence near to the 3' end, which encodes the APOE ε4 haplotype, harbors a CpG island which is heavily methylated. It is proposed that aberrant epigenetic control in this CpG island may contribute to LOAD pathology (Wang et al. 2008). Since the mere possession of an ε4 allele will not cause the disease, it would be of great interest to know if methylation status at this 3′ CpG site is altered in ε4 carriers who develop (or do not develop) AD. Similarly, a gene encoding another member of the apolipoprotein family, termed apolipoprotein J or clusterin (*APOJ* or *CLU*, respectively), which plays a role in the clearance of misfolded proteins, inflammation, and apoptosis, is considered to be the third most-significant genetic risk factor for the development of LOAD (Harold et al. 2009; Lambert et al. 2009). The promoter of *CLU* contains a CpG-rich methylation domain and the demethylation studies *in vitro* have been shown to enhance *CLU* expression (Rauhala et al. 2008; Suuronen et al. 2007). The majority of association studies have suggested *CLU* to be a risk factor, independent of the *APOE* genotype.

12.3.2 DNA Methylation Patterns in Other Genes Involved in AD

Recently, several genome-wide association studies have revealed *Triggering Receptor Expressed on Myeloid cells 2* (*TREM2*) to be a susceptibility gene associated with AD and other neurodegenerative diseases. *TREM2* expression was upregulated in the hippocampus of AD patients compared with controls and 5hmC was shown to play a role in the regulation of *TREM2* expression (Celarain et al. 2016). In the AD brain, increased DNA methylation in the superior temporal gyrus at a CpG site located 289 bp upstream of the transcription start site of the *TREM2* gene was reported in three independent study cohorts, and a meta-analysis across all three cohorts revealed a consistent AD-associated hypermethylation (Smith et al. 2016). Furthermore, hypomethylation at intron 1 showed higher *TREM2* mRNA expression in the peripheral leukocytes of AD subjects relative to controls (Ozaki et al. 2017). All these reports point toward *TREM2* serving as an epigenetically altered biomarker for predicting AD.

Brain-derived neurotropic factor (BDNF) is a neurotrophin, highly expressed in brain regions with a high degree of plasticity, such as the cortex, hippocampus, etc. Changes in BDNF expression have been reported in the brain as well as in blood of AD patients, which indicates a potential role for BDNF in the pathogenesis of AD. Emerging evidence indicates that *BDNF* promoter methylation is one of the most replicated epigenetic biomarkers of AD (Chang et al. 2014; Rao et al. 2012; Nagata et al. 2015). Hypermethylation of the *BDNF* promoter has been observed in the prefrontal cortex from AD and bipolar disorder patients (Rao et al. 2012), along with the hypermethylation of *CREB* and synaptophysin (*SYP*) genes, and hypomethylation of the cyclooxygenase-2 (*COX2*) and *NF-κB* genes. One study investigated the methylation of the *BDNF* promoter in the peripheral blood of AD patients and control but failed to observe any association (Carboni et al. 2015). However, another two reports suggested that elevation of methylation in the *BDNF* promoter from peripheral blood can be used as a potential epigenetic biomarker for predicting the progression from amnestic mild cognitive impairment (MCI) to AD (Xie et al. 2017a, b). Cao et al. demonstrated that, in rat models, the methylation changes in BDNF exon 4 and its differential expression is regulated by Aβ and SAM (Cao et al. 2018).

An investigation of the methylation status of DNA repair genes in AD subjects, compared with controls, did not find any increased promoter methylation in peripheral blood of AD patients (Coppedè et al. 2017). A cross-tissue analysis of methylomic variation in AD, using samples from four independent human post-mortem brain cohorts, identified a differentially hypermethylated region in the *Ankyrin 1* (*ANK1*) gene, that was associated with neuropathology in the entorhinal cortex (and also in the superior temporal gyrus and prefrontal cortex), the primary site of AD manifestation (Lunnon et al. 2014). A dynamic regulation of DNA methylation in the human cerebral cortex has been reported throughout the lifespan, with hypermethylation of vinexin (encoding a cell adhesion molecule expressed in neurons and glia) (Ito et al. 2007) and hypomethylation of S100A2 (a member of the S100 family of calcium-binding proteins), compared with other non-AD subjects older than 60 years (Siegmund et al. 2007). Hypomethylation of *CREB5*, encoding a transcription factor implicated in synaptic plasticity and cognition, was reported in the prefrontal cortex from AD and normal subjects (Zukin 2009). Hypomethylation of the mitochondrial DNA (mtDNA) D-loop region was reported in peripheral blood DNA of LOAD patients (Stoccoro et al. 2017). Another study reported hypermethylation in the opioid receptor delta 1 (OPRD1, a member of the opioid family of G-protein-coupled receptors) promoter region, and discussed its role in influencing the risk of AD.

Generally speaking, 5mC is associated with decreased gene expression and 5hmC has been associated with increased gene expression. Altered levels of 5mC and 5hmC are reported to play a role in the pathogenesis of AD. The levels of 5mC and 5hmC in the human middle frontal gyrus (MFG) and middle temporal gyrus (MTG) showed a global hypermethylation, along with significantly increased levels of 5hmC, which were positively correlated with each other and with markers of AD, including Aβ, tau, and ubiquitin loads in the MFG and MTG of AD subjects (Coppieters et al. 2014).

The role of 5hmC in the prefrontal cortex of post-mortem AD patients was studied through genome-wide analysis and RNA-sequencing (RNA-Seq) to correlate changes in 5hmC with transcriptional changes, and identified 325 genes (enriched with respect to pathways involved in neuron projection development and neurogenesis) containing differentially hydroxymethylated regions (DhMRs) in both discovery and replication datasets (Bernstein et al. 2016). Another study evaluated a genome-wide profiling of brain DNA hydroxymethylation in the dorsolateral prefrontal cortex of 30 deceased post-mortem brain samples and revealed that 517 DhMRs were significantly associated with neuritic plaques, and that 60 DhMRs were associated with neurofibrillary tangles (Zhao et al. 2017). A genome-wide hydroxymethylation study in an *APP-PSEN1* double transgenic mouse model of AD revealed a significant decrease in 5hmC in the hippocampus, but not in the cortex and cerebellum, as the mice aged, with DhMR-associated genes being highly enriched in multiple signaling pathways involving neuronal development/differentiation and neuronal function/survival (Shu et al. 2016).

Age-related differences of DNA methylation and hydroxymethylation were also studied in a range of animal models of AD, and their correlations with Aβ load in three transgenic mouse models (J20, APP/PS1dE9, and 3xTg-AD), as well as in a non-transgenic non-human primate AD model (Caribbean vervets) (Lardenoije et al. 2018). In the J20 mouse model, an age-related decrease in global DNA methylation was found in the dentate gyrus (DG) and a decrease in the ratio between DNA methylation and hydroxymethylation was found in the DG and cornu ammonis 3 (CA3). The hippocampal plaque load showed a significant negative correlation with DNA methylation in the DG, and a negative correlation with the 5mC: 5hmC ratio in the DG and CA3. In the 3xTg-AD mice, an age-related hypermethylation was found in the DG and CA1-2. No significant age-related alterations were found in the *APP/PS1dE9* mice and non-human primate models. For the APP/PS1dE9 model, a negative correlation between the ratio and the plaque load was observed in the CA3, as well as a negative correlation between DNMT3A levels and plaque load in the DG and CA3. None of the models showed age-related differences in levels of DNA hydroxymethylation and DNMT3A. These results warrant future studies to elucidate the contribution of different AD-related genetic variation to age-related epigenetic changes.

12.3.3 Histone Modifications in AD

Gene expression is controlled not only by DNA methylation but also by conformation of chromatin structure, mediated by histone modifications. Hence, histone modifications are also suggested to play an important role in pathogenesis of AD.

Among the histone acetylation marks, H4K16ac is a key modification because it regulates chromatin compaction, gene expression, stress responses, and DNA damage repair. In model organisms, modulators of H4K16ac play a role in whole-organism aging and cellular senescence. The first genome-wide profile of a histone modification in human brains affected with AD compared the genome-wide enrichment of H4K16ac (chromatin-state epigenetic marker) in the lateral temporal lobe of AD against both younger and elderly cognitively normal controls and found that, while normal aging leads to H4K16ac enrichment, AD entails dramatic loss of H4K16ac in the proximity of genes linked to aging and AD (Nativio et al. 2018). HDAC and Sirtuin expression levels in the frontal cortex of subjects with MCI, moderate AD or severe AD, compared with cognitively normal controls, found dysregulation of these epigenetic proteins contributing to the neuronal dysfunction and cognitive decline in the early stages of AD (Mahady et al. 2018). Animal model studies have suggested the contribution of histone tail modifications toward learning and memory processes. Administration of histone deacetylase inhibitors (HDACi) has been shown to ameliorate the cognitive deficit and to improve memory in animal models. HDAC2 levels were increased by AD-related neurotoxic insults *in vitro* in two mouse models and in post-mortem brain samples of patients with AD, whereby they reduced the histone acetylation of genes important for learning and memory, resulting in concomitant decrease in expression (Gräff et al. 2012). This implicates that HDAC2 might be involved in the pathogenesis of AD through chromatin modification of genes associated with synaptic plasticity and memory formation. A widespread loss of heterochromatin was reported in *tau* transgenic Drosophila and mice, whereas, in human AD patients, a widespread increase in the transcription of genes in AD brain, that were heterochromatically silenced in controls, as a result of the reduction of heterochromatin marks of H3K9me2 and heterochromatin protein 1 (HP1) (Frost et al. 2014).

Inhibitors of histone acetyltransferases also ameliorate the premature aging phenotypes of progeroid mice and extend their lifespan (Krishnan et al. 2011). Acetylation of the hippocampal histones, such as H2B, H3, and H4, were transiently increased in normal mice during learning processes, suggesting that histone acetylation is essential for memory consolidation (reviewed in Lu et al. 2015). Restoration of physiological H4 acetylation, through administration of HDACi, prevents the manifestation of age-associated memory impairment in mice (Peleg et al. 2010), indicating that reversion of epigenetic changes may have neuroprotective effects. Decreased H3K27 acetylation at regulatory regions of synaptic plasticity, as well as in immune response genes in the p25 transgenic model of AD, was found to correspond to the changes in transcription (Gjoneska et al. 2015). Whereas histone acetylation shows an overall decrease in the aged mice, the application of HDAC inhibitors reverses such decreases in the global histone acetylation and improves the memory deficits *in vivo* (Chuang et al. 2009; Gräff et al. 2012; Walker et al. 2013).

12.3.4 Alteration of Folate Metabolism in AD

AD individuals are characterized by decreased plasma folate values, as well as increased plasma homocysteine levels, and there is an indication of impaired SAM levels in AD brains, compared with healthy age-matched controls. Folate deficiency causes a decline in SAM and decreasing DNA methylation in AD and aging. Higher folate intake is related to lower AD risk in the elderly.

Polymorphisms in genes participating in one-carbon metabolism have been associated with increased AD risk and/or with increased homocysteine levels in AD individuals. The most studied gene associated with folate pathway is *MTHFR*. Two common single nucleotide polymorphisms (SNPs) present in *MTHFR*, namely 677C>T (Ala222Val) and 1298A>C (Glu429Ala), are known to reduce the enzyme's activity (Weisberg et al. 1998). Several studies have investigated the association of these SNPs in various cohorts, but the results were conflicting. Reduced folate carrier (RFC1) is a transport protein present in biological membranes to transport folate into the cells. Several studies have analyzed the association between *RFC1* 80G>A and its effect on folate and homocysteine levels, but obtained conflicting results. Another common SNP in *MTR*, 2756A>G (Asp919Gly), has been shown to influence homocysteine levels in some studies. The association analysis of this SNP in AD patients has also produced inconclusive results. Vitamin B_{12} serves as a coenzyme for MTR in the conversion of homocysteine to methionine. Transcobalamin (TC) is the transport protein required for cellular uptake of vitamin B_{12}. A common SNP in *TC*, 776C>G (Pro259Arg), is reported to alter vitamin B_{12} absorption and thereby increases plasma homocysteine levels. Risk factor assessment of this polymorphism in AD also provided inconclusive results (reviewed in Coppedè 2010). Another enzyme in the pathway, human cystathionine β-synthase (CBS), is a hemoprotein which catalyzes the condensation of homocysteine and serine to form cystathionine, which is then converted into glutathione (GSH). A common insertion polymorphism in *CBS*, 844ins68, has been investigated in several studies, but the results were again inconsistent (reviewed in Coppedè 2010). Interventions in this one-carbon metabolism pathway (Figure 12.2) could be achieved by supplementing with appropriate vitamins or nutritional factors to prevent or minimize the progression of AD pathology.

12.3.5 Non-Coding RNAs in AD

Increasing evidence has suggested that non-coding RNAs undergo aberrant expression in AD brains, which may affect the onset and progression of neurodegeneration occurring in AD. MicroRNAs (miRNAs) are the best-studied non-coding RNAs, playing an important role in the development, differentiation, and maturation of neurons. Several miRNAs have been shown to regulate the expression of AD-associated proteins, such as APP, PS1, BACE1, BDNF, etc. (Table 12.1).

12.4 EPIGENETIC MODIFIERS IN AD

Current medications provide only symptomatic relief to AD patients. There are no treatments which can prevent or reverse the neurodegeneration occurring in AD patients. Since epigenetic alterations have been reported in AD, therapies targeting epigenetic regulation have received a great deal of attention for their potential in AD treatment. The major epigenetic targets for therapeutic intervention include the regulation of DNA methylation, histone modification, and non-coding RNAs.

12.4.1 Therapies Targeting DNA Methylation

Hypermethylation of some pathogenic genes have been reported in the pathogenesis of AD. Hence, reducing the methylation has been suggested as an alternative therapy in AD. Inhibitors targeting DNMTs of specific genes may be effective epigenetic modifying drugs for AD. Alternatively, dietary supplementation with methyl donors such as folate, or administration with vitamin B_{12}, SAM, or L-methyl folate may help to prevent or reverse the pathogenesis associated with AD (Figure 12.2).

12.4.2 Therapies Targeting Histone Modification

Inhibitors targeting histone acetylation have been extensively studied in animal models of AD. HDAC inhibitors, such as valproic acid, trichostatin, sodium 4-phenylbutyrate, and vorinostat, have been shown to affect Aβ deposition and tau phosphorylation (Wang et al. 2013).

12.4.3 Therapies Targeting Non-Coding RNAs

Since abnormal levels of non-coding RNAs have been reported in the central nervous system, cerebrospinal fluid, and blood of AD patients they are regarded as ideal modifiers for AD therapy. The expression of *BACE*, *PTBP1*, *APP*, *PSEN1* and *PSEN2* genes were found to be regulated through non-coding RNAs, such as short interfering RNA (siRNA), miRNA, and short hairpin RNA (shRNA), through RNA interference. For example, miR124 and miR195 could be treated as targets for AD therapy by targeting *BACE1* since their overexpression is associated with decreased Aβ deposition (Fang et al. 2012; Zhu et al. 2012, Smith et al. 2011).

TABLE 12.1
Administration of MicroRNAs and Their Associated Target Effects in AD

MiRNA	Levels in AD	Locus	Target and Effect	Reference
miR-107	Downregulated	10q23.31	BACE1 downregulation	(Wang et al. 2008)
miR-29a/b-1	Downregulated	1q22/5q14.3/1	BACE1 downregulation	(Hebert et al. 2008)
miR-9	Downregulated	5q26.1		
miR-29c	Downregulated	1q32.2	BACE1 downregulation	(Yang et al. 2015)
miR188-3p	Downregulated	Xp11.23	BACE1 downregulation	(Zhang et al. 2014)
miR124	Downregulated	8p23.1, 8q12.3, and 20q13.33	BACE1 downregulation & PTBP1	(Smith et al. 2011) (Fang et al. 2012)
miR-339-5p	Downregulated	7p22.3	BACE1 downregulation	(Long et al. 2014)
miR-195	Downregulated	17p13.1	BACE1 & Tau downregulation	(Ai et al. 2013) (Sun et al. 2015; Zhu et al. 2012)
miR-186	Downregulated	1p31.1	BACE 1 downregulation	(Harold et al. 2009) (Jaekwang Kim et al. 2016)
miR-27a-3p	Downregulated	19p13.12	PSEN1	(Sala Frigerio et al. 2013)
miR-34a	Upregulated	1p36.22	Tau downregulation, γ-secretase upregulaton	(Dickson et al. 2013) (Jian et al. 2017)
miR-24	-	9q22.32	Nicastrin	(Delay et al. 2014)
miR-186	Downregulated	1p31.1	BACE1 downregulation	
miR-455	Upregulated	9q32	APP downregulation	
miR-132 & miR-212	Downregulated	17p13.3	GSK3, Tau PTEN, FOXO3a, and P300 downregulation	(Smith et al. 2015; Wong et al. 2013)
miR-125b, miR-138, miR-106b, miR-922	Upregulated	11q24.1/21q21.1	TAU	(Banzhaf-Strathmann et al. 2014; Liu et al. 2016; Wang et al. 2015)
	Upregulated	-		
	Downregulated	7q22.1		
	Downregulated	3q29		

(Continued)

TABLE 12.1 (CONTINUED)
Administration of MicroRNAs and Their Associated Target Effects in AD

MiRNA	Levels in AD	Locus	Target and Effect	Reference
miR-101	Downregulation		APP downregulation	(Barbato et al. 2014; Vilardo et al. 2010)
miR-16	Downregulated		APP downregulation	(Liu et al. 2012; Zhang et al. 2015)
miR-153	Downregulated		APP downregulation	(Long et al. 2012)
miR-147, miR-20a	-	9q33.2	APP downregulation	(Delay et al. 2011)
	-	13q31.3		
miR-15a and miR-16	Downregulated		ERK1 upregulation	(Hébert et al. 2010)
miR-15/107 family	Downregulated		CDK5R1 downregulation	(Moncini et al. 2017)
miR-33	-		ABCA1 and APOE lipidation	(Kim et al. 2015)
Let-7b		22q13.31		(Lehmann et al. 2012)
miR-146a	Upregulated	5q34	ROCK1	(Pogue et al. 2011; Wang et al. 2016)
miR-148a	Downregulated	7p15.2		(Cogswell et al. 2008)
miR-200b/c	Downregulated	1p36.33	Reduction of Aβ secretion	(Higaki et al. 2018)
miR-200c	Upregulated	12p13.31	PTEN downregulation	(Wu et al. 2016)
miR-219-5p	Downregulated		Tau downregulation	(Santa-Maria et al. 2015)
miR-135b	Downregulated	1q32.1	BACE1 downregulation	(Zhang et al. 2016)
miR-1229-3p	-	-	SORL1 downregulation	(Ghanbari et al. 2016)
miR-603	Upregulated	10p12.2	LRPAP1 downregulation	(Zhang et al. 2016)
miR-193b	Downregulated	16p13.12	APP downregulation	(Liu et al. 2014)
miR-30a-5p	Upregulated	6q13	BDNF downregulation	(Croce et al. 2013)
miR-206	Upregulated	6p12.2	BDNF downregulation	(Tian et al. 2014)
miR126	Upregulated	9q34.3	IRS-1 and PIK3R2 downregulation	(Kim et al. 2016)

12.4.4 Alternative Approaches to the Prevention of AD

AD is a multifactorial disorder, as evidenced from the involvement of multiple genetic, cellular, biochemical, and environmental factors in its pathogenesis. Potential targets for developing interventions include Aβ formation, abnormal tau phosphorylation, inflammation, excitotoxicity, oxidative stress, etc. Current medications for AD include acetylcholinesterase inhibitors (e.g. donepezil, rivastigmine, galantamine), N-methyl-D-aspartate (NMDA) antagonists (e.g. memantine), antihypertensive drugs, anti-inflammatory drugs, secretase inhibitors, etc. These are only symptomatic treatment strategies that may improve the cognitive dysfunction associated with AD, but would not reverse the neurodegeneration occurring in AD. Other therapeutic agents that have been shown to improve cognitive function in AD include administration of insulin and BDNF, antioxidant therapies, vaccination against Aβ, etc.

Other than these, natural therapies employing extracts from herbal medicinal plants have been widely used for the treatment of the memory deficits seen in AD. Some plant compounds, such as curcumin and resveratrol, may be promising therapeutic agents for AD therapy. Curcumin shows neuroprotective effects such as anti-inflammatory and antioxidant effects, as well as inhibition of Aβ formation, Aβ clearance, etc. Resveratrol has anti-inflammatory, anti-oxidant, and antiapoptotic properties, and it seems to reduce Aβ formation, decrease learning impairment and thereby reduce the risk of developing AD.

Some dietary nutrients have been suggested to prevent the cognitive deterioration occurring in AD. These include polyunsaturated fatty acids (omega-3 fatty acids such as docosahexaenoic acid (DHA), eicosapentaenoic acid (EPA), polyphenols (green tea, resveratrol, curcumin, ginkgolides, etc.) and some vitamins (vitamin A, D, E, and Bs). Since hyperhomocysteinemia associated with lower vitamin B levels has been reported in AD patients, B vitamins, such as B_6, B_{12} and folic acid, have been suggested as nutritional supplements to treat cognitive impairments in AD.

Since AD is an age-associated disorder, increased life expectancy will result in increased exposure to environmental risk factors that can induce adverse epigenetic modifications. The different environmental factors that can modulate epigenetic alterations include pollutants, nutrients, lifestyle, physical activities, mental stress, etc. Some brain stimulatory therapies, such as physical and mental exercises, have been suggested to improve cognitive functioning in AD. Therefore, in order to prevent neurodegeneration, it is important to maintain proper physical and mental health by appropriate exercise and good nutrition, including the use of appropriate dietary supplements.

12.5 SUMMARY

The increasing incidence of AD worldwide, without treatments for stopping or reversing the pathogenesis, is indeed a matter of great concern. With increase in age, the probability of developing AD grows exponentially. AD could be a reflection of aging gone wrong, due to altered physiological conditions resulting from the accumulation of damage at the molecular level over a lifetime, based on an individual's genetic, epigenetic, environmental, and stochastic factors. Several aberrant epigenetic mechanisms, such as DNA methylation and histone modification, have been reported to be associated with neurodegeneration and AD. Reversing these epigenetic alterations are critical to prevent the neurodegenerative progression. The present article tries to suggest that, in order to prevent further neurodegeneration, it is important to maintain proper physical and mental health, and to complement it with appropriate vitamin and nutritional supplementation based on the genetic and epigenetic background of the subject.

ACKNOWLEDGMENTS

The authors thank the Department of Biotechnology, Ministry of Science and Technology, New Delhi and RGCB for financial support, and APM thanks DST-SERB for the NPDF fellowship

REFERENCES

Ai, Jing, Li-Hua Sun, Hui Che, Rong Zhang, Tian-Zhu Zhang, Wan-Chen Wu, Xiao-Lin Su, et al. 2013. "MicroRNA-195 Protects against Dementia Induced by Chronic Brain Hypoperfusion via Its Anti-Amyloidogenic Effect in Rats." *The Journal of Neuroscience* 33 (9). Society for Neuroscience: 3989–4001. doi:10.1523/JNEUROSCI.1997-12.2013.

Banzhaf-Strathmann, J., E. Benito, S. May, T. Arzberger, S. Tahirovic, H. Kretzschmar, A. Fischer, and D. Edbauer. 2014. "MicroRNA-125b Induces Tau Hyperphosphorylation and Cognitive Deficits in Alzheimer's Disease." *The EMBO Journal* 33 (15): 1667–1680. doi:10.15252/embj.201387576.

Barbato, Christian, Silvia Pezzola, Cinzia Caggiano, Martina Antonelli, Paola Frisone, Maria Teresa Ciotti, and Francesca Ruberti. 2014. "A Lentiviral Sponge for MiR-101 Regulates RanBP9 Expression and Amyloid Precursor Protein Metabolism in Hippocampal Neurons." *Frontiers in Cellular Neuroscience* 8 (February). Frontiers: 37. doi:10.3389/fncel.2014.00037.

Barrachina, Marta, and Isidre Ferrer. 2009. "DNA Methylation of Alzheimer Disease and Tauopathy-Related Genes in Postmortem Brain." *Journal of Neuropathology & Experimental Neurology* 68 (8). Oxford University Press: 880–891. doi:10.1097/NEN.0b013e3181af2e46.

Bernstein, Alison I., Yunting Lin, R. Craig Street, Li Lin, Qing Dai, Li Yu, Han Bao, et al. 2016. "5-Hydroxymethylation-Associated Epigenetic Modifiers of Alzheimer's Disease Modulate Tau-Induced Neurotoxicity." *Human Molecular Genetics* April: ddw109. doi:10.1093/hmg/ddw109.

Bowman, Gregory D., and Michael G. Poirier. 2015. "Post-Translational Modifications of Histones That Influence Nucleosome Dynamics." *Chemical Reviews* 115 (6). American Chemical Society: 2274–2295. doi:10.1021/cr500350x.

Brohede, Jesper, Mia Rinde, Bengt Winblad, and Caroline Graff. 2010. "A DNA Methylation Study of the Amyloid Precursor Protein Gene in Several Brain Regions from Patients with Familial Alzheimer Disease." *Journal of Neurogenetics* 24 (4): 179–181. doi:10.3109/01677063.2010.503978.

Cao, Dandan, Jing Cui, Dandan Cao, Chenjia Guo, Guowen Min, Min Liu, and Liang Li. 2018. "S-Adenosylmethionine Reduces the Inhibitory Effect of Aβ on BDNF Expression through Decreasing Methylation Level of BDNF Exon IV in Rats." *Biochemical and Biophysical Research Communications* 495 (4). Academic Press: 2609–2615. doi:10.1016/J.BBRC.2017.12.166.

Carboni, Lucia, Francesca Lattanzio, Sanzio Candeletti, Elisa Porcellini, Elena Raschi, Federico Licastro, and Patrizia Romualdi. 2015. "Peripheral Leukocyte Expression of the Potential Biomarker Proteins Bdnf, Sirt1, and Psen1 Is Not Regulated by Promoter Methylation in Alzheimer's Disease Patients." *Neuroscience Letters* 605 (September): 44–48. doi:10.1016/j.neulet.2015.08.012.

Celarain, Naiara, Javier Sánchez-Ruiz de Gordoa, María Victoria Zelaya, Miren Roldán, Rosa Larumbe, Laura Pulido, Carmen Echavarri, and Maite Mendioroz. 2016. "TREM2 Upregulation Correlates with 5-Hydroxymethycytosine Enrichment in Alzheimer's Disease Hippocampus." *Clinical Epigenetics* 8. BioMed Central: 37. doi:10.1186/s13148-016-0202-9.

Chang, Lan, Yunliang Wang, Huihui Ji, Dongjun Dai, Xuting Xu, Danjie Jiang, Qingxiao Hong, et al. 2014. "Elevation of Peripheral BDNF Promoter Methylation Links to the Risk of Alzheimer's Disease." Edited by Lorenzo Chiariotti. *PLoS ONE* 9 (11): e110773. doi:10.1371/journal.pone.0110773.

Chapuis, J., F. Hansmannel, M. Gistelinck, A. Mounier, C. Van Cauwenberghe, K. V. Kolen, F. Geller, et al. 2013. "Increased Expression of BIN1 Mediates Alzheimer Genetic Risk by Modulating Tau Pathology." *Molecular Psychiatry* 18 (11): 1225–1234. doi:10.1038/mp.2013.1.

Chen, Kun-Lin, Steven Sheng-Shih Wang, Yi-Yuan Yang, Rey-Yue Yuan, Ruei-Ming Chen, and Chaur-Jong Hu. 2009. "The Epigenetic Effects of Amyloid-B1–40 on Global DNA and Neprilysin Genes in Murine Cerebral Endothelial Cells." *Biochemical and Biophysical Research Communications* 378 (1): 57–61. doi:10.1016/j.bbrc.2008.10.173.

Chuang, De-Maw, Yan Leng, Zoya Marinova, Hyeon-Ju Kim, and Chi-Tso Chiu. 2009. "Multiple Roles of HDAC Inhibition in Neurodegenerative Conditions." *Trends in Neurosciences* 32 (11): 591–601. doi:10.1016/j.tins.2009.06.002.

Cogswell, John P., James Ward, Ian A. Taylor, Michelle Waters, Yunling Shi, Brian Cannon, Kevin Kelnar, et al. 2008. "Identification of MiRNA Changes in Alzheimer's Disease Brain and CSF Yields Putative Biomarkers and Insights into Disease Pathways." *Journal of Alzheimer's Disease* 14 (1): 27–41.

Coppedè, Fabio. 2010. "One-Carbon Metabolism and Alzheimer's Disease: Focus on Epigenetics." *Current Genomics* 11 (4). Bentham Science Publishers: 246–260. doi:10.2174/138920210791233090.

Coppedè, Fabio, Pierpaola Tannorella, Andrea Stoccoro, Lucia Chico, Gabriele Siciliano, Ubaldo Bonuccelli, and Lucia Migliore. 2017. "Methylation Analysis of DNA Repair Genes in Alzheimer's Disease." *Mechanisms of Ageing and Development* 161 (January). Elsevier: 105–111. doi:10.1016/J.MAD.2016.04.003.

Coppieters, Natacha, Birger V. Dieriks, Claire Lill, Richard L. M. Faull, Maurice A. Curtis, and Mike Dragunow. 2014. "Global Changes in DNA Methylation and Hydroxymethylation in Alzheimer's Disease Human Brain." *Neurobiology of Aging* 35 (6): 1334–1344. doi:10.1016/j.neurobiolaging.2013.11.031.

Croce, Nicoletta, Francesca Gelfo, Maria Teresa Ciotti, Giorgio Federici, Carlo Caltagirone, Sergio Bernardini, and Francesco Angelucci. 2013. "NPY Modulates MiR-30a-5p and BDNF in Opposite Direction in an in Vitro Model of Alzheimer Disease: A Possible Role in Neuroprotection?" *Molecular and Cellular Biochemistry* 376 (1–2): 189–195. doi:10.1007/s11010-013-1567-0.

Delay, Charlotte, Frédéric Calon, Paul Mathews, and Sébastien S. Hébert. 2011. "Alzheimer-Specific Variants in the 3′UTR of Amyloid Precursor Protein Affect MicroRNA Function." *Molecular Neurodegeneration* 6 (1): 70. doi:10.1186/1750-1326-6-70.

Delay, Charlotte, Véronique Dorval, Alice Fok, Benjamin Grenier-Boley, Jean-Charles Lambert, G.-Y. Hsiung, and Sébastien S. Hébert. 2014. "MicroRNAs Targeting Nicastrin Regulate Aβ Production and Are Affected by Target Site Polymorphisms." *Frontiers in Molecular Neuroscience* 7. Frontiers Media SA: 67. doi:10.3389/fnmol.2014.00067.

Dickson, John R., Carla Kruse, Daniel R. Montagna, Bente Finsen, and Michael S. Wolfe. 2013. "Alternative Polyadenylation and MiR-34 Family Members Regulate Tau Expression." *Journal of Neurochemistry* 127 (6): 739–749. doi:10.1111/jnc.12437.

Dokmanovic, M., C. Clarke, and P. A. Marks. 2007. "Histone Deacetylase Inhibitors: Overview and Perspectives." *Molecular Cancer Research* 5 (10): 981–989. doi:10.1158/1541-7786.MCR-07-0324.

Fang, Marong, Jing Wang, Xiaobing Zhang, Yu Geng, Zhiying Hu, John A. Rudd, Shucai Ling, Wei Chen, and Shu Han. 2012. "The MiR-124 Regulates the Expression of BACE1/β-Secretase Correlated with Cell Death in Alzheimer's Disease." *Toxicology Letters* 209 (1): 94–105. doi:10.1016/j.toxlet.2011.11.032.

Frost, Bess, Martin Hemberg, Jada Lewis, and Mel B. Feany. 2014. "Tau Promotes Neurodegeneration through Global Chromatin Relaxation." *Nature Neuroscience* 17 (3): 357–366. doi:10.1038/nn.3639.

Fuso, Andrea, Vincenzina Nicolia, Alessia Pasqualato, Maria Teresa Fiorenza, Rosaria A. Cavallaro, and Sigfrido Scarpa. 2011. "Changes in Presenilin 1 Gene Methylation Pattern in Diet-Induced B Vitamin Deficiency." *Neurobiology of Aging* 32 (2): 187–199. doi:10.1016/j.neurobiolaging.2009.02.013.

Fuso, Andrea, Laura Seminara, Rosaria A. Cavallaro, Fabrizio D'Anselmi, and Sigfrido Scarpa. 2005. "S-Adenosylmethionine/Homocysteine Cycle Alterations Modify DNA Methylation Status with Consequent Deregulation of PS1 and BACE and Beta-Amyloid Production." *Molecular and Cellular Neuroscience* 28 (1): 195–204. doi:10.1016/j.mcn.2004.09.007.

GBD 2016 Dementia Collaborators. 2019 Jan. "Global, Regional, and National Burden of Alzheimer's Disease and Other Dementias, 1990–2016: A Systematic Analysis for the Global Burden of Disease Study 2016." *Lancet Neurology* 18 (1): 88–106. doi: 10.1016/S1474-4422(18)30403-4

Ghanbari, Mohsen, M. Arfan Ikram, Hans W. J. de Looper, Albert Hofman, Stefan J. Erkeland, Oscar H. Franco, and Abbas Dehghan. 2016. "Genome-Wide Identification of MicroRNA-Related Variants Associated with Risk of Alzheimer's Disease." *Scientific Reports* 6 (1): 28387. doi:10.1038/srep28387.

Gjoneska, Elizabeta, Andreas R. Pfenning, Hansruedi Mathys, Gerald Quon, Anshul Kundaje, Li-Huei Tsai, and Manolis Kellis. 2015. "Conserved Epigenomic Signals in Mice and Humans Reveal Immune Basis of Alzheimer's Disease." *Nature* 518 (7539). Nature Publishing Group: 365–369. doi:10.1038/nature14252.

Gräff, Johannes, Damien Rei, Ji-Song Guan, Wen-Yuan Wang, Jinsoo Seo, Krista M. Hennig, Thomas J. F. Nieland, et al. 2012. "An Epigenetic Blockade of Cognitive Functions in the Neurodegenerating Brain." *Nature* 483 (7388). Nature Publishing Group: 222–226. doi:10.1038/nature10849.

Guan, Ji-Song, Stephen J. Haggarty, Emanuela Giacometti, Jan-Hermen Dannenberg, Nadine Joseph, Jun Gao, Thomas J. F. Nieland, et al. 2009. "HDAC2 Negatively Regulates Memory Formation and Synaptic Plasticity." *Nature* 459 (7243). Nature Publishing Group: 55–60. doi:10.1038/nature07925.

Hanes, Steven D. 2015. "Prolyl Isomerases in Gene Transcription." *Biochimica et Biophysica Acta* 1850 (10). Elsevier: 2017–2034. doi:10.1016/J.BBAGEN.2014.10.028.

Harold, Denise, Richard Abraham, Paul Hollingworth, Rebecca Sims, Amy Gerrish, Marian L. Hamshere, Jaspreet Singh Pahwa, et al. 2009. "Genome-Wide Association Study Identifies Variants at CLU and PICALM Associated with Alzheimer's Disease." *Nature Genetics* 41 (10): 1088–1093. doi:10.1038/ng.440.

Hebert, S. S., K. Horre, L. Nicolai, A. S. Papadopoulou, W. Mandemakers, A. N. Silahtaroglu, S. Kauppinen, A. Delacourte, and B. De Strooper. 2008. "Loss of MicroRNA Cluster MiR-29a/b-1 in Sporadic Alzheimer's Disease Correlates with Increased BACE1/-Secretase Expression." *Proceedings of the National Academy of Sciences* 105 (17): 6415–6420. doi:10.1073/pnas.0710263105.

Hébert, Sébastien S., Aikaterini S. Papadopoulou, Pascal Smith, Marie-Christine Galas, Emmanuel Planel, Asli N. Silahtaroglu, Nicolas Sergeant, Luc Buée, and Bart De Strooper. 2010. "Genetic Ablation of Dicer in Adult Forebrain Neurons Results in Abnormal Tau Hyperphosphorylation and Neurodegeneration." *Human Molecular Genetics* 19 (20): 3959–3969. doi:10.1093/hmg/ddq311.

Higaki, Sayuri, Masashi Muramatsu, Akio Matsuda, Kenji Matsumoto, Jun-ichi Satoh, Makoto Michikawa, and Shumpei Niida. 2018. "Defensive Effect of MicroRNA-200b/c against Amyloid-Beta Peptide-Induced Toxicity in Alzheimer's Disease Models." Edited by Giuseppe Pignataro. *PLOS One* 13 (5): e0196929. doi:10.1371/journal.pone.0196929.

Huse, Jason T., Kangning Liu, Donald S. Pijak, Dan Carlin, Virginia M.-Y. Lee, and Robert W. Doms. 2002. "β-Secretase Processing in the trans-Golgi Network Preferentially Generates Truncated Amyloid Species That Accumulate in Alzheimer's Disease Brain." *Journal of Biological Chemistry* 277 (18): 16278–16284. doi:10.1074/jbc.M111141200.

Ito, Hidenori, Nobuteru Usuda, Kimie Atsuzawa, Ikuko Iwamoto, Kaori Sudo, Ritsuko Katoh-Semba, Kosuke Mizutani, et al. 2007. "Phosphorylation by Extracellular Signal-Regulated Kinase of a Multidomain Adaptor Protein, Vinexin, at Synapses." *Journal of Neurochemistry* 100 (2). Wiley/Blackwell (10.1111): 545–554. doi:10.1111/j.1471-4159.2006.04222.x.

Iwata, Nobuhisa, Satoshi Tsubuki, Yoshie Takaki, Kaori Watanabe, Misaki Sekiguchi, Emi Hosoki, Maho Kawashima-Morishima, et al. 2000. "Identification of the Major Aβ1–42-Degrading Catabolic Pathway in Brain Parenchyma: Suppression Leads to Biochemical and Pathological Deposition." *Nature Medicine* 6 (2): 143–150. doi:10.1038/72237.

Jaenisch, Rudolf, and Adrian Bird. 2003. "Epigenetic Regulation of Gene Expression: How the Genome Integrates Intrinsic and Environmental Signals." *Nature Genetics* 33 (S3): 245–254. doi:10.1038/ng1089.

Jager, Philip L. De, Gyan Srivastava, Katie Lunnon, Jeremy Burgess, Leonard C. Schalkwyk, Lei Yu, Matthew L. Eaton, et al. 2014. "Alzheimer's Disease: Early Alterations in Brain DNA Methylation at ANK1, BIN1, RHBDF2 and Other Loci." *Nature Neuroscience* 17 (9): 1156–1163. doi:10.1038/nn.3786.

Jeon, Yesu, Kavitha Sarma, and Jeannie T. Lee. 2012. "New and Xisting Regulatory Mechanisms of X Chromosome Inactivation." *Current Opinion in Genetics & Development* 22 (2). NIH Public Access: 62–71. doi:10.1016/j.gde.2012.02.007.

Jian, Chongdong, Mengru Lu, Zhao Zhang, Long Liu, Xianfeng Li, Fang Huang, Ning Xu, Lina Qin, Qian Zhang, and Donghua Zou. 2017. "MiR-34a Knockout Attenuates Cognitive Deficits in APP/PS1 Mice through Inhibition of the Amyloidogenic Processing of APP." *Life Sciences* 182 (August): 104–111. doi:10.1016/j.lfs.2017.05.023.

Kim, J., H. Yoon, T. Horie, J. M. Burchett, J. L. Restivo, N. Rotllan, C. M. Ramirez, et al. 2015. "MicroRNA-33 Regulates ApoE Lipidation and Amyloid – Metabolism in the Brain." *Journal of Neuroscience* 35 (44): 14717–14726. doi:10.1523/JNEUROSCI.2053-15.2015.

Kim, Jaekwang, Hyejin Yoon, Dah-eun Chung, Jennifer L. Brown, Krystal C. Belmonte, and Jungsu Kim. 2016. "MiR-186 Is Decreased in Aged Brain and Suppresses BACE1 Expression." *Journal of Neurochemistry* 137 (3): 436–445. doi:10.1111/jnc.13507.

Kim, Woori, Haneul Noh, Yenarae Lee, Jeha Jeon, Arthi Shanmugavadivu, Donna L. McPhie, Kwang-Soo Kim, Bruce M. Cohen, Hyemyung Seo, and Kai C. Sonntag. 2016. "MiR-126 Regulates Growth Factor Activities and Vulnerability to Toxic Insult in Neurons." *Molecular Neurobiology* 53 (1). Springer US: 95–108. doi:10.1007/s12035-014-8989-x.

Krishnan V, Chow MZ, Wang Z, Zhang L, Liu B, Liu X, and Zhou Z. (2011). Histone H4 Lysine 16 Hypoacetylation is Associated with Defective DNA Repair and Premature Senescence in Zmpste24-Deficient Mice. *Proceedings of the National Academy of Sciences of the United States of America 108*(30): 12325–12330. https://doi.org/10.1073/pnas.1102789108

Kurochkin, I. V., and S. Goto. 1994. "Alzheimer's Beta-Amyloid Peptide Specifically Interacts with and Is Degraded by Insulin Degrading Enzyme." *FEBS Letters* 345 (1): 33–37. http://www.ncbi.nlm.nih.gov/pubmed/8194595.

Lambert, Jean-Charles, Simon Heath, Gael Even, Dominique Campion, Kristel Sleegers, Mikko Hiltunen, Onofre Combarros, et al. 2009. "Genome-Wide Association Study Identifies Variants at CLU and CR1 Associated with Alzheimer's Disease." *Nature Genetics* 41 (10): 1094–1099. doi:10.1038/ng.439.

Lardenoije, Roy, Daniël L. A. van den Hove, Monique Havermans, Anne van Casteren, Kevin X. Le, Roberta Palmour, Cynthia A. Lemere, and Bart P. F. Rutten. 2018. "Age-Related Epigenetic Changes in Hippocampal Subregions of Four Animal Models of Alzheimer's Disease." *Molecular and Cellular Neuroscience* 86 (January). Academic Press: 1–15. doi:10.1016/J.MCN.2017.11.002.

Lehmann, Sabrina M., Christina Krüger, Boyoun Park, Katja Derkow, Karen Rosenberger, Jan Baumgart, Thorsten Trimbuch, et al. 2012. "An Unconventional Role for MiRNA: Let-7 Activates Toll-like Receptor 7 and Causes Neurodegeneration." *Nature Neuroscience* 15 (6): 827–835. doi:10.1038/nn.3113.

Lisch, Damon. 2012. "Regulation of Transposable Elements in Maize." *Current Opinion in Plant Biology* 15 (5). Elsevier Current Trends: 511–516. doi:10.1016/J.PBI.2012.07.001.

Liu, Chen-Geng, Jing Song, Yue-Qi Zhang, and Pei-Chang Wang. 2014. "MicroRNA-193b Is a Regulator of Amyloid Precursor Protein in the Blood and Cerebrospinal Fluid Derived Exosomal MicroRNA-193b Is a Biomarker of Alzheimer's Disease." *Molecular Medicine Reports* 10 (5): 2395–2400. doi:10.3892/mmr.2014.2484.

Liu, Wei, Chang Liu, Jingxi Zhu, Pengcheng Shu, Bin Yin, Yanhua Gong, Boqin Qiang, Jiangang Yuan, and Xiaozhong Peng. 2012. "MicroRNA-16 Targets Amyloid Precursor Protein to Potentially Modulate Alzheimer's-Associated Pathogenesis in SAMP8 Mice." *Neurobiology of Aging* 33 (3). Elsevier: 522–534. doi:10.1016/J.NEUROBIOLAGING.2010.04.034.

Liu, Wei, Jingya Zhao, and Guangxiu Lu. 2016. "MiR-106b Inhibits Tau Phosphorylation at Tyr18 by Targeting Fyn in a Model of Alzheimer's Disease." *Biochemical and Biophysical Research Communications* 478 (2): 852–857. doi:10.1016/j.bbrc.2016.08.037.

Long, Justin M., Balmiki Ray, and Debomoy K. Lahiri. 2012. "MicroRNA-153 Physiologically Inhibits Expression of Amyloid-β Precursor Protein in Cultured Human Fetal Brain Cells and Is Dysregulated in a Subset of Alzheimer Disease Patients." *The Journal of Biological Chemistry* 287 (37). American Society for Biochemistry and Molecular Biology: 31298–31310. doi:10.1074/jbc.M112.366336.

Long, Justin M., Balmiki Ray, and Debomoy K. Lahiri. 2014. "MicroRNA-339-5p Down-Regulates Protein Expression of β-Site Amyloid Precursor Protein-Cleaving Enzyme 1 (BACE1) in Human Primary Brain Cultures and Is Reduced in Brain Tissue Specimens of Alzheimer Disease Subjects." *Journal of Biological Chemistry* 289 (8): 5184–5198. doi:10.1074/jbc.M113.518241.

Lopatina, Nadejda, Joyce F. Haskell, Lucy G. Andrews, Joseph C. Poole, Sabita Saldanha, and Trygve Tollefsbol. 2002. "Differential Maintenance and de Novo Methylating Activity by Three DNA Methyltransferases in Aging and Immortalized Fibroblasts." *Journal of Cellular Biochemistry* 84 (2): 324–334. http://www.ncbi.nlm.nih.gov/pubmed/11787061.

Lu, Xi, Li Wang, Caijia Yu, Daohai Yu, and Gang Yu. 2015. "Histone Acetylation Modifiers in the Pathogenesis of Alzheimer's Disease." *Frontiers in Cellular Neuroscience* 9 (June). Frontiers: 226. doi:10.3389/fncel.2015.00226.

Lunnon, Katie, Rebecca Smith, Eilis Hannon, Philip L. De Jager, Gyan Srivastava, Manuela Volta, Claire Troakes, et al. 2014. "Methylomic Profiling Implicates Cortical Deregulation of ANK1 in Alzheimer's Disease." *Nature Neuroscience* 17 (9): 1164–1170. doi:10.1038/nn.3782.

Mahady, Laura, Muhammad Nadeem, Michael Malek-Ahmadi, Kewei Chen, Sylvia E. Perez, and Elliott J. Mufson. 2018. "Frontal Cortex Epigenetic Dysregulation During the Progression of Alzheimer's Disease." *Journal of Alzheimer's Disease* 62 (1). IOS Press: 115–131. doi:10.3233/JAD-171032.

Mastroeni, Diego, Andrew Grover, Elaine Delvaux, Charisse Whiteside, Paul D. Coleman, and Joseph Rogers. 2011. "Epigenetic Mechanisms in Alzheimer's Disease." *Neurobiology of Aging* 32 (7). Elsevier: 1161–1180. doi:10.1016/J.NEUROBIOLAGING.2010.08.017.

Moncini, Silvia, Marta Lunghi, Alice Valmadre, Margherita Grasso, Valerio Del Vescovo, Paola Riva, Michela Alessandra Denti, and Marco Venturin. 2017. "The MiR-15/107 Family of MicroRNA Genes Regulates CDK5R1/P35 with Implications for Alzheimer's Disease Pathogenesis." *Molecular Neurobiology* 54 (6): 4329–4342. doi:10.1007/s12035-016-0002-4.

Mueller-Steiner, Sarah, Yungui Zhou, Hideaki Arai, Erik D. Roberson, Binggui Sun, Jennifer Chen, Xin Wang, et al. 2006. "Antiamyloidogenic and Neuroprotective Functions of Cathepsin B: Implications for Alzheimer's Disease." *Neuron* 51 (6): 703–714. doi:10.1016/j.neuron.2006.07.027.

Nagata, Tomoyuki, Nobuyuki Kobayashi, Jumpei Ishii, Shunichiro Shinagawa, Ritsuko Nakayama, Nobuto Shibata, Bolati Kuerban, et al. 2015. "Association between DNA Methylation of the BDNF Promoter Region and Clinical Presentation in Alzheimer's Disease." *Dementia and Geriatric Cognitive Disorders Extra* 5 (1): 64–73. doi:10.1159/000375367.

Nativio, Raffaella, Greg Donahue, Amit Berson, Yemin Lan, Alexandre Amlie-Wolf, Ferit Tuzer, Jon B. Toledo, et al. 2018. "Dysregulation of the Epigenetic Landscape of Normal Aging in Alzheimer's Disease." *Nature Neuroscience* 21 (4). Nature Publishing Group: 497–505. doi:10.1038/s41593-018-0101-9.

Ozaki, Yuki, Yuta Yoshino, Kiyohiro Yamazaki, Tomoko Sao, Yoko Mori, Shinichiro Ochi, Taku Yoshida, Takaaki Mori, Jun-ichi Iga, and Shu-ichi Ueno. 2017. "DNA Methylation Changes at TREM2 Intron 1 and TREM2 MRNA Expression in Patients with Alzheimer's Disease." *Journal of Psychiatric Research* 92 (September). Pergamon: 74–80. doi:10.1016/J.JPSYCHIRES.2017.04.003.

Patterson, C. World Alzheimers Report, 2018. The state of the art of dementia research: New frontiers. Alzheimer's Disease International (ADI), London. (September 2018).

Peleg, Shahaf, Farahnaz Sananbenesi, Athanasios Zovoilis, Susanne Burkhardt, Sanaz Bahari-Javan, Roberto Carlos Agis-Balboa, Perla Cota, et al. 2010. "Altered Histone Acetylation Is Associated with Age-Dependent Memory Impairment in Mice." Science (New York, N.Y.) 328 (5979). American Association for the Advancement of Science: 753–756. doi:10.1126/science.1186088.

Pogue, Aileen I., Maire E. Percy, Jian-Guo Cui, Yuan Yuan Li, S. Bhattacharjee, James M. Hill, Theodore P. A. Kruck, Yuhai Zhao, and Walter J. Lukiw. 2011. "Up-Regulation of NF-KB-Sensitive MiRNA-125b and MiRNA-146a in Metal Sulfate-Stressed Human Astroglial (HAG) Primary Cell Cultures." *Journal of Inorganic Biochemistry* 105 (11): 1434–1437. doi:10.1016/j.jinorgbio.2011.05.012.

Rao, J. S., V. L. Keleshian, S. Klein, and S. I. Rapoport. 2012. "Epigenetic Modifications in Frontal Cortex from Alzheimer's Disease and Bipolar Disorder Patients." *Translational Psychiatry* 2: 132. doi:10.1038/tp.2012.55.

Rauhala, Hanna E., Kati P. Porkka, Outi R. Saramäki, Teuvo L. J. Tammela, and Tapio Visakorpi. 2008. "Clusterin Is Epigenetically Regulated in Prostate Cancer." *International Journal of Cancer* 123 (7): 1601–1609. doi:10.1002/ijc.23658.

Sala Frigerio, C., P. Lau, E. Salta, J. Tournoy, K. Bossers, R. Vandenberghe, A. Wallin, et al. 2013. "Reduced Expression of Hsa-MiR-27a-3p in CSF of Patients with Alzheimer Disease." *Neurology* 81 (24): 2103–2106. doi:10.1212/01.wnl.0000437306.37850.22.

Sanchez-Mut, Jose V., and Johannes Gräff. 2015. "Epigenetic Alterations in Alzheimer's Disease." *Frontiers in Behavioral Neuroscience* 9 (December): 347. doi:10.3389/fnbeh.2015.00347.

Sanchez-Mut, Jose Vicente, Ester Aso, Holger Heyn, Tadashi Matsuda, Christoph Bock, Isidre Ferrer, and Manel Esteller. 2014. "Promoter Hypermethylation of the Phosphatase DUSP22 Mediates PKA-Dependent TAU Phosphorylation and CREB Activation in Alzheimer's Disease." *Hippocampus* 24 (4). Wiley-Blackwell: 363–368. doi:10.1002/hipo. 22245.

Santa-Maria, Ismael, Maria E. Alaniz, Neil Renwick, Carolina Cela, Tudor A. Fulga, David Van Vactor, Thomas Tuschl, et al. 2015. "Dysregulation of MicroRNA-219 Promotes Neurodegeneration through Post-Transcriptional Regulation of Tau." *Journal of Clinical Investigation* 125 (2): 681–686. doi:10.1172/JCI78421.

Shu, Liqi, Wenjia Sun, Liping Li, Zihui Xu, Li Lin, Pei Xie, Hui Shen, et al. 2016. "Genome-Wide Alteration of 5-Hydroxymenthylcytosine in a Mouse Model of Alzheimer's Disease." *BMC Genomics* 17 (1): 381. doi:10.1186/s12864-016-2731-1.

Siegmund, Kimberly D., Caroline M. Connor, Mihaela Campan, Tiffany I. Long, Daniel J. Weisenberger, Detlev Biniszkiewicz, Rudolf Jaenisch, Peter W. Laird, and Schahram Akbarian. 2007. "DNA Methylation in the Human Cerebral Cortex Is Dynamically Regulated throughout the Life Span and Involves Differentiated Neurons." Edited by Thomas Reh. *PLoS One* 2 (9): e895. doi:10.1371/journal.pone.0000895.

Smith, Adam R., Rebecca G. Smith, Daniel Condliffe, Eilis Hannon, Leonard Schalkwyk, Jonathan Mill, and Katie Lunnon. 2016. "Increased DNA Methylation near TREM2 Is Consistently Seen in the Superior Temporal Gyrus in Alzheimer's Disease Brain." *Neurobiology of Aging* 47 (November): 35–40. doi:10.1016/j.neurobiolaging.2016.07.008.

Smith, Pascal, Amelle Al Hashimi, Johanne Girard, Charlotte Delay, and Sébastien S. Hébert. 2011. "In Vivo Regulation of Amyloid Precursor Protein Neuronal Splicing by MicroRNAs." *Journal of Neurochemistry* 116 (2): 240–247. doi:10.1111/j.1471-4159.2010.07097.x.

Smith, Pascal Y., Julia Hernandez-Rapp, Francis Jolivette, Cynthia Lecours, Kanchan Bisht, Claudia Goupil, Veronique Dorval, et al. 2015. "MiR-132/212 Deficiency Impairs Tau Metabolism and Promotes Pathological Aggregation in Vivo." *Human Molecular Genetics* 24 (23). Oxford University Press: 6721–6735. doi:10.1093/hmg/ddv377.

Stoccoro, Andrea, Gabriele Siciliano, Lucia Migliore, and Fabio Coppedè. 2017. "Decreased Methylation of the Mitochondrial D-Loop Region in Late-Onset Alzheimer's Disease." *Journal of Alzheimer's Disease* 59 (2). IOS Press: 559–564. doi:10.3233/JAD-170139.

Strahl, Brian D., and C. David Allis. 2000. "The Language of Covalent Histone Modifications." *Nature* 403 (6765). Nature Publishing Group: 41–45. doi:10.1038/47412.

Sun, Li-Hua, Tao Ban, Cheng-Di Liu, Qing-Xin Chen, Xu Wang, Mei-Ling Yan, Xue-Ling Hu, et al. 2015. "Activation of Cdk5/P25 and Tau Phosphorylation Following Chronic Brain Hypoperfusion in Rats Involves MicroRNA-195 down-Regulation." *Journal of Neurochemistry* 134 (6): 1139–1151. doi:10.1111/jnc.13212.

Suuronen, Tiina, Tapio Nuutinen, Tuomas Ryhänen, Kai Kaarniranta, and Antero Salminen. 2007. "Epigenetic Regulation of Clusterin/Apolipoprotein J Expression in Retinal Pigment Epithelial Cells." *Biochemical and Biophysical Research Communications* 357 (2): 397–401. doi:10.1016/j.bbrc.2007.03.135.

Tian, Ning, Zeyuan Cao, and Yan Zhang. 2014. "MiR-206 Decreases Brain-Derived Neurotrophic Factor Levels in a Transgenic Mouse Model of Alzheimer's Disease." *Neuroscience Bulletin* 30 (2): 191–197. doi:10.1007/s12264-013-1419-7.

Tognini, Paola, Debora Napoli, and Tommaso Pizzorusso. 2015. "Dynamic DNA Methylation in the Brain: A New Epigenetic Mark for Experience-Dependent Plasticity." *Frontiers in Cellular Neuroscience* 9 (August): 331. doi:10.3389/fncel.2015.00331.

Tohgi, Hideo, Kimiaki Utsugisawa, Yuriko Nagane, Masahiro Yoshimura, and Yasuko Genda. 1999a. "The Methylation Status of Cytosines in a Tau Gene Promoter Region Alters with Age to Downregulate Transcriptional Activity in Human Cerebral Cortex." *Neuroscience Letters* 275 (2): 89–92. doi:S0304-3940(99)00731-4 [pii].

Tohgi, Hideo, Kimiaki Utsugisawa, Yuriko Nagane, Masahiro Yoshimura, Yasuko Genda, and Miyuki Ukitsu. 1999b. "Reduction with Age in Methylcytosine in the Promoter Region −224∼−101 of the Amyloid Precursor Protein Gene in Autopsy Human Cortex." *Molecular Brain Research* 70 (2). Elsevier: 288–292. doi:10.1016/S0169-328X(99)001631.

Vilardo, Elisa, Christian Barbato, Mariateresa Ciotti, Carlo Cogoni, and Francesca Ruberti. 2010. "MicroRNA-101 Regulates Amyloid Precursor Protein Expression in Hippocampal Neurons." *The Journal of Biological Chemistry* 285 (24). American Society for Biochemistry and Molecular Biology: 18344–18351. doi:10.1074/jbc.M110.112664.

Walker, Michael P., Frank M. LaFerla, Salvador S. Oddo, and Gregory J. Brewer. 2013. "Reversible Epigenetic Histone Modifications and Bdnf Expression in Neurons with Aging and from a Mouse Model of Alzheimer's Disease." *AGE* 35 (3): 519–531. doi:10.1007/s11357-011-9375-5.

Wang, Gang, Yue Huang, Li-Ling Wang, Yong-Fang Zhang, Jing Xu, Yi Zhou, Guinevere F. Lourenco, et al. 2016. "MicroRNA-146a Suppresses ROCK1 Allowing Hyperphosphorylation of Tau in Alzheimer's Disease." *Scientific Reports* 6. Nature Publishing Group: 26697. doi:10.1038/srep26697.

Wang, Sun-Chong, Beatrice Oelze, and Axel Schumacher. 2008. "Age-Specific Epigenetic Drift in Late-Onset Alzheimer's Disease." Edited by Amanda Ewart Toland. *PLoS One* 3 (7). Public Library of Science: e2698. doi:10.1371/journal.pone.0002698.

Wang, W.-X., B. W. Rajeev, A. J. Stromberg, N. Ren, G. Tang, Q. Huang, I. Rigoutsos, and P. T. Nelson. 2008. "The Expression of MicroRNA MiR-107 Decreases Early in Alzheimer's Disease and May Accelerate Disease Progression through Regulation of – Site Amyloid Precursor Protein-Cleaving Enzyme 1." *Journal of Neuroscience* 28 (5): 1213–1223. doi:10.1523/JNEUROSCI.5065-07.2008.

Wang, Xiong, Lu Tan, Yanjun Lu, Jing Peng, Yaowu Zhu, Yadong Zhang, and Ziyong Sun. 2015. "MicroRNA-138 Promotes Tau Phosphorylation by Targeting Retinoic Acid Receptor Alpha." *FEBS Letters* 589 (6): 726–729. doi:10.1016/j.febslet.2015.02.001.

Watson, Corey T., Panos Roussos, Paras Garg, Daniel J. Ho, Nidha Azam, Pavel L. Katsel, Vahram Haroutunian, and Andrew J. Sharp. 2016. "Genome-Wide DNA Methylation Profiling in the Superior Temporal Gyrus Reveals Epigenetic Signatures Associated with Alzheimer's Disease." *Genome Medicine* 8 (1): 5. doi:10.1186/s13073-015-0258-8.

Weisberg, Ilan, Pamela Tran, Benedicte Christensen, Sahar Sibani, and Rima Rozen. 1998. "A Second Genetic Polymorphism in Methylenetetrahydrofolate Reductase (MTHFR) Associated with Decreased Enzyme Activity." *Molecular Genetics and Metabolism* 64 (3): 169–172. doi:10.1006/mgme.1998.2714.

West, Roger L., John M. Lee, and Leonard E. Maroun. 1995. "Hypomethylation of the Amyloid Precursor Protein Gene in the Brain of an Alzheimer's Disease Patient." *Journal of Molecular Neuroscience* 6 (2): 141–146. doi:10.1007/BF02736773.

Wong, Hon-Kit Andus, Tatiana Veremeyko, Nehal Patel, Cynthia A. Lemere, Dominic M. Walsh, Christine Esau, Charles Vanderburg, and Anna M. Krichevsky. 2013. "De-Repression of FOXO3a Death Axis by MicroRNA-132 and -212 Causes Neuronal Apoptosis in Alzheimer's Disease." *Human Molecular Genetics* 22 (15): 3077–3092. doi:10.1093/hmg/ddt164.

Wu, Qi, Xiaoyang Ye, Yi Xiong, Haili Zhu, Jianting Miao, Wei Zhang, and Jun Wan. 2016. "The Protective Role of MicroRNA-200c in Alzheimer's Disease Pathologies Is Induced by Beta Amyloid-Triggered Endoplasmic Reticulum Stress." *Frontiers in Molecular Neuroscience* 9. Frontiers Media SA: 140. doi:10.3389/fnmol.2016.00140.

Xie, Bing, Yao Xu, Zanchao Liu, Wenxuan Liu, Lei Jiang, Rui Zhang, Dongsheng Cui, Qingfu Zhang, and Shunjiang Xu. 2017a. "Elevation of Peripheral BDNF Promoter Methylation Predicts Conversion from Amnestic Mild Cognitive Impairment to Alzheimer's Disease: A 5-Year Longitudinal Study." Edited by Ling-Qiang Zhu. *Journal of Alzheimer's Disease* 56 (1): 391–401. doi:10.3233/JAD-160954.

Xie, Bing, Zanchao Liu, Wenxuan Liu, Lei Jiang, Rui Zhang, Dongsheng Cui, Qingfu Zhang, and Shunjiang Xu. 2017b. "DNA Methylation and Tag SNPs of the BDNF Gene in Conversion of Amnestic Mild Cognitive Impairment into Alzheimer's Disease: A Cross-Sectional Cohort Study." Edited by Ling-Qiang Zhu. *Journal of Alzheimer's Disease* 58 (1): 263–274. doi:10.3233/JAD-170007.

Xu, Yan-Ming, Ji-Ying Du, and Andy T. Y. Lau. 2014. "Posttranslational Modifications of Human Histone H3: An Update." *Proteomics* 14 (17–18): 2047–2060. doi:10.1002/pmic.201300435.

Yang, Guoshuai, Yanmin Song, Xiaoyan Zhou, Yidong Deng, Tao Liu, Guohu Weng, Dan Yu, and Suyue Pan. 2015. "MicroRNA-29c Targets β-Site Amyloid Precursor Protein-Cleaving Enzyme 1 and Has a Neuroprotective Role in Vitro and in Vivo." *Molecular Medicine Reports* 12 (2): 3081–3088. doi:10.3892/mmr.2015.3728.

Yu, Lei, Lori B. Chibnik, Gyan P. Srivastava, Nathalie Pochet, Jingyun Yang, Jishu Xu, James Kozubek, et al. 2015. "Association of Brain DNA Methylation in *SORL1, ABCA7, HLA-DRB5, SLC24A4*, and *BIN1* With Pathological Diagnosis of Alzheimer Disease." *JAMA Neurology* 72 (1): 15. doi:10.1001/jamaneurol.2014.3049.

Zhang, B., C.-F. Chen, A.-H. Wang, and Q.-F. Lin. 2015. "MiR-16 Regulates Cell Death in Alzheimer's Disease by Targeting Amyloid Precursor Protein." *European Review for Medical and Pharmacological Sciences* 19 (21): 4020–4027.

Zhang, Chi, Jie Lu, Bing Liu, Qinghua Cui, and Yun Wang. 2016. "Primate-Specific MiR-603 Is Implicated in the Risk and Pathogenesis of Alzheimer's Disease." *Aging* 8 (2): 272–290. doi:10.18632/aging.100887.

Zhang, J., M. Hu, Z. Teng, Y.-P. Tang, and C. Chen. 2014. "Synaptic and Cognitive Improvements by Inhibition of 2-AG Metabolism Are through Upregulation of MicroRNA-188-3p in a Mouse Model of Alzheimer's Disease." *Journal of Neuroscience* 34 (45): 14919–14933. doi:10.1523/JNEUROSCI.1165-14.2014.

Zhang, Yi, Hongxia Xing, Shuangxi Guo, Zhiyong Zheng, Haoliang Wang, and Dawei Xu. 2016. "MicroRNA-135b Has a Neuroprotective Role via Targeting of β-Site APP-Cleaving Enzyme 1." *Experimental and Therapeutic Medicine* 12 (2): 809–814. doi:10.3892/etm.2016.3366.

Zhao, Jinying, Yun Zhu, Jingyun Yang, Lin Li, Hao Wu, Philip L. De Jager, Peng Jin, and David A. Bennett. 2017. "A Genome-Wide Profiling of Brain DNA Hydroxymethylation in Alzheimer's Disease." *Alzheimer's & Dementia* 13 (6): 674–688. doi:10.1016/j.jalz.2016.10.004.

Zhu, Hong-Can, Li-Mei Wang, Miao Wang, Bo Song, Song Tan, Jun-Fang Teng, and Dong-Xiao Duan. 2012. "MicroRNA-195 Downregulates Alzheimer's Disease Amyloid-β Production by Targeting BACE1." *Brain Research Bulletin* 88 (6): 596–601. doi:10.1016/j.brainresbull.2012.05.018.

Zukin, Suzann. 2009. "Epigenetics." *Alzheimer's & Dementia* 5 (4). Elsevier: P146–P147. doi:10.1016/j.jalz.2009.05.502.

13 Mechanistic Aspects of Neurodegeneration in Alzheimer's Disease and the Role of Phytochemicals as Restorative Agents

Anindita Kundu, Vivekananda Mandal, Sujata Wangkheirakpam, and Subhash C. Mandal

CONTENTS

ABBREVIATIONS

Ach	acetylcholine
AChE	acetylcholinesterase
AD	Alzheimer's Disease
ALA	alinolenic Acid

AMPA	α-amino-3-hydroxy-5-methyl-4-isoxazolepropionic Acid
ATP	Adenosine Triphosphate
AV	Autophagic Vacuole
Aβ	Amyloid Beta
BAX	BCL2-Associated X Protein
Bcl2	B Cell Lymphoma2
BDNF	Brain-Derived Neurotrophic Factor
CAM	Cell Adhesion Molecule
CCL2	Chemokine (c-c motif) Ligand 2
CCP	Clathrin-Coated Pit
CNS	Central Nervous System
c-Raf	Cellular Rapidly Accelerated Fibrosarcoma
CREB	cAMP Response Element Binding Protein
DAT	Dopamine Reuptake Transporter
DNA	Deoxyribonucleic Acid
Drp1	Dynamin-related protein-1
EAAT	Excitatory Amino Acid Transporter
ECM	Extracellular Matrix
ERK	Extracellular Signal–Regulated Kinase
F-actin	Filament Actin
FasL	Fas Ligand
GABA	Gamma Amino Butyric Acid
GFAP	Glial Fibrillary Acidic Protein
GSK-3β	Glycogen Synthase Kinase- 3β
IL-1β	Interleukin-1 β
iNOS	Inducible Nitric Oxide Synthase
JNK	c-Jun N-terminal Protein Kinase
LA	Linoleic Acid
MAPK	Mitogen-Activated Protein Kinase
nAChR	Nicotinic Acetylcholine Receptor
NADPH	Nicotinamide Adenine Dinucleotide Phosphate
NCAM	Neural Cell Adhesion Molecule
NFκB	Nuclear Factor Kappa B
NGF	Nerve Growth Factor
NMDA	N-Methyl-D-Aspartate
NO	Nitric Oxide
OXPHOS	Oxidative Phosphorylation
$PI(4,5)P_2$	Phosphatidylinositol-4,5-bisphosphate
PI3K	Phosphoinositide 3-Kinase
PIs	Phosphoinositide
PKA	Protein Kinase A
PKC	Protein Kinase C
PS	Phosphatidylserine
PUFA	Poly-Unsaturated Fatty Acid
ROS	Reactive Oxygen Species
SERT	Serotonin Reuptake Transporter
TNF	Tumor Necrosis Factor
TRP	Transient Receptor Potential
VAChT	Vesicular Acetylcholine Transporter
VGLUT	Vesicular Glutamate Transporter

13.1 INTRODUCTION

Neurodegenerative diseases are traditionally defined as chronic, progressive disorders with selective loss of neurons, with symptoms related to the topography of the lesions, and with distinct involvement of functional systems defining the clinical presentation. Mutation and some infectious pathogens may cause alteration of the physicochemical properties of protein structure which is characterized by accumulation of abnormal protein structures, eventually leading to protein conformational changes and ultimately neurodegenerative disorders. Furthermore, neurodegenerative disorders are associated with mainly hereditary metabolic diseases and immune-mediated (autoimmune) etiology, where the loss of astroglial function also has a contributory role. Among the many different mechanisms underlying neurodegenerative disorders, the aggregation and deposition of misfolded proteins may be a major cause of neurodegenerative disease. This mechanism is characterized by the insidious accumulation of insoluble filamentary aggregates of normally soluble proteins in the central nervous system (CNS). The major pathological lesions are accumulations of insoluble filamentary aggregates, which are composed of a normal, soluble protein or peptide that has been misfolded ultimately to form amyloids. In different types of neurodegenerative diseases, the different constituents of the amyloidogenic protein are typically expressed systemically but accumulate in the CNS only during the early lifetime of the individual and manifest clinically in the middle or late stages of the lifespan.

Most Alzheimer's disease (AD) cases are sporadic, but genetic (e.g. familial) forms can be caused by a mutant gene encoding the amyloidogenic protein, that makes it more prone to misfolding and aggregation. Synaptic loss, nerve cell loss (primarily in the cerebral cortex, hippocampus, and amygdala), the deposition of extracellular amorphous amyloid-A protein, and the intracellular precipitation of hyperphosphorylated tau proteins are the major histopathological hallmarks of AD.

Several milestones in drug therapy against AD have been explored from different sources of ethnomedicinal information; they may also be useful as a starting point for the discovery of new drugs for the treatment of AD and cognitive impairments. Many of the hundreds of thousands of plant species growing throughout the world, which have a direct pharmacological action on the body, do not have any detrimental side effects. For that reason, plants may be a good promising alternative source as compared with conventional synthetic drugs. The aim of this review is to summarize the mechanisms of neurodegeneration and the role of phytochemicals as possible restorative agents.

13.2 MECHANISTIC PATHWAYS OF NEURODEGENERATION

13.2.1 Intracellular Mechanisms

13.2.1.1 Apoptosis

Apoptosis is a form of programed cell death, triggered by the activation of intrinsic cellular signaling cascades in response to various environmental signals. A wide variety of stimuli and conditions, both physiological and pathological, can initiate apoptosis as a defense mechanism. A consequence of those responses is DNA damage to some cells, eventually leading to apoptotic death through a p53-dependent pathway *via* Fas ligand (FasL) -binding and protein cross linking through FasL or tumor necrosis factor (TNF) receptors, where some other cells have a default death pathway, which must be blocked by a survival factor-like hormone or growth factor (Norbury and Hickson, 2001). The particular type of stimulus or the degree of stimulation determines the cell death mechanism, which is either by apoptosis or necrosis, two mechanisms which can occur independently, sequentially, or simultaneously (Hirsch et al., 1997; Zeiss, 2003). Finally, apoptosis is coordinated, whereby an energy-dependent physiological process is involved to energize a group of cysteine proteases called "caspases", and to induce a complex signaling cascade of events linked to the trigger stimulus, leading to the death of the cell. A number of mechanisms of apoptoses of nucleated cells has been presented in the platelet, such as activation and mitochondrial translocation of Bax, activation of caspase-3, -8 and -9, collapse of the mitochondrial inner membrane potential, B-cell lymphoma-2 (Bcl2) family protein expression, and phosphatidylserine (PS) exposure (Cattabeni et al., 2004; Haroutunian et al., 2009; Leytin and Freedman, 2003). It is now generally accepted that massive neuronal death, due to apoptosis, is a common characteristic of the brains of patients suffering from neurodegenerative diseases, and apoptotic cell death has been found in neurons and glial cells in AD. Four different genes, encoding the amyloid precursor protein, apolipoprotein E, or presenilins 1 and 2, have been implicated in the etiology of familial AD. The existence of senile plaques, neurofibrillary tangles, massive loss of neuronal cells, and synaptic loss in the cerebral cortex and the hippocampus lead to deterioration of cognition and memory, the major symptom of the most common human neurodegenerative disorder, AD.

13.2.1.2 Autophagy

Autophagy is a lysosome-degradative process, dealing with maintaining homeostasis or normal cell function by protein degradation and turnover of damaged cell organelles, to achieve new cell synthesis. During different cellular stresses, the autophagy process is initiated and proteins are eliminated by selective targeting to the lysosomes (DeDuve and Wattiaux, 1966). Autophagy is essential for neuron survival and is considered to be a neuroprotective process, induced to alleviate cellular stresses, such as nutrient deprivation states and protein aggregate accumulation. In addition, the expression of many components of the lysosomal system is regulated, and upregulation is sustained, even at late stages of neurodegeneration, when the expression of most other transcripts has declined (Nixon and Yang, 2012; Callahan et al., 1999; Ginsberg et al., 2000). Accumulation of autophagic vacuoles (AVs) in progressively affected neurons and the predominant organelles within grossly swollen dystrophic neurites are the major characteristics of AD neuropathology. The selectively impaired axonal transport of autophagy/lysosome-related compartments is responsible for inhibition of lysosomal proteolysis, which leads to the accumulation of amyloid-beta (Aβ)-containing AVs within affected neurons (Lee et al., 2011). The extensive neuronal dystrophy in AD and characteristically grossly distended neurites, filled almost fully with AVs, are not typical in neurodegenerative diseases that do not generate β-amyloid. The formation of a specialized large burden of autophagy-related compartments in the AD brain is the robust pathological effect of autophagic disruption in AD (Benzing et al., 1993).

13.2.1.3 Mitochondrial Dysfunction

Mitochondria, aptly termed the powerhouses of the cell, are responsible for production of most of the cell's energy currency, in the form of adenosine triphosphate (ATP), which is the end product of a series of successive pathways, having a role in oxidation of substrates, mainly carbohydrates and fat, in the cytosol (glycolysis) and mitochondria [pyruvate decarboxylation, tricarboxylic acid cycle (Krebs cycle), and oxidative phosphorylation (OXPHOS/respiratory chain complex)]. Mitochondria are also the site for many cellular functions, like housekeeping functions of the cell, and including the biosynthesis of amino acids and steroids, β-oxidation of fatty acids, and maintenance of the homeostatic balance of cytosolic calcium, buffering of calcium fluctuations, and production and regulation of reactive oxygen species (ROS), as well as playing a pivotal role in apoptosis (Davis and Williams, 2012). Considering the intense energy demands and limited regenerative capacity of neurons, the improper functioning of mitochondria can be the cause of damage to neurons, leading to neurodegeneration. Some reports have proposed that mitochondrial dysfunction may be responsible for Aβ deposition, synaptic degeneration, formation of extracellular neuronic plaques, and formation of neurofibrillary tangles, which are the fundamental characteristic features of sporadic AD (Swerdlow et al., 2010). Aβ peptides are the major component of the plaque, and tangles are composed of hyperphosphorylated tau proteins. Impaired activities of key enzymes, such as tricarboxylic acid cycle complexes, pyruvate dehydrogenase, isocitrate dehydrogenase, α-ketoglutarate dehydrogenase, and OXPHOS complexes I, III, IV, and abnormal expression of Drp1 negatively affects mitochondrial biogenesis, with diminished glucose/energy metabolism at an advanced age being the greatest risk factor for AD (Bubber et al., 2005) (Figure 13.1).

13.2.1.4 Oxidative Damage/Repair

Several normal cellular functions (mitochondrial respiratory chain, phagocytosis, arachidonic acid metabolism, ovulation, fertilization, and some pathological conditions) may cause generation of highly reactive molecules capable of independent existence, collectively known as reactive oxygen species (ROS), including superoxide (O_2 $^{\bullet-}$), hydrogen peroxide (H_2O_2), hydroxyl ($OH^{\bullet}$), peroxyl ($ROO^{\bullet}$), alkoxy (RO $^{\bullet}$) ions, and nitric oxide (NO), until they are completely reduced to H_2O molecules. Some specific enzymes, such as xanthine oxidase, tryptophan dioxygenase together accelerate the release of ROS when various pathological noxious stimuli attack the cerebral tissues, and are believed to be involved in the toxicity of xenobiotics, as well as in cognitive impairment. ROS-mediated injury, resulting in increased levels of malondialdehyde and 4-hydroxynonenal in the brain and cerebrospinal fluid, may be the cause of progressive neuronal loss, associated with aggregation of proteins as extracellular Aβ plaques and intracellular tau tangles, leading to AD brain (Lovell et al., 1995; Ghosh et al., 2009, 2011). It is well documented that elevated levels of protein and lipid peroxidation in the cortex and hippocampus, and protein carbonyl moieties in the hippocampus and in both the frontal and parietal cortices, and increased levels of hydroxylated guanine occur prior to the appearance of plaques or tangles ultimately leading to AD

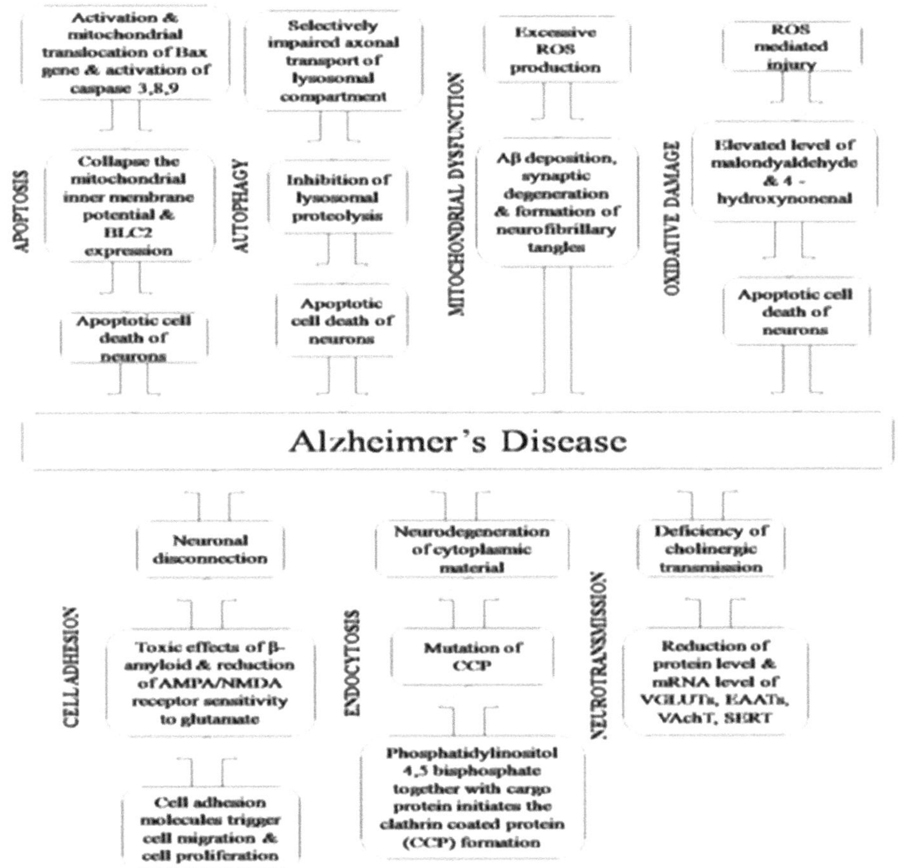

FIGURE 13.1 Diagrammatic representation of the mechanisms and steps involved in Alzheimer's disease. The mechanistic pathways of neurodegeneration depicted here are a) apoptosis, b) autophagy, c) mitochondrial dysfunction, d) oxidative damage, e) cell adhesion, f) endocytosis, and g) neurotransmission.

(Hensley et al., 1996, 1995; Mecocci et al., 1997, 1998; Pratico, 2008). Among the various neurodegeneration mechanisms (protein misfolding and aggregation, abnormal kinase-signaling pathways, neuronal calcium dysregulation, and impaired synaptic transmission), some interact with the different inducers of oxidative stress, mounting robust evidence for the oxidative damage of brain tissues (Kundu et al., 2016).

13.2.2 Local Tissue Environment

13.2.2.1 Cell Adhesion

Homophilic and heterophilic adhesion of cells in the brain can be initiated in an integrated, conventional manner to perform a significant and precise structural role through the specialized junctions, consisting of clustered cell adhesion molecules. To hold cells into a tissue by connecting the internal cytoskeleton directly to the cell exterior, either another cell or the extracellular matrix, *via* one or more cell adhesion molecules (CAMs), such as cadherins, selectins and integrins, play a contributory role in synaptic plasticity. Interaction of the CAMs with membrane receptors, matrix proteins, and signaling molecules influences the synaptic strength. As a result, the CAMs; such as integrins, neural CAMs get activated and associated with extracellular matrix (ECM) proteins, which triggers various cellular effects, including cell migration and proliferation *via* the F-actin signal transduction pathway, and can also participate in the toxic effects of Aβ in AD (Hoffman and Edelman, 1983; Dityatev et al., 2000; Cotman et al., 1998; Zhang et al., 1996). Among the various molecules involved, some participate in the formation of neuronal networks by producing neural cell adhesion molecule (NCAM) and its polysialylated derivative, which have been proposed to participate in the neuroprotective response (promoting dendritic/spine re-growth) in neurodegeneration, by reducing the sensitivity of AMPA (α-amino-3-hydroxy-5-methyl-4-isoxazolepropio nic acid)/NMDA (N-methyl-D-aspartate) receptors to glutamate, and facilitating disconnection of cell–cell interactions (Wielgat and Braszko, 2012).

13.2.2.2 Endocytosis

The internalization and subsequent endosomal trafficking of proteins and membranes along the endocytic pathway is a fundamental cellular process. This was shown to be subject to extensive regulation by phosphoinositides (PIs), phosphorylated derivatives of the minor membrane phospholipid, phosphatidylinositol. The most abundant PI, phosphatidylinositol-4,5-bisphosphate [PI(4,5) P_2], serves as an indicator of plasma membrane identity and, combined with cargo proteins, is instrumental in the initiation of clathrin-coated pit (CCP) formation.

Mutations in the clathrin-mediated endocytosis regulator PI-converting enzymes are linked to a wide spectrum of disorders, including mental retardation, neurodegeneration which may occur by throwing out the cytoplasmic material to the extracellular space and in turn lead to cell demise, and may cause acute inflammatory responses, associated with necrosis, unlike apoptosis (York et al., 2015). Depletion of the main endocytic machinery components, namely dynamin, synaptotagmin, and endophilin, suppresses necrotic neurodegeneration induced by diverse genetic and environmental insults (Troulinaki and Tavernarakis, 2012). Interfering with kinesin-mediated endosome trafficking prevents cell death. Synergistically, endocytosis and autophagy and, individually, the lysosomal-proteolytic mechanisms facilitate this necrotic neurodegeneration.

13.2.2.3 Neurotransmission

Neurotransmitters, also known as endogenous chemical messengers, enable neurotransmission of signals across the chemical synapses. To maintain the homeostatic balance of neural circuits, diverse sets of inhibitory interneurons regulate the activity of excitatory neurons in the CNS. Impaired co-activation of excitatory and inhibitory neurons, such as substantial loss of gamma amino butyric acid (GABA)-ergic interneurons, dysfunction of interneurons due to loss of their afferent excitatory input, changes in their receptors, and an imbalance of the different neurotransmitters, like glutamate, acetylcholine, dopamine, and serotonin, have been proposed in many neurobiological disorders like AD. AD is a neurodegenerative disorder which is characterized by memory loss, and behavioral and psychological symptoms of dementia (Southwell et al., 2014). It is hypothesized that altered reuptake of neurotransmitters by vesicular glutamate transporters (VGLUTs), excitatory amino acid transporters (EAATs), the vesicular acetylcholine transporter (VAChT), the serotonin reuptake transporter (SERT), or the dopamine reuptake transporter (DAT), are involved in the neurotransmission imbalance in AD. Compared with control subjects, the protein and mRNA levels of VGLUTs, EAAT1–3, VAChT, and SERT are reduced significantly in AD subjects; playing a contributory role to the recognized cholinergic deficiency, alteration in glutamatergic recycling and reduced SERT levels could exacerbate depressive symptoms in AD (Isaacson and Scanziani, 2011).

13.3 ROLE OF PHYTOCHEMICALS IN NEUROPROTECTION

13.3.1 Phenols

Phenolic compounds in foods and various dietary plants, such as vitamin C, gallic acid, quercetin, and many more, have attracted great research interest in terms of various beneficial effects evident in human health, like antiaging, antioxidant, anti-inflammatory, and anticarcinogenic properties, and neuroprotective effects (Rolls, 1990; Ercisli and Orhan, 2007; Rashid et al., 2018a, b). Cyanidin-3-*O*-β-glucopyranoside, a member of the anthocyanin family, and catechins and epicatechins, the two active constituents present in green tea, can achieve their neuroprotective activities by hampering glycogen synthase kinase-3β (GSK-3β) in the phosphoinositide 3-kinase (PI3K) pathway, and through the activation of protein kinase C (PKC), respectively. The transcription factor-induced expression of cell survival genes are capable of protecting neurons against a range of neurotoxicities, mediated *via* oxidative and metabolic insults, and some protein misfolding (Peng et al., 2011; Chen et al., 2009; Ehrnhoefer et al., 2006). Furthermore, various phenolic compounds and their metabolites can activate multiple signaling pathways. These are mediated through NGF (nerve growth factor) secretion *via* PI3K-mediated ERK1/2 (extracellular signal–regulated kinase) and CREB (cAMP response element-binding protein) activation, which can exert cell survival and anti-inflammatory actions, including altering the expression of pro-apoptotic and anti-apoptotic proteins, and upregulating antioxidant defense mechanisms, which have been suggested to suppress the pathogenesis of AD (Mandel et al., 2005).

13.3.2 Flavonoids

Activation of glial cells (microglia and astrocytes) increases production of cytokines (interleukin1β [IL1β], tumor necrosis factor alpha [TNFα]), inducible nitric oxide synthase (iNOS), and nitric oxide (NO). Increased levels of reduced nicotinamide adenine dinucleotide phosphate (NADPH) oxidase activation, controlled by mitogen-activated protein kinase (MAPK) signaling, mediates both the transcriptional and post-transcriptional regulation of iNOS and cytokines, and ultimately contributes to the apoptotic cell death of neurons observed in many neurodegenerative diseases (Sutherland et al., 2005; Bhat et al., 1998; Maiti et al., 2017). Flavonoids are capable of preventing the progressive neuronal loss resulting from neuroinflammation *via* direct modulation of protein and lipid kinase signaling pathways, for instance *via* the inhibition of MAPK signaling cascades, such as p38 or ERK1/2, which regulate both iNOS and TNFα expression in activated glial cells. The action of flavonoids on these kinases may influence the downstream proinflammatory nuclear factor Kappa B (NFκB), in response to p38 signaling, and is involved in induction of the iNOS transcription factor, suggesting an interplay between signaling pathways, transcription factors, and cytokine production in the determination of the neuroinflammatory response of the CNS (Marcus et al., 2003). The effective potential of isoflavones to exert positive effects on cognitive function occurs by altering the biosynthesis of acetylcholine and neurotrophic factors, such as the brain-derived neurotrophic factor (BDNF) and nerve growth factor (NGF) in the hippocampus and frontal cortex (Bhat et al., 2002; Pan et al., 1999b). Flavonoid-rich foods interact with the cellular and molecular architecture responsible for memory and learning, including those involved in long-term potentiation and synaptic plasticity, likely to lead to the enhanced neuronal connection and communication, and thus provide a greater capacity for memory acquisition, storage, and retrieval which ultimately improves neurocognitive function and, in turn, significantly lowers the risk for the onset of AD (Pan et al., 1999a; Spencer, 2008a, b; Amenta and Tayebati, 2008).

13.3.3 Alkaloids

Galantamine exerts its effect by inhibiting acetylcholinesterase (AChE) and modulates nicotinic neurotransmission *via* allosteric potentiation of pre- and postsynaptic nicotinic acetylcholine receptors (nAChR). This results in increased release of acetylcholine (ACh) and other neurotransmitters, such as glutamate and dopamine, which play important roles in normal brain function and are thought to responsible for the neuroprotective effect in the hippocampus (Jia et al., 2012).

Recent research indicates that berberine limits the production of proinflammatory cytokines, such as interleukin-6 and C-C motif chemokine 2 (CCL2), *via* inhibition of the NFκB, phosphoinositide 3-kinase, and MAPK-signaling pathways in Aβ-stimulated primary microglia and in a murine microglial cell line (BV-2), and also reduces the expression of cyclooxygenase-2 and iNOS (Zeitlin et al., 2011). A plethora of reports collectively indicate that berberine and galantamine are both promising antioxidants against oxidative stress involved in AD, exhibiting their activity by quenching the ROS, leading to an effective increment of neuronal survival rate and cognitive improvement.

Furthermore, caffeine decreases the levels of β-secretase, caspase-3 expression and soluble Aβ in the hippocampus, limiting the extent of Aβ deposition in the hippocampus and entorhinal cortex, and can stimulate the survival pathway by increasing protein kinase A (PKA) activity and phospho-CREB levels. On the other hand, caffeine inhibits phospho-JNK (c-Jun N-terminal protein kinase) and phospho-ERK expression in the striatum, promoting neuronal survival in AD pathogenesis (Arendash et al., 2009). The caffeine-induced reduction of β-secretase activity in the brain, mediated by the downregulation of the cRaf-1/NF-kB pathway, may have contributory beneficial effects on AD (McCann and Ames, 2005).

13.3.4 Miscellaneous Phytochemicals

Diets deficient in n23 fatty acids, like the monounsaturated fatty acids, such as oleic acid, and polyunsaturated fatty acids (PUFAs), such as linoleic acid (LA) and alinolenic acid (ALA), can impair cognitive functioning in animals and in humans (Yehuda et al., 2002). The effect depends upon the structure and functionality of neurons, as the cells must maintain appropriate electrical gradients across the membrane, with normal anchor receptors and the ion channels at the proper position to communicate with other cells, and to be able to release and reabsorb unmetabolized neurotransmitters. Whereas the essential fatty acids and PUFAs improve membrane fluidity, aging and the phospholipids in neuronal membranes can also directly participate in signaling cascades to modulate neuronal function, synaptic plasticity, and neuroprotective action (Marambaud et al., 2005). The food-derived phytochemicals sulforaphane, diferuloylmethane (curcumin), and resveratrol have been reported to protect neurons against oxidative stress and mitochondrial toxins, resulting in reduced levels of brain damage, brain edema, as well as protected retinal pigment epithelium and enhanced neurogenesis in the hippocampus *via* an increased expression of brain-derived neurotrophic factor (BDNF). They can also protect neuronal cells from being killed by the amyloid β-peptide; which ultimately play a pivotal role in prevention and treatment of AD (Winkler et al., 1995).

13.4 PHYTOCHEMICALS IN RECEPTOR-BINDING ACTIVITY

Of the 50 or so different neurotransmitters identified to be present in the brain, acetylcholine (ACh) is one of the most significant, determined to be essential for learning and memory (Johnston, 2005). Deficiency of ACh has been held to be responsible for senile dementia and other degenerative cognitive disorders, leading to AD. Numerous phytochemicals can modulate neuronal excitability by activating or inhibiting specific receptors or ion channels; for example, GABA activation through the specific Ca^{2+} channels called vanilloid receptors. A wide range of phytochemicals are able to cross the blood–brain barrier and influence brain function by lowering the activity of glutamate receptors, enhancing synaptic plasticity, and protecting neurons against dysfunction and degeneration, in part, by inducing the expression of the neurotrophic factor. In addition, because of their actions on the nervous system by activating transient receptor potential (TRP) calcium channels in the nerve cell, some phytochemicals, like capsaicin, allicin, and tetrahydrocannabinol, may be targeted to minimize the risk of AD (Malarkey and Parpura, 2008).

13.5 ROLE OF ASTROCYTES IN NEURODEGENERATIVE DISORDER

Within the territorial domains, astroglial membranes cover the majority of synaptic contacts and neurons; these astroglial membranes carry numerous pumps and transporters, and are responsible for releasing neurotransmitters (e.g. ATP, glutamate, or GABA), neuromodulators (such as D-serine or kynurenic acid), trophic factors (such as growth factors or tumor necrosis factor-α, TNF-α) and ions, metabolites, and ROS, all of which affect various aspects of synaptic plasticity and information processing in the CNS. Astroglial secretion employs several mechanisms, including exocytotic vesicular release, diffusion through plasmalemmal channels, or solute carrier transporters, whereas the "glymphatic" system promotes the removal of metabolites from the CNS parenchyma (Parpura et al., 2011; Heneka et al., 2005). The reactive astrocytes are recognized in brain parenchyma of transgenic mice over-expressing the amyloid precursor protein long before any detectable Aβ deposits; these reactive astrocytes produce proinflammatory factors and upregulated expression of iNOS, and arguably prepare the ground for future senile plaque which is present in the brains of AD animal models. In subjects of a more advanced age, reactive glial fibrillary acidic protein (GFAP)-positive astrocytes, associated with senile plaques, perivascular Aβ deposits, and abnormally frequent Ca^{2+} oscillations, have also been observed in the context of AD-type pathology (Verkhratsky et al., 2010; Rodriguez and Verkhratsky, 2011).

13.6 CONCLUSION

Empirically, societies all over the world have regarded various natural products as food for medicine, although this reductionist approach to the prevention or amelioration of ailments was deemed to be a relic of the past. The consumption of herbal medicinal principles throughout life has the potential to restrict neurodegeneration, and to slow down or reverse age-dependent deterioration in cognitive performances. However, due to the intense interest in the development of drugs capable of enhancing brain function, medicinal plants may represent important lead molecules in the quest to develop a new generation of brain communication-enhancing drugs. Specific targeting of astroglial homeostatic cascades suggests another novel therapeutic strategy, whereby the expression of astroglial glutamate uptake transporters was found to be augmented by a neuroprotective drug. Such a drug would be considered to be a powerful tool for the reversal of the progression of neurodegerative diseases. Nowadays, through multidisciplinary studies, research can investigate the mode-of action of herbal bioactives targeted at neurodegeneration, using the lances of a modern scientific approach.

CONFLICT OF INTEREST

The authors declared that there are no conflicts of interest.

ACKNOWLEDGMENTS

Research and infrastructural support given by Jadavpur University, Kolkata, India is gratefully acknowledged. The authors are also thankful to the Department of Biotechnology (DBT), New Delhi for financial assistance to Prof. (Dr.) Subhash C Mandal under DBT's Twinning Program for the North East (Grant no. DBT-NER/AGRI/29/2015 (Group 2).

REFERENCES

Amenta, F., Tayebati, S. K. 2008. Pathways of acetylcholine synthesis, transport and release as targets for treatment of adult-onset cognitive dysfunction. *Current Medical Chemistry* 15:488–498.

Arendash, G. W., Mori, T., Cao, C., et al. 2009. Caffeine reverses cognitive impairment and decreases brain amyloid-beta levels in aged Alzheimer's disease mice. *Journal of Alzheimer's Disease* 17(3):661–680.

Benzing, W. C., Mufson, E. J., Armstrong, D. M. 1993. Alzheimer's disease-like dystrophic neurites characteristically associated with senile plaques are not found within other neurodegenerative diseases unless amyloid beta-protein deposition is present. *Brain Research* 606:10–18.

Bhat, N. R., Feinstein, D. L., Shen, Q., et al. 2002. p38 MAPK mediated transcriptional activation of inducible nitric oxide synthase in glial cells. Roles of nuclear factors, nuclear factor kappa B, cAMP response element binding protein, CCAAT/enhancer binding protein beta, and activating transcription factor 2. *The Journal of Biological Chemistry* 277:29584–29592.

Bhat, N. R., Zhang, P., Lee, J. C., et al. 1998. Extracellular signal regulated kinase and p38 subgroups of mitogen activated protein kinases regulate inducible nitric oxide synthase and tumor necrosis factor alpha gene expression in endotoxin stimulated primary glial cultures. *Journal of Neuroscience* 18:1633–1641.

Bubber, P., Haroutunian, V., Fisch, G., et al. 2005. Mitochondrial abnormalities in Alzheimer brain: mechanistic implications. *Annals of Neurology* 57:695–703.

Callahan, L. M., Vaules, W. A., Coleman, P. D. 1999. Quantitative decrease in synaptophysin message expression and increase in cathepsin D message expression in Alzheimer disease neurons containing neurofibrillary tangles. *Journal of Neuropathology and Experimental Neurology* 58:275–287.

Cattabeni, F., Colciaghi, F., DiLuca, M. 2004. Platelets provide human tissue to unravel pathogenic mechanisms of Alzheimer disease. *Progress in Neuro-psychopharmacology and Biological Psychiatry* 28:763–770.

Chen, G., Bower, K. A., Xu, M., et al. 2009. Cyanidin-3-glucoside reverses ethanol-induced inhibition of neurite outgrowth: role of glycogen synthase kinase 3 beta. *Neurotoxicity Research* 15:321–331.

Cotman, C. W., Hailer, N. P., Pfister, K. K., et al. 1998. Cell adhesion molecules in neural plasticity and pathology: similar mechanisms, distinct organizations? *Progress in Neurobiology* 55:659–669.

Davis, R. E., Williams, M. 2012. Mitochondrial function and dysfunction: an update. *Journal of Pharmacology and Experimental Therapeutics* 342:598–607.

DeDuve, C., Wattiaux, R. 1966. Functions of lysosomes. *Annual Review of Physiology* 28:435–492.

Dityatev, A., Dityateva, G., Schachner, M. 2000. Synaptic strength as a function of post-versus presynaptic expression of the neural cell adhesion molecule NCAM. *Neuron* 26:207–217.

Ehrnhoefer, D. E., Duennwald, M., Markovic, P., et al. 2006. Green tea (–)-epigallocatechin gallate modulates early events in huntingtin misfolding and reduces toxicity in Huntington's disease models. *Human Molecular Genetics* 15:2743–2751.

Ercisli, S., Orhan, E. 2007. Chemical composition of white (*Morus alba*), red (*Morus rubra*) and black (*Morus nigra*) mulberry fruits. *Food Chemistry* 103:1380–1384.

Ghosh, N., Ghosh, R., Mandal S. C., et al. 2009. *In vitro* antioxidant study of livosyp: a polyherbal formulation. *Pharmacologyonline* 1:903–912.

Ghosh, N., Ghosh, R., Mandal, S. C. 2011. Antioxidant protection: a promising therapeutic intervention in neurodegenerative disease. *Free Radical Research* 45:888–905.

Ginsberg, S. D., Hemby, S. E., Lee, V. M., et al. 2000. Expression profile of transcripts in Alzheimer's disease tangle-bearing CA1 neurons. *Annals of Neurology* 48:77–87.

Haroutunian, V., Hoffman, L. B., Beeri, M. S. 2009. Is there a neuropathology difference between mild cognitive impairment and dementia? *Dialougesin Clinical Neuroscience* 11:171–179.

Heneka, M. T., Sastre, M., Dumitrescu-Ozimek, L., et al. 2005. Focal glial activation coincides with increased BACE1 activation and precedes amyloid plaque deposition in APP[V717I] transgenic mice. *Journal of Neuroinflammation* 2:22.

Hensley, K., Butter, D. A., Hall, N., et al. 1996. Reactive oxygen species as causal agents in the neurotoxicity of the Alzheimer's disease associated amyloid beta peptide. *Annals of the New York Academy of Science* 786:120–134.

Hensley, K., Hall, N., Subramaniam, R., et al. 1995. Brain regional correspondence between Alzheimer's disease histopathology and biomarkers of protein oxidation. *Journal of Neurochemistry* 65:2146–2156.

Hirsch, T., Marchetti, P., Susin, S. A., et al. 1997. The apoptosis necrosis paradox. Apoptogenic proteases activated after mitochondrial permeability transition determine the mode of cell death. *Oncogene* 15:1573–1581.

Hoffman, S., Edelman, G. M. 1983. Kinetics of hemophilic binding by embryonic and adult forms of the neural cell adhesion molecule. *Proceedings of the National Academy of Sciences of the United States of America* 80:5762–5766.

Isaacson, J. S., Scanziani, M. 2011. How inhibition shapes cortical activity. *Neuron* 72:231–243.

Jia, L., Liu, J., Song, Z., et al. 2012. Berberine suppresses amyloid-beta-induced inflammatory response in microglia by inhibiting nuclear factor-kappa B and mitogen-activated protein kinase signalling pathways. *Journal of Pharmacy and Pharmacology* 64(10):1510–1521.

Johnston, G. A. 2005. GABAA receptor channel pharmacology. *Current Pharmaceutical Design* 11:1867–1885.

Kundu, A., Mandal, V., Mandal, S. C. 2016. An overview on neurodegenerative diseases and possible leads from natural products. *The Pharma Review* 14:66–70.

Lee, S., Sato, Y., Nixon, R. A. 2011. Lysosomal proteolysis inhibition selectively disrupts axonal transport of degradative organelles and causes an Alzheimer's like axonal dystrophy. *Journal of Neuroscience* 31:7817–7830.

Leytin, V., Freedman, J. 2003. Platelet apoptosis in stored platelet concentrates and other models. *Transfusion and Apheresis Science* 28:285–295.

Lovell, M. A., Ehmann, W. D., Butler, S. M., et al. 1995. Elevated thiobarbituric acid-reactive substances and antioxidant enzyme activity in the brain in Alzheimer's disease. *Neurology* 45:1594–1601.

Maiti, P. P., Ghosh, N., Kundu, A., Panda, S., et al. 2017. Evaluation of anti-inflammatory and antinociceptive activity of methanol extract of *Calotropis gigantea* root. *International Journal of Green Pharmacy* 11:198–205.

Malarkey, E. B., Parpura, V. 2008. Mechanisms of glutamate release from astrocytes. *Neurochemistry International* 52:142–154.

Mandel, S. A., Avramovich-Tirosh, Y., Reznichenko, L., et al. 2005. Multifunctional activities of green tea catechins in neuroprotection. Modulation of cell survival genes, iron dependent oxidative stress and PKC signaling pathway. *Neurosignals* 14:46–60.

Marambaud, P., Zhao, H., Davies, P. 2005. Resveratrol promotes clearance of Alzheimer's disease amyloid beta peptides. *The Journal of Biological Chemistry* 280:37377–37382.

Marcus, J. S., Karackattu, S. L., Fleegal, M. A. 2003. Cytokine stimulated inducible nitric oxide synthase expression in astroglia: role of Erk mitogen activated protein kinase and NfkappaB. *Glia* 41:152–160.

McCann, J. C., Ames, B. N. 2005. Is docosahexaenoic acid, an n23 longchain polyunsaturated fatty acid, required for development of normal brain function? An overview of evidence from cognitive and behavioral tests in humans and animals. *The American Journal of Clinical Nutrition* 82:281–295.

Mecocci, P., Cherubini, A., Polidori, M. C., et al. 1997. Oxidative stress and dementia: new perspectives in AD pathogenesis. *Aging* 9 Supplement:51–52.

Mecocci, P., Polidori, M. C., Ingegni, T., et al. 1998. Oxidative damage to DNA in lymphocytes from AD patients. *Neurology* 51:1014–1017.

Nixon, R. A., Yang, D. S. 2012. Autophagy and neuronal cell death in neurological disorders. *Cold Spring Harbor Perspectives in Biology* 4(10):a008839.

Norbury, C. J., Hickson, I. D. 2001. Cellular responses to DNA damage. *Annual Review Pharmacology and Toxicology* 41:367–401.

Pan, Y., Anthony, M., Clarkson, T. B. 1999a. Effect of estradiol and soy phytoestrogens on choline acetyltransferase and nerve growth factor mRNAs in the frontal cortex and hippocampus of female rats. *Proceedings of the Society for Experimental Biology and Medicine* 221:118–125.

Pan, Y., Anthony, M., Clarkson, T. B. 1999b. Evidence for upregulation of brain derived neurotrophic factor mRNA by soy phytoestrogens in the frontal cortex of retired breeder female rats. *Neuroscience Letters* 261:17–20.

Parpura, V., Grubisic, V., Verkhratsky, A. 2011. Ca2+ sources for the exocytotic release of glutamate from astrocytes. *Biochimica et Biophysica Acta* 1813:984–991.

Peng, C. H., Liu, L. K., Chuang, C. M., et al. 2011. Mulberry water extracts possess an anti-obesity effect and ability to inhibit hepatic lipogenesis and promote lipolysis. *Journal of Agricultural and Food Chemistry* 59:2663–2671.

Pratico, D. 2008. Evidence of oxidative stress in Alzheimer's disease brain and antioxidant therapy: lights and shadows. *Annals of the New York Academy of Sciences* 1147:70–78.

Rashid, M. H. A., Bharadwaj, P. V. P. D., Majumder, S., et al. 2018a. Antioxidant and anticancer activity of extract and fractions obtained from *Diospyros melanoxylon* roxb. leaves and correlation with their polyphenolic profiles. *International Journal of Pharmacy and Pharmaceutical Sciences* 10:6–16.

Rashid, M. H. A., Majumder, S., Mandal, V., et al. 2018b. In search of suitable extraction technique for large scale commercial production of bioactive fraction for the treatment of diabetes: the case Diospyros melanoxylon Roxb. *Journal of Traditional and Complementary Medicine* xxx:1–13.

Rodriguez, J. J., Verkhratsky, A. 2011. Neuroglial roots of neurodegenerative diseases? *Molecular Neurobiology* 43:87–96.

Rolls, E. T. A. 1990. Theory of emotion, and its application to understanding the neural basis of emotion. *Cognition and Emotion* 4:161–190.

Southwell, D. G., Nicholas, C. R., Basbaum, A. I., et al. 2014. Interneurons from embryonic development to cell-based therapy. *Science* 344:1240622.

Spencer, J. P. 2008a. Flavonoids: Modulators of brain function? *British Journal of Nutrition* 99:ES60–ES77.

Spencer, J. P. 2008b. Food for thought: The role of dietary flavonoids in enhancing human memory, learning and neuro cognitive performance. *Proceedings of the Nutrition Society* 67:238–252.

Sutherland, B. A., Rahman, R. M., Appleton, I. 2005. Mechanisms of action of green tea catechins, with a focus on ischemia-induced neurodegeneration. *The Journal of Nutritional Biochemistry* 17:291–306.

Swerdlow, R. H., Burns, J. M., Khan, S. M. 2010. The Alzheimer's disease mitochondrial cascade hypothesis. *Journal of Alzheimer's Disease* 20 Supplement 2:S265–S279.

Troulinaki, K., Tavernarakis, N. 2012. Endocytosis and intracellular trafficking contribute to necrotic neurodegeneration in *C. elegans*. *The EMBO Journal* 31(3):654–666.

Verkhratsky, A., Olabarria, M., Noristani, H. N., et al. 2010. Astrocytes in Alzheimer's disease. *Neurotherapeutics* 7:399–412.

Wielgat, P., Braszko, J. J. 2012. Significance of the cell adhesion molecules and sialic acid in neurodegeneration. *Advances in Medical Sciences* 57:23–30.

Winkler, J., Suhr, S. T., Gage, F. H., et al. 1995. Essential role of neocortical acetylcholine in spatial memory. *Nature* 375:484–487.

Yehuda, S., Rabinovitz, S., Carasso, R. L. 2002. The role of polyunsaturated fatty acids in restoring the aging neuronal membrane. *Neurobiology of Aging* 23:843–853.

York, P., Marielle, E. G., Volker, H. 2015. Phosphoinositides in endocytosis. *Biochimica et Biophysica Acta* 1851:794–804.

Zeiss, C. J. 2003. The apoptosis necrosis continuum: insights from genetically altered mice. *Veterinary Pathology* 40:481–495.

Zeitlin, R., Patel, S., Burgess, S., et al. 2011. Caffeine induces beneficial changes in PKA signaling and JNK and ERK activities in the striatum and cortex of Alzheimer's transgenic mice. *Brain Research* 1417:127–136.

Zhang, C., Qiu, H. E., Krafft, G. A., et al. 1996. Protein kinase C and F-actin are essential for stimulation of neuronal FAK tyrosine phosphorylation by G-proteins and amyloid beta protein. *FEBS Letters* 386:185–188.

14 Pre-Clinical Approaches and Methods on Alzheimer's Disease

In Vivo and *In Vitro*

S. R. Chandra and Pooja Mailankody

CONTENTS

ABBREVIATIONS

AD Alzheimer's Disease
MCI Mild Cognitive Impairment
SCD Subjective Cognitive Dysfunction

14.1 INTRODUCTION

The incidence of dementia in the community is expected to double every 20 years, with a predicted population of about 115.4 million patients worldwide by 2050. AD is the most common type of degenerative dementia (Alzheimer 2015; Bennett et al. 2015). By the time the disease becomes overtly symptomatic, the options for improving quality of life are very limited. In spite of huge investments, dementia research has not been rewarded, in terms of either diagnosis or treatment. The medicines which work in mouse models do not work in humans (Borchelt et al. 1997; Brayne and Calloway 1988).

On 4 November, 1906, Alois Alzheimer described the first case. However, it still remains an enigma. Approximately 10% of patients with AD develop symptoms before 65 years of age and belong to the category of early-onset AD. The familial cases are linked to amyloid precursor protein and presenilin-1 and -2. There is progressive impairment of recent memory, visuospatial orientation, executive functions, language, and behavior. It is believed that there is a long, preclinical period, during which phase, if diagnosed, lifestyle modifications might delay the stage of dependency. This can be based on clinical or other laboratory evaluations. Mild cognitive impairment (MCI) is the term applied to the clinical state of early impairment. About 10 to 15% of these patients convert to MCI annually. The questions we need to address in this chapter are: 1) What is MCI? 2) How early can we diagnose AD? 3) How early can treatment start? 4) Will it be possible to stop the progression? 5) Will there be a cure and what are the current options? We shall approach these questions one by one. Such an understanding is important as, the earlier the diagnosis is made, the better the quality of life can be achieved.

14.2 WHAT IS SUBJECTIVE COGNITIVE DYSFUNCTION (SCD)?

SCD is a complex disorder, where there is a perceived decline in cognition in the absence of objective evidence. Though most patients fall into the category of suffering from mood disorders, older persons show altered hippocampal volume, AD biomarkers, and an increased risk of progression to dementia.

The Subjective Cognitive Decline Initiative working group is an established international consortium to create research criteria for evaluation of persons with SCD. There are different acronyms for SCD, such as SCI (subjective cognitive impairment) and SCC (subjective cognitive complaint).

The term SCD refers to everyday cognitive concerns raised by persons without objective evidence of dementia. The grouping is etiologically heterogeneous and therefore interventions might help some individuals. Irrespective of the nature, quality of life is affected. SCD is considered to be probably the earliest sign of dementia, but many unanswered questions remain. Decline is defined as a change to MCI or dementia over a follow-up interval. Which mental process impairment, biomarker, or functional neuroanatomy causes this decline? A lot of research has taken place in the past decade in this area. A widely accepted approach is lacking, and the heterogeneity is due to a lack of understanding of the mode of administration, number of terms, response options, domains to be tested, etc. But suspicion of this being pre-MCI is based on reports that amyloid-beta (Aβ) deposition correlates with SCD but not with objective cognitive impairment. Amyloid status, however, predicts future decline. Tau proteins are associated with SCD, cortical volume, medial temporal atrophy, and white matter changes, and indicate decreased structural integrity in the memory system.

Reisberg (1985), using a global deterioration scale (GDS), predicted that SCD + grade 2 GDS is not normal and grade 3 MCI, grade 4 MCI and higher were associated with dementia. SCD is associated more with depression (Bolla et al.), and depression influences hippocampal volume (Gurvits et al.), suggesting a complex interaction between these three states. The outcome studies have limitation in terms of early dementias, and whether MCI were excluded or not is not clear. Geerlings reported three times greater risk of developing dementia within 3.5 years of being diagnosed as MCI, whereas John and Montgomery and Wang et al. reported that it does not. Cross-sectional studies revealed a greater decline with MCI. Cognitive tests are difficult to quantify between SCD and non-SCD. Biological assessment with quantitative encephalography (qEEG) showed increased θ, whereas voxel-based morphometric studies reported grey matter differences in medial temporal, frontal, and other neocortices. A smaller hippocampus in SCD was reported by van den Filler. Positron emission tomography (PET) studies reported decreased cerebral metabolism of glucose in the parietotemporal and parahippocampal regions. Subjects who had SCD in conjunction with the apolipoprotein E ε4 (*APOEε4*) allele had greater changes. Higher cortisol levels were reported by Wolf et al. Functional magnetic resonance imaging (fMRI) studies have revealed no change in performance during tasks but observed differences in functional brain activation between SCD and non-SCD subjects. When semantically related words were used, increased activation of the lateral prefrontal cortex was seen and led to compensatory theory, classifying it to be compensation for decay of the hippocampal memory system elsewhere. Testing of the episodic memory and valuation system revealed decreased preference for future-oriented tasks, attenuating attention, and subjective evaluation systems. The phenomenon of "Negative Subsequent" is postulated to be the cause of increased activation of failed recall. Dedifferentiation theory argues that loss of specialization results in diffuse brain activation, but how this hyperactivity contributes to SCD is not clear. Homeostasis breakdown theory says that it could be associated with loss of comprehensive temporal dynamics. Prediction error theory describes brain functions as a statistical optimization engine, and makes implicit predictions of inputs actively making inferences, instead of passively recording. Predictive coding is the principle by which there is a comparison of internally generated predictions with external reality. Awareness of subtle errors can occur in multiple domains, causing SCD. Homeostasis breakdown occurs and compensatory functions act for some time. but these can lead to glutamate excitotoxicity and cell death. Depression is a common characteristic of SCD and there is probably a complex interaction between depression, SCD, MCI, and dementia. Outcome studies are not clear if MCI were excluded. The longer the follow-up, the longer the conversion period.

Is it time to separate SCD from MCI? MCI includes SCD as a core feature but how many normal elderly people have SCD? Does SCD affect MCI prevention? The Steel Valley study revealed that 6.3% persons without SCD qualified for MCI, whereas only 3.2% qualified from the SCD group. The Canadian Study of Health and Ageing (CSHA) evaluated how this relationship adversely affected MCI.

The relationship between subjective and objective cognitive impairment is not straightforward, and people can be categorized as group 1, where both impairments are present; group 2, where neither is present; group 3, where there is subjective impairment alone; and group 4, where there is objective impairment alone. The risk is greatest if both are present, with the next-greatest risk occurring with objective impairment alone, subjective impairment alone, and neither, in that order. Accurate risk profiling was not possible, in spite of ten years' research. Both subjective and objective tests are important. The use of other features with SCD increases specificity and positive predictive value and decreases sensitivity and negative predictive value. In the absence of any other clinically relevant features or association with other markers, the available data are controversial with respect to the significance of SCD as a harbinger of dementia.

14.3 WHAT IS MILD COGNITIVE IMPAIRMENT (MCI)?

MCI represents the early, incipient stage of dementia. This needs to be differentiated from minor changes associated with normal aging, where a person's experience of mild retrieval defect is manifested as a "tip-of-the-tongue" phenomenon (Burton 2004). Age-associated memory impairment (AAMI) is another term which manifests as memory performance being poorer than in younger persons, and aging-associated cognitive decline (AACD), when other cognitive domains, beside memory, are also affected (Busse et al. 2006). The term cognitive impairment non-demented (CIND) indicates that a subject is more deficient but cannot be called demented (Chandra 2017). When the term MCI is introduced, it points to abnormal processes, which are more likely to be the prodromal of the progress toward dementia (Chandra et al. 2016). Approximately 12 to 18% of persons above 65 years of age suffer from MCI (Chao et al. 2010). However, there are gross differences in the tools used to evaluate this parameter, and therefore the data also vary (Citron et al. 1992). Petersen (2004) proposed the following evaluation for non-demented subjects: memory complaint qualified by an informant; memory impairment normalized for age and education; general cognitive function preserved; and activities of daily living intact.

A neuroimaging initiative was proposed by Mueller et al. and Cruts et al. (2012). The patients thus identified undergo neuropsychological testing to decide whether it is only single- domain memory impairment, or whether there are other domains, such as language, executive function, and visuospatial functions, which are affected (Di Carlo et al. 2007). If there is no significant memory impairment, the other domains affected are tested to decide whether it is a non-amnestic MCI; if so, are single-domain or multi-domain cognitive abilities affected? This distinction is important to categorize the phenotype.

Following this work-up, assessment should be carried out to determine whether it is degenerative (gradual in onset and has insidious progression) or non-degenerative and vascular (abrupt in onset). Other medical disorders which should be looked for in association with MCI include depressive features and depression, co-morbid systemic features of endocrine metabolic diseases, and nutritional diseases. Some 5% of people diagnosed with MCI normalize and are categorized as unstable MCI, of which 10 to 15% progress to dementia per year (Fratiglioni et al. 1999). A major concern, with reference to MCI, is the ability to identify those who are likely to progress toward dementia. The predictors seen in clinically more symptomatic patients with amnestic multi-domain involvement are hippocampal atrophy in MRI, *APOEε4* carrier status, cerebrospinal fluid (CSF) showing increased tau and decreased Aβ levels, fluorodeoxyglucose (FDG)-PET showing temporoparietal hypometabolism, and positive amyloid imaging (Gauthier et al. 2006). Entorhinal cortex volume, whole-brain volume, and ventricular volume are other, useful markers (Huded et al. 2015). The *APOEε4* allele is associated not only with increased risk of AD but also with increased conversion of MCI to dementia (Hunderfund et al. 2006). Metabolic brain changes may precede actual disease manifestation and are therefore useful in predicting conversion to dementia. Pittsburg compound B (PIB) imaging is believed to differentiate normal, MCI, and AD patients (Issac et al. 2017). Autopsy studies have indicated early pathological changes but whether they were really MCI or advanced patients is not very clear (Issac et al. 2013).

14.4 HOW EARLY CAN WE DIAGNOSE AD FROM GENETIC TESTING?

Early symptoms in the preclinical phase can be suspected by applying the criteria to patients with subtle features, and this sensitization may be useful when treatment options become available, although tools are arbitrary. How ethical and how early are questions to be answered with reference to genetics? Three proteases, α, β and γ, process amyloid precursor protein. When acted upon by β-secretase, Aβ is generated, which is pathogenic. Presenilin-1 and -2 are involved in familial AD. The insoluble Aβ causes senile plaques. Tau hyperphosphorylation causes neurofibrillary tangles. In isolation, allele *APOEε4* cannot produce AD, but, when there is vascular compromise, trauma, anesthetic events, or excitotoxicity, interaction with Aβ leads to pathogenicity (Jack et al. 1999).

The allele of the *APOE* gene on chromosome 19 is associated with late-onset AD, and genes for sortilin-related receptor 1 (SORL1) and ubiquilin 1 on chromosome 1 are associated with recycling of amyloid precursor peptide (APP). There is overlap of major proteins, like amyloid and tau, in AD, with amyloid and α-synuclein in diffuse Lewy body disease (DLBD) causing problems in specificity. The amyloid hypothesis states that Aβ production and degradation is the pathology common to all types of AD and the causative genes for APP are on chromosome 9. The presenelin-1 gene on chromosome 14 causes severe, very early disease with features of parkinsonism, and is associated with about 60% of inherited AD cases. The presenelin-2 gene on chromosome 1 is a less common cause and is also involved in other diseases. APP is a part of neuronal synapses, and the corresponding gene is located on chromosome 21. Proteolysis of APP by α- or β-secretase leads to secretion of soluble fragments of amyloid alpha or beta peptide. These are subsequently cleaved by γ-secretase to generate either a gamma fragment. In early-onset AD, there is an imbalance between the $A\beta_{42}$, which increases, and the $A\beta_{40}$, which decreases, resulting in a propensity for aggregation (Klunk et al. 2004; Kumar et al. 2017). In screening for familial AD cases, it is better to look for presenilin-1 and APP, as they are the most common indicators. *APOEε4*, located on chromosome 19, is responsible for both familial and sporadic late-onset AD. Other genes which might play a role are *ABCA7*, *CLU*, which regulates the clearance of Aβ from the brain, *CR1*, *PLD3*, and *TREM2*, which contribute to chronic inflammation in the brain, and SORL1 and PICALM, which are involved in synaptic connectivity.

14.5 OTHER USEFUL TOOLS IN EARLY RECOGNITION

14.5.1 Transcranial Motor Stimulation

The resting motor threshold is reduced in AD, with normal central motor conduction (Larrieu et al. 2002; Petersen and Knopman 2006). This may serve as a biomarker in AD patients and may also open new therapeutic options, such as gamma aminobutyric acid (GABA) agonist. With the rationale that acetylcholine (ACh) is depleted in AD, autonomic functions were analyzed and parasympathetic suppression was found in AD (Pistollato et al. 2016). Our study on balance and gait found that patients with AD have problems of balance in limits of stability (Sinclair et al. 2012).

14.5.2 Dual-Task Gait Assessments

This is based on changes which can serve as an early differentiating tool. Our study, comparing quantitative voxel-based volumetric assessment of the brain with visual quantification of electroencephalography, showed significant correlation between grand total EEG score (GTES) and dementia severity and global grey matter volume (Tuokko and McDowell 2013).

14.5.3 Molecular Biomarkers Utilizing Cerebrospinal Fluid Analysis

In asymptomatic people, molecular biomarkers, utilizing CSF analysis, suggest that reduced levels of $A\beta_{42}$, and high CSF concentrations of tau proteins are of great sensitivity and specificity for preclinical AD. A radioactive tracer, which binds to fibrillar forms of $A\beta_{42}$, is injected and the radioactive tracer can be evaluated, using PET.

14.6 DISCUSSION

Early diagnosis of AD is considered to be important, keeping in mind the possibility of influencing at least some of the factors which lead to advanced disease. However, using various tools, it is understood that even diagnosis of MCI happens when the disease is quite advanced. Hence, criteria incorporating biomarkers and neuroimaging findings are considered. The search for biomarkers is based on the amyloid cascade as well as on domains and regions identified as being abnormal. The International Conference on AD and Related Disorders (ICAD) in Hawaii proposed criteria for diagnosis of preclinical AD (Velayutham et al. 2017). Living to the full length of life without dementia is important if control over other diseases is to be considered useful.

14.7 CONCLUSION

Though several biomarkers are being tested, their sensitivity and specificity are not good as stand-alone tests and involve high costs. But they are very important for searching for new preventive tools, using drugs, vaccines, stem cells, or genetic manipulation. However, compared with symptomatic patients, the question to be answered before carrying out these tests in asymptomatic persons carries ethical constraints, when we are not sure of their sensitivity and specificity in disease causation, more so when definite treatments are not available. Therefore, the decision for preclinical testing remains a personal choice.

CONFLICT OF INTEREST

We have no conflict of interest or any source of funding.

ACKNOWLEDGMENTS

We acknowledge with gratitude our patients, their families, and our Director, for encouraging our search for new biomarkers for early diagnosis and differential diagnosis in our Institute (NIMHANS).

REFERENCES

Alzheimer's Assoc. Alzheimer's disease facts and figures. *Alz Dement* 2015 Mar; 11(3): 332.

Bennett DA, Schneider JA, Bienias JL, Evans DA, Wilson RS. Mild cognitive impairment is related to Alzheimer disease pathology and cerebral infarctions. *Neurology* 2005 Mar 8; 64(5): 834–841.

Borchelt DR, Ratovitski T, Van Lare J, Lee MK, Gonzales V, Jenkins NA, Copeland NG, Price DL, Sisodia SS. Accelerated amyloid deposition in the brains of transgenic mice coexpressing mutant presenilin 1 and amyloid precursor proteins. *Neuron* 1997 Oct 1; 19(4): 939–945.

Brayne C, Calloway P. Normal ageing, impaired cognitive function, and senile dementia of the Alzheimer's type: a continuum? *Lancet* 1988 Jun 4; 331(8597): 1265–1267.

Burton A. 9th International Conference on AD and related disorders (ICAD). *Lancet Neurol* 2004 Sep 1; 3(9): 510.

Busse A, Hensel A, Gühne U, Angermeyer MC, Riedel-Heller SG. Mild cognitive impairment: long-term course of four clinical subtypes. *Neurology* 2006 Dec 26; 67(12): 2176–2185.

Chandra SR. Alzheimer's disease: An alternative approach. *Ind J Med Res* 2017 Jun; 145(6): 723.

Chandra SR, Issac TG, Nagaraju BC, Philip M. A study of cortical excitability, central motor conduction, and cortical inhibition using single pulse transcranial magnetic stimulation in patients with early frontotemporal and Alzheimer's dementia. *Indian J Psychol Med* 2016; 38: 25–30.

Chao LL, Mueller SG, Buckley ST, Peek K, Raptentsetseng S, Elman J, Yaffe K, Miller BL, Kramer JH, Madison C, Mungas D. Evidence of neurodegeneration in brains of older adults who do not yet fulfill MCI criteria. *Neurobiol Aging* 2010 Mar 1; 31(3): 368–377.

Citron M, Oltersdorf T, Haass C, McConlogue L, Hung AY, Seubert P, Vigo-Pelfrey C, Lieberburg I, Selkoe DJ. Mutation of the β-amyloid precursor protein in familial Alzheimer's disease increases β-protein production. *Nature* 1992 Dec; 360(6405): 672.

Cruts M, Theuns J, Van Broeckhoven C. Locus-specific mutation databases for neurodegenerative brain diseases. *Hum Mutat* 2012 Sep; 33(9): 1340–1344.

Di Carlo A, Lamassa M, Baldereschi M, Inzitari M, Scafato E, Farchi G, Inzitari D. CIND and MCI in the Italian elderly: frequency, vascular risk factors, progression to dementia. *Neurology* 2007 May 29; 68(22): 1909–1916.

Fratiglioni L, De Ronchi D, Agüero-Torres H. Worldwide prevalence and incidence of dementia. *Drugs Aging* 1999 Nov 1; 15(5): 365–375.

Gauthier S, Reisberg B, Zaudig M, Petersen RC, Ritchie K, Broich K, Belleville S, Brodaty H, Bennett D, Chertkow H, Cummings JL. Mild cognitive impairment. *Lancet* 2006 Apr 15; 367(9518): 1262–1270.

Huded CB, Bharath S, Chandra SR, Sivakumar PT, Varghese M, Subramanian S. Supportive CSF biomarker evidence to enhance the National Institute on Aging-Alzheimer's Association criteria for diagnosis of Alzheimer's type dementia – a study from Southern India. *Asian J Psychiatr* 2015 Feb 1; 13: 44–47.

Hunderfund AL, Roberts RO, Slusser TC, Leibson CL, Geda YE, Ivnik RJ, Tangalos EG, Petersen RC. Mortality in amnestic mild cognitive impairment: a prospective community study. *Neurology* 2006 Nov 28; 67(10): 1764–1768.

Issac TG, Chandra SR, Gupta N, Rukmani MR, Deepika S, Sathyaprabha TN. Autonomic dysfunction: a comparative study of patients with Alzheimer's and frontotemporal dementia – a pilot study. *J Neurosci Rural Pract* 2017; 8: 84–88.

Issac TG, Chandra SR, Nagaraju BC. Transcranial magnetic stimulation in patients with early cortical dementia: a pilot study. *Ann Indian Acad Neurol* 2013; 16: 619–622.

Jack CR, Petersen RC, Xu YC, O'Brien PC, Smith GE, Ivnik RJ, Boeve BF, Waring SC, Tangalos EG, Kokmen E. Prediction of AD with MRI-based hippocampal volume in mild cognitive impairment. *Neurology* 1999 Apr 1; 52(7): 1397.

Klunk WE, Engler H, Nordberg A, Wang Y, Blomqvist G, Holt DP, Bergström M, Savitcheva I, Huang GF, Estrada S, Ausén B. Imaging brain amyloid in Alzheimer's disease with Pittsburgh Compound-B. *Ann Neurol* 2004 Mar; 55(3): 306–319.

Kumar RK, Chandra SR, Kulkarni GB, Bharath RD. Use of Jonkman et al. Score for visual quantification of electroencephalography as a tool to assess disease severity in cortical dementias. *Ind J Psychol Med* 2017 Mar; 39(2): 122.

Larrieu S, Letenneur L, Orgogozo JM, Fabrigoule C, Amieva H, Le Carret N, Barberger-Gateau P, Dartigues JF. Incidence and outcome of mild cognitive impairment in a population-based prospective cohort. *Neurology* 2002 Nov 26; 59(10): 1594–1599.

Petersen RC, Knopman DS. MCI is a clinically useful concept. *Int Psychogeriatr* 2006 Sep; 18(3): 394–402.

Pistollato F, Ohayon EL, Lam A, Langley GR, Novak TJ, Pamies D, Perry G, Trushina E, Williams RS, Roher AE, Hartung T. Alzheimer disease research in the 21st century: past and current failures, new perspectives and funding priorities. *Oncotarget* 2016 Jun 28; 7(26): 38999.

Sinclair AJ, Morley JE, Vellas B, editors. *Pathy's Principles and Practice of Geriatric Medicine*. John Wiley & Sons; 2012 Mar 13.

Tuokko HA, McDowell I. An overview of mild cognitive impairment. In *Mild Cognitive Impairment* 2013 May 13 (pp. 12–37). Psychology Press.

Velayutham SG, Chandra SR, Bharath S, Shankar RG. Quantitative balance and gait measurement in patients with frontotemporal dementia and Alzheimer diseases: a pilot study. *Ind J Psychol Med* 2017 Mar; 39(2): 176.

15 Ethanolic Extracts of *Dysphania ambrosioides* Alleviates Scopolamine-Induced Amnesia in Experimental Animals

Rajashri Bezbaruah, Chandana C. Barua, Lipika Buragohain, Pobitra Borah, Iswar Chandra Barua, and Ghanshyam Panigrahi

CONTENTS

ABBREVIATIONS

AChE	Acetylcholinesterase
AD	Alzheimer's Disease
Aβ	Amyloid β
CPCSEA	Committee for the Purpose of Control and Supervision of Experiments on Animals
D. ambrosioides	*Dysphania ambrosioides*
DA	*Dysphania Ambrosioides*
Dys100	Ethanolic extract of DA at a concentration of 100 mg/kg bodyweight
Dys200	Ethanolic extract of DA at a concentration of 200 mg/kg bodyweight
EPM	Elevated Plus Maze
$GABA_A$	Gamma-Aminobutyric Acid A Receptor
I. P.	Intraperitoneal
IAEC	Institutional Animal Ethical Committee
LD_{50}	Median half-maximal Lethal Dose
MWM	Morris Water Maze
NFT	Neurofibrillary Tangles
NO	Nitric Oxide
OECD	Organization for Economic Co-operation and Development
P. O.	Per os
TL	Transfer Latency

15.1 INTRODUCTION

The complex process of memory formation involves many neurotransmitters and multiple neural pathways, where the cholinergic neural system plays a crucial role (Joshi and Malviya, 2017). The word "memory" can be defined as the ability of an individual to record previous sensations, information, experiences, and ideas, to retain them for a period of time, and then to retrieve the same, when required (Richardson and Zucco, 1989).

Some specific psychiatric and neurodegenerative disorders like Alzheimer's disease (AD), vascular dementia, schizophrenia, normal aging, and stress may cause impairment of memory (amnesia). Physical injury or ingestion of toxic substances that affect the brain may also lead to amnesia (Abiola et al., 2019). Amnesia is a core symptom of dementia (Hirai, 2001). According to the World Alzheimer's Report 2018, 50 million of people were suffering from dementia in 2018, a figure which is expected to reach 82 million in 2030, and about 152 million in 2050 (Patterson, 2018).

AD is a subtype of dementia and is the most common progressive neurodegenerative disorder with a slow onset. Alongside cognitive decline, it often shows non-cognitive symptoms like psychosis, depression, apathy, etc., which, if they remain untreated, may lead to death (Joshi and Malviya, 2017; Abiola et al., 2019). Pathologically, AD is characterized by atrophy of the cortex and hippocampus due to deposition of amyloid β (Aβ), as well as formation of senile plaques and neurofibrillary tangles (NFT). Senile plaques are collections of sinuous and decaying nerve terminals around an amyloid core. Formation of Aβ occurs as a result of enzymatic cleavage and improper processing of amyloid precursor protein. NFT contain hyperphosphorylated tau proteins. Abnormal accumulation of Aβ and tau proteins initiates neurotoxicity, which is facilitated by oxidative stress. Hence, oxidative stress plays an important role in the pathogenesis of AD. Acetylcholinesterase also plays an important role in the development of AD. Lack of acetylcholinesterase (AChE) causes damage to the central cholinergic system, which results in cognitive deficits, leading ultimately to AD (Dhingra and Kumar, 2012; Kim et al., 2016; Uddin et al., 2016). Reduction in the hippocampal nitric oxide- (NO-) containing neurons and decreased synthesis of NO are consequences of neuronal damage associated with AD. Moreover, loss of gamma aminobutyric acid A receptor ($GABA_A$) and functional abnormality of the GABAergic system are also implicated in AD (Abiola et al., 2019).

AChE inhibitors, such as donepezil, rivastigmine or galantamine, are prescribed for the treatment of AD patients. Memantine, an N-methyl-D-aspartate (NMDA) receptor blocker, is also prescribed in more severe cases (Kim et al., 2016). Antihyperlipidemic drugs, like statins, anti-inflammatory, and antioxidant drugs, are also used to prevent neurotoxicity or the formation of senile plaques (Kamila et al., 2015). However, these drugs may only delay disease progression, and are often associated with many severe side effects, like somnolence, diarrhea, headache, vomiting, and loss of appetite. Therefore, there is an urgent need to find more effective and safer agents for the treatment of AD. Herbal remedies from medicinal plants are presumed to be less toxic and to exhibit fewer side effects than the synthetic drugs. *Hibiscus rosa-sinensis, Ocimum sanctum, Ginkgo biloba, Santalum album, Bacopa monnieri, Convolvulus pluricaulis, Huperzia serrata* and *Avena sativa* are well-known natural cognitive enhancers used in the treatment of AD (Kim et al., 2016). *Terminalia arjuna* and *Abelmoschus esculentus* act as nootropic agents by reducing the concentrations of free radicals (Tongjaroenbuangam et al., 2011).

Dysphania ambrosioides (DA) (syn. *Chenopodium ambrosioides*) belongs to the family Amaranthaceae (Pereira et al., 2010). In Assamese, DA is known as Jilmil Sak (Patiri and Borah, 2007) and it is also popularly known as American wormseed, mastruz, epazote, paico, Mexican tea, and erva-de-santa-maria (Kliks 1985; Sá et al., 2016).

DA is a short-lived perennial or annual undershrub, growing up to 1 m in height, with irregular branching, oblong-lanceolate leaves, and small green flowers that are produced in a branched panicle at the apex of the stem (Sá et al., 2016). Flowering and fruiting occur almost throughout the year (Patiri and Borah, 2007). DA is found abundantly in warm temperate to subtropical areas of Central America, South America, and Southern Mexico. In India, locations of DA include Maharashtra (Pune, Raigad, Satara), Karnataka (Chikmagalur, Coorg, Hassan, Mysore), Kerala (Idukki, Kannur, Palakkad, Pathanamthitta), Tamil Nadu (Coimbatore, Dharmapuri, Dindigul, Nilgiri, Salem, Theni, Tiruvannamalai, Tiruchchirappalli), and throughout Assam (Renu).

The plant is rich in essential oils, containing terpenes such as ascaridole (55.38%), *p*-cymene (16.2%), α-terpinene (9.7%), isoascaridole (4.3%), and limonene (3.8%) (Kumar et al., 2007). Among these, ascaridole is the major constituent of the plant oil (Zohra et al., 2019; Gadano et al., 2002). DA also contains minor components such as *trans*-pinocarveol, aritasone, β-pynene, myrcene, phellandrene, alcanphor, and terpineol (Gadano et al., 2002).

In traditional medicine, DA leaves, roots, and inflorescences have been used for centuries in the form of decoctions and infusions. Moreover, the World Health Organisation (WHO) has considered this plant to be one of the most-used traditional medicinal plants (Sá et al., 2016). In Assam, young leaves and shoots of DA are eaten as a vegetable, and the essential oil produced by the plant is considered to be an antispasmodic and tonic (Patiri and Borah, 2007). Ethnomedicinally, the leaves are used as anthelmintic and antifungal preparations (Sá et al., 2016). Other properties identified are anti-inflammatory, antitumor, antiulcer, antipyretic, analgesic, antinociceptive, antiprotozoal, and antioxidant (Barros et al., 2013; Gadano et al., 2002; Kumar et al., 2007; Nascimento et al., 2006; Sá et al., 2016; Zohra et al., 2019; Kliks, 1985). The plant is also used to treat digestive disorders, bone fractures, and muscle pain. This species is widely used in Brazil, where the leaves are blended with milk and administered as a treatment against influenza (Sá et al., 2016). Various bioactive compounds isolated from DA are used in the treatment of respiratory diseases, rheumatism, tuberculosis, and uterine hemorrhages (Zohra et al., 2019). It has also been reported that, in Peru, DA is traditionally used as a memory enhancer (Potawale et al., 2008). Studies have confirmed the antioxidant activity of DA, but no scientific investigation has been performed to evaluate its memory-enhancing activity, a finding which formed the basis of our present study. This study was designed to investigate the memory-enhancing activity of ethanolic extracts of DA on scopolamine-induced amnesia in universally used rodent models.

15.2 MATERIAL AND METHODS

15.2.1 Drugs and Reagents

Scopolamine hydrobromide and tacrine hydrochloride were obtained from Sigma-Aldrich, St. Louis, Missouri. All other chemicals and reagents used in the present work were of analytical grade.

15.2.2 Plant Material

Dysphania ambrosioides was collected from the medicinal garden of Assam Agricultural University, Jorhat, India. The plant was authenticated by Dr. I. C. Barua, Principal Scientist, Department of Agronomy, Assam Agricultural University, Jorhat. A voucher specimen has been deposited in the Herbarium with ref. no 5166/ 12.02.201.

15.2.3 Preparation of Ethanolic Extract

The collected plant materials were washed thoroughly and dried in the shade for 15 d. The dried materials were segregated and pulverized, using a mechanical grinder. Powdered material was allowed to pass through sieve (mesh size 60) and stored in an air-tight container. Subsequently, the crude powder was subjected to a cold maceration process, i.e. 500 g of dried powder was suspended in 750 ml of ethanol for one week with continuous stirring after every 18 h, using a sterile glass rod. The filtrate was obtained by treating the suspension with ethanol three times and filtering through Whatman filter paper No. 1, and the solvent was removed from the filtrate by rotary evaporation (R-210; BÜCHI Labortechnik AG, Flawil, Switzerland) under reduced pressure, below 50°C, to obtain a dark brown residue. This residue was stored in an air-tight container at 4°C until use. The recovery percentage, of the dried ethanolic extract of the DA powder relative to the dried DA powder, was found to be 21.3% w/w.

15.2.4 Acute DA Toxicity Studies

According to the Organization of Economic Co-operation and Development (OECD) Guidelines No. 425, the acute toxicity studies of ethanolic extract of DA were performed using Swiss albino mice of either sex (20–30 g). Mice were selected randomly and divided into four groups, each group consisting of three animals. The extract was prepared by using 0.9% normal saline. After 3 to 4 h of fasting, different doses (i.e. 5, 50, 300, or 2000 mg/kg Per os) of ethanolic extract were administered orally to the different groups of animals. Food was withdrawn for 1–2 h and any behavioral changes in the animals were recorded for the next 24 h. For the next 14 d, the animals were kept under observation to record mortality or gross abnormality in response to the given doses.

15.2.5 Effect of DA Extract on Scopolamine-Induced Amnesia

Male Swiss albino mice (20–30 g) and Wistar rats (150–200 g) were selected for different models of this study. The animals were housed in polypropylene cages, with clean bedding materials, and maintained at room temperature (25± 0.5°C) with a 12-h light/dark cycle. They were supplied with standard rodent pellet diet and drinking water *ad libitum*. Animals were acclimated to the testing room before starting each experiment. All experiments were performed in accordance with the guidelines recommended by Committee for the Purpose of Control and Supervision of Experiments on Animals (CPCSEA), Ministry of Social Justice and Empowerment, Government of India. All the protocols were approved by Institutional Animal Ethical Committee (IAEC) of the College of Veterinary Sciences, Assam Agricultural University, with registration number IAEC approval no: 770/ac/CPCSEA/ FVSc.AAU/ IAEC/ 367, Date: 10/4/15.

15.2.6 Treatment Schedule

The animals were divided into five groups ($n = 6$)

Group I: Control, received the vehicle (normal saline 10 ml/kg bodyweight p.o.).

Group II: Standard group, received tacrine at 3 mg/kg bodyweight, by intraperitoneal (i.p.) injection + scopolamine 0.4 mg/kg (i.p.)

Group III: Scopolamine (negative control) group, received scopolamine 0.4 mg/kg, i.p.

Group IV: Dys100 group, received ethanolic extract of DA 100 mg/kg p.o. + scopolamine 0.4 mg/kg i.p.

Group V: Dys200 group, received ethanolic extract of DA 200 mg/kg p.o. + scopolamine 0.4 mg/kg i.p.

Dys100 and Dys200 groups were subjected to their respective treatments once daily for 14 consecutive days. On day 15, 45 min after extract administration, scopolamine (0.4 mg/kg, i.p.) was injected into all the groups of animals, except the saline control group. The negative control group (Group III) received only scopolamine, on day 15. After one hour of scopolamine challenge, the behavioral tests were performed.

15.2.7 Behavioral Tests

15.2.7.1 Elevated Plus Maze (EPM)

To investigate memory and learning, the EPM model is extensively used in mice. The main principle of the EPM model is the innate aversion of rodents to open and high spaces. The EPM consists of two open arms (16 cm × 5 cm) and two closed arms (16 cm × 5 cm × 12 cm), bisecting each other to form a central platform of 5 cm^2, and the maze is elevated to a height of 25 cm above the ground (Ramadas et al., 2016; Joshi and Malviya, 2017).

Transfer latency (TL) was measured as a parameter reflecting enhancement of memory. Transfer latency is the time taken by a mouse to enter either of the closed arms from the open arm with all four paws (Dhingra et al., 2004). Each mouse was placed at the end of an open arm, facing away from the central platform, and allowed to explore the maze. The animal will then try to enter one of the enclosed arms as a result of thigmotaxis. A decrease in TL will indicate the enhancement of memory.

The experiment was set up in three phases. In the acclimatization phase (1 d), animals were transferred to the maze and allowed to explore it for 5 min without administering the drug. This phase was followed by a training phase (14 d) in which animals were treated with the respective treatments. Then, the animals were allowed to explore the maze, and TL was recorded manually. If an animal failed to enter the enclosed arms within 90 s, it was gently pushed into one of the two enclosed arms, using a glass beaker, and TL was recorded as 90 s. The mouse was allowed to explore the maze for 10 s and then returned to its home cage. The 15th day was the probe phase (the last phase), in which animals were subjected to the trial and TL was measured, using Anymaze software (Stoelting Co, Wood Dale, IL).

15.2.7.2 Barnes Maze Model

The Barnes maze model was first developed by Dr. Carol Barnes in 1979 to measure spatial learning and memory in rodents, such as mice or rats (Barnes, 1979). The fundamental purpose of the Barnes maze model is to evaluate the potential of a rodent to recognize the location of a target zone with the help of an arrangement of distal visual cues located around the testing area. This function is based on the ability of the animal to run away from an aversive environment. The Barnes maze model is widely used by neuroscientists for evaluating the effect of novel chemical entities on the cognitive deficit model for diseases, like AD, and also to determine the effect on retention of learning and spatial memory of a mild traumatic brain injury. The maze is a circular surface consisting of 20 circular holes around its circumference. Different-colored shapes are placed around the table as visual cues in plain sight of the animal, and radiant light is used to light the table surface. An "escape box", with some food, is placed under one of the holes. A rodent's aversion to open environments prompts the animal to look for shelter in the escape box. Within four to five trials, a normal rodent will learn to find the escape box (Gawel et al., 2019; Paul et al., 2009).

The experimental setup consisted of three phases. The first phase was the acclimatization phase (1 d), where the rats were placed at the center of the maze beneath a glass beaker for 30 s and, by slowly moving the glass beaker, the animals were directed to the target hole that leads to the escape box. Then, the rats were allowed to explore the maze freely for 5 min and to find the escape box through the target hole. If any rat failed to enter the escape box during the specified time, the rats were directed to enter with the help of the beaker. The animals were allowed to stay in the escape box for 1 min; after completing the session, the animals were returned to their home cage. During the second (training) phase (14 d), an opaque cardboard cylinder, 25 cm tall and 17.5 cm in diameter, was used to place the rats at the center of the maze for 15 s, in order to enable the rats to face in a random direction when the cylinder was lifted. As soon as the cylinder lifted, the trial began and the rats were allowed to move freely in the maze for 5 min. The time taken for the animal to enter the escape box was recorded as the escape latency. If the animals could not find the target hole, it was directed to the target hole using the glass beaker and allowed to freely enter the escape box, and stay there for 1 min, before being returned to the home cage. If, within 3 min, the animal did not go inside the escape box, it was directed to do that by nudging it with the help of the beaker. After 1 min of nudging, if a mouse did not enter the escape box, the mouse was manually put into the escape box.

The last phase was the probe phase (1 d), where the trial set-up was the same as for the training phase except that manual nudging was excluded. The escape latency and poke error values were noted for each animal. Anymaze software was used to record the escape latency, whereas poke error (the number of times the animal entered its head inside an incorrect hole) was counted manually.

15.2.7.3 Morris Water Maze (MWM)

The MWM test is one of the widely used tests by which to evaluate spatial learning and memory. Richard G. Morris, in 1981, designed the MWM test, which depends on visual cues to direct the test animals from the starting point to swim around the circumference of an open swimming arena and to locate a submerged escape platform. The MWM took place in a circular tank, 150 cm in diameter and 45 cm in height. The tank was filled with water and maintained at 25°C. The water was made non-transparent by adding milk. The pool was divided into four imaginary quadrants, marked as Q1, Q2, Q3, and Q4. Different-colored strips were attached to different quadrants as visual cues. A rectangular white platform, 20 cm × 10 cm, was placed in Q4, which is considered to be the target quadrant. The height of the platform was 28 cm, so that it presents 2 cm underneath the level of the water surface. Constant positions for visual cues and for the platform were maintained throughout the experiment (Dhingra and Kumar, 2012; Kim et al., 2016; Parameshwari et al., 2018; Bromley-Brits et al., 2011).

As in the other two behavioral models, MWM also composed of three phases. In the habituation phase (1 d), the mice were allowed to explore the water-filled maze for 60 s without installing the platform. During the training phase (14 d), each animal was subjected to four consecutive trials with an interval of 5 min between trials. During each trial, mice were allowed to detect the hidden platform and allowed to remain there for 20 s, before being returned to the home cage. The start point was different for each of the four trials (Q1, Q2, Q3, or Q4). The animals were guided to the platform with a stick if they were unable to locate the hidden platform. Following the completion of the training phase, the 15th day was considered to be the probe phase, with parameters, like the time required by the animal to reach the hidden platform, i.e. escape latency, and the distance traveled to locate the platform from the initiation point, being recorded, retaining the platform in a consistent position. Another parameter, time spent in the target quadrant, was recorded after removing the platform from its location. On the probe day, the site of initiation of the trial for each mouse was the same i.e. quadrant Q1. Each animal was allowed to explore the pool for 60 s and parameters were recorded by Anymaze software.

15.2.8 Statistical Analysis

Statistical analysis was performed using Graph Pad Prism software version 5.0 (GraphPad Software, San Diego, CA, USA). The statistical significance of differences among various experimental groups were calculated by one-way ANOVA, followed by Dunnett's multiple comparison tests. All the values were expressed as mean ± standard error of the mean (SEM) and the results were considered to be statistically significant at $P < 0.05$.

15.3 RESULTS

15.3.1 Phytochemical Analysis

The dried powder of DA was green, bitter, and had no specific odor. Phytochemical screening of the ethanolic extract of DA revealed the presence of glycosides, flavonoids, tannins, and steroids in the extract (Table 15.1).

15.3.2 Acute Toxicity Study

According to OECD guidelines no. 425, an oral dose of the ethanolic extract of up to 2000 mg/kg bodyweight did not cause any untoward effect in the mice. No changes were observed in behavior,

TABLE 15.1
Results of Phytochemical Screening of an Ethanolic Extract of *Dysphania ambrosioides*

Chemical Test	Results
A) Carbohydrates	
1) Molisch's Test	−ve
2) Benedict Test	−ve
B) Alkaloids	
1) Mayer's Test	−ve
2) Wagner's Test	−ve
C) Glycosides	
1) Modified Borntrager's Test	+ve
2) Legal's Test:	+ve
D) Proteins and amino acids	
1) Xanthoproteic Test	−ve
2) Ninhydrin Test	−ve
E) Flavonoids	
1) Shinoda Test	+ve
2) Lead acetate Test	+ve
F) Phytosterols	
1) Salkowski's Test	+ve
2) Liebermann Burchard's Test	+ve
G) Tannin	
1) Gelatin Test	

TABLE 15.2
Transfer Latency of Mice in Different Treatment Groups on the Probe Day

Group	Treatment	Dose (mg/kg)	Transfer latency (s)
I	Control (normal saline)	10 ml/kg, p.o.	6.500 ± 0.6455*
II	Scopolamine control	0.4 (i.p.)	11.500 ± 1.323 #
III	Standard (tacrine)	3 (i.p.)	4.500 ± 1.041**
IV	Dys100	100 (p.o.)	6.000 ± 1.581*
V	Dys200	200 (p.o.)	5.250 ± 0.8539**

All the values represent the mean ± standard error of the mean (SEM) (n = 6). # denotes $P < 0.5$, ## denotes $P < 0.01$ and ### denotes $P < 0.001$ when compared with the control, and * denotes $P < 0.05$, ** denotes $P < 0.01$ and *** denotes $P < 0.001$ when compared with the scopolamine control, as a result of one-way analysis of variance (ANOVA), followed by Dunnett's test.

motor, or neuronal functions. The extract did not cause any anatomical changes. Hence, 100 and 200 mg/kg oral doses of the extract were used in the study.

15.3.3 EPM

15.3.3.1 Effect on Transfer Latency (TL)

On the probe day, the effects of the vehicle (saline), tacrine, scopolamine, Dys100 and Dys200 on TL were recorded. The scopolamine-treated group showed a significant increase in TL ($P < 0.05$) when compared with the saline control group, indicating memory impairment in the mice, whereas tacrine (the standard drug) caused reduced TL in mice ($P < 0.01$), indicating amelioration of scopolamine-induced amnesia in the animals. Treatment with Dys100 or Dys200 before exposure to scopolamine also exhibited decreased TL in the mice, compared with the scopolamine-treated group (Table 15.2 and Figure 15.1).

15.3.4 Barnes Maze

15.3.4.1 Effect on Escape Latency and Poke Error

All the animals showed a decrease in escape latencies and poke errors across the trials. Mice in the scopolamine-treated group showed longer ELs and made more errors, compared with the untreated control group ($P < 0.01$). Mice in the tacrine-treated group exhibited the shortest ELs and made fewer poke errors ($P < 0.01$) in the trials. A significant decrease in ELs ($P < 0.01$) and poke errors ($P < 0.05$) were also observed in the case of animals treated with Dys100 and Dys200, prior to scopolamine treatment, when compared with the scopolamine-treated group (See , Figure 15.1, and Table 15.3).

15.3.5 MWM

15.3.5.1 Effect on Escape Latency and Path Length

Mice In the scopolamine-treated group showed a significant increase in EL, when compared with the untreated control group ($P < 0.01$), whereas mice in the standard group showed a significant decrease ($P < 0.001$), in the EL than the scopolamine induced group. Consecutive training sessions of 14 d in the MWM revealed significant retention of memory in the test groups. Dys100- and Dys200-treated mice rapidly learned the location of the hidden platform as reflected by a

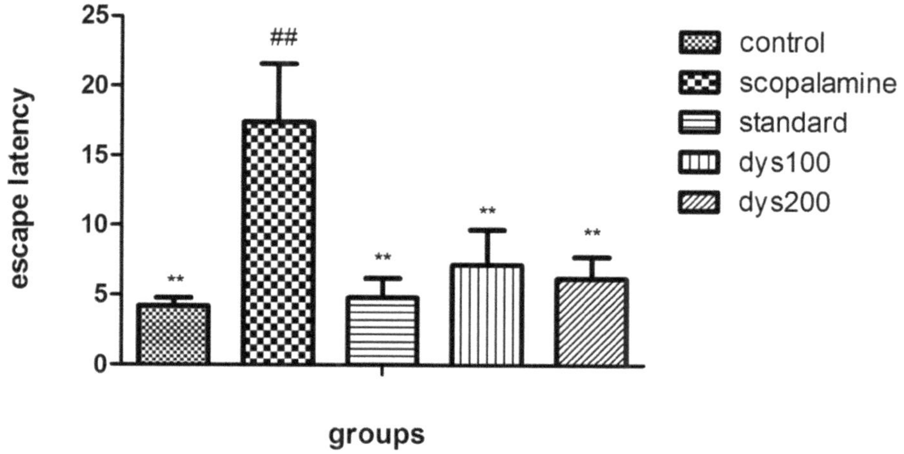

FIGURE 15.1 Effect on escape latency shown by mice in different treatment groups in the Barnes maze model. All the values represent the mean ± standard error of the mean, SEM (n=6). # denotes P < 0.05, ## denotes P < 0.01 and ### denotes P < 0.001 when compared with the control and * denotes P < 0.05, ** denotes P < 0.01 and *** denotes P < 0.001 when compared with the scopolamine control, as a result of one-way analysis of variance (ANOVA), followed by Dunnett's test.

TABLE 15.3
Effect on Numbers of Poke Errors (Barnes Maze Model) Made by Different Treatment Groups on the Probe Day

Group	Treatment	Dose (mg/kg)	Number of poke errors
I	Control (Normal saline)	10 ml/kg, p.o.	1.400 ± 0.5099**
II	Scopolamine	0.4 (i.p.)	7.000 ± 1.378 ##
III	Standard (tacrine)	3 (i.p.)	2.000 ± 0.8944**
IV	Dys100	100 (p.o.)	2.600 ± 1.249*
V	Dys200	200 (p.o.)	2.800 ± 0.8602*

All the values represent the mean ± standard error of the mean (SEM) (n=6), # denotes ***P*** < 0.05, ## denotes P < 0.01 and ### denotes P < 0.001 when compared with the control, and * denotes P < 0.05, ** denotes P < 0.01 and *** denotes P < 0.001 when compared with the scopolamine control, as a result of one-way analysis of variance (ANOVA), followed by Dunnett's test.

decrease in their latencies from day 1 to day 15, indicating the normal acquisition behavior. On the probe day, mice treated with Dys100 or Dys200 prior to treatment ($P < 0.001$) with scopolamine revealed significant decreases in EL, indicating alleviation of scopolamine-induced amnesia (Figure 15.2).

Mice in the scopolamine-treated group showed a longer path length ($P < 0.05$), compared with the control group, whereas mice in the standard group ($P < 0.01$) showed a significant decrease in the path length, compared with those in the scopolamine-treated group. Similarly, the path length (distance travel to reach the platform) was significantly shorter in both Dys100- and Dys200-treated groups ($P < 0.05$) compared with scopolamine treated group (Table 15.4 and Figure 15.5).

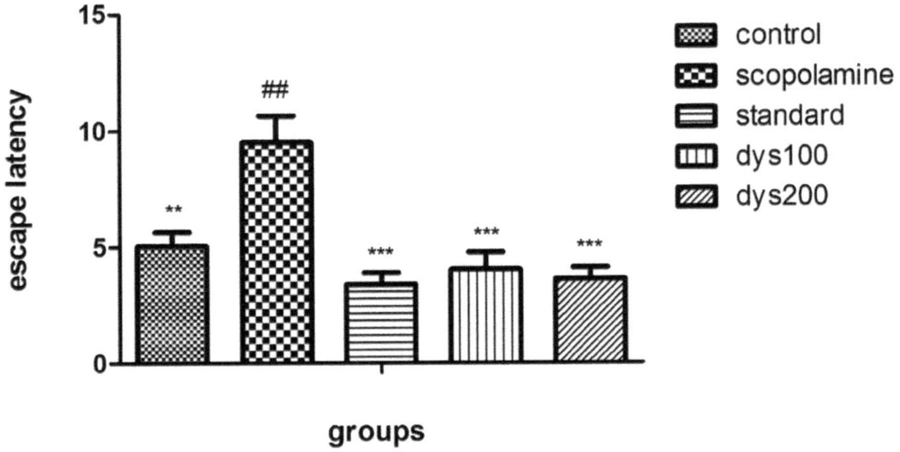

FIGURE 15.2 Effect on escape latency showed by different treatment groups of rats in the MWM model. All the values represent the mean ± standard error of the mean (SEM) (n=6). #denotes P < 0.05, ##denotes P < 0.01 and ### denotes P < 0.001 when compared with the control, and *denotes P < 0.05, **denotes P < 0.01 and ***denotes P < 0.001when compared with the scopolamine control, as a result of one-way analysis of variance (ANOVA), followed by Dunnett's test.

TABLE 15.4
Path Lengths of Different Treatment Groups on the Probe Day (MWM)

Group	Treatment	Dose (mg/kg)	Path length (m)
I	Control (normal saline)	10 ml/kg, p.o.	0.1945±0.0319*
II	Scopolamine	0.4 (i.p.)	0.3803±0.05008 #
III	Standard (tacrine)	3 (i.p.)	0.1485±0.04831**
IV	Dys100	100 (p.o.)	0.1993±0.03424*
V	Dys200	200 (p.o.)	0.1643±0.05006*

All the values represent the mean ± standard error of the mean (SEM) (n=6), # denotes ***P***<0.05, ## denotes P<0.01 and ### denotes P<0.001 when compared with the control, and * denotes P<0.05, ** denotes P<0.01 and *** denotes P<0.001 when compared with the scopolamine control, as a result of one-way analysis of variance (ANOVA), followed by Dunnett's test.

TABLE 15.5
Total Time Spent in the Target Quadrant by Different Treatment Groups on the Probe Day (MWM)

Group	Treatment	Dose (mg/kg)	Time spent in target quadrant (s)
I	Control (normal saline)	10 ml/kg, p.o.	29.48±5.795
II	Scopolamine	0.4 (i.p.)	24.68±5.773
III	Standard (tacrine)	3 (i.p.)	43.00±4.282
IV	Dys100	100 (p.o.)	32.08±7.014
V	Dys200	200 (p.o.)	33.33±3.659

All the values represent the mean±standard error of the mean (SEM) (n=6). # denotes ***P***<0.05 when compared with the saline control, and * denotes P<0.05 when compared with the scopolamine control, as a result of one-way analysis of variance (ANOVA), followed by Dunnett's test.

15.3.5.2 Effect on Total Time Spent in the Target Quadrant

The total time spent in the target quadrant was measured by removing the platform from the target quadrant (Q4) and then allowing the animals to explore the maze. Analysis of the swimming performance during the probe trial revealed that animals which had received scopolamine spent less time in the target quadrant, whereas mice which had received Dys100 or Dys200 prior to scopolamine treatment spent comparatively more time in the target zone (Table 15.5 and Figure 15.6).

15.4 DISCUSSION

AD is a debilitating neurodegenerative disorder, the incidence of which continues to rise worldwide (Kulkarni et al., 2011). AD involves progressive loss of memory and cognition, characterized by aphasia, apraxia, and agnosia (Saikia et al., 2018). Despite the availability of a number of allopathic medicines for the treatment of AD, searches for herbal remedies with high potency and fewer side effects than the allopathic drugs is going on. The present study investigated the therapeutic efficacy of an ethanolic extract of *D. ambrosioides* for memory enhancement. Scopolamine was used to induce the impairment of memory in the experimental animals. In the acute toxicity study, no death was observed up to a dose of 2000 mg/kg. The mice were physically active, indicating that the median half-maximal lethal dose (LD_{50}) could be higher than 2000 mg/kg in mice.

The elevated plus maze, Morris water maze, and Barnes maze models were employed to assess the memory-enhancing effects of the ethanolic extract of *D. ambrosioides*. These models are commonly used for assessment of anti-amnesic property of drugs.

The results of the EPM task revealed that mice, after oral treatment with Dys100 or Dys200, prior to scopolamine treatment, showed a significant decline in TL quite similar to the effects observed after administration of the standard nootropic drug, tacrine. This suggests the possible memory-enhancing property of both Dys100 and Dys200. Moreover, both the extracts were assessed for their cognitive enhancement effect on mice against scopolamine-induced amnesia, using MWM. Reversal of scopolamine-induced amnesic parameters in the MWM test reflected increased retention of memory in the animals. Both the Dys100 and Dys200 groups showed remarkable reductions in EL and path lengths, when compared with the scopolamine group. In addition to this, the animals also spent more time in the target quadrant searching for the platform removed from the target quadrant, which is an indicator of cognitive improvement. The Barnes maze test was performed on rats in order to assess the retention of memory in animals. EL and the number of poke errors were recorded as markers of memory enhancement. The two test groups, Dys100 and Dys200, each took comparatively less time to find the target hole and made fewer poke errors, in contrast with the scopolamine-treated group.

Hence, it was revealed from the study that administration of an ethanolic extract of *D. ambrosioides* (15 d oral administration) showed a pronounced effect on reversal of scopolamine-induced memory loss in rodents. Comparatively, the higher dose (200 mg/kg) of DA extract showed greater activity than the lower dose (100 mg/kg) of the extract. This is the first preclinical study investigating the memory-enhancing activity of the ethanolic extract of DA. In Peru, the plant is also reported to be used ethnomedicinally as a memory enhancer (Potawale et al., 2008). Oxidative stress plays an important role in aggravating the pathogenesis of AD. It facilitates abnormal accumulation of Aβ- and tau protein-initiated neurotoxicity (Dhingra and Kumar, 2012; Kim et al., 2016; Uddin et al., 2016). Scopolamine causes memory impairment in experimental animals by blocking the cholinergic neurotransmission (Pushpalatha et al., 2013), whereas oxidative stress induced by scopolamine can also lead to a decline in memory (Fan et al., 2005). An antioxidant property of DA has also been reported (Barros et al., 2013; Nascimento et al., 2006). Thus, the memory-enhancing activity of the ethanolic extract of DA might be due to multiple factors in the extract, with properties such as antioxidant and elevated cholinergic neurotransmission.

15.5 CONCLUSION

The reversal of the amnesic behaviors in the behavioral models, following administration of scopolamine, suggest the increased memory retention capacity of the ethanolic extract of DA. The amelioration of scopolamine-induced amnesia by the extracts may be associated with the antioxidant properties of the plant. This study supports the traditional claim of the plant as a memory enhancer. However, biochemical analysis and insight into the probable underlying mechanism(s) will be required in order to understand the clinical efficacy of the plant extract.

ACKNOWLEDGMENTS

The authors express their deep gratitude to the Dean and the Director of Research (Vety), College of veterinary science, Assam Agricultural University, Khanapara, Assam, for providing us with the facilities with which to carry out this research work.

REFERENCES

Abiola AL, Medinat AO, Julius OI, Emmanuel OG, Gbola O. Anti-amnesic and cognitive enhancing effects of ethanol leaf extract of *Milicia excelsa* (Moraceae) in mice. *International Journal of Neuroscience and Behavioral Science.* 2019;7(1):1–11.

Barnes CA. Memory deficits associated with senescence: a neurophysiological and behavioral study in the rat. *Journal of Comparative and Physiological Psychology.* 1979;93(1):74.

Barros L, Pereira E, Calhelha RC, Dueñas M, Carvalho AM, Santos-Buelga C, Ferreira IC. Bioactivity and chemical characterization in hydrophilic and lipophilic compounds of *Chenopodium ambrosioides* L. *Journal of Functional Foods.* 2013;5(4):1732–1740.

Bromley-Brits K, Deng Y, Song W. Morris water maze test for learning and memory deficits in Alzheimer's disease model mice. *Journal of Visualized Experiments.* 2011(53):e2920.

Dhingra D, Kumar V. Memory-enhancing activity of palmatine in mice using elevated plus maze and Morris water maze. *Advances in Pharmacological Sciences.* 2012;2012:1–7.

Dhingra D, Parle M, Kulkarni S. Memory enhancing activity of *Glycyrrhiza glabra* in mice. *Journal of Ethnopharmacology.* 2004;91(2–3):361–365.

Fan Y, Hu J, Li J, Yang Z, Xin X, Wang J, Ding J, Geng M. Effect of acidic oligosaccharide sugar chain on scopolamine-induced memory impairment in rats and its related mechanisms. *Neuroscience Letters.* 2005;374(3):222–226.

Gadano A, Gurni A, López P, Ferraro G, Carballo M. In vitro genotoxic evaluation of the medicinal plant *Chenopodium ambrosioides* L. *Journal of Ethnopharmacology.* 2002;81(1):11–16.

Gawel K, Gibula E, Marszalek-Grabska M, Filarowska J, Kotlinska JH. Assessment of spatial learning and memory in the Barnes maze task in rodents—methodological consideration. *Naunyn-Schmiedeberg's Archives of Pharmacology.* 2019;392(1):1–18.

Hirai S. Distinction between dementia and memory decline. *Japan Medical Association Journal.* 2001;44(6):274–278.

Joshi A, Malviya N. Memory enhancing activity of hydroalcoholic extract of *Terminalia catappa* leaves. *Journal of Drug Delivery and Therapeutics.* 2017;7(7):197–199.

Kamila S, Madhav NVS, Sarkar CN. Screening of novel polyphyto formulations, natural remedies for learning and memory enhancing properties in rat. *International Journal of Nutrition, Pharmacology, Neurological Diseases.* 2015;5(1):13.

Kim E, Ko HJ, Jeon SJ, Lee S, Lee HE, Kim HN, Woo ER, Ryu JH. The memory-enhancing effect of erucic acid on scopolamine-induced cognitive impairment in mice. *Pharmacology Biochemistry and Behavior.* 2016;142:85–90.

Kliks MM. Studies on the traditional herbal anthelmintic *Chenopodium ambrosioides* L.: ethnopharmacological evaluation and clinical field trials. *Social Science & Medicine.* 1985;21(8):879–886.

Kulkarni PD, Ghaisas MM, Chivate ND, Sankpal PS. Memory enhancing activity of *Cissampelos pariera* in mice. *International Journal of Pharmacy and Pharmaceutical Sciences.* 2011;3(2):206–211.

Kumar R, Mishra AK, Dubey N, Tripathi Y. Evaluation of *Chenopodium ambrosioides* oil as a potential source of antifungal, antiaflatoxigenic and antioxidant activity. *International journal of Food Microbiology.* 2007;115(2):159–164.

Nascimento FR, Cruz GV, Pereira PVS, Maciel MC, Silva LA, Azevedo APS, Barroqueiro ESB, Guerra RN. Ascitic and solid Ehrlich tumor inhibition by *Chenopodium ambrosioides* L. treatment. *Life Sciences.* 2006;78(22):2650–2653.

Patiri B., Borah A. *Wild Edible Plants of Assam.* Guwahati: Geetakhi Printers and Publishers. 2007.

Parameshwari K, Neeta C, Prathima C. Investigation on learning and memory-enhancing activity of *Saraca asoca* flower (Roxb.) Wilde in experimental mice. *National Journal of Physiology, Pharmacy and Pharmacology.* 2018;8(9):1250–1255.

Patterson C. *World Alzheimer Report 2018: The State of the Art of Dementia Research: New Frontiers.* London, UK: Alzheimer's Disease International (ADI). 2018.

Paul C-M, Magda G, Abel S. Spatial memory: theoretical basis and comparative review on experimental methods in rodents. *Behavioural Brain Research.* 2009;203(2):151–164.

Pereira WS, Ribeiro BP, Sousa AI, Serra IC, Mattar NS, Fortes TS, Reis AS, Silva LA, Barroqueiro ES, Guerra RN, Nascimento FR. Evaluation of the subchronic toxicity of oral treatment with *Chenopodium ambrosioides* in mice. *Journal of Ethnopharmacology.* 2010;127(3):602–605.

Potawale SE, Luniya KP, Mantri RA, Mehta UK, Waseem MD, Sadiq MD, Vetal YD, Deshmukh RS. *Chenopodium ambrosioides*: an ethnopharmacological review. *Pharmacology online.* 2008;2:272–286.

Pushpalatha B, Venumadhav N, Swathi M, Raju AB. Neuroprotective effect of resveratrol against scopolamine-induced cognitive impairment and oxidative stress in rats. *Archives of Biological Sciences.* 2013;65:1381–1386.

Ramadas D, Ravishankar M, Shwetha S, Srinivas L. The learning and memory enhancing properties of *Bacopa monnieri* plant leaves protein: a systematic study in Wistar Albino rats model system. *Scholars Academic Journal of Biosciences.* 2016;4(2):179–184.

Renu G, Thilakar SJ, Narasimhan D. *Chenopodium ambrosioides L. Synonym of Dysphania ambrosioides(L.) Mosyakin & Clemants.* accessed 15 May. https://indiabiodiversity.org/biodiv/species/show/266344.

Richardson JT, Zucco GM. Cognition and olfaction: a review. *Psychological Bulletin.* 1989;105(3):352.

Sá RD, Santana AS, Silva FC, Soares LAL, Randau KP. Anatomical and histochemical analysis of *Dysphania ambrosioides* supported by light and electron microscopy. *Revista Brasileira de Farmacognosia.* 2016;26(5):533–543.

Saikia B, Barua CC, Sarma J, Haloi P, Tamuli SM, Kalita DJ, Purkayastha A, Barua AG. *Zanthoxylum alatum* ameliorates scopolamine-induced amnesia in rats: behavioral, biochemical, and molecular evidence. *Indian Journal of Pharmacology.* 2018;50(1):30.

Tongjaroenbuangam W, Ruksee N, Chantiratikul P, Pakdeenarong N, Kongbuntad W, Govitrapong P. Neuroprotective effects of quercetin, rutin and okra (*Abelmoschus esculentus* Linn.) in dexamethasone-treated mice. *Neurochemistry International.* 2011;59(5):677–685.

Uddin MS, Al Mamun A, Hossain MS, Akter F, Iqbal MA, Asaduzzaman M. Exploring the effect of *Phyllanthus emblica* L. on cognitive performance, brain antioxidant markers and acetylcholinesterase activity in rats: promising natural gift for the mitigation of Alzheimer's disease. *Annals of Neurosciences.* 2016;23(4):218–229.

Zohra T, Ovais M, Khalil AT, Qasim M, Ayaz M, Shinwari ZK. Extraction optimization, total phenolic, flavonoid contents, HPLC-DAD analysis and diverse pharmacological evaluations of *Dysphania ambrosioides* (L.) Mosyakin & Clemants. *Natural Product Research.* 2019;33(1):136–142.

16 Neuroprotective Role of Quercetin in Alzheimer's Disease

Magisetty Obulesu

CONTENTS

ABBREVIATIONS

AD	Alzheimer's Disease
APP	Amyloid Precursor Protein
APP/PS1	Amyloid Precursor Protein/Presenilin-1
Aβ	Amyloid-Beta
BBB	Blood–Brain Barrier
CURC	Curcumin
ISR	Integrated Stress Response
NaR	Sodium Salt of Rutin

16.1 INTRODUCTION

The number of AD patients has increased remarkably in developed countries (Maher and Schubert, 2009; Huang et al., 2019). Epidemiological studies have shown that diabetic patients have an enhanced risk of developing AD (Kopf and Frolich, 2009; Han and Li, 2010; Huang et al., 2019). Quercetin, a plant flavonoid, is abundantly available in a wide range of foods, such as red onions, tea, broccoli, and apples (Nijveldt et al., 2001; Li et al., 2019). With its known antioxidant, anti-inflammatory, and antiapoptotic effects, quercetin shows substantial efficacy in the treatment of diabetes and its associated complications (Youl et al., 2010; Eid et al., 2015; Peng et al., 2017; Li et al., 2019). Quercetin also shows anticancer, antithrombotic, antiatherosclerotic, and antihypertensive activities, in addition to its potential to control resistance to various drugs (Bischoff, 2008; Chen et al., 2010; Larson et al., 2010; Kressler et al., 2011; Russo et al., 2012; Paula et al., 2019). Quercetin was found to ameliorate cognitive function in mice supplied with a high-fat diet, probably by intervening in the Nrf2 signaling pathway (Xia et al., 2015; Li et al., 2019).

The biological and neuroprotective roles of quercetin have been extensively studied and reviewed (Pocernich et al., 2011; Babaei et al., 2018; Nakagawa and Ohta, 2019). The neuroprotective roles of quercetin against AD have been corroborated in a plethora of cell and animal models (Ansari et al., 2009; Sabogal-Guaqueta et al., 2015; Kong et al., 2016; Li et al., 2019). Although pretreatment with quercetin improved amyloid-β_{1-42} ($A\beta_{1-42}$)-initiated protein oxidation, cytotoxicity, lipid peroxidation, and apoptosis, increased doses showed toxicity and failed to show neuroprotection in cultured neurons (Ansari et al., 2009; Li et al., 2019). Quercetin probably plays a positive role in neurogenesis and brain-derived neurotrophic factor (BDNF) expression, and consequently delays the progression of early-stage AD (Nakagawa et al., 2016, 2019). A few studies have shown that quercetin protects neurons against cytotoxicity, lipid peroxidation, protein oxidation, and apoptosis induced by amyloid-beta (Aβ), and mediates the activity of antioxidant genes (Paula et al., 2019).

Since quercetin has similar bioavailability characteristics in both rats and humans, and shows no gender-based variation, its treatment is highly effective in AD patients (Burak et al., 2017; Paula et al., 2019). Studies have also shown that natural powder extracts of food containing quercetin show higher bioavailability of quercetin than the pure dihydrate powder and this also acts as a robust food matrix (Kashino et al., 2015; Paula et al., 2019). Quercetin has been found to have 3.5-fold higher antioxidant activity than curcumin (Zhang et al., 2011; Saleem et al., 2019). Despite the scant knowledge about the mechanisms of the neuroprotective action by quercetin, its neural effects have been proven in both *in-vitro* and *in-vivo* models (Mercer et al., 2005; Arredondo et al., 2010; Paula et al., 2019).

16.2 QUERCETIN-3-RUTINOSIDE

Rutin (quercetin-3-rutinoside), a natural flavonoid, has had its various biological functions confirmed in a number of pathological conditions (Habtemariam, 2016; Pan et al., 2019). It is abundantly available in plants, fruits, and vegetables, and has no toxic effect even if consumed as a supplement along with a daily diet (Yuan et al., 2017; Pan et al., 2019). It specifically offers antioxidative and anti-inflammatory effects in the treatment of obesity, diabetes, and AD (Xu et al., 2014; Yuan et al., 2017; Pan et al., 2019). Although it shows appreciable biological activity, its low aqueous solubility (0.125 g/l at room temperature) and low bioavailability significantly impede its usage (Samsonowicz et al., 2015; Pan et al., 2019). A number of strategies have been developed to overcome problems of low solubility and bioavailability in other such compounds (Mauludin et al., 2009; Sato et al., 2015; Pan et al., 2019); salt formation has been extensively used to enhance the solubility and dissolution rates of drugs (Serajuddin, 2007; Samsonowicz et al., 2015; Pan et al., 2019). In line with this, the sodium salt of rutin, NaR, showed appreciable solubility and bioavailability, and ameliorated learning and memory dysfunction in amyloid precursor protein/presenilin-1 (APP/PS1) and 5xFAD mouse models of AD (Pan et al., 2019).

NaR administration has been found to inhibit neuroinflammation and to increase mitochondrial oxidative phosphorylation and microglia-regulated Aβ scavenging, improving synaptic plasticity, spatial learning, and memory dysfunction (Pan et al., 2019). While microglial phagocytosis requires large amounts of energy, TREM-2 deficiency results in a remarkable reduction in adenosine 5'-triphosphate (ATP) production (Engl and Attwell, 2015; Ulland et al., 2017; Pan et al., 2019). Moreover, metabolic impairment has been reported in the etiopathogenesis of sporadic AD (Hoyer, 2002; Pan et al., 2019). A metabolic switch from mitochondrial oxidative phosphorylation to anaerobic glycolysis has been found in activated microglia in AD subjects and in M1 macrophages initiated by lipopolysaccharide (LPS), bacteria, or interferon-γ (Galvan-Pena and O'Neill, 2014; Ulland et al., 2017; Wendeln et al., 2018; Pan et al., 2019).

Being the local immune cells of the brain, microglia detect Aβ aggregation and induce phagocytosis (Fu et al., 2016; Pan et al., 2019). Nevertheless, phagocytic efficacy of microglia deteriorates with age and impedes the Aβ scavenging during AD progression (Hickman et al., 2008;

Pan et al., 2019). It is understood that phagocytosis regulates brain homeostasis by eliminating undesirable cellular debris and misfolded proteins (Diaz-Aparicio et al., 2016; Pan et al., 2019). Studies have shown that perturbation in the expression of multiple phagocytic receptors results in neurodegeneration (Lucin et al., 2013; Pan et al., 2019). Therefore, upregulation of these receptors ameliorates the phagocytosis of accumulated pathological proteins such as Aβ, and slows the progression of neuropathology (Jiang et al., 2014; Lee et al., 2018; Pan et al., 2019). Pan et al. (2019) showed that NaR substantially enhanced the expression of these receptors and combated Aβ-mediated pathology.

16.3 INTEGRATED STRESS RESPONSE (ISR) SIGNALING

Mounting evidence has shown that enhanced endoplasmic reticulum (ER) stress contributes to AD pathology, both in mouse models and in AD patients (O'Connor et al., 2008; Hoozemans et al., 2009; Segev et al., 2013; Endres and Reinhardt, 2013; Lourenco et al., 2015; Nakagawa and Ohta 2019). Studies have shown that ISR regulates memory dysfunction in AD, which is linked with APOE4 (Oliveira and Lourenco, 2016; Nakagawa and Ohta 2019). Quercetin plays a pivotal role in ameliorating pathological conditions like diabetes and AD, by mediating antioxidative stress enzymes through the action of Nrf2 and the antioxidant effect of *PON2* expression (Kobori et al., 2009; Costa et al., 2016; Zaplatic et al., 2019; Nakagawa and Ohta 2019). In line with this, several studies have shown the neuroprotective action of quercetin in memory amelioration through ISR regulation (Lu et al., 2010; Hayakawa et al., 2015; Nakagawa et al., 2017, Nakagawa and Ohta 2019). Combating ISR signaling with quercetin offers appreciable therapeutic benefit by attenuating Aβ production and averting cognitive dysfunction (Nakagawa and Ohta 2019).

16.4 ANIMAL MODELS

Several lines of evidence have shown that quercetin increases the life span of *Drosophila* and also climbing ability in AD flies. Studies have also shown that quercetin protects cell cycle proteins, which are perturbed due to Aβ aggregation (Kong et al., 2016; Li et al., 2019). A three-month quercetin treatment significantly reduced extracellular β-amyloidosis and improved microglial and astroglial activation in the brain, as observed by reduced levels of $A\beta_{1\text{-}40}$, $A\beta_{1\text{-}42}$ and beta-amyloid cleaving enzymel (BACE1) -induced cleavage of APP in a triple transgenic AD mouse model (Sabogal-Guaqueta et al., 2015; Li et al., 2019). With robust antioxidant action, quercetin mitigated Aβ plaque accumulation and interleukin-1β (IL-1β)/ cyclooxygenase-2 (COX-2)/ inducible nitric oxide synthase (iNOS) proinflammatory signaling in the hippocampal CA-1 region of triple transgenic AD mice (Vargas-Restrepo et al., 2018; Li et al., 2019).

The neuroprotective role of quercetin has been studied in a number of species (Wang et al., 2014; Sabogal-Guaqueta et al., 2015; Kong et al., 2016; Moreno et al., 2017; Rishitha and Muthuraman, 2018; Vargas-Restrepo et al., 2018; Karimipour et al., 2019; Nakagawa et al., 2019). Quercetin showed significant amelioration of learning impairment and memory loss, and instigated neurogenesis in $A\beta_{1\text{-}42}$ treated rats (Karimipour et al., 2019; Nakagawa et al., 2019). It has also been shown that quercetin ameliorates cognitive dysfunction in the APP/PS1dE9 mouse model by mitigating mitochondrial dysfunction through the control of 5' AMP-activated protein kinase (AMPK) activity (Wang et al., 2014; Nakagawa et al., 2019). Oral administration of 0.5% quercetin for 5 weeks decreased the levels of activating transcription factor-4 (ATF-4) expression in the amygdala, hippocampus, and cerebral cortex of the brain of APP23/$Lepr^{db/db}$ mice (Nakagawa et al., 2017, 2019). This reduction in ATF-4 expression has been found in the brain of APP23 mice to which quercetin was administered for more than one year (Hayakawa et al., 2015; Nakagawa et al., 2019). Furthermore, chronic (12 months) oral administration of quercetin profoundly combated tauopathy in the hippocampus and amygdala, thus decreasing β-amyloidosis in the triple transgenic Alzheimer's Disease mouse (3x-Tg-AD) model (Paula et al., 2019).

16.5 THERAPEUTIC ROLE OF QUERCETIN-CONTAINING PLANT EXTRACTS

Abelmoschus esculentus (AE), commonly known as okra, is a vegetable which is well known for its antidiabetic effect (Chiu and Chang, 1995; Council, 2006; Huang et al., 2019). AE extracts F1 (with high concentrations of quercetin glucosides and the triterpene ester) and F2 (with a high concentration of polysaccharides) substantially inhibited dipeptidyl peptidase-4 (DPP-4)-mediated apoptosis (Huang et al., 2019). F1 inhibited Aβ-instigated caspase-3 expression at a concentration of 25 μg/mL, whereas F2 inhibited caspase-3 activation at 1 μg/mL (Huang et al., 2019). Both fractions reduced Aβ-increased DPP-4 activity but increased Aβ-reduced phospho-AMPK (p-AMPK) concentration and phosphorylation of phosphatidylinositol 3-kinase (p-PI3K) (Peng et al., 2016; Huang et al., 2017, 2019).

Albizia lebbek seed extract (ALE), which contains quercetin, has shown substantial protection against cognitive dysfunction by improving cholinergic deficits, probably by attenuating hyperactive acetylcholinesterase (AChE) (Saleem et al., 2019). *A. lebbek* belongs to the family Fabaceae (Saleem et al., 2019). It is a deciduous tree with bipinnate leaves and white odorous flowers, with each fruit containing 6–12 seeds (Saleem et al., 2019). The seeds have long been used in the treatment of various diseases, such as leukoderma, diarrhea, gonorrhea, and piles (Verma et al., 2013; Srivastav Neeti et al., 2016; Saleem et al., 2019). They are also known for their neuropharmacological activity (Islam et al., 2018; Saleem et al., 2019). ALE administration ameliorated spatial, associative, and working cognition and memory, and enabled the patients to return to the social interactions of life, which had been suppressed in AD (Jheng and Pai, 2009; Schiller et al., 2015; Saleem et al., 2019).

16.6 NANOTECHNOLOGY

Nanotechnology plays an important role in targeted delivery of therapeutic molecules and their controlled release. Oral administration of quercetin-loaded nanoparticles (NPs) significantly alleviated cognitive and memory impairments in senescence accelerated mouse-prone 8 (SAMP8) mice (Moreno et al., 2017; Nakagawa et al., 2019). In another study, concave cubic quercetin-modified and gold–palladium tethered NPs were designed, which enhanced the autophagy of SH-SY5Y cells, and induced the binding of autophagosomes and lysosomes, thus augmenting Aβ scavenging (Liu et al., 2019). Indeed, the autophagous lysosomal pathway primarily guards cells from misfolded and aggregated proteins, and necrotic organelles, thereby substantially scavenging protein aggregates and organelles involved in cell death (Moreau et al., 2014; Vilchez et al., 2014; Issa et al., 2018; Liu et al., 2019). Since autophagy impairment has been the underlying cause of neurodegenerative diseases such as AD and Parkinson's Disease (PD) (Maulik et al., 2015; Martini-Stoica et al., 2016; Kerr et al., 2017; Zhu et al., 2017), the nanoformulation developed by Liu et al. (2019) significantly facilitates the treatment of these diseases.

16.7 LIPOSOMES

Liposomes have long been used to encapsulate both hydrophilic and hydrophobic drugs, due to their bilayer structure and their ability to offer controlled release of drugs (Spuch and Navarro, 2011; Kuo et al., 2019). Although liposomes loaded with multiple pharmaceutical compounds show substantial therapeutic activity against neurodegenerative diseases, inadequate nerve-targeting ability and low traversing ability of liposomes through the blood–brain barrier (BBB) significantly impede their success (Kuo et al., 2019). To overcome these challenges, a recent study has shown the development of liposomes containing cardiolipin and phosphatidic acid to target tau hyperphosphorylation, and a transactivator of a transcription factor (TAT) to span the BBB for nerve growth factor, rosmarinic acid, curcumin, and quercetin. Interestingly, these liposomes showed enhanced cell viability in SK-N-MC cells treated with Aβ fibrils, and averted hyperphosphorylation of tau proteins in the Wistar rat brain (Kuo et al., 2019). The TAT peptide facilitates BBB ferrying and localization of the formulation around neuronal nuclei, thereby enhancing its therapeutic ability (Liu et al., 2008; Torchilin, 2008; Qin et al., 2011; Kuo et al., 2019).

16.8 CONCLUSIONS AND FUTURE PERSPECTIVES

Quercetin exhibits important biological roles, as well as an antioxidant capacity higher than that of curcumin. Research has overcome the water solubility issue of quercetin by making a salt form of it. In addition, other studies have employed nanotechnological methods to overcome the solubility, bioavailability, and side effect issues associated with quercetin. However, there is still significant ambiguity about the neuroprotective role of quercetin since the *in-vitro* results showed neuroprotection, whereas several *in-vivo* studies failed to show neuroprotection after chronic oral administration (Dajas et al., 2015; Paula et al., 2019). There is also a substantial need to optimize the daily doses of quercetin, since side effects, such as renal dysfunction and breast cancer vulnerability, have been reported (Andres et al., 2018; Paula et al., 2019). Based on the above findings, it can be concluded that there is a pressing need to develop more appropriate methods to combat neurodegeneration, using quercetin or its nanotechnological formulations.

REFERENCES

Andres S, Pevny S, Ziegenhagen R, Bakhiya N, Schafer B, Hirsch-Ernst KI, Lampen A. Safety aspects of the use of quercetin as a dietary supplement. *Mol Nutr Food Res.* 2018;62:1700447.

Ansari MA, Abdul HM, Joshi G, Opii WO, Butterfield DA. Protective effect of quercetin in primary neurons against Aβ(1–42): relevance to Alzheimer's disease. *J Nutr Biochem.* 2009;20:269–275.

Arredondo F, Echeverry C, Abin-Carriquiry JA, Blasina F, Antunez K, Jones DP, Go YM, Liang YL, Dajas F. After cellular internalization, quercetin causes Nrf2 nuclear translocation, increases glutathione levels, and prevents neuronal death against an oxidative insult. *Free Radic Biol Med.* 2010;49:738–747.

Babaei F, Mirzababaei M, Nassiri-Asl M. Quercetin in food: possible mechanisms of its effect on memory. *J Food Sci.* 2018;83:2280–2287.

Bischoff SC. Quercetin: potentials in the prevention and therapy of disease. *Curr Opin Clin Nutr Metab Care.* 2008;11:733–740.

Burak C, Brull V, Langguth P, Zimmermann BF, Stoffel-Wagner B, Sausen U, Stehle P, Wolffram S, Egert S. Higher plasma quercetin levels following oral administration of an onion skin extract compared with pure quercetin dihydrate in humans. *Eur J Nutr.* 2017;56:343–353.

Chen C, Zhou J, Ji C. Quercetin: a potential drug to reverse multidrug resistance. *Life Sci.* 2010;87:333–338.

Chiu N, Chang K. *The Illustrated Medicinal Plants in Taiwan.* Volume I. SMC Publ. Inc., Taipei (In Chinese), 1995.

Costa LG, Garrick JM, Roque PJ, Pellacani C. Mechanisms of neuroprotection by quercetin: counteracting oxidative stress and more. *Oxid Med Cell Longev.* 2016;2016:2986796.

Council NR. *Lost Crops of Africa: Volume II: Vegetables.* National Academies Press, 2006.

Dajas F, Abin-carriquiry JA, Arredondo F, Echeverry C, Martinez M, Rivera F, Vaamonde L. Quercetin in brain diseases: potential and limits. *Neurochem Int.* 2015;89:140–148.

Diaz-Aparicio I, Beccari S, Abiega O, Sierra A. Clearing the corpses: regulatory mechanisms, novel tools, and therapeutic potential of harnessing microglial phagocytosis in the diseased brain. *Neural Regen Res.* 2016;11:1533–1539.

Eid HM, Nachar A, Thong F, Sweeney G, Haddad PS. The molecular basis of the antidiabetic action of quercetin in cultured skeletal muscle cells and hepatocytes. *Pharmacogn Mag.* 2015;11:74–81.

Endres K, Reinhardt S. ER-stress in Alzheimer's disease: turning the scale? *Am J Neurodegener Dis.* 2013;2:247–265.

Engl E, Attwell D. Non-signalling energy use in the brain. *J Physiol.* 2015;593:3417–3429.

Fu AKY, Hung KW, Yuen MYF, Zhou X, Mak DSY, Chan ICW, Cheung TH, Zhang B, Fu WY, Liew FY, Ip NY. IL-33 ameliorates Alzheimer's disease-like pathology and cognitive decline. *Proc Natl Acad Sci USA.* 2016;113:E2705–E2713.

Galvan-Pena S, O'Neill LAJ. Metabolic reprograming in macrophage polarization. *Front Immunol.* 2014;5:420.

Habtemariam S. Rutin as a natural therapy for Alzheimer's disease: insights into its mechanisms of action. *Curr Med Chem.* 2016;23:860–873.

Han W, Li C. Linking type 2 diabetes and Alzheimer's disease. *Proc Natl Acad Sci.* 2010;107:6557–6558.

Hayakawa M, Itoh M, Ohta K, Li S, Ueda M, Wang MX, Nishida E, Islam S, Suzuki C, Ohzawa K, Kobori M, Inuzuka T, Nakagawa T. Quercetin reduces eIF2alpha phosphorylation by GADD34 induction. *Neurobiol Aging.* 2015;36:2509–2518.

Hickman SE, Allison EK, El Khoury J. Microglial dysfunction and defective β-amyloid clearance pathways in aging Alzheimer's disease mice. *J Neurosci.* 2008;28:8354–8360.

Hoozemans JJ, van Haastert ES, Nijholt DA, Rozemuller AJ, Eikelenboom P, Scheper W. The unfolded protein response is activated in pretangle neurons in Alzheimer's disease hippocampus. *Am J Pathol.* 2009;174:1241–1251.

Hoyer S. The brain insulin signal transduction system and sporadic (type II) Alzheimer disease: an update. *J Neural Transm.* 2002;109:341–360.

Huang CN, Wang CJ, Lee YJ, Peng CH. Active subfractions of *Abelmoschus esculentus* substantially prevent free fatty acid-induced β cell apoptosis via inhibiting dipeptidyl peptidase-4. *PloS One.* 2017;12:e0180285.

Huang CN, Wang CJ, Lin CL, Yen AT, Li HH, Peng CH. *Abelmoschus esculentus* subfractions attenuate beta amyloid-induced neuron apoptosis by regulating DPP-4 with improving insulin resistance signals. *PLoS One.* 2019;14:e0217400.

Islam S, Shajib MS, Datta BK, Rashid MA. Neuropharmacological activities of methanol extract of *Albizia lebbeck* (L.) Benth. *Bangladesh Pharm J.* 2018;21:7.

Issa AR, Sun J, Petitgas C, Mesquita A, Dulac A, Robin M, Mollereau B, Jenny A, Cherif-Zahar B, Birman S. The lysosomal membrane protein LAMP2A promotes autophagic flux and prevents SNCA-induced Parkinson disease-like symptoms in the drosophila brain. *Autophagy* 2018;14:1898–1910.

Jheng SS, Pai MC. Cognitive map in patients with mild Alzheimer's disease: a computer-generated arena study. *Behav Brain Res.* 2009;200:42–47.

Jiang T, Tan L, Zhu XC, Zhang QQ, Cao L, Tan MS, Gu LZ, Wang HF, Ding ZZ, Zhang YD, Yu JT. Upregulation of TREM2 ameliorates neuropathology and rescues spatial cognitive impairment in a transgenic mouse model of Alzheimer's disease. *Neuropsychopharmacology.* 2014;39:2949–2962.

Karimipour M, Rahbarghazi R, Tayefi H, Shimia M, Ghanadian M, Mahmoudi J, Bagheri HS. Quercetin promotes learning and memory performance concomitantly with neural stem/progenitor cell proliferation and neurogenesis in the adult rat dentate gyrus. *Int J Dev Neurosci.* 2019;74:18–26.

Kashino Y, Murota K, Matsuda N, Tomotake M, Hamano T, Mukai R, Terao J. Effect of processed onions on the plasma concentration of quercetin in rats and humans. *J Food Sci.* 2015;80:H2597–H2602.

Kerr JS, Adriaanse BA, Greig NH, Mattson MP, Cader MZ, Bohr VA, Fang E. Mitophagy and Alzheimer's disease: cellular and molecular mechanisms. *Trends Neurosci.* 2017;40:151–166.

Kobori M, Masumoto S, Akimoto Y, Takahashi Y. Dietary quercetin alleviates diabetic symptoms and reduces streptozotocin-induced disturbance of hepatic gene expression in mice. *Mol Nutr Food Res.* 2009;53:859–868.

Kong Y, Li K, Fu T, Wan C, Zhang D, Song H, Zhang Y, Liu N, Gan Z, Yuan L. Quercetin ameliorates Aβ toxicity in Drosophila AD model by modulating cell cycle-related protein expression. *Oncotarget.* 2016;7:67716–67731.

Kopf D, Frolich L. Risk of incident Alzheimer's disease in diabetic patients: a systematic review of prospective trials. *J Alzheimer's Dis.* 2009;16:677–685.

Kressler J, Millard-Stafford M, Warren GL. Quercetin and endurance exercise capacity: a systematic review and meta-analysis. *Med Sci Sports Exerc.* 2011;43:2396–2404.

Kuo YC, Chen CL, Rajesh R. Optimized liposomes with transactivator of transcription peptide and anti-apoptotic drugs to target hippocampal neurons and prevent tau hyperphosphorylated neurodegeneration. *Acta Biomateria.* 2019;87:207–222.

Larson AJ, Symons JD, Jalili T. Quercetin: a treatment for hypertension?—a review of efficacy and mechanisms. *Pharmaceuticals.* 2010;3:237–250.

Lee CYD, Daggett A, Gu X, Jiang LL, Langfelder P, Li X, Wang N, Zhao Y, Park CS, Cooper Y, Ferando I, Mody I, Coppola G, Xu H, Yang XW. Elevated TREM2 gene dosage reprograms microglia responsivity and ameliorates pathological phenotypes in Alzheimer's disease models. *Neuron* 2018;97:1032–1048.e5.

Li R, Zhang Y, Rasool S, Geetha T, Ramesh Babu J. Effects and underlying mechanisms of bioactive compounds on type-2 diabetes mellitus and Alzheimer's disease. *Oxid Med Cell Longev.* 2019 (In Press).

Liu L, Guo K, Lu J, Venkatraman SS, Luo D, Ng KC, Ling EA, Moochhala S, Yang YY. Biologically active core/shell nanoparticles self-assembled from cholesterol-terminated PEG-TAT for drug delivery across the blood–brain barrier. *Biomaterials.* 2008;29:1509–1517.

Liu Y, Zhou H, Yin T, Gong Y, Yuan G, Chen L, Liu J. Quercetin modified gold-palladium nanoparticles as a potential autophagy inducer for the treatment of Alzheimer's disease. *J Colloid Interface Sci.* 2019;552:388–400.

Lourenco MV, Ferreira ST, De Felice FG. Neuronal stress signaling and eIF2 alpha phosphorylation as molecular links between Alzheimer's disease and diabetes. *Prog Neurobiol.* 2015;129:37–57.

Lu J, Wu DM, Zheng YL, Hu B, Zhang ZF, Shan Q, Zheng ZH, Liu CM, Wang YJ. Quercetin activates AMP-activated protein kinase by reducing PP2C expression protecting old mouse brain against high cholesterol-induced neurotoxicity. *J Pathol.* 2010;222:199–212.

Lucin KM, O'Brien CE, Bieri G, Czirr E, Mosher KI, Abbey RJ, Mastroeni DF, Rogers J, Spencer B, Masliah E, Wyss-Coray T. Microglial beclin 1 regulates retromer trafficking and phagocytosis and is impaired in Alzheimer's disease. *Neuron.* 2013;79:873–886.

Maher PA, Schubert DR. Metabolic links between diabetes and Alzheimer's disease. *Expert Rev. Neurother.* 2009;9:617–630.

Martini-Stoica H, Xu Y, Ballabio A, Zheng H. The autophagy-lysosomal pathway in neurodegeneration: a TFEB perspective. *Trends Neurosci.* 2016;39:221–234.

Maulik M, Kar S, Chung J, Wang Y, Vance JE, Peake K. APP overexpression in the absence of NPC1 exacerbates metabolism of amyloidogenic proteins of Alzheimer's disease. *Hum Mol Genet.* 2015;24:7132–7150.

Mauludin R, Muller RH, Keck CM. Development of an oral rutin nanocrystal formulation. *Int J Pharm.* 2009;370:202–209.

Mercer LD, Kelly BL, Horne MK, Beart PM. Dietary polyphenols protect dopamine neurons from oxidative insults and apoptosis: investigations in primary rat mesencephalic cultures. *Biochem Pharmacol.* 2005;69:339–345.

Moreau K, Fleming A, Imarisio S, Lopez Ramirez A, Mercer JL, Jimenez-Sanchez M, Bento CF, Puri C, Zavodszky E, Siddiqi F, Lavau CP, Betton M, O'Kane CJ, Wechsler DS, Rubinsztein DC. PICALM modulates autophagy activity and tau accumulation. *Nat Commun.* 2014;5:4998.

Moreno L, Puerta E, Suarez-Santiago JE, Santos-Magalhaes NS, Ramirez MJ, Irache JM. Effect of the oral administration of nanoencapsulated quercetin on a mouse model of Alzheimer's disease. *Int J Pharm.* 2017;517:50–57.

Nakagawa K, Ueda M, Itoh M, Islam S, Tana Nakagawa T. Dietary quercetin ameliorates memory impairment in a murine model of Alzheimer's disease with obesity and diabetes, suppressing ATF4 expression. *J Neurol Neurosci.* 2017;8:234.

Nakagawa T, Itoh M, Ohta K, Hayashi Y, Hayakawa M, Yamada Y, Akanabe H, Chikaishi T, Nakagawa K, Itoh Y, Muro T, Yanagida D, Nakabayashi R, Mori T, Saito K, Ohzawa K, Suzuki C, Li S, Ueda M, Wang MX, Nishida E, Islam S, Tana, Kobori M, Inuzuka T. Improvement of memory recall by quercetin in rodent contextual fear conditioning and human early-stage Alzheimer's disease patients. *Neuroreport.* 2016;27:671–676.

Nakagawa T, Ohta K. Querceting regulates the integrated stress response to improve memory. *Int J Mol Sci.* 2019;20:2761.

Nijveldt RJ, van Nood E, van Hoorn DEC, Boelens PG, van Norren K, van Leeuwen PAM. Flavonoids: a review of probable mechanisms of action and potential applications. *Am J Clin Nutr.* 2001;74:418–425.

O'Connor T, Sadleir KR, Maus E, Velliquette RA, Zhao J, Cole SL, Eimer WA, Hitt B, Bembinster LA, Lammich S, Lichtenthaler SF, Hébert SS, De Strooper B, Haass C, Bennett DA, Vassar R. Phosphorylation of the translation initiation factor eIF2alpha increases BACE1 levels and promotes amyloidogenesis. *Neuron.* 2008;60:988–1009.

Oliveira MM, Lourenco MV. Integrated stress response: connecting ApoE4 to memory impairment in Alzheimer's disease. *J Neurosci.* 2016;36:1053–1055.

Pan RY, Ma J, Kong XX, Wang XF, Li SS, Qi XL, Yan YH, Cheng J, Liu Q, Jin W, Tan CH, Yuan Z. Sodium rutin ameliorates Alzheimer's disease like pathology by enhancing microgliala amyloid β clearance. *Sci Adv.* 2019;5:eaau6328.

Paula PC, Angelica Maria SG, Luis CH, Gloria Patricia CG. Preventive effect of quercetin in a triple transgenic Alzheimer's disease mice model. *Molecules.* 2019;24:12.

Peng CH, Chyau CC, Wang CJ, Lin HT, Huang CN, Ker YB. Abelmoschus esculentus fractions potently inhibited the pathogenic targets associated with diabetic renal epithelial to mesenchymal transition. *Food Funct.* 2016;7:728–740.

Peng J, Li Q, Li K, Zhu L, Lin X, Lin X, Shen Q, Li G, Xie X. Quercetin improves glucose and lipid metabolism of diabetic rats: involvement of Akt signaling and SIRT1. *J Diabetes Res.* 2017;2017:3417306.

Pocernich CB, Lange ML, Sultana R, Butterfield DA. Nutritional approaches to modulate oxidative stress in Alzheimer's disease. *Curr Alzheimer Res.* 2011;8:452–469.

Qin Y, Chen H, Zhang Q, Wang X, Yuan W, Kuai R, Tang J, Zhang L, Zhang Z, Zhang Q, Liu J, He Q. Liposome formulated with TAT-modified cholesterol for improving brain delivery and therapeutic efficacy on brain glioma in animals. *Int J Pharm.* 2011;420:304–312.

Rishitha N, Muthuraman A. Therapeutic evaluation of solid lipid nanoparticle of quercetin in pentylenetetrazole induced cognitive impairment of zebrafish. *Life Sci.* 2018;199:80–87.

Russo M, Spagnuolo C, Tedesco I, Bilotto S, Russo GL. The flavonoid quercetin in disease prevention and therapy: facts and fancies. *Biochem Pharmacol.* 2012;83:6–15.

Sabogal-Guaqueta AM, Munoz-Manco JI, Ramirez-Pineda JR, Lamprea-Rodriguez M, Osorio E, Cardona-Gomez GP. The flavonoid quercetin ameliorates Alzheimer's disease pathology and protects cognitive and emotional function in aged triple transgenic Alzheimer's disease model mice. *Neuropharmacology.* 2015;93:134–145.

Saleem U, Raza Z, Anwar F, Ahmad B, Hira S, Ali T. Experimental and computational studies to characterize and evaluate the therapeutic effect of *Albizia lebbeck* (L.) seeds in Alzheimer's disease. Medicina (Kaunas). 2019;55 (In Press).

Samsonowicz M, Kaminska I, Kalinowska M, Lewandowski W. Alkali metal salts of rutin—synthesis, spectroscopic (FT-IR, FT-Raman, UV–VIS), antioxidant and antimicrobial studies. *Spectrochim Acta A Mol Biomol Spectrosc.* 2015;151:926–938.

Sato H, Fujimori M, Suzuki H, Kadota K, Shirakawa Y, Onoue S, Tozuka Y. Absorption improvement of tranilast by forming highly soluble nano-size composite structures associated with α-glucosyl rutin via spray drying. *Eur J Pharm Biopharm.* 2015;92:49–55.

Schiller D, Eichenbaum H, Buffalo EA, Davachi L, Foster DJ, Leutgeb S, Ranganath C. Memory and space: towards an understanding of the cognitive map. *J Neurosci Off J Soc Neurosci.* 2015;35:13904–13911.

Segev Y, Michaelson DM, Rosenblum K. ApoE epsilon4 is associated with eIF2alpha phosphorylation and impaired learning in young mice. *Neurobiol Aging.* 2013;34:863–872.

Serajuddin ATM. Salt formation to improve drug solubility. *Adv Drug Deliv Rev.* 2007;59:603–616.

Spuch C, Navarro C. Liposomes for targeted delivery of active agents against neurodegenerative diseases. *J Drug Deliv.* 2011;2011:469679.

Srivastav Neeti SS, Vijay J, Tiwari Brijesh K. Anti-convulsant activity of leaf extracts of *Albizia lebbeck* Linn in experimental rats. *Int J Pharm Sci Rev Res.* 2016;41:173–176.

Torchilin VP. TAT peptide-mediated intracellular delivery of pharmaceutical nanocarriers. *Adv Drug Deliv Rev.* 2008;60:548–558.

Ulland TK, Song WM, Huang SCC, Ulrich JD, Sergushichev A, Beatty WL, Loboda AA, Zhou Y, Cairns NJ, Kambal A, Loginicheva E, Gilfillan S, Cella M, Virgin HW, Unanue ER, Wang Y, Artyomov MN, Holtzman DM, Colonna M. TREM2 maintains microglial metabolic fitness in Alzheimer's disease. *Cell.* 2017;170:649–663.e13.

Vargas-Restrepo F, Sabogal-Guaqueta AM, Cardona-Gomez GP. Quercetin ameliorates inflammation in CA1hippocampal region in aged triple transgenic Alzheimer's disease mice model. *Biomedica.* 2018;38:69–76.

Verma SC, Singh VE, Kumari A, Meena AK, Pant P, Bhuyan GC, Padhi MM. A review on parts of *Albizia lebbeck* (L.) Benth. used as Ayurvedic drugs. *Res J Pharm Technol.* 2013;6:1307–1313.

Vilchez D, Saez I, Dillin A. The role of protein clearance mechanisms in organismal ageing and age-related diseases. *Nat Commun.* 2014;5:5659.

Wang DM, Li SQ, Wu WL, Zhu XY, Wang Y, Yuan HY. Effects of long-term treatment with quercetin on cognition and mitochondrial function in a mouse model of Alzheimer's disease. *Neurochem Res.* 2014;39:1533–1543.

Wendeln AC, Degenhardt K, Kaurani L, Gertig M, Ulas T, Jain G, Wagner J, Hasler LM, Wild K, Skodras A, Blank T, Staszewski O, Datta M, Centeno TP, Capece V, Islam MR, Kerimoglu C, Staufenbiel M, Schultze JL, Beyer M, Prinz M, Jucker M, Fischer A, Neher JJ. Innate immune memory in the brain shapes neurological disease hallmarks. *Nature.* 2018;556:332–338.

Xia SF, Xie ZX, Qiao Y, Li LR, Cheng XR, Tang X, Shi YH, Le GW. Differential effects of quercetin on hippocampus-dependent learning and memory in mice fed with different diets related with oxidative stress. *Physiol Behav.* 2015;138:325–331.

Xu PX, Wang SW, Yu XL, Su YJ, Wang T, Zhou WW, Zhang H, Wang YJ, Liu RT. Rutin improves spatial memory in Alzheimer's disease transgenic mice by reducing Aβ oligomer level and attenuating oxidative stress and neuroinflammation. *Behav Brain Res.* 2014;264:173–180.

Youl E, Bardy G, Magous R, Cros G, Sejalon F, Virsolvy A, Richard S, Quignard JF, Gross R, Petit P, Bataille D, Oiry C. Quercetin potentiates insulin secretion and protects INS-1 pancreatic β-cells against oxidative damage via the ERK1/2 pathway. *Brit J Pharmacol.* 2010;161:799–814.

Yuan X, Wei G, You Y, Huang Y, Lee HJ, Dong M, Lin J, Hu T, Zhang H, Zaplatic E, Bule M, Shah SZA, Uddin MS, Niaz K. Molecular mechanisms underlying protective role of quercetin in attenuating Alzheimer's disease. *Life Sci.* 2019;224:109–119.

Yuan X., Wei G., You Y., Huang Y., Lee H. J., Dong M., Lin J., Hu T., Zhang H., Zhang C., Zhou H., Ye R., Qi X., Zhai B., Huang W., Liu S., Xie W., Liu Q., Liu X., Cui C., Li D., Zhan J., Cheng J., Yuan Z., Jin W., Rutin ameliorates obesity through brown fat activation. *FASEB J.* 31, 333–345 (2017).

Zaplatic E, Bule M, Ali Shah SZ, Uddin MS, Niaz K. Molecular mechanisms underlying protective role of quercetin in attenuating Alzheimer's disease. *Life Sci.* 2019;224:109–119.

Zhang S, Zhang SB, Ju K, Olek S, DJ Jr, Schwartz L, Keng PC, Howell R, Zhang L, Okunieff P. Antioxidant properties of quercetin. *Adv Exp Med Biol.* 2011;701:283–290.

Zhu MW, Zhang S, Tian XL, Wu CL. Mask mitigates MAPT- and FUS-induced degeneration by enhancing autophagy through lysosomal acidification. *Autophagy.* 2017;13:1924–1938.

17 Plant Alkaloids and Their Derivatives Relevant to Alzheimer's Disease

Atanu Bhattacharjee and Akula Ramakrishna

CONTENTS

ABBREVIATIONS

ACh	Acetylcholine
AChE	Acetylcholinesterase
AD	Alzheimer's Disease
APP	Amyloid Precursor Protein
Aβ PP	Aβ Precursor Protein
Aβ	Amyloid β
BACE	β-site of APP Cleaving Enzyme
BChE	Butyrylcholinesterase
FDA	Food and Drug Administration
IC_{50}	Half-maximal Inhibitory Concentration
MAO	Monoamine Oxidase
NMDA	N-methyl-D-aspartate
NMDAR	N-methyl-D-aspartate Receptor
PPAR	Peroxisome Proliferator-Activated Receptors
SAR	Structure-Activity Relationship
UV	Ultraviolet
WHO	World Health Organization

17.1 INTRODUCTION

Alzheimer's disease (AD) is an irreversible age-related form of dementia that slowly damages the brain, robs the person of memory and cognitive skills, and causes changes in personality and behavior (George, 2016). Formation of extracellular amyloid β (Aβ) plaque, with drastic neuronal and synaptic reduction in the cholinergic system of the brain is considered to be the major pathological hallmark of AD (Puchchakayala et al., 2012). During the past decade, significant growth in the incidence of Alzheimer's disease has stimulated research into the search for new medicines.

One of the major clinical advances in the treatment of AD have been the use of acetylcholinesterase (AChE) and butyrylcholinesterase (BChE) inhibitors to increase the ACh levels in the brain, although cholinergic compounds with nicotinic and muscarinic agonist properties have also attracted some interest (Mahesh et al., 2014; Ferri et al., 2006). Several synthetic compounds are available, but they may cause several other health issues. Therefore, natural molecules from plants or other sources are valuable resources with which to replace available medicines as they are considered to be safe and relatively inexpensive. The structural diversity of phytochemicals makes them a valuable source of novel lead compounds in the quest for drugs to treat AD (Bush, 2003; Fariba et al., 2012).

Alkaloids exhibit a range of structures and also show an extraordinary spectrum of pharmacological activities. Since time immemorial, plant- derived alkaloids have played an important role in the treatment of various cognitive and neurological disorders (Skovronsky et al., 2006; Harvey, 2008). Alkaloids play positive roles in ameliorating the pathophysiology of AD by functioning as muscarinic and adenosine receptor agonists, antioxidants, antiamyloids and monoamine oxidase (MAO) inhibitors, acetylcholinesterase (AChE) and butyrylcholinesterase (BChE) inhibitors, inhibitors of α-synuclein aggregation, dopaminergic and nicotine agonists, and N-methyl-D-aspartic acid (NMDA) antagonists (Houghton et al., 2004; Williams et al., 2011). Therefore, systematic ethnopharmacological screening of plant alkaloids as lead molecules may identify useful avenues in the search for new drugs for AD therapy. This chapter represents a systematic review to update the available knowledge on various alkaloids and their derivatives, along with their predicted mechanism of action to interfere with AD progression.

17.2 CURRENT STRATEGIES FOR ALZHEIMER'S DISEASE

Existing pharmacological treatments for AD act by relieving symptoms rather than targeting the etiological mechanisms. The US Food and Drug Administration (FDA)-approved medications for AD include acetylcholinesterase (AChE) inhibitors and N-methyl-D-aspartic acid receptor (NMDAR) antagonists (Rinne et al., 2003; Brinton et al., 1998). As the loss of cognitive function in AD patients is strongly correlated with the reduction in cholinergic neurotransmission in the brain, rebalancing cholinergic input should theoretically increase memory and cognition in AD patients. Cholinergic transmission is mediated by the neurotransmitter acetylcholine (ACh) through the activation of nicotinic and muscarinic ACh receptors (Orhan et al., 2009; Kim et al., 2002). AChE inhibitors can increase cholinergic transmission by limiting degradation of ACh. In fact, the first FDA-approved medication for AD was an AChE inhibitor; tacrine (Cognex™) was approved in 1993 but withdrawn from the market in 2012 because of its hepatotoxicity (National Institute on Aging, 2015). The three most-commonly prescribed AChE inhibitors are donepezil (Aricept™), rivastigmine (Exelon™), and galantamine (Reminyl™), which were approved in 1996, 2000, and 2001, respectively. Donepezil is the only AChE inhibitor approved for the treatment of all stages of AD (Orhan et al., 2007).

The second class of FDA-approved medications acts by blocking NMDAR (Tariot et al., 2004). In AD, excess glutamate released from damaged cells causes a massive influx of calcium into neurons *via* NMDAR activation; this results in excitotoxicity, ultimately leading to neuronal death (Salloway et al., 2008). Memantine (Namenda™), a neuroprotective agent that blocks NMDAR, was approved for the treatment of moderate to severe AD in 2003. Memantine can be used alone or in combination with AChE inhibitors, such as donepezil (Szwajgier et al., 2013). Furthermore, antioxidants and free radical scavengers act as natural protectors to reduce the level of free radical accumulation and thereby slow down Aβ aggregation (Sarna et al., 2010; Hyun et al., 2009). Probable mechanisms of plant-derived alkaloids against AD progression are shown in Figure 17.1. A summary of current treatment strategies for AD is described in Table 17.1.

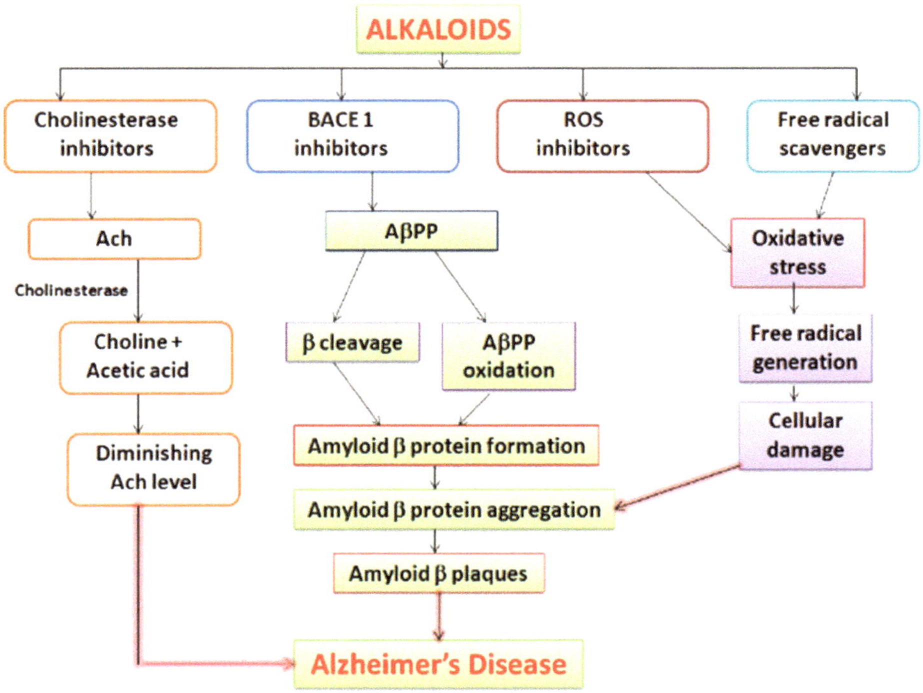

FIGURE 17.1 Mechanism of plant-derived alkaloids for treatment against AD progression (Adopted and modified from Hyun et al., 2009).

TABLE 17.1
Current Treatment Strategies for AD (Modified from Yu et al., 2015)

Treatment Strategy	Mechanism of Action	Stages of AD
Modulation of neurotransmitter (existing/approved therapy)	**1. AChE inhibitor** **2. NMDA antagonist**	Early stage of AD
Disease-modifying therapies (under investigation)	**1. Amyloid cascade** • Modulation of α-, β-, γ- Secretase • β amyloid inhibitor • Promoting β amyloid clean-up **2. Tau protein modulation** • Inhibition of tau hyperphosphorylation • Degradation of tau proteins • Inhibition of tau oligomerization	Mild to moderate stage of AD
Immunotherapy (under investigation)	**1. Passive immunization** • Solanezumab • Crenezumab **2. Active immunization CAD106**	Mild to moderate stage of AD
Gene-based therapy (under investigation)	**1. Modulation of expression of presenilin**	Mild to moderate stage of AD
Antioxidants (existing/approved therapy)	**1. Oxidative stress reduction** **2. Free radical scavenger**	Mild to moderate stage of AD
Anti-inflammatory agents (existing/approved therapy)	**1. Caspase inhibitors** **2. Metal chelators** **3. Statins** **4. PPAR-γ**	Mild to moderate stage of AD

17.3 MECHANISTIC APPROACHES OF PLANT-DERIVED ALKALOIDS AGAINST AD

17.3.1 Alkaloids as AChE Inhibitors

The central role of the neurotransmitter Ach, with respect to cognitive function, is clinically well established now (Bush, 2003). One of the hallmarks of AD pathology is the loss of cholinergic cells in the basalis of Meynert and the hippocampus, resulting in diminished levels of ACh in the brain (Kwon et al., 2003). Hence, the replenishment of ACh levels has been exploited therapeutically over the past few decades to achieve symptomatic relief in AD (Schneider et al., 1996; Orhan et al., 2009). Based on these etiologies, several pharmacological strategies with multiple possible targets are under investigation (Brinton et al., 1998) and the first-line therapeutic approach involves re-establishment of ACh levels by the inhibition of cholinesterases, namely AChE and BChE, and of monoamine oxidase (MAO) enzymes (Senol et al., 2012; Kim et al., 2002).

AChE principally acts by termination of nerve impulse at the cholinergic synapses by rapid hydrolysis of ACh to choline and acetic acid. This action shortens the half-life of ACh, thereby decreasing its concentration at the synapse (Adewusi et al., 2011). The AChE inhibitory activity of alkaloids is thought to be due to the positively charged nitrogen moiety, which binds to an anionic aspartate residue and a region separated by a lipophillic area from the positive charge, which can form a hydrogen bond with tyrosine or serine residues. On the other hand, this does not explain the binding characteristics of other natural products, such as terpenoids, flavanoids, and derived compounds, with AChE inhibitory activity (Mankil et al., 2007). As most of the synthetic drugs used for

AD are AChE inhibitors, extensive searches have been carried out in the past few years to screen for potential AChE inhibitors from plant sources. Like galantamine, many plant alkaloids have AChE inhibitory activity and are discussed below. The different alkaloids effective in AD and their current status are shown in Table 17.2.

17.3.2 Alkaloids as Anti-Amyloid Agents

According to the 'β-amyloid cascade', deposition of the Aβ peptide triggers the neurotoxic cascade and promotes neuroinflammation, which ultimately results in neurodegeneration (Keyvan et al., 2006; Wang et al., 2009). Aβ is derived from sequential proteolytic cleavage of the amyloid precursor protein (APP) by β- and γ-secretases. Initial cleavage by β-secretase (β-site of APP cleaving enzyme, BACE), a membrane-anchored aspartic protease, generates a soluble N-terminal fragment and a membrane-associated C-terminal fragment (Peter et al., 2005; Lee et al., 2005; Urbain et al., 2004). The C-terminal fragment then undergoes proteolysis by γ-secretase to give the Aβ peptide. BACE has been shown to be a promising therapeutic target as it initiates the first step in Aβ production (Orhan et al., 2004; Gulachi et al., 2014). Abnormal processing of the APP is responsible for amyloid deposition. The two enzymes, β-secretase and γ-secretase, which catalyze the cleavage of the Aβ peptide, are important targets in the treatment of AD. Until recently, these approaches had not been explored, but recent studies have shown that the anti-amyloid strategy can be a powerful approach to halting the progression of AD. Berberine has gained attention in this direction as it can ameliorate Aβ pathology in AD (Durairajan et al., 2012). *In-vitro* studies have shown that nicotine can prevent the precipitation of the $A\beta_{1-42}$ peptide as an amyloid-like deposit (Salomon et al., 1996).

17.3.3 Alkaloids as NMDA Antagonists

It has been confirmed that NMDA-induced neurotoxicity and glutamate-induced exo-cytotoxicity play roles in neurodegenerative diseases. Overactivity of NMDA receptors results in production of free radicals, which are responsible for neuronal damage and cell death (Bonfoco et al., 1995; Popik et al., 1995; Zhang et al., 2001). Therefore, inhibition of NMDA and glutamate toxicity is a powerful therapeutic approach for treatment of neurodegenerative diseases. Studies have shown that plant alkaloids, like huperzine-A and ibogaine, have inhibitory effects against NMDA and glutamate toxicity.

17.3.4 Alkaloids as Antioxidants

It has been widely established that oxidative stress plays an important role in the pathophysiology of neurodegeneration. The major pathological changes involved in AD and Parkinson's disease (PD) are accumulation of free radicals, oxidative damage to neuronal cells, and diminished cellular antioxidant pool. Therefore, natural antioxidants have important roles to play in such diseases, as they can reduce the oxidative stress. Plenty of natural compounds with antioxidant potential are being investigated for treatment of AD (Cardoso et al., 2004). The antioxidant activities of various alkaloids, such as berberine and huperzine-A, have been widely demonstrated.

17.4 POTENTIAL ALKALOIDAL LEAD MOLECULES FOR AD

Bioactive phytochemicals, resulting from the isolation and characterization of the natural flora and fauna, have always been an important reservoir of drugs. The majority of the alkaloids examined to date to slow down the progression of AD and to aid protection against AD are primarily derived from plant sources. Various types of alkaloids, with significant activity against AD and structures of these compounds are shown in Figure 17.2.

TABLE 17.2
Alkaloids as AChE Inhibitors

Chemical Nature of Phytoconstituents	Alkaloid				
	Class	Source	Family	Activity on AChE	References
Assoanine	Steroidal alkaloid	*Narcissus assoanus*	Amaryllidaceae	IC_{50} value at 3.87 ± 0.24 pM	Lopez et al. (2002)
Buxamine B	Steroidal alkaloid	*Buxus hyrcana*	Buxaceae	IC_{50} value at 7.56 ± 0.008 pM	Khalid et al. (2005)
Epinorgalantamine	Steroidal alkaloid	*Narcissus confusus*	Amaryllidaceae	IC_{50} value at 9.60 ± 0.65 pM	Lopez et al. (2002)
Galantamine	Steroidal alkaloid	*Galanthus nivalis*	Amaryllidaceae	IC_{50} value at 1.07 ± 0.18 pM	Rhee et al. (2001)
Sanguinine	Steroidal alkaloid	*Eucharis grandiflora*	Amaryllidaceae	IC_{50} value at 0.10 ± 0.01 pM	Lopez et al. (2002)
Oxoassoanine	Steroidal alkaloid	*Narcissus assoanus*	Amaryllidaceae	IC_{50} value at 47.21 ± 1.13 pM	Lopez et al. (2002)
N, N-dimethyl buxapapine	Steroidal alkaloid	*Buxus papillosa*	Buxaceae	IC_{50} value of7.28 ± 0.06 pM	Rahman and Choudhary (2001)
Sarsalignone	Steroidal alkaloid	*Sarcococca saligna*	Buxaceae	44.3% inhibition at 10 pM	Rahman and Choudhary (2001)
Homomoenjodaramine	Steroidal alkaloid	*Buxus sempervirens*	Buxaceae	IC_{50} value of 19.2 mM (1 mg/ml)	Rahman A-ur et al. (1998)
Moenjodaramine	Steroidal alkaloid	*Buxus sempervirens*	Buxaceae	IC_{50} value of 50.8 mM (1 mg/ml)	Rahman A-ur et al. (1998)
α-Solanine	Glycoalkaloid	*Sarcococca saligna*	Buxaceae	IC_{50} value at 8.59 ± 0.155 pM	Rahman and Choudhary (2001)
Vaganine	Steroidal alkaloid	*Solanum tuberosum*	Solanaceae	IC_{50} value at 7.028 ± 0.007 pM	Natarajan et al. (2000)
Physostigmine	Indole alkaloid	*Physostigtna venenosiun*	Fabaceae	IC_{50} value at 6 ± 1.0 pM	Peter et al. (2005)
Coronaridine	Indole alkaloid	*Tabernaernontana austral*	Apocynaceae	Minimum concentration of 25 pM to produce detectable spot on TLC	Andrade et al. (2005)
Voacangine	Indole alkaloid	*Tabernaentontana australis*	Apocynaceae	Minimum concentration of 25pM to produce detectable spot on TLC	Andrade et al. (2005)
Rupicoline	Indole alkaloid	*Tabernaetnontana australis*	Apocynaceae	Minimum concentration of 25μM to produce detectable spot on TLC	Andrade et al. (2005)
Retamine	Quinolizidine alkaloid	*Genista aucheri*	Fabaceae	AchE and BchE inhibition (%) at 1 mg/ml of 15.0 ± 1.08 & 66.3 ± 0.88 respectively	Orhan et al. (2007)
Corynoline	Isoquinoline alkaloid	*Corydalis incisa*	Papaveraceae	IC_{50} value at 30.6 pM	Keyvan et al. (2007)
Palmatine	Isoquinoline alkaloid	*Corydalis speciosa*	Papaveraceae	IC_{50} value at 5.8 pM	Keyvan et al. (2007)
Protopine	Isoquinoline alkaloid	*Corydalis speciosa*	Papaveraceae	IC_{50} value at 16.1μM	Keyvan et al. (2007)
(-)-Huperzine A	Quinolizidine alkaloid	*Huperzia serrata*	Lycopodiaceae	IC_{50} value at 10.1 pM	Wang et al. (2009)
Retamine	Quinolizidine alkaloids	*Genista aucheri*	Fabaceae	IC50 value 15.0 for AchE inhibition and 66.3 for BchE inhibition	Orhan et al. (2007)
Stepharanine	Protoberberine alkaloids	*Stephania venosa*	Menispermaceae	IC_{50} value of 14.10 ± 0.81 mM	Ingkaninan et al. (2006)
Cyclanoline	Protoberberine alkaloids	*Stephania venosa*	Menispermaceae	IC_{50} value of 9.23 ± 3.47 μM	Ingkaninan et al. (2006)
N- methyl stepholidine	Protoberberine alkaloids	*Stephania venosa*	Menispermaceae	IC_{50} value of 31.30 ± 3.67 μM	Ingkaninan et al. (2006)

17.4.1 Indole Alkaloids

17.4.1.1 Physostigmine

Physostigmine [Figure 17.2(i)] is a reversible AChE inhibitor, originally isolated from the seed of *Physostigma venenosum* (Family: Fabaceae). It enhances short-term memory in dementia patients and is used to treat mild to moderate AD (Urbain et al., 2004).

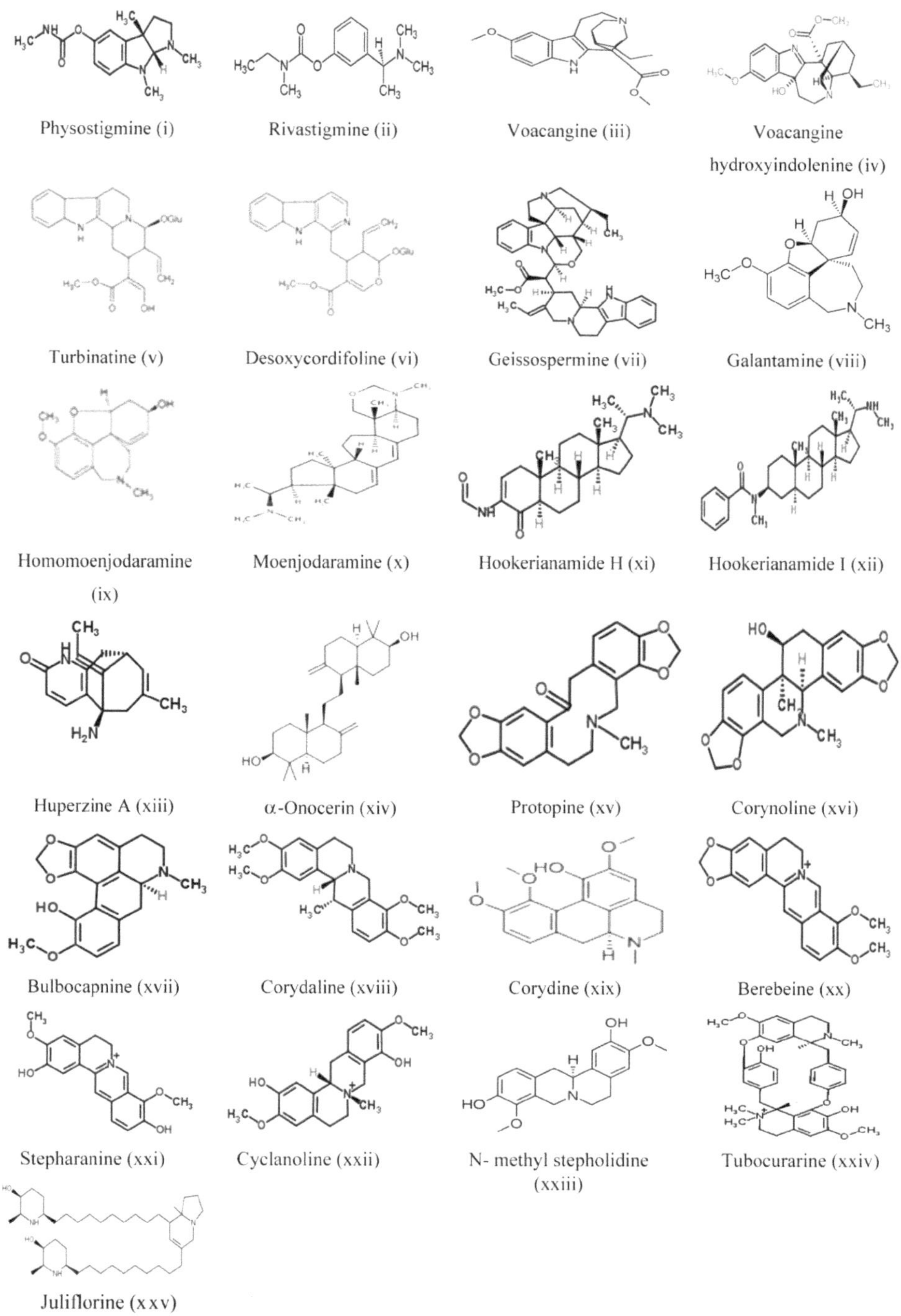

FIGURE 17.2 Structure of various potential alkaloids for AD.

17.4.1.2 Rivastigmine

Rivastigmine [Figure 17.2(ii)], an analog of physostigmine, is a potent AChE inhibitor, used for the symptomatic treatment of mild to moderately severe AD. Rivastigmine is reported to inhibit AChE in the cortex and hippocampus, brain areas involved in cognition (Thomas et al., 2007).

17.4.1.3 Voacangine and Voacangine Hydroxyindolenine

Thin-layer chromatography (TLC) analysis of AChE inhibitory activity (using Ellman's method) of voacangine and voacangine hydroxyindolenine [Figure 17.2(iii & iv)] isolated from *Tabernaemontana australis* (Family: Apocynaceae) showed a detectable spot at the minimum concentration of 25 μM (Andrade et al., 2005).

17.4.1.4 Turbinatine and Desoxycordifoline

Turbinatine and desoxycordifoline [Figure 17.2(v & vi)] isolated from *Chimarrhis turbinata* (Family: Rubiaceae) bark and leaves showed moderate AchE inhibitory activity, with values of half-maximal inhibitory concentration (IC_{50}) of 0.1 μM and 1.0 μM, respectively (Cardoso et al., 2004).

17.4.1.5 Legucin A

Legucin A, isolated from the Ayurvedic medicinal plant Shalaparni (*Desmodium gangeticum*; family Fabaceae) showed activity against AChE with an IC_{50} of 27.0 μM (Houghton et al., 2006).

17.4.1.6 Geissospermine

Bioactivity-guided fractionation of an extract of *Geissospermum vellosii* (Family: Apocynaceae) detected the presence of geissospermine [Figure 17.2(vii)], which exhibited inhibitory activity to rat brain AChE and horse serum BChE in a concentration-dependent manner, with mean IC_{50} values of 39.3 and 1.6 μg/ml, respectively. *In-vivo* experiments also supported the AchE inhibitory activity of geissospermine, which can thereby ameliorate cognitive deficits in a model of cholinergic hypofunction (Lima et al., 2009).

17.4.2 Steroidal Alkaloids

17.4.2.1 Galantamine

Galantamine [Figure 17.2 (viii)] and epinorgalantamine, isolated from *Galanthus nivalis* and *Leucojum aestivum* (Family: Amaryllidaceae), respectively, are reversibly competitive AChE inhibitors and also modulate nicotinic ACh receptors (Vladimir-Knezevic et al., 2014). Both the phytoconstituents have recently been introduced in practice in the treatment of AD.

17.4.2.2 Homomoenjodaramine and Moenjodaramine

Homomoenjodaramine and moenjodaramine [Figure 17.2 (ix & x)], isolated from *Buxus hyrcana* (Family: Buxaceae), show non-competitive AChE inhibitory activity, with IC_{50} values of 19.2 and 50.8 mM, respectively (Lee et al., 2004).

17.4.3 Pregnane-Type Steroidal Alkaloids

17.4.3.1 Hookerianamides H and I

Bioactivity-guided fractionation of an extract of *Sarcococca hookeriana* (Family: Buxaceae) resulted in the isolation of two new pregnane-type steroidal alkaloids, hookerianamide H and hookerianamide I [Figure 17.2 (xi & xii)], as well as three other alkaloids, namely N-α-methyl-epipachysamine D, sarcovagine C, and dictyophlebine. All compounds showed significant inhibitory activities against AChE and BChE, with IC_{50} values in the ranges 2.9–34.1 mM and 0.3–3.6 mM, respectively (Gulacti et al., 2014).

Salignenamides C, E, and F, axillarine-C, saligcinnamide, vaganine-A, 5,6-dehydrosarconidine, 2-hydroxysalignarine-E, salignamine, 2-hydroxysalignamine-E, epipachysamine-D, dictyophlebine, iso-N-formylchone-morphine, and axillaridine-A were isolated from *Sarcococca saligna* (Family: Buxaceae), and inhibited both AChE and BChE non-competitively, with IC_{50} values in the range 2.65–250.0 μM against AChE and 1.63–30.0 μM against BuChE (Jing et al., 1999)

17.4.4 Quinolizidine Alkaloids

17.4.4.1 Huperzine A

Huperzine A [Figure 17.2 (xiii)], isolated from the clubmoss *Lycopodium serratum* (Family: Lycopodiaceae), showed AchE inhibitory activity *in vivo.* Alpha-onocerin [Figure 17.2 (xiv)], a triterpene-type compound, from *Lycopodium clavatum* also showed inhibitory activity against AChE (Orhan et al., 2003). Huperzine A is also a NMDA receptor antagonist, which protects the brain against glutamate-induced damage, and increases nerve growth factor levels (Eduardo et al., 2012).

17.4.5 Isoquinoline Alkaloids

17.4.5.1 Protopine

Bioactivity-guided fractionation of extracts from tubers of *Corydalis ternata* (Family: Papaveraceae) isolated protopine [Figure 17.2 (xv)], which exhibited reversible competitive AChE inhibition, with an IC_{50} value of 30.5 μM. This finding was supported by *in-vivo* experiments (Keyvan et al., 2007).

17.4.5.2 Corynoline

Corynoline [Figure 17.2 (xvi)], isolated from *Corydalis incisa*, exhibited reversible non-competitive inhibition of AChE, with an IC_{50} value of 50 μM (Ma et al., 1999).

17.4.5.3 Bulbocapnine, Corydaline, and Corydine

Bulbocapnine, corydaline, and corydine [Figure 17.2 (xvii, xviii & xix)] were isolated from *Corydalis cava* as bioactive constituents. Bulbocapnine inhibited AChE and BChE in a dose-dependent manner with mean ± standard deviation IC_{50} values of 40 ± 2.0 and 83 ± 3.0 μM, respectively whereas corydaline inhibited AChE and BChE in a dose-dependent manner, with IC_{50} values of 15 ± 3.0 μM and 52 ± 4.0 μM, respectively (Adsersen et al., 2007).

17.4.5.4 Berberine and Its Derivatives

Bioactivity-guided fractionation of *Corydalis turtschaninovii* extracts led to the isolation of five alkaloids, namely 7-epiberberine, pseudocopsitine, berberine, pseudoberberine, and pseudodehydrocorydaline [Figure 17.2 (xx)], which exhibited AChE inhibitory activity, with IC_{50} values of 6.5 ± 0.5, 8.4 ± 0.5, 4.7 ± 0.2, 4.3 ± 0.3, and 4.5 ± 0.2 μM, respectively (Hung et al., 2008).

17.4.6 Protoberberine Alkaloids

17.4.6.1 Stepharanine, Cyclanoline, and N-Methyl Stepholidine

Bioactivity-guided fractionation of a tuber extract of *Stephania venosa* (Family: Menispermaceae) isolated stepharanine, cyclanoline, and N-methyl stepholidine [Figure 17.2 (xxi, xxii) & (xxiii)], which exhibited inhibitory activity toward AChE, with IC_{50} values of 14.10 ± 0.81, 9.23 ± 3.47 and 31.30 ± 3.67 μM, respectively (Cousin et al., 1996).

17.4.6.2 Tubocurarine

Tubocurarine [Figure 17.2 (xxiv)], obtained from *Chondodendron tomentosum* (Family: Menispermaceae), showed AChE inhibitory activity *in vivo* (Thandla, 2002).

TABLE 17.3
Preclinical and Clinical Development of Plant-Derived Alkaloids (Adapted and modified from Mona et al., 2012)

Drug	Derivatives	Manufacturing Company	Present Status
Physostigmine	Rivastigmine	Novartis	First drug investigated; however, due to side effects, short half-life, and better treatment options, it is no longer in use. Failed in phase III
	Phenserine	QR Pharma	In phase I
	Posiphen	QR Pharma	In phase I
	Bisnorcumserine	National Institute of Aging; Cheisi Farmaceutisi	Failed in phase I; discontinued
	Tolserine	QR Pharma	A promising physostigmine derivative, suggested from clinical trials
	Esolerine	QR Pharma	Another physostigmine derivative in pipeline, with AChE and BChE inhibitory activities
Donepezil	Aricept	United States Food and Drug Administration (USFDA)	Highly selective anticholinesterase. Approved for mild, moderate, and severe AD
Galantamine	Memogain	Neurodyn Inc.	Lower AChE inhibitory potency with allosteric nicotinic receptor modulation properties compared with parent molecule galantamine
Metrifonate	Trichlorfon	Bayer (Germany)	A highly selective AChE inhibitor but was abandoned after Phase III randomised control trails (RCTs) because of risk of neuromuscular dysfunction
Huperzine A	ZT-1	Debiopharm International	A selective ChE inhibitor and used as a supplement in the US and China. Phase II trials in the US showed significant effect on improved cognition in AD
Anabaseine	GTS-21	CoMentis	A selective ChE inhibitor and used as a supplement in the US and China. Phase II trials in the US showed significant effect on improved cognition in AD

17.4.7 Piperidine Alkaloids

17.4.7.1 Juliflorine

Juliflorine [Figure 17.2 (xxv)] has been isolated from the leaves of *Prosopis juliflora* (Family: Fabaceae), and it non-competitively inhibits both AChE (IC_{50} = 0.42 μM) and BChE (IC_{50} = 0.12 μM) (Choudhary et al., 2005).

17.5 CURRENT STATUS OF PLANT-DERIVED ALKALOIDS IN CLINICAL TRIALS

Up to now, a number of alkaloids have been investigated for the treatment of AD. A summary of potential phytoextracts and their lead molecules, which slow down the progress of AD, and their current status of preclinical and clinical development is given in Table 17.3.

17.6 CONCLUSION

During the past decade, research efforts on ethnomedicinal plants affecting cholinergic neurotransmission have generated substantial data and thus provided a rationale for them to be used either as mainstream or complementary medicines, to provide symptomatic relief in AD. Up to the present day, cholinomimetics, such as tacrine, along with other AChE inhibitors, have made substantial progress in AD therapy (Howes et al., 2003; Natalia et al., 2010), but resulting side effects, with high toxicity, short duration of action, low bioavailability, etc. have limited their usefulness. Hence, from a patient safety point-of-view, a search for new drugs, with low toxicity profiles and greater potency, has become essential. With this in mind, an array of phytoextracts and bioactive phytochemicals from those species with AchE and BchE inhibitory activity have been screened to treat AD and other neurodegenerative disorders (Perry et al., 2002; Mukherjee et al., 2007b).

Natural alkaloids with AChE inhibitory activity, namely physostigmine, huperzine-A, and galantamine, have been successfully tested to determine their effect on the progression of AD. Stilbene oligomers, such as α-viniferin, and triterpenoids, like ursolic acid, are other highly potential lead molecules with AChE inhibitory activity. The other major classes of phytochemicals reported to have such activity are the flavonoids, glycosides, and coumarins. Plants belonging to diverse families, such as Acanthaceae, Apocynaceae, Amaryllidaceae, Araceae, Asteraceae, Berberidaceae, Buxaceae, Combretaceae, Cyperaceae, Ericaceae, Fabaceae, Fumariaceae, Gentianaceae, Lamiaceae, Lycopodiaceae, Magnoliaceae, Menispermaceae, Moraceae, Papaveraceae, Pinaceae, Piperaceae, Rubiaceae, Rutaceae, Solanaceae, Tamaricaceae, and Zingiberaceae, have been reported to possess AChE inhibitory activity (Mukherjee et al., 2007a; Kennedy et al., 2011; Ingkaninan et al., 2003). Although structure-activity relationships (SAR) of a few isolated bioactive compounds have been established, after considerable effort, most such relationships are yet to be elucidated. Moreover, cell-based mechanisms of action, clinical efficacy, and toxicity profiles of these phytoextracts and their derivatives require further assessment, before proceeding towards clinical trials and final approval to treat AD.

ACKNOWLEDGMENTS

The author is grateful to Assam Down Town University, Assam for providing the necessary support for preparation of this manuscript.

REFERENCES

Adewusi EA, Steenkamp V. *In vitro* screening for acetylcholinesterase inhibition and antioxidant activity of medicinal plants from southern Africa. *Asian Pac J Trop Med.* 2011; 5(2): 829–835.

Adsersen A, Kjolbye A, Dall O, Jaager AK. Acetylcholinesterase and butyrylcholinesterase inhibitory compounds from *Corydalis cava. J Ethanophramacol.* 2007; 113: 179–182.

Andrade MT, Lima JA, Pinto AC, Rezende CM, Carvalho MP, Epifanio RA. Indole alkaloids from *Tabernaemontana australis* (Muell. Arg) Miers that inhibit acetylcholinesterase enzyme. *Bioorg Med Chem.* 2005; 13: 4092–4095.

Bonfoco E, Krainc D, Ankarcrona M, Nicotera P, Lipton SA. Apoptosis and necrosis: two distinct events induced, respectively, by mild and intense insults with N-methyl-D-aspartate or nitric oxide/superoxide in cortical cell cultures. *Proc Natl Acad Sci.* 1995; 92(16): 7162–7166.

Brinton RD, Yamazaki RS. Advances and challenges in the prevention and treatment of Alzheimer's disease. *Pharmaceut Res.* 1998; 15: 386–398.

Bush AI. The metallobiology of Alzheimer's disease. *Trends Neurosci.* 2003; 26(4): 207–214.

Cardoso CL, Castro-Gamboa I, Silva DH, Furlan M, Epifanio Rde A, Pinto Ada C, et al. Indole glucoalkaloids from *Chimarrhis turbinata* and their evaluation as antioxidant agents and acetylcholinesterase inhibitors. *J Nat Prod.* 2004; 67(11): 1882–1885.

Choudhary MI, Nawaz SA, Zaheer-ul-Haq, Azim MK, Ghayur MN, Lodhi MA, et al. Juliflorine: a potent natural peripheral anionic-site-binding inhibitor of acetylcholinesterase with calcium-channel blocking potential, a leading candidate for Alzheimer's disease therapy. *Biochem Biophys Res Commun.* 2005; 332(4): 1171–1177.

Cousin SB, Duval N, Bassoulie J, Bon C. Cloning and expression of acetylcholinesterase from *Bungarus fasciatus* venom: a new type of COOH-terminal domain; involvement of a positively charged residue in the peripheral site. *J Biol Chem.* 1996; 271: 15099–15108.

Durairajan SS, Liu LF, Lu JH, Chen LL, Yuan Q, Chung SK. Berberine ameliorates beta-amyloid pathology, gliosis, and cognitive impairment in an Alzheimer's disease transgenic mouse model. *Neurobiol Aging.* 2012; 33(12): 2903–2919.

Eduardo LK, Bruna MN, Paula SL, Carolina dos S. Investigation of the in vitro and ex vivo acetylcholinesterase and antioxidant activities of traditionally used Lycopodium species from South America on alkaloid extracts. *J Ethnopharmacol.* 2012; 139(1): 58–67.

Fariba S, Mansour M, Mohammad JA, Ehsan Z. Essential oil and methanolic extract of *Zataria multiflora* Boiss with anticholinesterase effect. *Pak J Biol Sci.* 2012; 15(1): 49–53.

Ferri CP, Prince M, Brayne C, Brodaty H, Fratiglioni L, Ganguli M, et al. Global prevalence of dementia: a Delphi consensus study. *Lancet.* 2006; 366: 2112–2117.

George A. A role for the regulation of the melatonergic pathways in Alzheimer's disease and other neurodegenerative and psychiatric conditions. In: Gokhare AR, Akula R, editors. *Seratonin and Melatonin: Their Functional Role in Plants, Food, Phytomedicine, and Human Health.* New York, NY: Taylor & Francis Group, 2016.

Gulacti T, Tuba K. Lamiaceae family plants as a potential anticholinesterase source in the treatment of Alzheimer's disease. *Bezmialem Sci.* 2014; 1: 1–25.

Harvey AL. Natural products in drug discovery. *Drug Discov Today.* 2008; 13: 894–901.

Houghton PJ, Howes MJ. Natural products and derivatives affecting neurotransmission relevant to Alzheimer's and Parkinson's disease. *Neurosignals.* 2004; 14: 6–22.

Houghton PJ, Ren Y, Howes MJ. Acetylcholinesterase inhibitors from plants and fungi. *Nat Prod Rep.* 2006; 23: 181–199.

Howes MJ, Houghton PJ. Plants used in Chinese and Indian traditional medicine for improvement of memory and cognitive function. *Pharmacol Biochem Behav.* 2003; 75: 513–527.

Hung TM, Na MK, Dat NT, Ngoc TM, Youn UJ, Kim HJ, et al. Cholinesterase inhibitory and anti-amnesic activity of alkaloids from *Corydaliss turtschaninovii. J Ethanophramacol.* 2008; 119: 74–80.

Hyun AJ, Byung-Sun M, Takako Y, Je-Hyun L, Yeong SK, Jae SC. Anti-Alzheimer and antioxidant activities of *Coptidis Rhizoma* alkaloids. *Biol Pharm Bull.* 2009; 32(8): 1433–1438.

Ingkaninan K, Phengpa P, Yuenyongsawad S, Khorana N. Acetylcholinesterase inhibitors from *Stephania venosa* tuber. *J Pharm Pharmacol.* 2006; 58: 695–700.

Ingkaninan K, Temkitthawon P, Chuenchom K, Yuyaem T, Thongnoi W. Screening for acetylcholinesterase inhibitory activity in plants used in Thai traditional rejuvenating and neurotonic remedies. *J Ethnopharmacol.* 2003; 89: 261–264.

Jing L, Zhang HY, Wang LM, Tang XC. Inhibitory effects of huperzine B on cholinesterase activity in mice. *Acta Pharmacol Sin.* 1999; 20: 141–145.

Kennedy DO, Dodd FL, Robertson BC, Okello EJ, Reay JL, Scholey AB, et al. Monoterpenoid extract of sage (*Salvia lavandulaefolia*) with cholinesterase inhibiting properties improves cognitive performance and mood in healthy adults. *J Psychopharmacol.* 2011; 25(8): 1088–1100.

Keyvan D, Damien Dorman HJ, Heikki V, Raimo H. Plants as potential sources for drug development against Alzheimer's disease. *Int J Biomed Pharm Sci.* 2007; 1(2): 83–104.

Khalid A, Azim MK, Parveen S, Atta-ur-Rahman, Choudhary MI. Structural basis of acetylcholinesterase inhibition by triterpenoidal alkaloids. *Biochem Biophys Res Commun.* 2005; 331(4): 1528–1532.

Khalid A, Zaheer-ul-Haq, Anjum S, Khan MR, Atta-ur-Rahman, Choudhary MI. Kinetics and structure-activity relationship studies on steroidal alkaloids that inhibit cholinesterases. *Bioorg Med Chem.* 2004; 12: 1995–2003.

Kim WG, Cho KM, Lee CK, Yoo ID. Terreulactone A, a novel meroterpenoid with antiacetylcholinesterase activity from *Aspergillus terreus. Tetrahedron Lett.* 2002; 43: 3197–3198.

Kwon J, Seo YH, Lee JE, Seo EK, Li S, Guo Y, et al. Spiroindole alkaloids and spiroditerpenoids from *Aspergillus duricaulis* and their potential neuroprotective effects. *J Nat Prod.* 2015; 78(11): 2572–2579.

Lee JH, Lee KT, Yang JH, Baek NL, Kim DK. Acetylcholinesterase inhibitors from the twigs of *Vaccinium oldhami* Miquel. *Arc Pharmacal Res.* 2004; 27: 53–56.

Lee KY, Yoon JS, Kim ES, Kang SY, Kim YC. Anti-acetylcholinesterase and anti-amnesic activities of a pregnane glycoside, cynatroside B, from *Cynanchum atratum. Planta Med.* 2005; 71: 7–11.

Lima J, Costa RS, Epifanio RA, Castro NG, Rocha MS, Pinto AC. *Geissospermum vellosii* stem bark: anticholinesterase activity and improvement of scopolamine-induced memory deficits. *Pharmacol Biochem Behav.* 2009; 92: 508–513.

Lopez S, Bastida J, Viladomat F, Codina C. Acetylcholinesterase inhibitory activity of some Amaryllidaceae alkaloids and Narcissus extracts. *Life Sci.* 2002; 71: 2521–2529.

Ma WG, Fukushi Y, Tahara S. Fungitoxic alkaloids from Hokkaido; a *Corydalis* species. *Fitoter.* 1999; 70: 258–265.
Mahesh G, Tasneem S. Biomarker controversies and diagnostic difficulties in Alzheimer's disease. *Am J Phytomed Clin Therap.* 2014; 2(4): 463–468.
Mankil J, Moonsoo P. Acetylcholinesterase inhibition by flavonoids from *Agrimonia pilosa*. *Molecules.* 2007; 12: 2130–2139.
Mona M, Abdu A, Marwan S. New acetylcholinesterase inhibitors for Alzheimer's disease. *Int J Alz Dis.* 2012; 2012: 1–8.
Mukherjee PK, Kumar V, Houghton PJ. Screening of Indian medicinal plants for acetylcholinesterase inhibitory activity. *Phytother Res.* 2007a; 21: 1142–1145.
Mukherjee PK, Kumar V, Mal M, Houghton PJ. Acetylcholinesterase inhibitors from plants. *Phytomedicine.* 2007b; 14: 289–300.
Natalia W, Agnieszka K, Anna KK. Screening of traditional European herbal medicines for acetylcholinesterase and butyrylcholinesterase inhibitory activity. *Acta Pharm.* 2010; 60: 119–128.
Natarajan S, Shunmugiahthevar KP, Kasi PD. Cholinesterase inhibitors from plants: possible treatment strategy for neurological disorders – a review. *Int J Biomed Pharm Sci.* 2009; 3(1): 87–103.
Orhan I, Aslan M. Appraisal of scopolamine-induced antiamnesic effect in mice and in vitro antiacetylcholinesterase and antioxidant activities of some traditionally used Lamiaceae plants. *J Ethnopharmacol.* 2009; 122(2): 327–332.
Orhan I, Kartal M, Naz Q, Ejaz A, Yilmaz G, Kan Y, et al. Antioxidant and anticholinesterase evaluation of selected Turkish *Salvia* species. *Food Chem.* 2007; 103: 1247–1254.
Orhan I, Qamar N, Murat K, Fatma T, Bilge S, Iqbal CM. *In vitro* anticholinesterase activity of various alkaloids. *Z Naturforsch.* 2007; 62c: 684–688.
Orhan I, Salih T, Bilge S. An acetylcholinesterase inhibitor from *Lycopodium clavatum*. *Planta Med.* 2003; 69: 1–3.
Orhan I, Sener B, Choudhary MI, Khalid A. Acetylcholinesterase and butyrylcholinesterase inhibitory activity of some Turkish medicinal plants. *J Ethnopharmacol.* 2004; 91: 57–60.
Perry NS, Houghton PJ, Jenner P, Keith A, Perry EK. *Salvia lavandulaefolia* essential oil inhibits cholinesterase *in vivo*. *Phytomedicine.* 2002; 9: 48–51.
Peter JH, Melanie-Jayne H. Natural products and derivatives affecting neurotransmission relevant to Alzheimer's and Parkinson's disease. *Neurosignals.* 2005; 14: 6–22.
Popik P, Layer RT, Fossom LH, Benveniste M, Geter-Douglass B, Witkin JM, Skolnick P. NMDA antagonist properties of the putative antiaddictive drug, ibogaine. *J Pharmacol Exp Ther.* 1995; 275(2): 753–760.
Puchchakayala G, Akina S, Thati M. Neuroprotective effects of meloxicam and selegiline in scopolamine-induced cognitive impairment and oxidative stress. *Int J Alzheimer Dis.* 2012; 12: 1–8.
Rahman AU, Choudhary MI. Bioactive natural products as a potential source of new pharmacophores a theory of memory. *Pure Appl Chem.* 2001; 73: 555–560.
Rahman A-ur, Parveen S, Khalid A, Farooq A, Ayattollahi SAM, Choudhary MI. Acetylcholinesterase inhibiting triterpenoidal alkaloids from *Buxus hyrcana*. *Heterocycle.* 1998; 49: 481–488.
Rhee IK, Meent MV, Ingkaninan K, Verpoorte R. Screening for acetylcholinesterase inhibitors from Amaryllidaceae using silica gel thin-layer chromatography in combination with bioactivity staining. *J Chromatogr.* 2001; 915: 217–223.
Rinne JO, Kaasinen V, Jarvenpaa T, Någren K, Roivainen A, Yu M, et al. Brain acetylcholinesterase activity in mild cognitive impairment and early Alzheimer's disease. *Neurol Neurosurg Psychiatr.* 2003; 74: 113–115.
Salloway S, Mintzer J, Weiner MF, Cummings JL. Disease-modifying therapies for Alzheimer's disease. *Alzheimer Dement.* 2008; 4: 65–79.
Salomon AR, Marcinowski KJ, Friedland RP, Zagorski MG. Nicotine inhibits amyloid formation by the beta-peptide. *Biochemistry.* 1996; 35(42): 13568–13578.
Sarna LK, Wu N, Hwang SY, Siow YLOK. Berberine inhibits NADPH oxidase mediated superoxide anion production in macrophages. *Can J Physiol Pharmacol.* 2010; 88(3): 369–378.
Schneider LS. New therapeutic approaches to Alzheimer's disease. *Psychiatry.* 1996; 57 Supplement 14: 30–36.
Senol FS, Orhan I, Yilmaz G, Cic ek M, Sener B. Acetylcholinesterase, butyrylcholinesterase, and tyrosinase inhibition studies and antioxidant activities of 33 *Scutellaria* L. taxa from Turkey. *Food Chem Toxicol.* 2010; 48: 781–788.
Skovronsky DM, Lee VMY, Trojanowsky JQ. Neurodegenerative diseases: new concepts of pathogenesis and their therapeutic implications. *Annu Rev Pathol.* 2006; 1: 151–170.

Szwajgier D, Maria W, Edyta W, Zdzislaw T. Anticholinesterase and antioxidant activities of commercial preparations from *Ginkgo biloba* leaves. *Acta Sci Pol Hortorum Cultus*. 2013; 12(5): 111–125.

Tariot PN, Farlow MR, Grossberg GT, Graham SM, McDonald S, Gergel I. Memantine treatment in patients with moderate to severe Alzheimer disease already receiving donepezil: a randomized controlled trial. *JAMA*. 2004; 291(3): 317–324.

Thandla R. Neuromuscular blocking drugs: discovery and development. *J R Soc Med*. 2002; 95(7): 363–367.

Thomas M. Rivastigmine in the treatment of patients with Alzheimer's disease. *Neuropsychiatr Dis Treat*. 2007; 3(2): 211–218.

Urbain A, Marston A, Queiroz EF, Ndjoko K, Hostettmann K. Xanthones from *Gentiana campestris* as new acetylcholinesterase inhibitors. *Planta Med*. 2004; 70: 1011–1014.

Vladimir-Knezevic S, Biljana B, Marija K, Jelena V, Agnieszka DL, Adelheid HB. Acetylcholinesterase inhibitory, antioxidant and phytochemical properties of selected medicinal plants of the Lamiaceae family. *Molecules*. 2014; 19: 767–782.

Wang BS, Wang H, Wei ZH, Song YY, Zhang L, Chen HZ. Efficacy and safety of natural acetylcholinesterase inhibitor huperzine A in the treatment of Alzheimer's disease: an updated meta-analysis. *J Neural Transm*. 2009; 116(4): 457–465.

Williams P, Sorribas A, Howes MJ. Natural products as a source of Alzheimer's drug leads. *Nat Prod Rep*. 2011; 28(1): 48–77.

Yu PN, Terry CTO, Nancy YI. Plant alkaloids as drug leads for Alzheimer's disease. *Neurochem Int*. 2015; 89: 260–270.

Zhang JM, Hu GY. Huperzine A, a nootropic alkaloid, inhibits N-methyl-D-aspartate-induced current in rat dissociated hippocampal neurons. *Neuroscience*. 2001; 105(3): 663–669.

18 Epigallocatechin-3-Gallate in Alzheimer's Disease

Khaleel Pasha Md and Magisetty Obulesu

CONTENTS

ABBREVIATIONS

AA	Ascorbic Acid
AChE	Acetylcholinesterase
AD	Alzheimer's Disease
$AlCl_3$	Aluminum Chloride
APP	Amyloid Precursor Protein
ATP	Adenosine Triphosphate
Aβ	Amyloid Beta
BACE1	Beta Amyloid Cleaving Enzyme1
BBB	Blood–Brain Barrier
BChE	Butyrylcholinesterase
EC	Epicatechin
ECG	Epicatechin Gallate
EGCG	Epigallocatechin Gallate
ER	Estrogen Receptor
ERK	Extracellular Signal-Regulated Kinase
GCG	Gallocatechin Gallate
GTC	Green Tea Catechins
GTP	Green Tea Polyphenols
iNOS	interleukin 6 (IL-6) Orinducible Nitric Oxide Synthase
LPS	Lipopolysaccharide
mRNA	Messenger ribonucleic Acid
N2a	Murine Neuron-like Cells
NDs	Neurodegenerative Diseases

NEP	Neprilysin
NFTs	Neurofibrillary Tangles
NMDA	N-methyl-D-aspartate
NMR	Nuclear Magnetic Resonance
NO	Nitric Oxide
NPs	Nanoparticles
OA	Okadaic Acid
PEG	Poly (Ethylene Glycol)
PEP	Prolyl Endopeptidase
PLA	Poly D, L-lactic Acid
PLGA	Poly (Lactic-co-Glycolic Acid)
PPAR γ	Peroxisome Proliferator-Activated Receptor γ
RCMkappa-CN	Carboxymethylated kappa-casein
ROS	Reactive Oxygen Species
SAMP8	Senescence Accelerated Mouse Prone 8
TNF-α	Tumor Necrosis Factor-α

18.1 INTRODUCTION

Tea has long been the widely-used beverage in the world. Green tea, black tea, and oolong tea are derived from the same plant, *Camellia sinensis*, but treated in different ways, based on the degree of fermentation (Miyoshi et al., 2015; Suzuki et al., 2016; Pervin et al., 2018). Of these, green tea plays a vital role in providing health benefits, and has attracted the attention of researchers (Pervin et al., 2018). Green tea contains valuable chemical ingredients such as green tea catechins (GTC), caffeine, and theanine, which all play a key role in ameliorating neurodegeneration (Chen et al., 2018; Pervin et al., 2018). GTC were found to target several events, such as unusual aggregation of fibrous proteins like amyloid-beta (Aβ) and α-synuclein, enhanced expression of pro-apoptotic proteins, inflammation, and oxidative stress, the latter being linked to neuronal cell death in the cerebral cortex (Pervin et al., 2018). Daily tea intake has been found to lower AD risk, despite ambiguity regarding its beneficial effect (Ma et al., 2016; Pervin et al., 2018).

Preclinical and clinical trials of AD have shown that epigallocatechin-3-gallate (EGCG) reduces Tau aggregation and tumor necrosis factor alpha (TNF-α), inhibits Aβ aggregation, interleukin-6 (IL-6) or inducible nitric oxide synthase (iNOS) expression, and increases mitochondrial function (Mandel et al., 2008; Wobst et al., 2015; Wei et al., 2016; Awasthi et al., 2016; Cano et al., 2019). In addition to its antioxidant and metal chelation properties, EGCG intervenes in Aβ pathways and potentially decreases its accumulation (Singh et al., 2016, 2018). A wealth of studies has shown that the dysregulated blood–brain barrier (BBB) in AD makes it permeable to numerous molecules which cannot normally pass through the BBB under healthy conditions (Minogue et al., 2014; Yamazaki and Kanekiyo, 2017; Zenaro et al., 2017; Cano et al., 2019).

Despite the availability of approved drugs to treat AD, such as the acetylcholinesterase inhibitors donepezil, galantamine, rivastigmine, and the NMDA receptor antagonist memantine, these approved pharmaceuticals do not show sufficient potential to curb progression of AD (Ballard et al., 2011; Cummings et al., 2015; Cano et al., 2019). Therefore, innovative therapeutic approaches are currently in high demand. Within the past decade, EGCG has attracted the attention of researchers as a potential AD therapeutic (Singh et al., 2018). EGCG has exhibited robust therapeutic efficacy against the symptoms of a plethora of diseases such as cancer, Down syndrome, and various neurological disorders, and has been found to be a safe molecule (Chowdhury et al., 2016; de la Torre et al., 2016; Cascella et al., 2017; Cano et al., 2019). Although EGCG consumption of more than 800 mg/d was associated with liver damage in a few cases, this side effect may be due to idiosyncratic reactions (Younes et al., 2018; Cano et al., 2019).

Studies have shown that GTCs and black tea theaflavins positively influence verbal memory and language (Kesse-Guyot et al., 2012; Polito et al., 2018). A few other studies have also emphasized the positive role of tea consumption in averting neurodegenerative diseases (NDs) such as AD (Liu et al., 2011; Feng et al., 2015; Polito et al., 2018). A Growing number of studies has paid closer attention to effects of tea catechins such as oxidation, microglia activation, iron chelation, and control of intracellular neuronal signal transduction pathways (Weinreb et al., 2009; Singh et al., 2016; Fernando et al., 2017; Polito et al., 2018). Green tea polyphenols (GTPs) markedly decreased okadaic acid (OA)-induced neuronal damage and improved AD symptoms in mice (Li et al., 2014; Polito et al., 2018). Specific endoplasmic reticulum (ER) alterations were considered to be a potential AD therapeutic event, and EGCG was found to be an adequately tolerated substitute for estrogen therapy in the prophylaxis and treatment of AD (Fernandez et al., 2010; Polito et al., 2018).

EGCG attenuates *in vitro* fibril formation through decreased Carboxymethylated kappa-casein (RCMkappa-CN) by averting RCMkappa-CN fibril formation (Hudson et al., 2009; Polito et al., 2018). Metal-chelating efficacy of EGCG substantially attenuated fibril formation (Polito et al., 2018). The oxidized EGCG formed Schiff bases by interacting with free amines of the amyloid fibrils, thus reducing the toxicity (Palhano et al., 2013; Polito et al., 2018). NMR studies also showed that EGCG conjugated nonspecifically to the Aβ monomer (Sinha et al., 2012; Polito et al., 2018).

18.2 INFLUENCE ON ENZYMES

Prolyl endopeptidase (PEP), a serine protease, has been found to show greater activity in AD subjects compared with people without AD (Aoyagi et al., 1991; Polito et al., 2018). EGCG, epicatechin gallate [(-)-ECG], and gallocatechin gallate (GCG), isolated from tea leaves, were potential PEP inhibitors and successfully achieved AD prevention (Kim et al., 2001; Polito et al., 2018). EGCG also inhibited acetylcholinesterase (AChE) and butyrylcholinesterase (BChE) activities, leading to increased cholinergic transmission (Ali et al., 2016; Polito et al., 2018).

18.3 NEPRILYSIN

When inhibited, neprilysin (NEP), a vital Aβ-degrading enzyme, induces Aβ aggregation in sporadic late-onset AD patients (Marr et al., 2003; Hama et al., 2004; Miners et al., 2006; Polito et al., 2018). Treatment with EGCG enhanced the degradation of Aβ by initiating extracellular signal-regulated kinase (ERK) activity, indicating a potential therapeutic effect of EGCG against AD (Yamamoto et al., 2017; Polito et al., 2018). EGCG administration also enhanced NEP activity in blood plasma, the hippocampus, and the cortex, as well as ameliorating memory loss in the 8-arm maze and object recognition tests (Zhuvarin et al., 2019).

18.4 MITOCHONDRIAL FUNCTION

EGCG showed substantial protective activity against AD by preventing mitochondrial dysfunction, which is an early event in disease pathology (Wu et al., 2014; Polito et al., 2018). In addition, its administration to amyloid precursor peptide/ presenilin-1 (APP/PS-1) double transgenic AD mice potentially improved mitochondrial respiratory rates, mitochondrial membrane potential, reactive oxygen species (ROS) damage, and ATP levels by 50-85% in mitochondria of the hippocampus, cortex, and striatum (Dragicevic et al., 2011; Polito et al., 2018). It also inhibited an Aβ-induced mitochondrial apoptotic bax increase, achieving protection from the Aβ-induced neurotoxicity through attenuation of the protein expression linked to the mitochondrion-dependent cell death pathway (Kim et al., 2005; Polito et al., 2018).

18.5 INFLUENCE ON PATHOLOGICAL AB AND TAU

GTPs, such as EGCG, EC, catechin, quercetin, myricetin, and kaempferol, offer protection from Aβ-induced neurotoxicity in a dose-dependent manner by attenuating Aβ fibril formation from fresh $A\beta_{1-40}$ and $A\beta_{1-42}$ through disruption of the fibrils (Ono et al., 2003; Polito et al., 2018). Oral uptake of epicatechin (EC) exhibited analogous effects on Aβ pathology by attenuating beta amyloid-cleaving enzymel (BACE1) (Cox et al., 2015; Polito et al., 2018). EGCG successfully scavenged phosphorylated tau protein species in a particular manner by enhancing adaptor protein expression (Chesser et al., 2016; Polito et al., 2018). It has also been shown that EGCG administration substantially recovers recognition and memory in senescence-accelerated mouse prone 8 (SAMP8) mice by decreasing Aβ and Tau hyperphosphorylation (Guo et al., 2017; Polito et al., 2018). EGCG also exhibits neuroprotective properties by inhibiting Aβ-mediated neuronal apoptosis by eliminating ROS accumulation and mitigating AD progression (Choi et al., 2001; Avramovich-Tirosh et al., 2007; Harvey et al., 2011; Polito et al., 2018). $A\beta_{25-35}$ administration (100 μmol/μL) into the cornu Ammonis (CA1) hippocampal area of mice induced a remarkable increase in lipid peroxidation, ROS accumulation, and memory dysfunction (Polito et al., 2018). However, EC (30 mg/kg) administration substantially reversed the $A\beta_{25-35}$ -induced oxidative stress damage (Cuevas et al., 2009; Polito et al., 2018). EGCG has been shown to bind to Aβ and to avert neurotoxicity by inhibiting formation of free radicals (Ehrnhoefer et al., 2008; Singh et al., 2018).

18.6 CLINICAL TRIALS

A study conducted on 1003 Japanese subjects aged 70 or older (in a group consisting of green tea consumers and low consumers of green tea) showed significantly decreased cognitive impairment (Kuriyama et al., 2006; Polito et al., 2018). Another cross-sectional study on 1143 Japanese subjects showed that lower intake of green tea was linked with increased incidence of cognitive impairment (Kitamura et al., 2016; Polito et al., 2018). Similarly, another cross-sectional study, on 2501 Singapore citizens aged 55 or older, demonstrated the lower incidence of cognitive impairment associated with tea consumption (Ng et al., 2008; Polito et al., 2018).

18.7 CHEMISTRY

Of the many pharmacological studies conducted in attempts to combat AD, those on the green tea polyphenol EGCG, a vital polyphenol of green tea plant *Camellia sinensis*, have been of considerable importance (Schimidt et al., 2017; Cano et al., 2019). EGCG showed substantial antioxidant and chelating activities, due to the presence of two gallocatechol rings that scavenge free radicals effectively (Braicu et al., 2013; Cano et al., 2019).

18.8 ANIMAL MODELS

Oral administration of EGCG (1.5 and 3 mg/kg bodyweight for three weeks) daily through drinking water improved a lipopolysaccharide (LPS) (1 μg/mouse, i.c.v.) –induced memory deficit in a dose-dependent manner (Lee et al., 2009; Polito et al., 2018). In another study, intake of 6 mg EGCG/kg/d profoundly decreased Aβ aggregation and neuronal injury in the hippocampus of the AD mouse model (He et al., 2012; Pervin et al., 2018). In another study, administration of EGCG (50 mg/kg/d) for four months showed improved cognition and decreased Aβ levels in TgCRND8 transgenic mice, compared with control mice (Walker et al., 2015; Pervin et al., 2018). EGCG inhibited Aβ production in both murine neuron-like cells (N2a) transfected with Swedish mutant APP mice and primary neurons obtained from Swedish mutant APP-overexpressing mice. EGCG induced marked cleavage of the α-C-terminal fragment of APP and increased the concentration of the N-terminal APP cleavage product, soluble APP- α (Polito et al., 2018). This cleavage is linked with increased α-secretase activity and increased hydrolysis of the TNF-α converting enzyme, an initial product of α-secretase (Polito et al., 2018). Studies on TgAPPsw transgenic mice demonstrated that EGCG administration reduced Aβ levels and plaques by inducing the non-amyloidogenic α-secretase proteolytic pathway (Rezai-Zadeh et al., 2005; Omar, 2017; Polito et al., 2018). Additionally, EGCG has been found to upregulate the nuclear receptor peroxisome proliferator-activated receptor γ (PPARγ) mRNA and protein expression to induce therapeutic activity for AD (Zhang et al., 2017; Polito et al., 2018).

18.9 DISADVANTAGES OF EGCG

Despite its remarkable therapeutic efficacy, EGCG has a few demerits, which include its instability and low bioavailability (Granja et al., 2017; Krupkova et al., 2016; Cano et al., 2019). EGCG degradation is essentially induced by oxidation of the polyphenolic structure (Cano et al., 2019). Therefore, robust antioxidants, such as ascorbic acid (AA), are often added to counter this effect (Cano et al., 2019). AA removes oxygen, guards double bonds, and also exhibits anti-inflammatory properties in the formulation (Zhang et al., 2018; Dey and Bishayi, 2018; Cano et al., 2019). AA, in association with EGCG, decreases the inflammatory response (Ellulu et al., 2015; Ohishi et al., 2016; Cano et al., 2019).

18.10 NANOTECHNOLOGY

Nanotechnology-based targeted drug delivery has been extensively used to treat diseases such as diabetes, cancer, and NDs (Saraiva et al., 2016; Elzoghby et al., 2016; Cano et al., 2019). Moreover, nano systems facilitate the conjugation of targeting ligands on their surface, indicating novel internalization pathways (El-Say and El-Sawy, 2017; Bahrami et al., 2017; Cano et al., 2019). Poly (lactic-co-glycolic acid) (PLGA) is a polymer extensively used in the preparation of nanoparticles (NPs) due to its biocompatibility, biodegradability, and non-toxicity (Salem et al., 2013; Sharma et al., 2015; Cano et al., 2019). Despite numerous studies showing improved drug transport to the brain, even with the use of non-ligand-coated PLGA NPs, the underlying mechanisms are still ambiguous (Li and Sabliov, 2013; Md et al., 2014; Kreuter, 2014; Chen et al., 2017; Zhou et al., 2018; Cano et al., 2019). In addition, surface poly(ethylene glycol) (PEG)ylation of NPs offers appreciable benefits, which include increased half-life, increased aqueous solubility, decreased aggregation, and lower immunogenicity (Kolate et al., 2014; El-Hammadi et al., 2017; Cano et al., 2019).

EGCG exerts enhanced therapeutic activity against AD. However, the instability and low bioavailability of EGCG impede its success as a potential therapeutic (Cano et al., 2019). Increased stability of EGCG was observed after formulation with dual drug-loaded PEGylated PLGA NPs (Cano et al., 2019). Oral administration of EGCG/ascorbic acid NPs showed increased aggregation of EGCG in all vital organs, such as the brain (Cano et al., 2019). EGCG/AA NPs showed 5-fold higher EGCG concentrations after a long duration (5–25 hours), although initial concentrations were similar in both free EGCG and EGCG/AA NPs, following oral administration (Cano et al., 2019). Interestingly, EGCG, unloaded NPs, and EGCG/AA NPs all induced tight junction destabilization and crossed the BBB *in vitro* and *ex vivo* (Cano et al., 2019). Oral administration of EGCG/AA NPs significantly augmented the synapses, and inhibited neuroinflammation and Aβ plaque burden in APPswe/PS1 dE9 (APP/PS1) mice (Cano et al., 2019). It has been proposed that free or nano-formulated EGCG crossed the BBB *via* the destabilized junctions (Cano et al., 2019).

In another study, nano EGCG reversed the neurobehavioural dysfunction in $AlCl_3$ -treated rats (Singh et al., 2018). Additionally, $AlCl_3$-induced pathological markers, such as neuritic plaques and NFTs, were absent from nano EGCG-treated rats (Singh et al., 2018). In this study, EGCG had been encapsulated into PLA and PEG polymer NPs, which substantially induced antioxidant and metal-chelating abilities and attenuated Al (III) initiated $A\beta_{42}$ fibrillation *in vitro* (Singh et al., 2018). It also led to significant decreases in ROS and NO levels in the cortex and hippocampus (Singh et al., 2018).

18.11 CONCLUSIONS AND FUTURE PERSPECTIVES

Although tea intake has shown profound health benefits, similar protective effects have not been observed in humans (Pervin et al., 2018). EGCG is a potential antioxidant and is extensively used in the treatment of several diseases, such as NDs. Nevertheless, a few demerits, such as instability and low bioavailability, limit its success. Therefore, numerous nanotechnological strategies have been used to overcome these issues. Interestingly, a few formulations, such as EGCG/AA NPs, showed appreciable activity in AD treatment. On the other hand, several studies have shown that tea intake has no link with the prevention or treatment of AD (Kim et al., 2015; Pervin et al., 2018). Based on the wide range of studies performed on EGCG and EGCG-based delivery systems, it can be concluded that the expertise gleaned from various biological, medical, and nanotechnological fields can lay a potential cornerstone, based around which vital and novel therapeutic strategies can be designed.

REFERENCES

Ali B, Jamal QMS, Shams S, Al-Wabel NA, Siddiqui MU, Alzohairy MA, Al Karaawi MA, Kesari KK, Mushtaq G, Kamal MA. In silico analysis of green tea polyphenols as inhibitors of AChE and BChE enzymes in Alzheimer's disease treatment. *CNS Neurol Disord Drug.* 2016;15:624–628.

Aoyagi T, Nagai M, Ogawa K, Gojima F, Okada M, Ikeda T, Hamada M, Takeuchi T. Poststatin, a new inhibitor of prolylendopeptidase, produced by Streptomyces viridochromogens MH534-30F3. I. Taxonomy, production, isolation, physico-chemical properties and biological activities. *J Antibiot.* 1991;44:949–955.

Avramovich-Tirosh Y, Rezrlichenko D, Amit T, Zheng H, Fridkin M, Weinreb O, Mandel S, Youdim MBH. Neurorescue activity, APP regulation and amyloid-β peptide reduction by novel multi-functional brain permeable iron- chelating- antioxidants, m-30 and green tea polyphenol, EGCG. *Curr Alzheimer Res.* 2007;4:403–411.

Awasthi M, Singh S, Pandey VP, Dwivedi UN. Alzheimer's disease: an overview of amyloid beta dependent pathogenesis and its therapeutic implications along with in silico approaches emphasizing the role of natural products. *J Neurol Sci.* 2016;361:256–271.

Bahrami A, Hojjat-farsangi M, Mohammadi H, Anvari E. Nanoparticles and targeted drug delivery in cancer therapy. *Immunol Lett.* 2017;190:64–83.

Ballard C, Gauthier S, Corbett A, Brayne C, Aarsland D, Jones E. Alzheimer's disease. *Lancet.* 2011;377:1019–1031.

Braicu C, Ladomery MR, Chedea VS, Irimie A. The relationship between the structure and biological actions of green tea catechins. *Food Chem.* 2013;141:3282–3289.

Cano A, Ettcheto M, Chang JH, Barroso E, Espina M, Kuhne BA, Barenys M, Auladell C, Folch J, Souto EB, Camins A, Turowski P, Garcia ML. Dual-drug loaded nanoparticles of Epigallocatechin-3-gallate (EGCG)/Ascorbic acid enhance therapeutic efficacy of EGCG in a APPswe/PS1dE9 Alzheimer's disease mice model. *J Control Rel.* 2019;301:62–75.

Cascella M, Bimonte S, Muzio M, Schiavone V, Cuomo A. The efficacy of Epigallocatechin-3-gallate (green tea) in the treatment of Alzheimer's disease: an overview of pre-clinical studies and translational perspectives in clinical practice. *Infect Agents Cancer.* 2017;12:1–7.

Chen SQ, Wang ZS, Ma YX, Zhang W, Lu JL, Liang YR, Zheng XQ. Neuroprotective effects and mechanisms of tea bioactive components in neurodegenerative diseases. *Molecules.* 2018;23:512.

Chen T, Li C, Li Y, Yi XR, Wang SM, Lee SM, Zheng Y. Small-sized mPEG-PLGA nanoparticles of Schisantherin A with sustained release for enhanced brain uptake and anti-parkinsonian activity. *ACS Appl Mater Interfaces.* 2017;9:9516–9527.

Chesser AS, Ganeshan V, Yang J, Johnson GVW. Epigallocatechin-3-gallate enhances clearance of phosphorylated tau in primary neurons. *Nutr Neurosci.* 2016;19:21–31.

Choi YT, Jung CH, Lee SR, Bae JH, Baek WK, Suh MH, Park J, Park CW, Suh SI. The green tea polyphenol (-)-epigallocatechin gallate attenuates β-amyloid-induced neurotoxicity in cultured hippocampal neurons. *Life Sci.* 2001;70:603–614.

Chowdhury A, Sarkar J, Chakraborti T, Pramanik PK, Chakraborti S. Protective role of epigallocatechin-3-gallate in health and disease: a perspective. *Biomed Pharmacother.* 2016;78:50–59.

Cox CJ, Choudhry F, Peacey E, Perkinton MS, Richardson JC, Howlett DR, Lichtenthaler SF, Francis PT, Williams RJ. Dietary (–)-epicatechin as a potent inhibitor of βγ-secretase amyloid precursor protein processing. *Neurobiol Aging.* 2015;36:178–187.

Cuevas E, Limon D, Perez-Severiano F, Diaz A, Ortega L, Zenteno E, Guevara J. Antioxidant effects of epicatechin on the hippocampal toxicity caused by amyloid-beta 25–35 in rats. *Eur J Pharmacol.* 2009;616:122–127.

Cummings J, Isaacson R, Schmitt F, Velting D. A practical algorithm for managing Alzheimer's disease: what, when, and why? *Ann Clin Transl Neurol.* 2015;2:307–323.

de la Torre R, de Sola S, Hernandez G, Farre M, Pujol J, Rodriguez J, Espadaler JM, Langohr K, Cuenca-Royo A, Principe A, Xicota L, Janel N, Catuara-Solarz S, Sanchez-Benavides G, Blehaut H, Duenas-Espin I, Del Hoyo L, Benejam B, Blanco-Hinojo L, Videla S, Fito M, Delabar JM, Dierssen M, TESDAD study group. Safety and efficacy of cognitive training plus epigallocatechin-3-gallate in young adults with Down's syndrome (TESDAD): a double-blind, randomised, placebo controlled, phase 2 trial. *Lancet Neurol.* 2016;15:801–810.

Dey S, Bishayi B. Killing of *S. aureus* in murine peritoneal macrophages by ascorbic acid along with antibiotics Chloramphenicol or Ofloxacin: correlation with inflammation. *Microb Pthog.* 2018;115:239–250.

Dragicevic N, Smith A, Lin XY, Yuan F, Copes N, Delic V, Tan J, Cao CH, Shytle RD, Bradshaw PC. Green tea epigallocatechin-3-gallate (EGCG) and other flavonoids reduce Alzheimer's amyloid-induced mitochondrial dysfunction. *J Alzheimers Dis.* 2011;26:507–521.

Ehrnhoefer DE, Bieschke J, Boeddrich A, Herbst M, Masino L, Lurz R, Engemann S, Pastore A, Wanker EE. EGCG redirects amyloidogenic polypeptides into unstructured, off-pathway oligomers. *Nat Struct Mol Biol.* 2008;15:558–566.

El-Hammadi MM, Delgado AV, Melguizo C, Prados JC, Arias JL. Folic acid decorated and PEGylated PLGA nanoparticles for improving the antitumour activity of 5-fluorouracil. *Int J Pharm.* 2017;516:61–70.

Ellulu M, Rahmat A, Patimah I, Khaza'ai H, Abed Y. Effect of vitamin C on inflammation and metabolic markers in hypertensive and/or diabetic obese adults: a randomized controlled trial. *Drug Des Dev Ther.* 2015;9:3405–3412.

El-Say KM, El-Sawy HS. Polymeric nanoparticles: promising platform for drug delivery. *Int J Pharm.* 2017;528:675–691.

Elzoghby AO, Hemasa AL, Freag MS. Hybrid protein-inorganic nanoparticles: from tumor-targeted drug delivery to cancer imaging. *J Control Rel.* 2016;243:303–322.

Feng L, Chong MS, Lim WS, Lee TS, Kua EH, Ng TP. Tea for Alzheimer prevention. *J Prev Alzheimer Dis.* 2015;2:136–141.

Fernandez JW, Rezai-Zadeh K, Obregon D, Tan J. EGCG functions through estrogen receptor-mediated activation of ADAM10 in the promotion of non-amyloidogenic processing of APP. *FEBS Lett.* 2010;584:4259–4267.

Fernando W, Somaratne G, Goozee KG, Williams S, Singh H, Martins RN. Diabetes and Alzheimer's disease: can tea phytochemicals play a role in prevention? *J Alzheimer Dis.* 2017;59:481–501.

Granja A, Frias I, Neves AR, Pinheiro M, Reis S. Therapeutic potential of Epigallocatechin gallate nanodelivery systems. *Biomed Res Int.* 2017;17:1–15.

Guo YF, Zhao Y, Nan Y, Wang X, Chen YL, Wang S. (–)-Epigallocatechin-3-gallate ameliorates memory impairment and rescues the abnormal synaptic protein levels in the frontal cortex and hippocampus in a mouse model of Alzheimer's disease. *Neuroreport.* 2017;28:590–597.

Hama E, Shirotani K, Iwata N, Saido TC. Effects of neprilysin chimeric proteins targeted to subcellular compartments on amyloid beta peptide clearance in primary neurons. *J Biol Chem.* 2004;279:30259–30264.

Harvey BS, Musgrave IF, Ohlsson KS, Fransson A, Smid SD. The green tea polyphenol (–)-epigallocatechin-3-gallate inhibits amyloid-β evoked fibril formation and neuronal cell death in vitro. *Food Chem.* 2011;129:1729–1736.

He M, Liu MY, Wang S, Tang QS, Yao WF, Zhao HS, Wei MJ. Research on EGCG improving the degenerative changes of the brain in AD model mice induced with chemical drugs. *Zhong Yao Cai.* 2012;35:1641–1644.

Hudson SA, Ecroyd H, Dehle FC, Musgrave IF, Carver J. (–)-Epigallocatechin-3-gallate (EGCG) maintains k-casein in its pre-fibrillar state without redirecting its aggregation pathway. *J Mol Biol.* 2009;392:689–700.

Kesse-Guyot E, Fezeu L, Andreeva VA, Touvier M, Scalbert A, Hercberg S, Galan P. Total and specific polyphenol intakes in midlife are associated with cognitive function measured 13 years later. *J Nutr.* 2012;142:76–83.

Kim JH, Kim SI, Song KS. Prolyl endopeptidase inhibitors from green tea. *Arch Pharm Res.* 2001;24:292–296.

Kim MS, Jung JY, Kim EC, Kim HJ, Kim WJ, Lee EJ, Kim SH. Inhibition of amyloid peptide-induced neuronal cytotoxicity by EGCG. *Korean J Phys Anthropol.* 2005;18:139–147.

Kim YS, Kwak SM, Myung SK. Caffeine intake from coffee or tea and cognitive disorders: a meta-analysis of observational studies. *Neuroepidemiology.* 2015;44:51–63.

Kitamura K, Watanabe Y, Nakamura K, Sanpei K, Wakasugi M, Yokoseki A, Onodera O, Ikeuchi T, Kuwano R, Momotsu T, Narita I, Endo N. Modifiable factors associated with cognitive impairment in 1143 Japanese outpatients: the project in Sado for total health (PROST). *Dement Geriatr Cogn Disord Extra.* 2016;6:341–349.

Kolate A, Baradia D, Patil S, Vhora I, Kore G, Misra A. PEG – a versatile conjugating ligand for drugs and drug delivery systems. *J Control Rel.* 2014;192:67–81.

Kreuter J. Drug delivery to the central nervous system by polymeric nanoparticles: what do we know? *Adv Drug Deliv Rev.* 2014;71:2–14.

Krupkova O, Ferguson SJ, Wuertz-Kozak K. Stability of (–)-epigallocatechin gallate and its activity in liquid formulations and delivery systems. *J Nutr Biochem.* 2016;37:1–12.

Kuriyama A, Hozawa SA, Ohmori K, Shimazu T, Matsui T, Ebihara S, Awata S, Nagatomi R, Arai H, Tsuji I. Green tea consumption and cognitive function: a cross-sectional study from the Tsurugaya project. *Am J Clin Nutr.* 2006;83:355–361.

Lee YK, Yuk DY, Lee JW, Lee SY, Ha TY, Oh KW, Yun YP, Hong JT. Epigallocatechin-3-gallate prevents lipopolysaccharide-induced elevation of beta-amyloid generation and memory deficiency. *Brain Res.* 2009;1250:167–174.

Li HY, Wu XK, Wu Q, Gong DZ, Shi MJ, Guan LL, Zhang J, Liu J, Yuan B, Han GZ, Zou Y. Green tea polyphenols protect against okadaic acid-induced acute learning and memory impairments in rats. *Nutrition.* 2014;30:337–342.

Li L, Sabliov C. PLA/PLGA nanoparticles for delivery of drugs across the blood brain barrier. *Nanotechnol Rev.* 2013;2:241–257.

Liu K, Liang X, Kuang W. Tea consumption may be an effective active treatment for adult attention deficit hyperactivity disorder (ADHD). *Med Hypotheses.* 2011;76:461–463.

Ma QP, Huang C, Cui QY, Yang DJ, Sun K, Chen X, Li XH. Meta-analysis of the association between tea intake and the risk of cognitive disorders. *PLoS One.* 2016;11:e0165861.

Mandel SA, Amit T, Kalfon L, Reznichenko L, Weinreb O, Youdim MBH. Cell signaling pathways and iron chelation in the neurorestorative activity of green tea polyphenols: special reference to Epigallocatechin Gallate (EGCG). *J Alzheimers Dis.* 2008;15:211–222.

Marr RA, Rockenstein E, Mukherjee A, Kindy MS, Hersh LB, Gage FH, Verma IM, Masliah E. Neprilysin gene transfer reduces human amyloid pathology in transgenic mice. *J Neurosci.* 2003;23:1992–1996.

Md S, Ali M, Baboota S, Sahni JK, Bhatnagar A, Ali J. Preparation, characterization, in vivo biodistribution and pharmacokinetic studies of donepezil-loaded PLGA nanoparticles for brain targeting. *Drug Dev Ind Pharm.* 2014;40:278–287.

Miners JS, Van Helmond Z, Chalmers K, Wilcock G, Love S, Kehoe PG. Decreased expression and activity of neprilysin in Alzheimer disease are associated with cerebral amyloid angiopathy. *J Neuropathol Exp Neurol.* 2006;65:1012–1021.

Minogue AM, Jones RS, Kelly RJ, McDonald CL, Connor TJ, Lynch MA. Age associated dysregulation of microglial activation is coupled with enhanced blood brain barrier permeability and pathology in APP/PS1 mice. *Neurobiol Aging.* 2014;35:1442–1452.

Miyoshi N, Pervin M, Suzuki T, Isemura M, Nakamura Y. Green tea catechins for well-being and therapy: prospects and opportunities. *Bot Targets Ther.* 2015;5:85–96.

Ng TP, Feng L, Niti M, Kua EH, Yap KB. Tea consumption and cognitive impairment and decline in older Chinese adults. *Am J Clin Nutr.* 2008;88:224–231.

Ohishi T, Goto S, Monira P, Isemura M. Anti-inflammatory action of green tea. *Antiinflamm Antiallergy Agents Med Chem.* 2016;15:74–90.

Omar SH. Biophenols pharmacology against the amyloidogenic activity in Alzheimer's disease. *Biomed Pharmacother.* 2017;89:396–413.

Ono K, Yoshiike Y, Takashima A, Hasegawa K, Naiki H, Yamada M. Potent anti-amyloidogenic and fibril-destabilizing effects of polyphenols in vitro: implications for the prevention and therapeutics of Alzheimer's disease. *J Neurochem.* 2003;87:172–181.

Palhano FL, Lee J, Grimster NP, Kelly JW. Toward the molecular mechanism(s) by which EGCG treatment remodels mature amyloid fibrils. *J Am Chem Soc.* 2013;135:7503–7510.

Pervin M, Unno K, Ohishi T, Tanabe H, Miyoshi N, Nakamura Y. Beneficial effects of green tea catechins on neurodegenerative diseases. *Molecules.* 2018;23:1297.

Polito CA, Cai ZY, Shi YL, Li X, Yang R, Shi M, Li Q, Ma S, Xiang L, Wang K, Ye J, Lu J, Zheng X, Liang Y. Association of tea consumption with risk of Alzheimer's disease and anti β amyloid effects of tea. *Nutrients.* 2018;10:E655.

Rezai-Zadeh K, Shytle D, Sun N, Mori T, Hou HY, Jeanniton D, Ehrhart J, Townsend K, Zeng J, Morgan D, Hardy J, Town T, Tan J. Green tea epigallocatechin-3-gallate (EGCG) modulates amyloid precursor protein cleavage and reduces cerebral amyloidosis in Alzheimer transgenic mice. *J Neurosci.* 2005;25:8807–8814.

Salem SA, Hwei NM, Bin Saim A, Ho CC, Sagap I, Singh R. Yusof MR, Md Zainuddin Z, Idrus RB. Polylactic-coglycolic acid mesh coated with fibrin or collagen and biological adhesive substance as a prefabricated, degradable, biocompatible, and functional scaffold for regeneration of the urinary bladder wall. *J Biomed Mater Res.* 2013;101:2237–2247.

Saraiva A, Praca C, Ferreira R, Santos T, Ferreira L, Bernardino L. Nanoparticle mediated brain drug delivery: overcoming blood–brain barrier to treat neurodegenerative diseases. *J Control Rel.* 2016;235:34–47.

Schimidt HL, Garcia A, Martins A, Mello-Carpes PB, Carpes FP. Green tea supplementation produces better neuroprotective effects than red and black tea in Alzheimer-like rat model. *Food Res Int.* 2017;100:442–448.

Sharma AS, Parmar A, Kori S, Sandhir R. PLGA-based nanoparticles: a new paradigm in biomedical applications. *TrAC Trends Anal Chem.* 2015;80:30–40.

Singh NA, Bhardwaj V, Ravi C, Ramesh N, Mandal AKA, Khan ZA. EGCG nanoparticles attenuate aluminum chloride induced neurobehavioral deficits, beta amyloid and tau pathology in a rat model of Alzheimer's disease. *Front Aging Neurosci.* 2018;10:244.

Singh NA, Mandal AKA, Khan ZA. Potential neuroprotective properties of epigallocatechin-3-gallate (EGCG). *Nutr J.* 2016;15:60.

Sinha S, Du ZM, Maiti P, Klarner FG, Schrader T, Wang CY, Bitan G. Comparison of three amyloid assembly inhibitors: the sugar scyllo-inositol, the polyphenol epigallocatechingallate, and the molecular Tweezer CLR01. *ACS Chem Neurosci.* 2012;3:451–458.

Suzuki T, Pervin M, Goto S, Isemura M, Nakamura Y. Beneficial effects of tea and the green tea catechin epigallocatechin-3-gallate on obesity. *Molecules.* 2016;21:1305.

Walker JM, Klakotskaia D, Ajit D, Weisman GA, Wood WG, Sun GY, Serfozo P, Simonyi A, Schachtman TR. Beneficial effects of dietary EGCG and voluntary exercise on behavior in an Alzheimer's disease mouse model. *J Alzheimer's Dis.* 2015;44:561–572.

Wei JC, Huang H, Chen W, Huang C, Peng C, Lin C. Epigallocatechin gallate attenuates amyloid β-induced inflammation and neurotoxicity in EOC 13.31 microglia. *Eur J Pharmacol.* 2016;770:16–24.

Weinreb O, Amit T, Mandel S, Youdim MBH. Neuroprotective molecular mechanisms of (–)-epigallocatechin-3-gallate: a reflective outcome of its antioxidant, iron chelating and neuritogenic properties. *Genes Nutr.* 2009;4:283–296.

Wobst HJ, Sharma A, Diamond MI, Wanker EE, Bieschke J. The green tea polyphenol (–)-epigallocatechin gallate prevents the aggregation of tau protein into toxic oligomers at substoichiometric ratios. *FEBS Lett.* 2015;589:77–83.

Wu ZF, Zhu YS, Cao XS, Sun SF, Zhao BL. Mitochondrial toxic effects of a beta through mitofusins in the early pathogenesis of Alzheimer's disease. *Mol Neurobiol.* 2014;50:986–996.

Yamamoto N, Shibata M, Ishikuro R, Tanida M, Taniguchi Y, Ikeda-Matsuo Y, Sobue K. Epigallocatechin gallate induces extracellular degradation of amyloid beta-protein by increasing neprilysin secretion from astrocytes through activation of ERK and PI3K pathways. *Neuroscience.* 2017;362:70–78.

Yamazaki Y, Kanekiyo T. Blood-brain barrier dysfunction and the pathogenesis of Alzheimer's disease. *Mol Sci.* 2017;18:1–19.

Younes M, Aggett P, Aguilar F, Crebelli R, Dusemund B, Filipi M. Scientific opinion on the safety of green tea catechins. *EFSA J.* 2018;16:5239.

Zenaro E, Piacentino G, Constantin G. The blood-brain barrier in Alzheimer's disease. *Neurobiol Dis.* 2017;107:41–56.

Zhang W, Wu Y, Dong H, Yin J, Zhang H, Wu HA, Song LN, Chong Y, Li ZX, Gu N, Zhang Y. Sparks fly between ascorbic acid and iron-based nanozymes: a study on Prussian blue nanoparticles. *Colloids Surf B Biointerfaces.* 2018;163:379–384.

Zhang ZX, Li YB, Zhao RP. Epigallocatechin gallate attenuates beta-amyloid generation and oxidative stress involvement of PPAR gamma in N2a/APP695 cells. *Neurochem Res.* 2017;42:468–480.

Zhou Y, Peng Z, Seven ES, Leblanc RM. Crossing the blood-brain barrier with nanoparticles. *J Control Rel.* 2018;270:290–303.

Zhuvarin IA, Dubrovskaya NM, Vasilev DS, Kozlova DI, Kochkina EG, Numanova NL, Nalivaeva NN. Regulation of neprilysin activity and cognitive functions in rats after prenatal hypoxia. *Neurochem Res.* 2019;44:1387–1398.

19 β-Secretase (BACE1) Inhibitors From Natural Products

Atanu Bhattacharjee

CONTENTS

19.1 INTRODUCTION

Alzheimer's disease (AD) is a progressive neurodegenerative disorder, an irreversible age-related form of dementia that slowly damages the brain and causes severe changes in memory, cognitive skills, personality, and behavior (Amod et al., 2005; Colucci et al., 2012). AD was first described in 1906 by German neuropsychiatrist Prof. Alois Alzheimer. It is a complex, multifactorial, progressive disorder, associated with diminished level of acetylcholine (ACh) in the brain (Dwivedi et al., 1978). AD is recognized by the World Health Organization (WHO) as a global public health priority. AD is the main cause of dementia in the elderly, with an average duration of around nine years between the onset of clinical side effects and death, and the incidence has risen to become one of the deadliest issues in developed countries. By 2040, World Health Organization (WHO) has estimated that around 71% of the dementia cases will happen in developing nations (Zhang et al., 2015). There are considerable financial, social, and emotional burdens associated with caring for patients with this disease. In fact, with the progress of medical science, the life expectancy has been increased to a great extent. But due to lack of proper medication and treatment facilty, this disease is a major cause of morbidity, and it imposes severe strains on the social welfare systems (Anderson, 2000). It is estimated that, in the USA alone, more than 5 million people are affected by AD whereas, in India, the disease has already emerged as one of the deadliest progressive threats to mankind, after diabetes, cancer, and cardiac disease (Gupta et al., 2013).

Formation of extracellular amyloid beta (Aβ) plaques, with drastic neuronal and synaptic reductions in the cholinergic system of the brain, is considered to be the major pathological hallmark of AD (Azimi et al., 2017; Berrino, 2002). According to the 'beta-amyloid cascade', deposition of the Aβ peptide triggers neuroinflammation, resulting in neurodegeneration. Aβ is derived from sequential proteolytic cleavage of the amyloid precursor protein (APP) by beta- and gamma-secretases. Initial cleavage by beta-secretase (beta-site of APP cleaving enzyme; BACE1), a membrane-anchored aspartic protease, generates a soluble N-terminal fragment and a membrane-associated C-terminal fragment. The C-terminal fragment then undergoes proteolysis by gamma-secretase to give the Aβ peptide (Skovronsky et al., 2006; Brinton et al., 1998). BACE1 has been proposed to be a promising therapeutic target as it initiates the first step in Aβ production (Barao et al., 2016). Neuroinflammation of AD likely starts as a host defense response to the damaging effects of the amyloid deposits in the brain. Hence, anti-inflammatory drugs could be another potential therapeutic target to delay progress of AD (Zhang et al., 2015).

Medicinal plants represent a great untapped reservoir of natural pharmacologically active chemicals and are a potential source of anti-inflammatory chemicals, and inhibitors of BACE or cholinesterases (Bachurin et al., 2017; Ben et al., 2016). Therefore, it is worthwhile to explore the utility of traditional medicinal plants in the early prevention of AD, as these plants and their extracts are considered to be safe and economical by the WHO. Consequently, systematic ethnopharmacological screening of these plants may give valuable leads in the identification of new chemical structures for AD treatment.

19.2 PATHOLOGY OF AD

The main characteristics of Alzheimer's pathology are the presence of amyloid plaques and neurofibrillary tangles (aggregates of hyperphosphorylated tau proteins) (Hardy and Selkoe, 2002; Tanzi and Bertram, 2005). In addition, neuropil threads, dystrophic neurites, associated astrogliosis, and microglial activation frequently coexist. The downstream consequences of these pathological processes include neurodegeneration, with synaptic and neuronal loss leading to macroscopic atrophy (Crouch et al., 2008). Research suggests that the brain changes associated with AD may begin 20 or more years before symptoms appear. When the initial changes occur, the brain compensates for them, enabling individuals to continue to function normally. As neuronal damage increases, the brain can no longer compensate for the changes, and individuals show subtle cognitive decline. Later, neuronal damage is so significant that individuals show obvious cognitive decline and behavioral changes with the progress of time (Selkoe, 2004; Armstrong, 2009).

19.3 CURRENTLY AVAILABLE TREATMENTS FOR AD

Currently, five drugs are approved for the treatment of AD. These include four acetylcholinesterase inhibitors (AChEi): tacrine (approved in 1993), donepezil (approved in 1996), rivastigmine (1998), and galantamine (approved in 2001). This class of drugs acts by blocking acetylcholinesterase (AChE) and thereby preventing hydrolysis of acetylcholine (Ach) at nerve terminals (Mahesh et al., 2014; Citron, 2004; Beher and Graham, 2005). Although tacrine was the first AChEi approved by Food and Drug Administration (FDA), it is currently not used due to its hepatotoxicity (Howes et al., 2003). Donepezil, rivastigmine, and galantamine belong to the same therapeutic class, but differ in their pharmacodynamic (PD) and pharmacokinetic (PK) profiles: donepezil is a noncompetitive reversible AChEi, galantamine is a selective reversible AChEi and a positive allosteric modulator of nicotinic ACh receptors, and rivastigmine acts as an inhibitor of both AChE and butyrylcholinesterase (BuChE) (Tariot et al., 2004; Scarpini et al., 2003; Parihar and Hemnani, 2004).

An alternative therapy to AChEi is the administration of memantine, a non-competitive antagonist of the N-methyl-D-aspartate (NMDA) receptor, approved in 2004 (Szwajgier et al., 2013). This drug regulates the activity of glutamate in the brain. Attachment of the neurotransmitter glutamate to the cell surface of NMDA receptors allows calcium to enter the cell. This is an important event in cell signaling, as well as in learning and memory. However, in AD patients, excess glutamate released from damaged cells leads to overexposure to calcium and accelerates cell damage. Memantine disrupts this chain of events by blocking the NMDA receptors (Shankar et al., 2007; Popik et al., 1995). The drugs currently used in the therapy of AD are listed in Table 19.1.

19.4 DISEASE-MODIFYING THERAPIES AND DRUG DEVELOPMENT

At present, solutions available to treat AD are restricted, and most of them are used either to delay the progress of symptoms or for symptomatic alleviation for a brief timeframe. Yet, adverse side effects, along with the high expense associated with these medications, have limited their application. There is an urgent need for the development of disease-modifying therapies or treatments (DMTs) targeting the primary pathophysiology of AD (Mei et al., 2012; Carlsson, 2008).

TABLE 19.1
Approved Drugs For the Treatment of AD (Adopted and modified from Miguel et al., 2019)

Name	Structure	Chemical Name	Trade Name	Reference
Tacrine	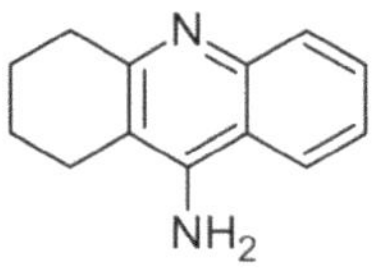	1,2,3,4-tetrahydroacridin-9-amine	Cognex	Mahesh et al., 2014
Donepezil	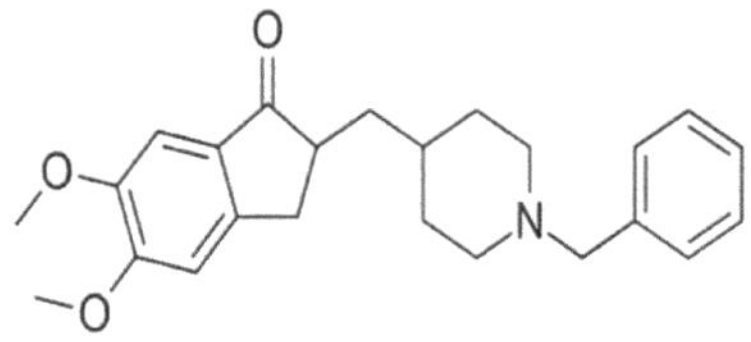	2-[(1-benzylpiperidin-4-yl)methyl]-5,6-dimethoxy-2,3-dihydroinden-1-one	Aricept	Tariot et al., 2004
Rivastigmine	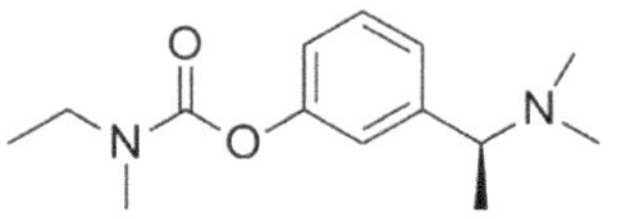	[3-[(1S)-1-(dimethylamino)ethyl[phenyl]N-ethyl-N-methylcarbamate	Exelon	Scarpini et al., 2003
Galantamine	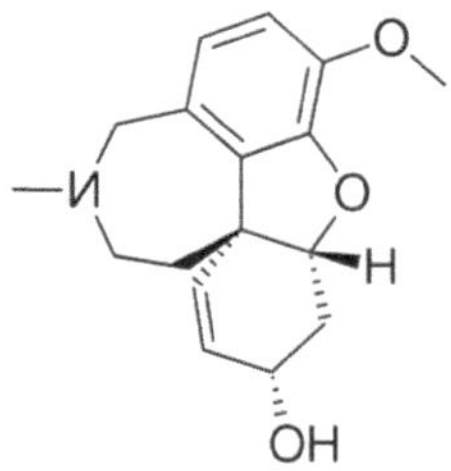	(1S,12S,14R)-9-methoxy-4-methyl-11-oxa-4-azatetracyclo heptadeca-6(17),7,9,15-tetraen-14-ol	Razadyne	Parihar and Hemnani, 2004
Memantine	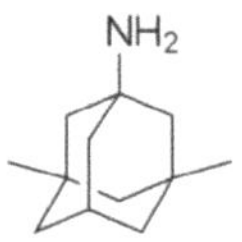	3,5-dimethyladamantan-1-amine	Axura	Shankar et al., 2007

TABLE 19.2
Current Treatment Strategies for AD (Modified from Yu et al., 2015)

Treatment Strategy	Mechanism of Action	Stages of AD
Modulation of neurotransmitter (existing/ approved therapy)	**1. AChE inhibitor** **2. NMDA antagonist**	Early stage of AD
Disease modifying therapies (under investigation)	**1. Amyloid cascade** • Modulation of α-,β-,γ- Secretase • β amyloid depleter • Promoting β-amyloid cleaning **2. Tau protein modulation** • Inhibition of tau hyperphosphorylation • Degradation of tau protein • Inhibition of tau oligomerization	Mild to moderate stage of AD
Immunotherapy (under investigation)	**1. Passive immunization** • Solanezumab • Crenezumab **2. Active immunization CAD106**	Mild to moderate stage of AD
Gene-based therapy (under investigation)	**1. Modulation of expression of presenilin**	Mild to moderate stage of AD
Antioxidants (existing/approved therapy)	**1. Oxidative stress reduction** **2. Free radical scavenger**	Mild to moderate stage of AD
Anti-inflammatory agents (existing/ approved therapy)	**1. Caspase inhibitors** **2. Metal chelators** **3. Statins** **4. PPAR-γ**	Mild to moderate stage of AD

Unfortunately, drug development for AD has proven to be very difficult. The high cost of drug development, the relatively long time needed to observe whether an experimental treatment affects disease progression, and the need for the drug to cross the blood–brain barrier (BBB) are some factors that contribute to the absence of new approved drugs for AD. Even considering the compounds that reach clinical trials, many of them fail to be demonstrably active or present unacceptable toxicity, both small molecules and immunotherapies (Paris et al., 2010; Hom et al., 2003). Over the past two decades, more than 200 compounds were assessed in 413 trials for AD treatment, out of which only memantine has been cleared phase III clinical trials (Volloch and Rits, 2018). This represents an overall success rate for approval of 0.4%, which is among the lowest for any therapeutic area. A summary of current treatment strategies for AD is listed in Table 19.2.

19.5 THE AMYLOID HYPOTHESIS

The amyloid hypothesis, the current prevalent theory underlying AD pathogenesis, suggests that the accumulation of pathological forms of Aβ, due to an increase of production and/or a decrease in clearance of Aβ, is the primary pathological process in AD (Dewachter and Van, 2002). The accumulation of Aβ peptides leads to their oligomerization and the formation of Aβ plaques. These plaques generate an anti-inflammatory response, causing oxidative stress in neurons and disrupting normal kinase and phosphatase activities, resulting in hyperphosphorylation of tau proteins and subsequent neurofibrillary tangle formation. This cascade of events leads to abnormal signaling and synaptic impairment, resulting ultimately in neuronal death and dementia in the AD patient (Choi et al., 2008; Jeon et al., 2008, 2005; Bhattacharjee, 2018) (Figure 19.1).

Aβ is produced by a two-step sequential cleavage of amyloid precursor protein (APP): first, beta-site APP-cleaving enzyme (BACE1) cleaves APP to generate soluble APPÁ (sAPPÁ) and a

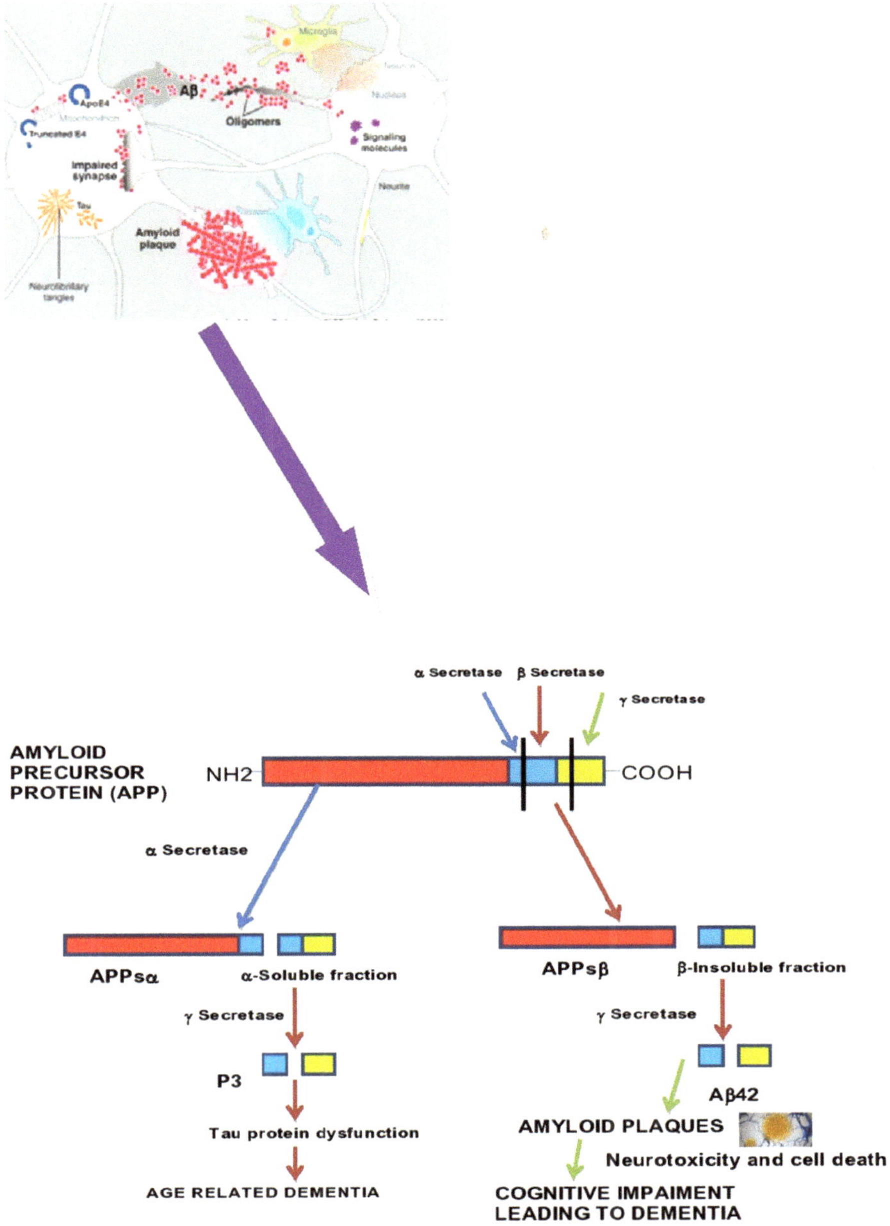

FIGURE 19.1 Mechanism of toxic amyloid-β formation, leading to cognitive impairment in AD (adopted and modified from Eric et al., 2016).

99-amino acid fragment (C99), which then suffers several cleavage events by γ-secretase to produce peptides of different lengths, from 38 to 43 amino acids, with AÁ40 and AÁ42 being the main products, and both playing a key role in the aggregation of neuritic plaques (Kinghorn, 2001; Balunas and Kinghorm, 2005). The longer peptide amyloid beta (Aβ) 42 has been shown to most prone to aggregation, with an increased amyloid beta Aβ42:Aβ40 ratio observed in the familial form of the disease (Gurib-Fakim, 2006; Huang and Mucke, 2012). The activity of β-cleavage is considered to determine the total amount of Aβ production, and the efficiency of the successive γ-cleavages impacts the production ratio of toxic Aβ42 to total Aβ (Eric and Bard, 2016).

19.6 B-SECRETASE (BACE1)

BACE1 is the transmembrane aspartyl protease that cleaves APP at the β-site. The sequential proteolytic cleavage of APP by BACE1 and γ-secretase leads to the production and release of Aβ peptide in the brain. Therefore, amyloidogenic secretases are key therapeutic targets being currently explored for AD-modifying intervention (Roberds et al., 2001). Several studies report that BACE1 inhibitors hold great potential as a potential strategy to decrease Aβ brain concentrations, thus preventing the progression of AD (Guo, 2006; Salloway, 2008). Since the identification of BACE1, inhibitors covering many different structural classes have been extensively reported in the literature (Vassar, 2004; McArdle and Quinn, 2007; Salloway, 2008). An overview of the recent advances in the identification of BACE1 inhibitor classes obtained from natural products is summarized below.

19.7 MEDICINAL PLANTS WITH BACE1 INHIBITORY EFFECTS

Despite the clear success of drug discovery from medicinal plants, future endeavors face many challenges. Pharmacognosists, phytochemists, and other natural product scientists will need to continuously improve the quality and quantity of compounds that enter the drug development phase to keep pace with other drug discovery efforts (Fenical and Jensen, 2006). Medicinal plants and their concentrates are assuming an indispensable part in the present treatment of psychological conditions, either as standard or integral drug, with specific reference to their ethnopharmacological perspectives (George, 2011). The history of drug discovery has shown that plants contain active compounds, which have become new sources to be investigated by the pharmaceutical industry. Plant constituents may act not only synergistically with other constituents from the same plant but may also enhance the activity of compounds or counteract toxic effects of compounds from other plant species. In traditional practices, numerous plants have been used to treat cognitive disorders, including neurodegenerative diseases and different neuropharmacological disorders (Perry et al., 1999; Vaidya, 1997). A list of medicinal plants used as sources of BACE1 inhibitors is summarized in Table 19.3.

19.8 PHYTOCONSTITUENTS WITH BACE1 INHIBITORY ACTIVITY

19.8.1 Phenylpropanoid Derivatives

Phenylpropanoids are widely distributed plant secondary metabolites, formed initially from phenylalanine by the action of phenylalanine ammonia-lyase (PAL). It has been observed that they inhibit protein aggregation in a non-stoichiometric fashion (Feng et al., 2006). Four bioactive compounds isolated from an ethanol extract of the fruit of *Cordia sebestena* (a plant from Hawaii) showed BACE1 inhibitory activity against the aspartic protease, which is a central blocker of the etiology of AD (Coan et al., 2009). New phenylpropanoids, namely sebestenoids A-D [Figure 19.2 (i)] had been isolated from bioactive fractions of the same plant and showed potent BACE1 inhibitory activity in a dose-dependent manner (Dai et al., 2010). *In-vitro* studies revealed that sebestenoids C and D were the most potent, with half-maximal inhibitory concentration (IC_{50}) values of 20 and 22 μM, respectively. In addition, sebestenoids C and D were investigated using a surrogate system. These compounds were assayed against the serine protease chymotrypsin in a standard chemiluminescent assay with and without the addition of detergent. The IC_{50} values of sebestenoids C and D showed them to be strongly inhibitory toward BACE1. These findings suggest that phenylpropanoid derivatives of sebestenoids A, B, C and D are potential agents for treatment of AD (Eglen et al., 2002; Gunasekera et al., 2010).

19.8.2 Flavonoid Derivatives

Flavonoids are among the most widely distributed and important groups of secondary metabolites, with a low toxicity profile, and are found in a variety of fruits, vegetables, and flowers, including

TABLE 19.3
Potential Phytoextracts and Their Derivatives to Treat AD (Adopted and modified from Abdul et al., 2018)

Plant Name	Extract	Extracted Compound(s)	Structure	Mechanism of Action	Pharmacological Study	Reference
Sophora flavescens	Chloroform extract of root	Lavandulyl flavanones (Saphoraflavones)	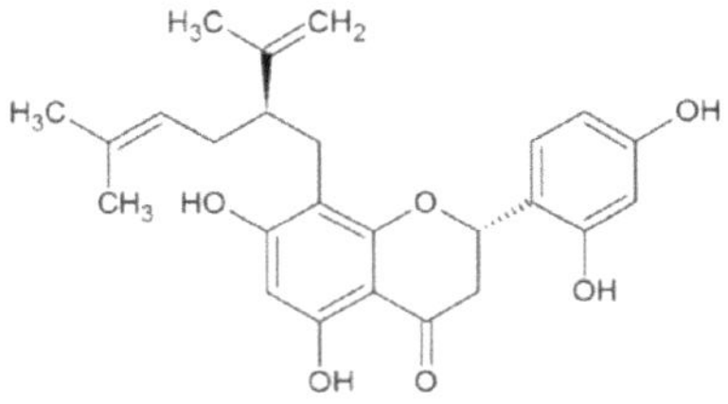	Inhibits the activity of BACE1 in a dose-dependent manner	*In-vitro* study	Hwang et al., 2008
Fructus gardeniae	Methanol extract of whole plant	Geniposide	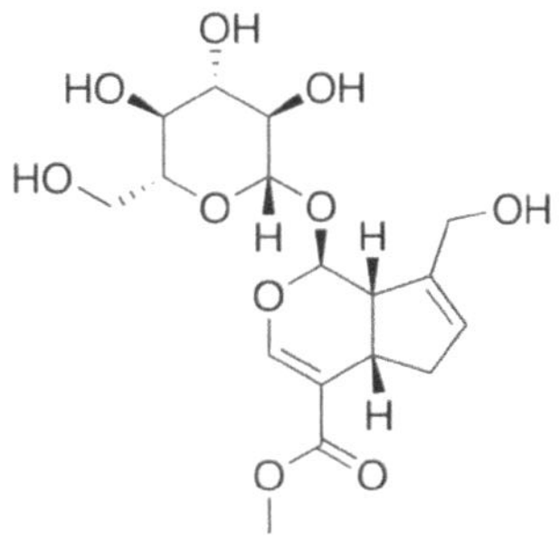	Inhibits acetylcholinesterase activity. Ameliorates scopolamine-induced memory impairment in amnesic mice	*In-vitro* study, *in-vivo* study	Nam and Lee, 2013
Paeonia lactiflora	Ethanol extract of of seeds	Resveratrol oligomer	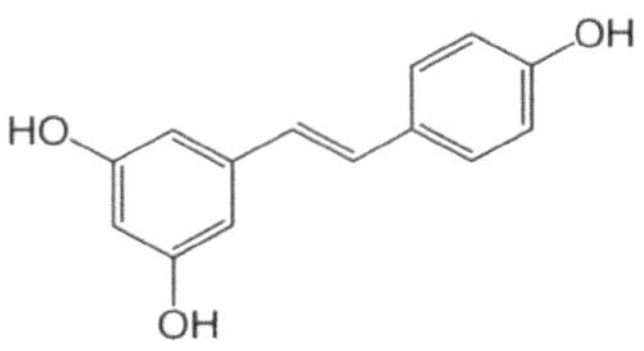	Exhibits a significant inhibitory effect on baculovirus-expressed BACE1	*In-vitro* study	Choi et al., 2011

(Continued)

TABLE 19.3 (CONTINUED)
Potential Phytoextracts and Their Derivatives to Treat AD (Adopted and modified from Abdul et al., 2018)

Plant Name	Extract	Extracted Compound(s)	Structure	Mechanism of Action	Pharmacological Study	Reference
Psoralea corylifolia	Methanol extract of seeds	Isoflavones	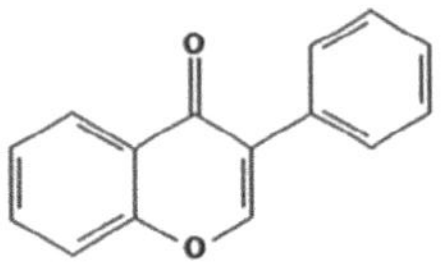	Exhibits a significant inhibitory effect on baculovirus-expressed BACE 1	*In-vitro* study	Choi et al., 2008
Cordia sebestena	Ethanolic extract of fruit	Sebestenoids	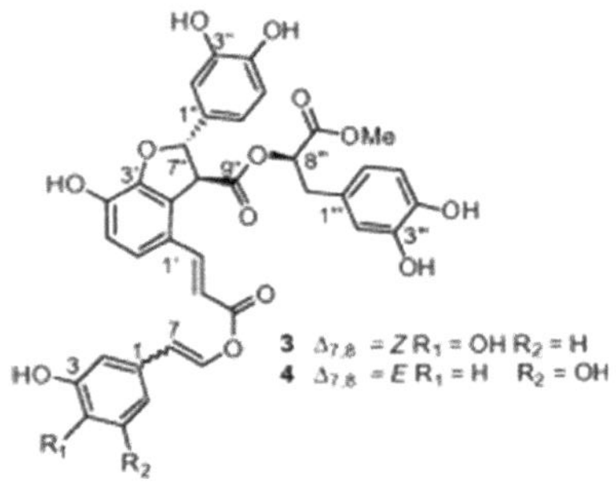	Exhibits moderate inhibition of the aspartic protease BACE1	*In-vitro* study	Dai et al., 2010
Perilla frutescens var. *acuta*	Methanol extract of leaves	Luteolin and rosmarinic acid	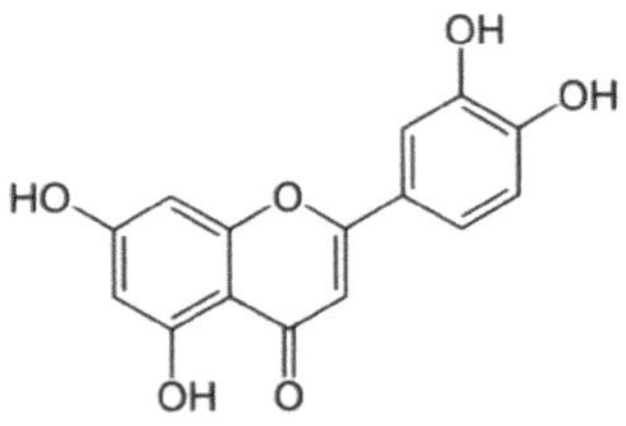 Luteolin	Inhibits the activity of BACE1 in a dose-dependent manner	*In-vitro* study	Choi et al., 2008

(Continued)

TABLE 19.3 (CONTINUED)
Potential Phytoextracts and Their Derivatives to Treat AD (Adopted and modified from Abdul et al., 2018)

Plant Name	Extract	Extracted Compound(s)	Structure	Mechanism of Action	Pharmacological Study	Reference
			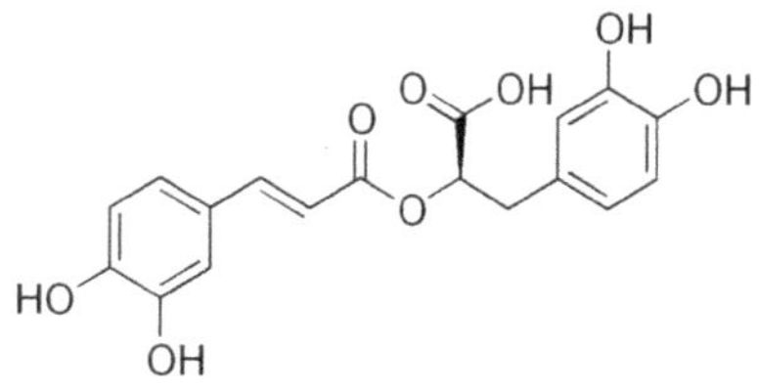 Rosmarinic acid			
Smilax china (Smilax Rhizoma)	Methanol extract of rhizomes	*Trans-/cis-* resveratrol mixture, oxyresveratrol, veraphenol, and cis-scirpusin A	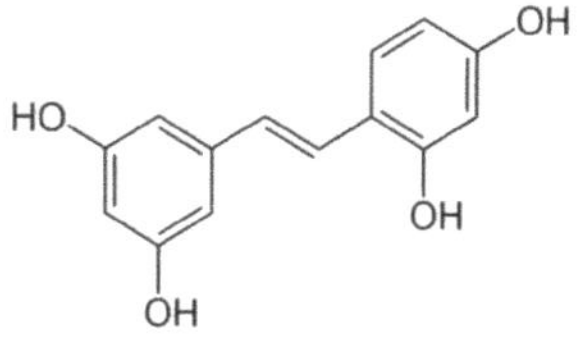 Oxyresveratrol 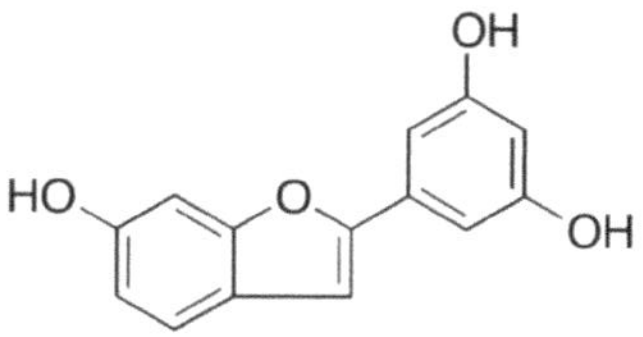 Veraphenol	Inhibits the activity of BACE1 in a dose-dependent manner	*In-vitro* study	Smit, 2004

(Continued)

TABLE 19.3 (CONTINUED)
Potential Phytoextracts and Their Derivatives to Treat AD (Adopted and modified from Abdul et al., 2018)

Plant Name	Extract	Extracted Compound(s)	Structure	Mechanism of Action	Pharmacological Study	Reference
			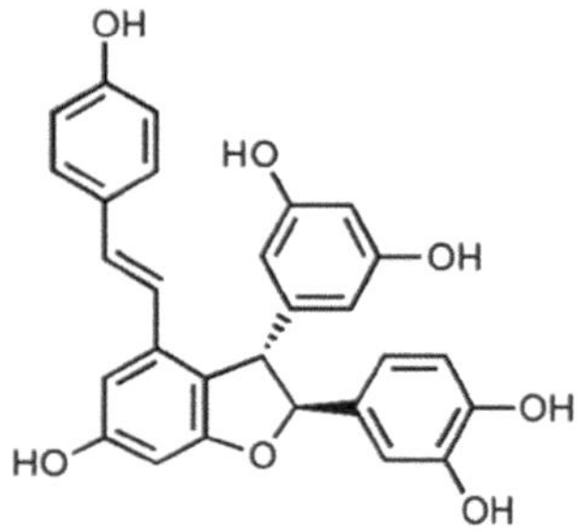 Scirpusin A			
Sanguisorba officinalis (Sanguisorbae Radix)	Methanol extract of roots	1,2,3-trigalloyl-4,6-hexahydroxydiphenoyl-β-D-glucopyranoside and 1,2,3,4,6-pentagalloyl-β-D-glucopyranoside	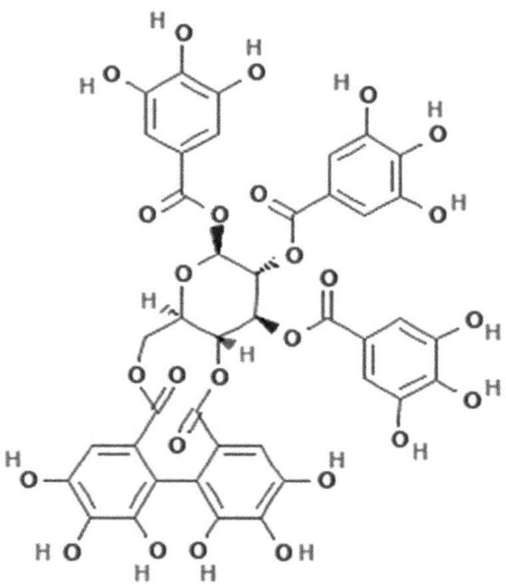	Inhibits the activity of BACE1 in a dose-dependent manner	*In-vitro* study	Lee et al., 2005

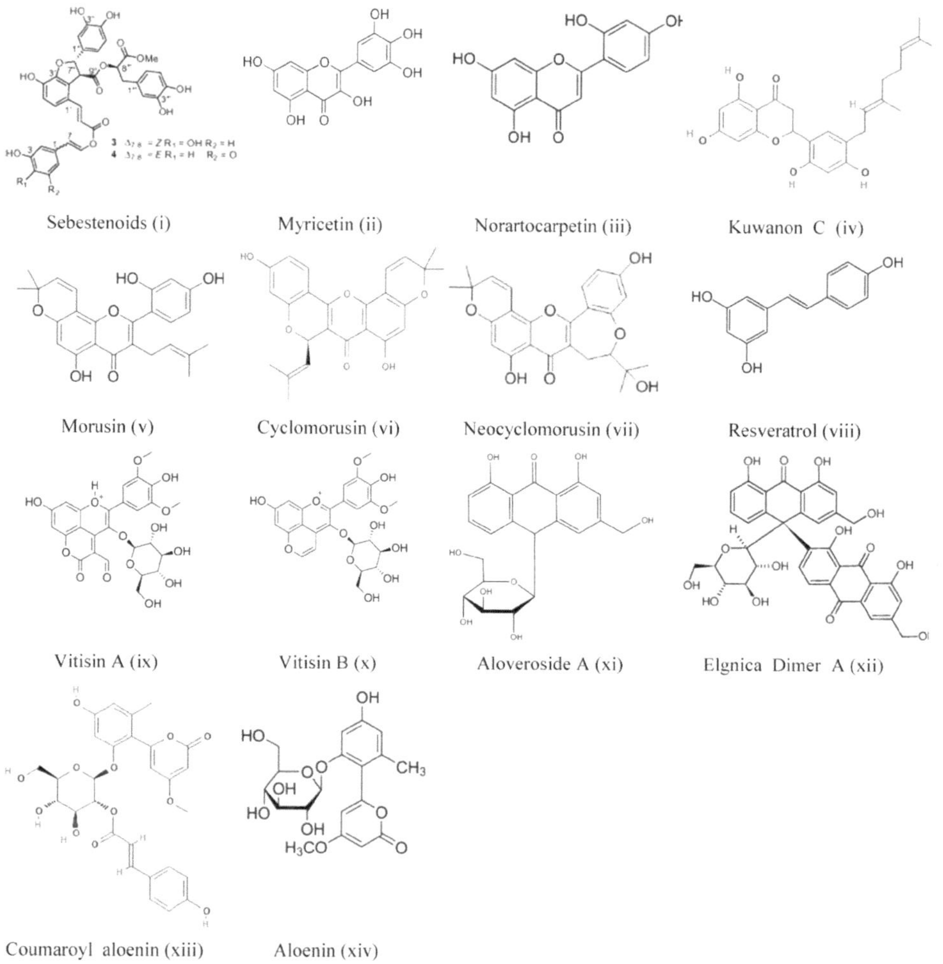

FIGURE 19.2 Structure of various potential phytoconstituents to treat AD.

citrus, garlic, tea, etc. Recent studies revealed that flavonoids are able to cross the BBB *in vivo* (Youdim et al., 2004). Numerous studies have reported protective effects of natural flavonoids, including flavonols and flavones, against various substances, such as Aβ. They significantly reduced Aβ1–40 and Aβ1–42 formation by inhibiting BACE1 enzyme activity *in vitro* and thereby decreased Aβ-induced neuronal cell death (Ross et al., 2002; Commenges et al., 2000). These flavonoids have strong antioxidant activity and inhibit Aβ oligomerization. The flavonoid myricetin [Figure: 19.2 (ii)] showed neuroprotective effect against Aβ-induced neuronal cell injury (Shimmyo et al., 2008). Methanolic extracts of *Morus lhou* stem bark exhibited significant BACE1 inhibitory activity, with an IC_{50} of 78.4 μg/ml (Ono et al., 2003). The bioactive fraction of the extract lead to the isolation of several compounds, namely norartocarpetin, kuwanon C, morusin, kuwanon A, morusinol, cyclomorusin, and neocyclomorusin [Figure: 19.2 (iii-vii)]. Each compound showed significant reversible BACE1 inhibition in a dose-dependent manner (Jeong et al., 2009; Kang et al., 2004).

19.8.2 Napthoquinone Derivatives

Napthoquinones (NQs) are a group of fat-soluble vitamins, with the molecular formula $C_{10}H_6O_2$. Novel 1,4-NQ derivatives have been identified as representing a new class of inhibitor of heat shock protein 90 (Hsp90), which might be useful for AD therapy (Muto et al., 1987). Different naphthoquinone-derivative ring structures have shown to activate the nuclear receptor gamma, a strategy which could be promising for the treatment of several neurological pathologies. In this regard, α-secretase activity increases with enhanced membrane fluidity, and processing of APP by β-secretase might be explained by alterations in cell membrane fluidity. The activity of BACE1 is sensitive to oxidative stress, and there is convincing evidence that oxidative stress results in Aβ accumulation (Tauraite et al., 2009). Therefore, BACE1 inhibition by NQ could contribute to an improvement in cell membrane fluidity., By inhibiting BACE1 activity, the active 1,4-NQs could make the α-secretase pathway the predominant metabolic route of APP, thus increasing the release of α-APP (Montenegro et al., 2010). The NQ derivative resveratrol [Figure: 19.2 (viii)] is an active compound and a potential biomarker for the treatment of AD. Resveratrol oligomers, isolated from the seed extract of *Paeonia lactiflora*, showed potent BACE1 inhibitory activity *in vitro* (Hadden et al., 2009).

Vitisin A and B [Figure: 19.2 (ix-x)] are promising lead candidates for the design of potential new BACE1 inhibitors. They have been reported to reduce amyloid-induced oxidative stress in PC12 cell lines. However, the mechanism is not yet clear (Ko et al., 2005).

19.8.3 Glycoside Derivatives

Nine glycosides from *Aloe vera* were isolated by bioassay-guided fractionation techniques, and structural characterization identified them as aloveroside A, elgnica dimer A, elgnica dimer B, *p*-coumaroyl aloenin and aloenin [Figure 19.2 (xi-xiv)]. The ability to cleave APP *via* inhibition of BACE1 was assessed using a fluorescent resonance energy transfer (FRET) peptide cleavage assay. Briefly, assays were performed in triplicate in 96-well plates with 100 µl aliquots of 50 mM sodium acetate buffer, containing 4 µM substrate, 2 µg/ml recombinant human BACE1, and different concentrations of the isolated compounds. Of these, coumaroyl aloenin showed the greatest BACE1 inhibitory activity, with an IC_{50} of 68.3 µg/ml (Speranza et al., 1986; Hyun et al., 1997; Jung et al., 2010).

19.9 FUTURE PERSPECTIVES

The therapeutic potential of BACE1 inhibition has been investigated in the past decade. However, even though inhibitors can efficiently lower brain Aβ levels, clinical trials still have not demonstrated improvements in cognitive function when inhibitors are administered to mild-to-moderate AD patients, calling into question the real worth of these potential anti-AD drugs and the clinical trials design (Bastianetto et al., 2006; Luvone et al., 2006). Emerging evidence suggests that the optimal timing for treatment with BACE1 inhibitors should be as early as possible. The optimal time point for treatment with BACE1 inhibitors is a crucial issue that possibly explains some of the previous failures. The advances in technological diagnostic tools, allowing better identification of patients at risk of developing AD, will enable clinical trials to be carried out at the preclinical stage, when BACE1 inhibitors are expected to have the largest impact on amyloid plaques (Hu et al., 2004; Yang et al., 2006). Moreover, taking into account the complexity of AD, recent studies have reported multitarget approaches centered on BACE1, using ligands developed as small molecules, that can modulate both BACE1 and other AD-related targets within synergistic pathways (Hardy, 2006; Shankar et al., 2008; Zhao et al., 2006). As BACE1 biological functions may be affected following inhibition, further studies are required to develop efficient strategies to minimize the side effects associated with long-term use of BACE1 inhibitors (Von et al., 2008). Indeed, although the design and development of BACE1 inhibitors have proved extremely challenging, there is a substantial body of evidence that BACE1 inhibitors can act as disease-modifying agents and their use should be pursued to achieve benefits for AD patients.

19.10 CONCLUSIONS

The discovery of disease-modifying agents for AD has proved to be very challenging for the health care community. Phytocompounds should display improved CNS access as a result of improved BBB porosity and decreased P-gp ER (P-glycoprotein effux ratio). It has now been clinically established that oxidative stress (OS) and Aβ are linked to each other since Aβ aggregation induces OS *in vivo* and *in vitro*, and oxidant agents increase the production of Aβ. (Tamagno et al., 2002; Apelt et al., 2004; Jeon et al., 2007). Furthermore, off-target impacts should also be identified, as such effects highlight one of the chief causes for the termination of clinical projects. Restorative medical groups have used high-throughput and virtual screening strategies, followed by substance modification, attempting to meet a few physico-synthetic subtleties, to find new molecules capable of improving cognitive prformance in AD subjects (Smit, 2004).

Taking into consideration the actual AD therapeutics pipeline, a special focus has been given to BACE1 as a target for a disease-modifying therapy for AD. The information currently available points to the inhibition of BACE1 as a safe and effective target for Aβ reduction. All the adverse effects identified to date in the use of BACE1 inhibitors were identified as off-target effects, confirming BACE1 to be a suitable target to explore. Nevertheless, pharmacological chemists should perform extended SAR studies, in terms not only of investigating potency and PK properties, but also for selectivity, targeting the discovery of compounds highly selective for BACE1, rather against being active against other, related proteases, such as Cat-D (Cathespin-D) (Bourguet et al., 2005; Perry et al., 2001).

Another issue involves the matching of the pharmacological therapy with the appropriate stage of AD. The use of disease-modifying therapies, such as BACE1 inhibitors, should be a suitable option for early stages of AD, where minimum neuronal loss and synaptic dysfunction are observed. On the other hand, in a mild-to-moderate AD scenario, it would possibly be too late in the disease process for BACE1 inhibition to be effective, and a symptomatically therapeutic strategy should be preferred. In summary, the future of AD treatments will rely on the development of potent, selective, and safe compounds able to delay AD progression and neuronal impairment. At the same time, it is essential to identify specific biomarkers to allow an early and efficacious pharmacological intervention (Shinichi et al., 2016; Miguel et al., 2019).

ACKNOWLEDGMENT

The author is grateful to Assam Down Town University, Assam for providing the support necessary for preparation of this manuscript.

REFERENCES

Abdul BAA, Vidhyavathi R, Magesh J, Vijaykumar M, et al. Synthesis and development of BACE 1 inhibitor for Alzheimer's diseases from medicinal plants. *Annu Res Rev Biol.* 2018;28(3):1–18.

Amod PK, Laurie AK, Girish JK. Herbal complement inhibitors in the treatment of neuroinflammation. *Ann NY Acad Sci.* 2005;1056:413–429.

Anderson RN. Deaths: leading causes for 2000. *Natl Vital Stat Rep.* 2002;50:1.

Apelt J, Bigi M, Wunderlich P, Schliebs R. Aging-related increase in oxidative stress correlates with developmental pattern of beta-secretase activity and beta-amyloid plaque formation in transgenic Tg2576 mice with Alzheimer-like pathology. *Int J Dev Neurosci.* 2004;22:475–484.

Armstrong RA. The molecular biology of senile plaques and neurofibrillary tangles in Alzheimer's disease. *Folia Neuropathol.* 2009;47:289–299.

Azimi S, Zonouzi A, Firuzi O, Iraji A, Saeedi M, Mahdavi M, et al. Discovery of imidazopyridines containing isoindoline-1,3-dione framework as a new class of BACE1 inhibitors: design, synthesis and SAR analysis. *Eur J Med Chem.* 2017;138:729–737. doi:10.1016/j.ejmech.2017.06.040.

Bachurin SO, Bovina EV, Ustyugov AA. Drugs in clinical trials for Alzheimer's disease: the major trends. *Med Res Rev.* 2017;37:1186–1225. doi:10.1002/med.21434.

Balunas MJ, Kinghorn AD. Drug discovery from medicinal plants. *Life Sci.* 2005;78:431–441.

Barao S, Moechars D, Lichtenthaler SF, De Strooper B. BACE1 physiological functions may limit its use as therapeutic target for Alzheimer's disease. *Trends Neurosci.* 2016;39:158–169. doi:10.1016/j.tins.2016.01.003.

Bastianetto S, Yao ZX, Papadopoulos V, Quirion R. Neuroprotective effects of green and black teas and their catechin gallate esters against beta-amyloid-induced toxicity. *Eur J Neurosci.* 2006;23:55–64.

Beher D, Graham SL. Protease inhibitors as potential disease-modifying therapeutics for Alzheimer's disease. *Expert Opin Invest Drugs.* 2005;14:1385–1409.

Ben Halima S, Mishra S, Raja KMP, Willem M, Baici A, Simon K, et al. Specific inhibition of β-secretase processing of the Alzheimer disease amyloid precursor protein. *Cell Rep.* 2016;14:2127–2141. doi:10.1016/j.celrep.2016.01.076.

Berrino F. Western diet and Alzheimer's disease. *Epidemiol Prev.* 2002;26:107.

Bhattacharjee A. Phytoextracts and their derivatives affecting neurotransmission relevant to Alzheimer's disease: an ethno-medicinal perspective. Akula R, Roshchina VV, Editors: *Neurotransmitters in Plants*: New Achievements and Perspectives. Taylor & Francis, USA, 2018, 357–386.

Bourguet-Kondracki ML, Kornprobst JM. Marine pharmacology: potentialities in the treatment of infectious diseases, osteoporosis and Alzheimer's disease. *Adv Biochem Eng/Biotechnol.* 2005;97:105–131.

Brinton RD, Yamazaki RS. Advances and challenges in the prevention and treatment of Alzheimer's disease. *Pharmaceut Res.* 1998;15:386–398.

Carlsson CM. Lessons learned from failed and discontinued clinical trials for the treatment of Alzheimer's disease: future directions. *J Alzheimer's Dis.* 2008;15:327–338.

Choi CW, Choi YH, Cha MR, Kim YS, Yon GH, Hong KS, et al. In vitro BACE 1 inhibitory activity of resveratrol oligomers from the seed extract of *Paeonia lactiflora. Planta Med.* 2011;77:374–376.

Choi SH, Hur JM, Yang EJ, Jun M, Park HJ, Lee KB, Moon E, Song KS. *Beta-secretase (BACE 1) inhibitors from Perilla frutescens var. acuta. Arch Pharmacal Res.* 2008;31:183–187.

Choi YH, Yon GH, Hong KS, Yoo DS, Choi CW, Park WK, Kong JY, Kim YS, Ryu SY. In vitro BACE 1 inhibitory phenolic components from the seeds of *Psoralea corylifolia. Planta Med.* 2008;74:1405–1408.

Citron M. Strategies for disease modification in Alzheimer's disease. *Nat Rev Neurosci.* 2004;5:677–685.

Coan KE, Maltby DA, Burlingame AL, Shoichet BK. Promiscuous aggregate-based inhibitors promote enzyme unfolding. *J Med Chem.* 2009;52:2067–2075.

Colucci L, Bosco M, Ziello AR, Rea R, Amenta F, Fasanaro AM. Effectiveness of nootropic drugs with cholinergic activity in treatment of cognitive deficit: a review. *J Exp Pharmacol.* 2012;4:163–172.

Commenges D, Scotet V, Renaud S, Jacqmin-Gadda H, Barberger-Gateau P, Dartigues JF. Intake of flavonoids and risk of dementia. *Eur J Epidemiol.* 2000;16:357–363.

Crouch PJ, Harding SM, White AR, Camakaris J, Bush AI, Masters CL. Mechanisms of a beta mediated neurodegeneration in Alzheimer's disease. *Int J Biochem Cell Biol.* 2008;40:181–198.

Dai J, Sorribas A, Yoshida WY, Williams PG. Sebestenoids A–D, BACE *1 inhibitors from Cordia sebestena. Phytochemistry.* 2010;71:2168–2173.

Dewachter I, Van LF. Secretases as targets for the treatment of Alzheimer's disease: the prospects. *Lancet Neurol.* 2002;1:409–416.

Dwivedi KK, Singh RH. A clinical study of medhya rasayana therapy in the management of convulsive disorder. *J Res Ayurveda Siddha.* 1978;13:97.

Eglen RM. Enzyme fragment complementation: a flexible high throughput screening assay technology. *Assay Drug Dev Technol.* 2002;1:97–104.

Eric K, Bard DS. The amyloid cascade hypothesis: are we poised for success or failure? *J Neurochem.* 2016;139(2) Supplement 2:237–252.

Feng BY, Shoichet BK. A detergent-based assay for the detection of promiscuous inhibitors. *Nat Protocol.* 2006;1:550–553.

Fenical WH, Jensen PJ. Developing a new resource for drug discovery: marine actinomycete bacteria. *Nat Chem Biol.* 2006;2:666–673.

George P. Concerns regarding the safety and toxicity of medicinal plants – an overview. *J Appl Pharm Sci.* 2011;1(6):40–44.

Gunasekera SP, Miller MW, Kwan JC, Luesch H, Paul VJ. Molassamide, a dipeptide serine protease inhibitor from the marine cyanobacterium *Dichothrix utahensis. J Nat Prod.* 2010;73:459–462.

Guo T, Hobbs DW. Development of BACE 1 inhibitors for Alzheimer's disease. *Curr Med Chem.* 2006;13:1811–1829.

Gupta BM, Bala A. Alzheimer's disease research in India: a scientometric analysis of publications output during 2002–11. *Res Neurol Int J.* 2013;2013. doi:10.5171/2013.204542.

Gurib-Fakim A. Medicinal plants: traditions of yesterday and drugs of tomorrow. *Mol Aspect Med.* 2006;27:1–93.

Hadden MK, Hill SA, Davenport J, Matts RL, Blagg BS. Synthesis and evaluation of Hsp90 inhibitors that contain the 1,4-naphthoquinone scaffold. *Bioorg Med Chem.* 2009;17:634–640.

Hardy J. Has the amyloid cascade hypo-thesis for Alzheimer's disease been proved? *Curr Alzheimer Res.* 2006;3:71–73.

Hardy J, Selkoe DJ. The amyloid hypothesis of Alzheimer's disease: progress and problems on the road to therapeutics. *J Sci.* 2002;297:353–356.

Hom RK, Fang LY, Mamo S, Tung JS, Guinn AC, Walker DE, Davis DL, Gailunas AF, Thorsett ED, Sinha S, Knops JE, Jewett NE, Anderson JP, John V. Design and synthesis of statine-based cell-permeable peptidomimetic inhibitors of human beta-secretase. *J Med Chem.* 2003;46:1799–1802.

Howes MJ, Houghton PJ. Plants used in Chinese and Indian traditional medicine for improvement of memory and cognitive function. *Pharmacol Biochem Behav.* 2003;75:513–527.

Hu B, Fan KY, Bridges K, Chopra R, Lovering F, Cole D, Zhou P, Ellingboe J, Jin G, Cowling R, Bard J. Synthesis and SAR of bis-statine based peptides as BACE 1 inhibitors. *Bioorg Med Chem Lett.* 2004;14:3457–3460.

Huang Y, Mucke L. Alzheimer mechanisms and therapeutic strategies. *Cell.* 2012;148(6):1204–1222.

Hwang EM, Ryu YB, Kim HY, Kim DG, Hong SG, Lee JH, Curtis-Long MJ, Jeong SH, Park JY, Park KH. BACE 1 inhibitory effects of lavandulyl flavanones from *Sophora flavescens*. *Bioorg Med Chem.* 2008;16:6669–6674.

Hyun SK, Sick WW, Sung LS, Sub SC, Sook CH, Kennelly EJ, Kinghorn AD. Elgonica-dimers A and B, two potent alcohol metabolism inhibitory constituents of *Aloe arborescens*. *J Nat Prod.* 1997;60:1180–1182.

Jeon SY, Kwon SH, Seong YH, Bae K, Hur JM, Lee YY, Suh DY, Song KS. Beta-secretase (BACE 1)-inhibiting stilbenoids from Smilax rhizoma. *Phytomedicine.* 2007;14:403–408.

Jeon YH, Heo YS, Kim CM, Hyun YL, Lee TG, Ro S, Cho JM. Phosphodiesterase: overview of protein structures, potential therapeutic applications and recent progress in drug development. *Cell Mol Life Sci.* 2005;62:1198–1220.

Jeong SH, Ryu YB, Curtis-Long MJ, Ryu HW, Baek YS, Kang JE, Lee WS, Park KH. Tyrosinase inhibitory polyphenols from roots of *Morus lhou*. *J Agric Food Chem.* 2009;57:1195–1203.

Jung HA, Jung YJ, Hyun HK, Min BS, Kim DW, Jung JH, Choi JS. Selective cholinesterase inhibitory activities of a new monoterpene diglycoside and other constituents from *Nelumbo nucifera* stamens. *Biol Pharmaceut Bull.* 2010;33:267–272.

Kang HS, Kim HR, Byun DS, Son BW, Nam TJ, Choi JS. Tyrosinase inhibitors isolated from the edible brown alga *Ecklonia stolonifera*. *Arch Pharmacol Res.* 2004;27:1226–1232.

Kinghorn AD. Pharmacognosy in the 21st century. *J Pharm Pharmacol.* 2001;53:135–148.

Ko PC, Higgins JA, Kilduff PT, Milberg WP, McGlinchey R. Evidence for intact selective attention in Alzheimer's disease patients using a location priming task. *Neuropsychology.* 2005;19:381–389.

Lee HJ, Seong YH, Bae KH, Kwon SH, Kwak HM, Nho SK, et al. β-Secretase (BACE 1) inhibitors from Sanguisorbae radix. *Arch Pharm Res.* 2005;28:799–803.

Luvone T, De Filippis D, Esposito G, D'Amico A, Izzo AA. The spice sage and its active ingredient rosmarinic acid protect PC12 cells from amyloid-β peptide-induced neurotoxicity. *J Pharmacol Exp Ther.* 2006;317:1143–1149.

Mahesh G, Tasneem S. Biomarker controversies and diagnostic difficulties in Alzheimer's disease. *Am J Phytomed Clin Ther.* 2014;2(4):463–468.

McArdle BM, Quinn RJ. Identification of protein fold topology shared between different folds inhibited by natural products. *Chem Biol Chem.* 2007;8:788–798.

Mei Z, Situ B, Tan X, Zheng S, Zhang F, Yan P, Liu P. Cryptotanshinione upregulates alpha-secretase by activation PI3K pathway in cortical neurons. *Brain Res.* 2010;12:165–173.

Miguel AM, Emília S. BACE-1 and γ-secretase as therapeutic targets for Alzheimer's disease. *Pharmaceuticals.* 2019;12(41):1–31.

Montenegro RC, Araujo AJ, Molina MT, Marinho Filho JD, Rocha DD, Lopez Montero E, et al. Cytotoxic activity of naphthoquinones with special emphasis on juglone and its 5-*O*-methyl derivative. *Chem-Biol Interact.* 2010;184:439–448.

Muto N, Inouye K, Inaba A, Nakanishi T, Liat T. Inhibition of cytochrome P-450-linked monooxygenase systems by naphthoquinones. *Biochem Biophys Res Commun.* 1987;146:487–494.

Nam Y, Lee D. Ameliorating effect of Zhizi (Fructus Gardeniae) extract and its glycosides on scopolamine-induced memory impairment. *J Tradit Chin Med.* 2013;15:223–227.

Ono K, Yoshiike Y, Takashima A, Hasegawa K, Naiki H, Yamada M. Potent anti-amyloidogenic and fibril-destabilizing effects of polyphenols in vitro: implications for the prevention and therapeutics of Alzheimer's disease. *J Neurochem.* 2003;7:172–181.

Parihar MS, Hemnani T. Alzheimer's disease pathogenesis and therapeutic interventions. *J Clin Neurosci.* 2004;11:456–467.15.

Paris D, Ganey NJ, Laporte V, Patel NS, Beaulieu-Abdelahad D, Bachmeier C, March A, Ait-Ghezala G, Mullan MJ. Reduction of beta-amyloid pathology by celastrol in a transgenic mouse model of Alzheimer's disease. *J Neuroinfla.* 2010;7:17.

Perry EK, Pickering AT, Wang WW, Houghton PJ, Perry NS. Medicinal plants and Alzheimer's disease: from ethnobotany to phytotherapy. *J Pharm Pharmacol.* 1999. 51:527–533.

Perry NSL, Houghton PJ, Sampson J, Theolad AE, Hart S, Lis-balchin M. *In vitro* activities of *Salvia lavandulaefolia* (Spanish Sage) relevant to treatment of Alzheimer's disease. *J Pharm Pharmacol.* 2001;53:1347–1356.

Popik P, Layer RT, Fossom LH, Benveniste M, Geter-Douglass B, Witkin JM, Skolnick P. NMDA antagonist properties of the putative antiaddictive drug, ibogaine. *J Pharmacol Exp Ther.* 1995;275(2):753–760.

Roberds SL, Anderson J, Basi G, Bienkowski MJ, McConlogue L. BACE knockout mice are healthy despite lacking the primary beta-secretase activity in brain: implications for Alzheimer's disease therapeutics. *Hum Mol Genet.* 2001;10:1317–1324.

Ross JA, Kasum CM. Dietary flavonoids: bioavailability, metabolic effects, and safety. *Ann Rev Nutr.* 2002;22:19–34.

Salloway S, Mintzer J, Weiner MF, Cummings JL. Disease-modifying therapies in Alzheimer's disease. *Alzheimer's Dement.* 2008;4:65–79.

Samuelsson G. *A Textbook of Pharmacognosy, Swedish Pharamaceutical Society*, 5th ed. Swedish Pharmaceutical Press, Stockholm, 2004, 259.

Scarpini E, Scheltens P, Feldman H. Treatment of Alzheimer's disease: current status and new perspectives. *Lancet Neurol.* 2003;2:539–547.

Selkoe DJ. Alzheimer's disease: mechanistic understanding predicts novel therapies. *Ann Intern Med.* 2004;140:627–638.

Shankar GM, Bloodgood BL, Townsend M, Walsh DM, Selkoe DJ, Sabatini BL. Natural oligomers of the Alzheimer amyloid-β protein induce reversible synapse loss by modulating an NMDA-type glutamate receptor-dependent signaling pathway. *J Neurosci.* 2007;27:2866–2875.

Shankar GM, Li S, Mehta TH, Garcia-Munoz A, Shepardson NE, Smith I, Brett FM, Farrell MA, Rowan MJ, Lemere CA, Regan CM, Walsh DM, Sabatini BL, Selkoe DJ. Amyloid-beta protein dimers isolated directly from Alzheimer's brains impair synaptic plasticity and memory. *Nat Med.* 2008;14:837–842.

Shimmyo Y, Kihara T, Akaike A, Niidome T, Sugimoto H. Multifunction of myricetin on Aβ: neuroprotection via a conformational change of Aβ and reduction of Aβ via the interference of secretases. *J Neurosci Res.* 2008;86:368–377.

Shinichi M, Kazuya M, Yuri Y, Hideaki M. Search for β-secretase inhibitors from natural spices show less. *Nat Prod Commun.* 2016;11(4):18–27.

Skovronsky DM, Lee VMY, Trojanowsky JQ. Neurodegenerative diseases: new concepts of pathogenesis and their therapeutic implications. *Annu Rev Pathol.* 2006;1:151–170.

Smit AJ. Medicinal and pharmaceutical uses of seaweed natural products: a review. *J Appl Phycol.* 2004;16:245–262.

Speranza G, Data G, Lunazzi L. Aloenin B, a new diglucosylated 6-phenyl-2-pyrone from Kenya *Aloe*. *J Nat Prod.* 1986;45:800–805.

Szwajgier D, Maria W, Edyta W, Zdzislaw T. Anticholinesterase and antioxidant activities of commercial preparations from *Ginkgo biloba* leaves. *Acta Sci Pol Hortorum Cultus.* 2013;12(5):111–125.

Tamagno E, Bardini P, Obbili A, Vitali A, Borghi R, Zaccheo D, et al. Oxidative stress increases expression and activity of BACE in NT2 neurons. *Neurobiol Dis.* 2002;10:279–288.

Tanzi RE, Bertram L. Twenty years of the Alzheimer's disease amyloid hypothesis: a genetic perspective. *Cell.* 2005;120:545–555.

Tariot PN, Farlow MR, Grossberg GT, Graham SM, McDonald S, Gergel I. Memantine treatment in patients with moderate to severe Alzheimer disease already receiving donepezil: a randomized controlled trial. *JAMA.* 2004;291(3):317–324.

Tauraite D, Razumas V, Butkus E. Lipophilic 1,4-naphthoquinone derivatives: synthesis and redox properties in solution and entrapped in the aqueous cubic liquid-crystalline phase of monoolein. *Chem Phys Lipids.* 2009;159:45–50.

Vaidya AB. The status and scope of Indian medicinal plants acting on the central nervous system. *Indian J Pharmacol.* 1997;29:S340:228–234.

Vassar R. BACE1: the beta-secretase enzyme in Alzheimer's disease. *J Mol Neurosci.* 2004;23(1–2):105–114.

Volloch V, Rita S. Results of beta secretase-inhibitor clinical trials support amyloid precursor protein-independent generation of beta amyloid in sporadic Alzheimer's disease. Med Sci (Basel). 2018;6(2):45–58.

Von Arnim CA, von Einem B, Weber P, Wagner M, Schwanzar D, Spoelgen R, Strauss WL, Schneckenburger H. Impact of cholesterol level upon APP and BACE proximity and APP cleavage. *Biochem Biophys Res Commun.* 2008;370:207–212.

Yang X, Dai G, Li G, Yang ES. Coenzyme Q10 reduces beta-amyloid plaque in an APP/PS1 transgenic mouse model of Alzheimer's disease. *J Mol Neurosci.* 2010;41:110–113.

Youdim KA, Qaiser MZ, Begley DJ, Rice-Evans CA, Abbott NJ. Flavonoid permeability across an *in-situ* model of the blood-brain barrier. *Free Rad Biol Med.* 2004;36:592–604.

Yu PN, Or TCT, Nancy YIP. Plant alkaloids as drug leads for Alzheimer's disease. *Neurochem Int.* 2015;32(4):1e–11.

Zhang F, Jiang L. Neuroinflammation in Alzheimer's disease. *Neuropsychiatr Dis Treat.* 2015;11:243–256.

Zhao X, Ou Z, Grotta JC, Waxham N, Aronowski J. Peroxisome-proliferator-activated receptor-gamma (PPARγ) activation protects neurons from NMDA excitotoxicity. *Brain Res.* 2006;1073–1074:460–469.

20 Carotenoids in Alzheimer's Disease

Magisetty Obulesu

CONTENTS

ABBREVIATIONS

AD	Alzheimer's Disease
ATRA	All-*trans* Retinoic Acid
Aβ	Amyloid Beta
BACE1	Beta Amyloid Cleaving Enzyme1
CNS	Central Nervous System
HD	Huntington's Disease
HT22	Hippocampal Neuronal Cell Line
LPS	Lipopolysaccharide
NLC	Nanostructured Lipid Carriers
NRF2	Nuclear Factor Erythroid 2-Related Factor2
PC12	Pheochromocytoma Cells
PD	Parkinson's Disease
PI3K/Akt	Phosphoinositide-3-kinase/Protein Kinase B
RA	Retinoic Acid
ROS	Reactive Oxygen Species
RXR	Retinoid X Receptor
SH-SY5y	Human Neuroblastoma Cell Lines

20.1 INTRODUCTION

Although identification of the molecular mechanisms involved in Azheimer's disease (AD) pathogenesis has proven elusive, oxidative stress and neuronal apoptosis play essential roles (Mines et al., 2011; Chen and Zhong, 2014; Wang et al., 2019). Whereas the potential risk factors include age, education, and family history of the disease, the presumed risk factors are smoking, social isolation, and physical inactivity (Alzheimer's Association, 2017; Livingston et al., 2017; Nolan et al., 2018). Although many drugs and bioactive compounds which have been tested for their efficacy against AD showed some symptomatic relief, substantial therapeutic compounds to combat AD have still to be discovered (Nolan et al., 2018).

Many plants used extensively in traditional medicine contain carotenoids, monoterpenes and polyphenol compounds, which all play pivotal roles in the amelioration of neurodegenerative diseases (Khazdair et al., 2019). Since more than 95% of sporadic AD patients were found to lack adequate amyloid-beta (Aβ) scavenging, a plethora of drugs have been targeted at Aβ scavenging (Yuan et al., 2019). *Hancornia speciosa*, a fruit tree extensively used in traditional medicine in Brazil, has been found to contain important carotenoids, such as β-carotene and lycopene (El-Agamey et al., 2004; Van den berg et al., 2000; Dos Santos et al., 2018). These have been found to show appreciable biological and physiological functions (Dos Santos et al., 2018). Mounting evidence recommends that dietary supplementation with specific nutritional compounds can mitigate the AD risk (Solfrizzi et al., 2017; Nolan et al., 2018). A healthy Japanese or Mediterranean diet significantly decreases the risk of AD (Scarmeas et al., 2006; Ozawa et al., 2013; Nolan et al., 2018). Nevertheless, the exact foodstuffs which decrease the risk of developing AD are still unclear (Scarmeas et al., 2009; Psaltopoulou et al., 2013; Sofi et al., 2014; Singh et al., 2014; Nolan et al., 2018).

20.2 XANTHOPHYLL CAROTENOIDS

Adequate intake of xanthophyll carotenoids, such as lutein, zeaxanthin, and meso- zeaxanthin, decreases AD risk (Loef and Walach, 2012; Min and Min, 2014; Feart et al., 2016; Nolan et al., 2018). In addition, lutein and zeaxanthin intake achieved marked cognitive improvements, even in non-AD people (Johnson et al., 2008a; Hammond et al., 2017; Power et al., 2018; Nolan et al., 2018). They were also found to enhance membrane integrity and to contribute to neural efficacy (Bovier and Hammond, 2015; Zamroziewicz et al., 2016; Lindbergh et al., 2017; Nolan et al., 2018). Lutein, zeaxanthin, and meso-zeaxanthin have been found in increased concentrations in the macula (retina), a part of the central nervous system (CNS). They are also found in brain regions such as the hippocampus, cerebellum, and the frontal, temporal, and occipital cortices (Craft et al., 2004; Johnson et al., 2013; Nolan et al., 2018).

Studies have shown that combination treatments between xanthophyll carotenoids (e.g. lutein) and omega-3 fatty acids improved retinal concentrations of xanthophyll in healthy female subjects (Johnson et al., 2008b; Nolan et al., 2018). This is due to the enhanced carotenoid uptake and bioavailability when carotenoids are administered in the presence of oils or cholesterol (Van Het Hof et al., 2000; Nolan et al., 2018). Although the combination intake of xanthophyll carotenoids and omega-3 fatty acids substantially ameliorated AD symptoms, further studies are needed to corroborate these findings (Nolan et al., 2018).

20.3 ASTAXANTHIN

Astaxanthin is a red-colored carotenoid pigment, abundantly found in many marine organisms, like crustaceans, microalgae, and krill (Higuera-Ciapara et al., 2006; Miki, 1991; Alghazwi et al., 2019). In addition, it is also present in a small number of plants and yeasts, and in the feathers of a few birds (Hussein et al., 2006; Alghazwi et al., 2019). Astaxanthin belongs to the xanthophyll family of carotenoids and is commercially offered isolated from the microalga *Haematococcus pluvialis* and the yeast *Phaffia rhodozyma* (Wu et al., 2015; Alghazwi et al., 2019). Astaxanthin, being a powerful antioxidant, showed substantial neuroprotective efficacy in the PC12 cell line, which includes neuroblastic cells, against $A\beta_{25-35}$-induced toxicity (Chang et al., 2010; Alghazwi et al., 2019). In another study, astaxanthin showed substantial inhibition of $A\beta_{25-35}$-induced toxicity in the SH-SY5Y human neuroblastoma cell line by reducing the Bcl–2:Bax ratio, decreasing the rate of apoptosis (Wang et al., 2010; Alghazwi et al., 2019). Antioxidant and anti-inflammatory properties of astaxanthin contribute substantially to the protective activity against AD (Zhang et al., 2014; Wu et al., 2015; Han et al., 2019). Astaxanthin has also demonstrated greater protective efficacy against $A\beta_{25-35}$-induced cytotoxicity, compared with that achieved by β-carotene and canthaxanthin (Chang et al., 2013; Alghazwi et al., 2019).

Astaxanthin has received approval from the United States Food and Drug Administration (FDA) as a food supplement (Guerin et al., 2003; Stewart et al., 2008; Alghazwi et al., 2019). In another study, astaxanthin showed reduced memory loss in mice (Han et al., 2019). Although astaxanthin has low bioavailability, co-intake of lipids may enhance its bioavailability (Alghazwi et al., 2019). The emulsifier polysorbate 80 also caused a 4-fold increase in the bioavailability of astaxanthin (Odeberg et al., 2003; Alghazwi et al., 2019). In another study, Wistar rats, to which 0.5 mg astaxanthin /kg bodyweight was administered, significantly ameliorated $A\beta_{1-42}$-induced cognitive impairment (Rahman et al., 2019). Since astaxanthin is not synthesized in humans, it has to be supplemented through diet (Guerin et al., 2003; Rodriguez-Ruiz et al., 2018).

20.4 FUCOXANTHIN

Fucoxanthin, a tetraterpenoid, is obtained from brown macro- and microalgae (Peng et al., 2011; Alghazwi et al., 2019). It is an orange-colored pigment. Members of the Haptophyta, Phaeophyceae, Bacillariophyceae, and Chrysophyceae are rich in fucoxanthin, which is found in low concentrations in members of the Raphidophyceae, Rhodophyta, and Dinophyta (Takaichi, 2011; Alghazwi et al., 2019). With oxygen in its functional group, fucoxanthin belongs to the xanthophyll class of carotenoids, distinct from the carotenes (Mikami and Hosokawa, 2013; Alghazwi et al., 2019). It has been shown to exert numerous health benefits, which include cardioprotective activity (Matsumoto et al., 2010), anticancer (Kumar et al., 2013), antioxidant (Sachindra et al., 2007), antidiabetic (Nishikawa et al., 2012), and antiobesity effects (Okada et al., 2008; Alghazwi et al., 2019). It has also been shown to attenuate $A\beta_{1-42}$ -induced toxicity in neurons of the cerebral cortex (Zhao et al., 2015; Alghazwi et al., 2019). In line with this, in another study, attenuation of $A\beta_{1-42}$ -aggregation was observed in SH-SY5Y cells in the presence of fucoxanthin (Xiang et al., 2017; Alghazwi et al., 2019). The primary protective mechanism of fucoxanthin against the Aβ oligomer was found to involve inhibition of the extracellular signal-regulated kinase (ERK) pathway and induction of the phosphoinositide-3-kinase/protein kinase B (PI3K/Akt) pathway (Lin et al., 2017; Alghazwi et al., 2019). Studies on the protective efficacy of marine carotenoids, such as astaxanthin and fucoxanthin, against Aβ aggregation showed that fucoxanthin is more effective than astaxanthin against $A\beta_{1-42}$ aggregation (Alghazwi et al., 2019).

20.5 CROCIN

Crocus sativus (saffron) belongs to the Iridaceae family and has been extensively cultivated and used in India, Iran, Morocco, Greece, Turkey, Italy, Spain, Azarbaijan, Pakistan, Egypt, and China (Bhat and Broker, 1953; Leone et al., 2018). The active components of saffron include crocin and crocetin, which are atypical carotenoids with a 20-carbon atom chain (unlike the 35–40 carbon atom chains of other carotenoid pigments), with two carboxylic groups on either side (Leone et al., 2018). Crocins are carotenoids, which exhibit high water solubility due to the occurrence of a sugar moiety (Leone et al., 2018). Crocetin is an important antioxidant that has been extensively studied for its numerous health benefits (Frank 1961; Leone et al., 2018). Crocin has shown substantial protection against L-glutamate-induced damage in the HT22 mouse hippocampal neuron cell line by reducing the apoptotic rate, decreasing mitochondrial impairment, and attenuating intracellular reactive oxygen species (ROS) accumulation (Wang et al., 2019). Therefore, crocin is a potential compound for the treatment of AD by intervening with the oxidative stress-associated apoptosis signaling pathway (Wang et al., 2019).

20.6 RETINOIC ACID

Retinoic acid (RA) plays an essential role in neuroprotection by impacting on the cell cycle genes. However, it may not avert the abnormal re-entry of neurons into the cell cycle (Ashok et al., 2019). RA shows substantial neuroprotective efficacy against AD due to its antioxidant, antiapoptotic, anti-inflammatory, Aβ-decreasing and acetylcholine (Ach) activating properties (Behairi et al., 2016; Chakrabarti et al., 2015; Lee et al., 2009; Moutinho and Landreth, 2017; Niewiadomska-Cimicka et al., 2017). Bexarotene, a retinoid X receptor (RXR) agonist, mitigated Aβ levels in the brain, and ameliorated cognitive function in AD mouse models following a 7-d treatment (Yuan et al., 2019). Nevertheless, several subsequent studies failed to reproduce these results (Fitz et al., 2013; Price et al., 2013; Tesseur et al., 2013; Veeraraghavulu et al., 2013; Yuan et al., 2019).

20.7 LYCOPENE

Lycopene, an aliphatic hydrocarbon carotenoid, is usually isolated from papayas, tomatoes, or watermelons (Heber and Lu, 2002; Mourvaki et al., 2005; Chen et al., 2019). It has a protective efficacy, through its substantial anti-inflammatory, antioxidative and antiproliferative activities (Chen et al., 2019). It also shows appreciable therapeutic efficacy against a number of CNS disorders, such as AD, Parkinson's disease (PD), Huntington's disease (HD), epilepsy, cerebral $_{\text{ischemia}}$, and depression (Sandhir et al., 2010; Qu et al., 2011; Yu et al., 2017; Chen et al., 2019). Lycopene showed remarkable recovery of cognition in transgenic mice with the P301L tau mutation and inhibited Aβ-instigated cellular toxicity in cultured neurons (Qu et al., 2011; Yu et al., 2017; Chen et al., 2019). The long-term intake of lycopene (5 mg/kg for 21 d) inhibited $A\beta_{1-42}$-induced caspase activation in the hippocampus of rats (Prakash and Kumar, 2014; Chen et al., 2019). In another study, lycopene pre-treatment (0.2–0.5 μM) successfully averted $A\beta_{1-42}$-initiated cellular apoptosis by decreasing ROS generation and mitochondrial impairment (Hwang et al., 2017; Chen et al., 2019). Long-term lycopene administration (0.03% w/w) inhibited lipopolysaccharide (LPS)-induced Aβ aggregation and BACE1 enhancement (Wang et al., 2018; Chen et al., 2019). Additionally, lycopene administration (5 mg/kg for 8 weeks) also inhibited tau hyperphosphorylation at Thr231, Ser235, Ser262, and Ser396 in brain tissues of P301 transgenic mice (Chen et al., 2019).

20.8 ALL-*TRANS* RETINOIC ACID (ATRA)

20.8.1 ATRA Physiology

Retinol introduced into cells is transformed to all-*trans* RA (ATRA) in the cytoplasm (Sandell et al., 2007; Lee et al., 2009). Despite the occurrence of RA in many stereoisomeric forms, it preferably occurs as ATRA (Lee et al., 2009). Components of the retinoid metabolic pathway available in adult brain tissues emphasize that ATRA can be synthesized in diverse regions of the adult brain, which include the amygdala, cortex, hypothalamus, hippocampus, striatum, and related brain regions (Kane et al., 2008; Lee et al., 2009). ATRA, a lipophilic molecule, can more readily span the cellular membrane, compared with other isoforms like 13-*cis* RA, possibly due to its cooperative configurations (Le Doze et al., 2000; Lee et al., 2009; Obulesu et al., 2011).

20.8.2 Treatment with ATRA

As neuroinflammation is one of the main factors involved in AD etiology, ATRA probably has an inhibitory effect on AD pathology (Lee et al., 2009). ATRA, being a principal antimitotic and differentiation-inducing agent, possibly reduces APP processing and tau hyperphosphorylation by inhibiting the cell cycle proteins (Lee et al., 2009). Subsequently, ATRA has the ability to impede the cell cycle and to induce apoptosis, with RA possibly acting as a proapoptotic agent in neoplastic and developing cells (Herget et al., 1998; Lee et al., 2009; Zheng et al., 1997). ATRA regulates the levels of Aβ peptides by increasing α-secretase expression and activity. In addition, ATRA treatment affects the localization of β-secretase (beta-site amyloid precursor protein cleaving enzyme 1; BACE1) and presenilin-1 (PS1), to inhibit APP cleavage (Koryakina et al., 2009; Lee et al., 2009). A few neurotrophic factors, such as phorbol ester, RA, staurosporine, or brain-derived neurotrophic factors play an essential role in the differentiation of human neuroblastoma (SH-SY5Y) cells into mature human neurons (Encinas et al., 1999; Shipley et al., 2016; Yuan et al., 2018).

20.9 NANOTECHNOLOGY

Although astaxanthin exhibits high efficacy, as a result of its potential antioxidant activity, its high lipophilicity and thermolability impede its antioxidant efficacy considerably. To overcome this problem, astaxanthin-encapsulated nanostructured lipid carriers (NLC) have been designed, using sunflower oil as a liquid lipid, *via* an environmentally friendly process (Guerin et al., 2003; Rodriguez-Ruiz et al., 2018). These NLCs protect the active component of the formulation and also facilitate its controlled release (Tamjidi et al., 2014, 2018; Rodriguez-Ruiz et al., 2018). A number of the astaxanthin-loaded NLC studies to date concentrated on the optimization of the formulations and the impact of lipid composition and physical parameters (Tamjidi et al., 2014, 2018; Zhu et al., 2015; Rodriguez-Ruiz et al., 2018). NLCs can achieve feasible scale-up and therefore are substantial drug delivery systems (Muchow et al., 2008; Krasodomska et al., 2016; Garces et al., 2018; Rodriguez-Ruiz et al., 2018).

20.10 CONCLUSIONS AND FUTURE PERSPECTIVES

Xanthophyll carotenoids, fucoxanthin, β-carotenes, lycopene, RA, ATRA, and their neuroprotective effects have been discussed. Although treatment with combinations of a xanthophyll carotenoid and omega-3 fatty acids showed significant improvement of cognition in both healthy and AD patients, a few limitations exist with the studies. The studies on patients involved only a few subjects. Therefore, there is a growing need to develop more, larger-scale studies to corroborate these findings. Most of the carotenoid compounds show therapeutic efficacy as a result of their antioxidant and anti-inflammatory effects. Antioxidants may decrease oxidative stress by decreasing ROS accumulation or by improving the body's antioxidant defense mechanisms (Hegazy et al., 2019). The latter effect is probably achieved by upregulating expression of genes encoding some antioxidant enzymes through the nuclear factor erythroid 2-related factor2 (Nrf2) pathway (Hegazy et al., 2019). Crocin, a vital ingredient of saffron, also plays an important role in the treatment of AD by influencing the apoptosis signaling pathways. A few limitations, such as its high lipophilicity and thermolability, have restricted the success of astaxanthin as a potential therapeutic. To overcome these challenges, NLCs were designed, which significantly improved the therapeutic efficacy of astaxanthin. In line with this, using nanotechnology, numerous formulations can be designed to overcome the issues concerning the bioavailability of the bioactive components. To develop a potential therapeutic with which to combat AD, substantial expertise from a number of different fields, such as biochemistry, medicine, and nanotechnology, is required.

REFERENCES

Alghazwi M, Smid S, Musgrave I, Zhang W. *In vitro* studies of the neuroprotective activities of astaxanthin and fucoxanthin against amyloid beta toxicity and aggregation. *Neurochem Int.* 2019;124:215–224.

Alzheimer's Association. *Alzheimer's Disease Facts and Figures*, Alzheimer's Association, Chicago, IL, USA, 2017.

Ashok A, Naaz S, Kota LN, Sen S, Purushottam M, Faruq M, Kumari R, Yadav V, Kannan R, Jain S, Panicker MM, Viswanath B. Does retinoic acid reverse cell cycle dysregulation in Alzheimer's disease lymphocytes? *Asian J Psychiatr.* 2019;39:174–177.

Behairi N, Belkhelfa M, Rafa H, Labsi M, Deghbar N, Bouzid N, Mesbah-Amroun H, Touil-Boukoffa C. All-trans retinoic acid (ATRA) prevents lipopolysaccharide-induced neuroinflammation, amyloidogenesis and memory impairment in aged rats. *J Neuroimmunol.* 2016;300:21–29.

Bhat JV, Broker R. Riboflavine and thiamine contents of saffron, Crocus sativus linn. *Nature.* 1953;172:544.

Bovier ER, Hammond BR. A randomized placebo controlled study on the effects of lutein and zeaxanthin on visual processing speed in young healthy subjects. *Arch Biochem Biophys.* 2015;572:54–57.

Chakrabarti M, McDonald AJ, Will Reed J, Moss MA, Das BC, Ray SK. Molecular signaling mechanisms of natural and synthetic retinoids for inhibition of pathogenesis in Alzheimer's disease. *J Alzheimers Dis.* 2015;50:335–352.

Chang CH, Chen CY, Chiou JY, Peng RY, Peng CH. Astaxanthin secured apoptotic death of PC12 cells induced by β-amyloid peptide 25–35: its molecular action targets. *J Med Food.* 2010;13:548–556.

Chang CS, Chang CL, Lai GH. Reactive oxygen species scavenging activities in a chemiluminescence model and neuroprotection in rat pheochromocytoma cells by astaxanthin, beta-carotene, and canthaxanthin. *Kaohsiung J Med Sci.* 2013;29:412–421.

Chen D, Huang C, Chen Z. A review for the pharmacological effect of lycopene in central nervous system disorders. *Biomed Pharmacother.* 2019;111:791–801.

Chen Z, Zhong C. Oxidative stress in Alzheimer's disease. *Neurosci Bull.* 2014;30:271–281.

Craft NE, Haitema TB, Garnett KM, Fitch KA, Dorey CK. Carotenoid, tocopherol, and retinol concentrations in elderly human brain. *J Nutr Health Aging.* 2004;8:156–162.

Dos Santos UP, Tolentino GS, Morais JS, de Picoli Souza K, Estevinho LM, Dos Santos EL. Physicochemical characterization, microbiological quality and safety, and pharmacological potential of *Hancornia speciosa* Gomes. *Oxid Med Cell Longev.* 2018;2018:2976985.

El-Agamey A, Lowe GM, McGarvey DJ, Mortensen A, Phillip DM, Truscott TG, Young AJ. Carotenoid radical chemistry and antioxidant/pro-oxidant properties. *Arch Biochem Biophys.* 2004;430:37–48.

Encinas M, Iglesias M, Llecha N, Comella JX. Extracellular regulated kinases and phosphatidylinositol 3-kinase are involved in brain-derived neurotrophic factor-mediated survival and neuritogenesis of the neuroblastoma cell line SH-SY5Y. *J Neurochem.* 1999;73:1409–1421.

Feart C, Letenneur L, Helmer C, Samieri C, Schalch W, Etheve S, Delcourt C. Plasma carotenoids are inversely associated with dementia risk in an elderly French cohort. *J Gerontol A Biol Sci Med Sci.* 2016;71:683–688.

Fitz NF, Cronican AA, Lefterov I, Koldamova R. Comment on "ApoE-directed therapeutics rapidly clear beta-amyloid and reverse deficits in AD mouse models, *Science.* 2013;340:924-c.

Frank A. Unusual purpura in artificial abortion. *Deut Med Wochenschr.* 1961;86:1618–1620.

Garces A, Amaral MH, Sousa Lobo JM, Silva AC. Formulations based on solid lipid nanoparticles (SLN) and nanostructured lipid carriers (NLC) for cutaneous use: a review. *Eur J Pharm Sci.* 2018;112:159–167.

Guerin M, Huntley ME, Olaizola M. *Haematococcus* astaxanthin: applications for human health and nutrition. *Trends Biotechnol.* 2003;21:210–216.

Hammond BR Jr, Miller LS, Bello MO, Lindbergh CA, Mewborn C, Renzi-Hammond LM. Effects of lutein/zeaxanthin supplementation on the cognitive function of community dwelling older adults: a randomized, double masked, placebo-controlled trial. *Front Aging Neurosci.* 2017;9:254.

Han JH, Lee YS, Im JH, Ham YW, Lee HP, Han SB. Astaxanthin ameliorates lipopolysaccharide-induced neuroinflammation, oxidative stress and memory dysfunction through inactivation of the signal transducer and activator of transcription 3 pathway. *Mar Drugs.* 2019;17:(in press).

Heber D, Lu QY. Overview of mechanisms of action of lycopene. Exp Biol Med (Maywood). 2002;227:920–923.

Hegazy AM, El-Sayed EM, Ibrahim KS, Abdel-Azeem AS. Dietary antioxidant for disease prevention corroborated by the Nrf2 pathway. *J Complement Integr Med.* 2019;16:3.

Herget T, Specht H, Esdar C, Oehrlein SA, Maelicke A. Retinoic acid induces apoptosis-associated neural differentiation of a murine teratocarcinoma cell line. *J Neurochem.* 1998;70:47–58.

Higuera-Ciapara I, Felix-Valenzuela L, Goycoolea F. Astaxanthin: a review of its chemistry and applications. *Crit Rev Food Sci Nutr.* 2006;46:185–196.

Hussein G, Sankawa U, Goto H, Matsumoto K, Watanabe H. Astaxanthin, a carotenoid with potential in human health and nutrition. *J Nat Prod.* 2006;69:443–449.

Hwang S, Lim JW, Kim H. Inhibitory effect of lycopene on amyloid-β-induced apoptosis in neuronal cells. *Nutrients.* 2017;9:883.

Johnson EJ, Chung HY, Caldarella SM, Snodderly DM. The influence of supplemental lutein and docosahexaenoic acid on serum, lipoproteins, and macular pigmentation. *Am J Clin Nutr.* 2008b;87:1521–1529.

Johnson EJ, McDonald K, Caldarella SM, Chung HY, Troen AM, Snodderly DM. Cognitive findings of an exploratory trial of docosahexaenoic acid and lutein supplementation in older women. *Nutr Neurosci.* 2008a;11:75–83.

Johnson EJ, Vishwanathan R, Johnson MA, Hausman DB, Davey A, Scott TM, Green RC, Miller LS, Gearing M, Woodard J, Nelson PT, Chung HY, Schalch W, Wittwer J, Poon LW. Relationship between serum and brain carotenoids, alpha-tocopherol, and retinol concentrations and cognitive performance in the oldest old from the Georgia Centenarian Study. *J Aging Res.* 2013;2013:951786.

Kane MA, Folias AE, Wang C, Napoli JL. Quantitative profiling of endogenous retinoic acid in vivo and in vitro by tandem mass spectrometry. *Anal Chem.* 2008;80:1702–1708.

Khazdair MR, Anaeigoudari A, Hashemzehi M, Mohebbati R. Neuroprotective potency of some spice herbs, a literature review. *J Tradit Complement Med.* 2018;9:98–105.

Koryakina A, Aeberhard J, Kiefer S, Hamburger M, Kuenzi P. Regulation of secretases by all=trans-retinoic acid. *FEBS J.* 2009;276:2645–2655.

Krasodomska O, Paolicelli P, Cesa S, Casadei MA, Jungnickel C. Protection and viability of fruit seeds oils by nanostructured lipid carrier (NLC) nanosuspensions. *J Colloid Interface Sci.* 2016;479:25–33.

Kumar SR, Hosokawa M, Miyashita K. Fucoxanthin: a marine carotenoid exerting anti-cancer effects by affecting multiple mechanisms. *Mar Drugs.* 2013;11:5130–5147.

Le Doze F, Debruyne D, Albessard F, Barre L, Defer GL. Pharmacokinetics of all-trans retinoic acid, 13-cis retinoic acid, and fenretinide in plasma and brain of Rat. *Drug Metab Dispos.* 2000;28:205–208.

Lee HP, Casadesus G, Zhu X, Lee HG, Perry G, Smith MA, Gustaw-Rothenberg K, Lerner A. All-trans retinoic acid as a novel therapeutic strategy for Alzheimer's disease. *Expert Rev Neurother.* 2009;9:1615–1621.

Leone S, Recinella L, Chiavaroli A, Orlando G, Ferrante C, Leporini L, Brunetti L, Menghini L. Phytotherapeutic use of *Crocus sativus* L (Saffron) and its potential applications: a brief overview. *Phytother Res.* 2018;32:2364–2375.

Lin J, Yu J, Zhao J, Zhang K, Zheng J, Wang J, Huang C, Zhang J, Yan X, Gerwick WH. Fucoxanthin, a marine carotenoid, attenuates β-amyloid oligomer-induced neurotoxicity possibly via regulating the PI3K/Akt and the ERK pathways in SH-SY5Y cells. *Oxid Med Cell Longev.* 2017;2017:1–10.

Lindbergh CA, Mewborn CM, Hammond BR, Renzi-Hammond LM, Curran-Celentano JM, Miller LS. Relationship of lutein and zeaxanthin levels to neurocognitive functioning: An fMRI study of older adults. *J Int Neuropsychol Soc.* 2017;23:11–22.

Livingston G, Sommerlad A, Orgeta V, Costafreda SG, Huntley J, Ames D, Ballard C, Banerjee S, Burns A, Cohen-Mansfield J, Cooper C, Fox N, Gitlin LN, Howard R, Kales HC, Larson EB, Ritchie K, Rockwood K, Sampson EL, Samus Q, Schneider LS, Selbæk G, Teri L, Mukadam N. Dementia prevention, intervention, and care. *Lancet.* 2017;390:2673–2734.

Loef M, Walach H. Fruit, vegetables and prevention of cognitive decline or dementia: a systematic review of cohort studies. *J Nutr Health Aging.* 2012;16:626–630.

Matsumoto M, Hosokawa M, Matsukawa N, Hagio M, Shinoki A, Nishimukai M, Miyashita K, Yajima T, Hara H. Suppressive effects of the marine carotenoids, fucoxanthin and fucoxanthinol on triglyceride absorption in lymph duct cannulated rats. *Eur J Nutr.* 2010;49:243–249.

Mikami K, Hosokawa M. Biosynthetic pathway and health benefits of fucoxanthin, an algae-specific xanthophyll in brown seaweeds. *Int J Mol Sci.* 2013;14:13763–13781.

Miki W. Biological functions and activities of animal carotenoids. *Pure Appl Chem.* 1991;63:141–146.

Min JY, Min KB. Serum lycopene, lutein and zeaxanthin, and the risk of Alzheimer's disease mortality in older adults. *Dement Geriatr Cogn Disord.* 2014;37:246–256.

Mines MA, Beurel E, Jope RS. Regulation of cell survival mechanisms in Alzheimer's disease by glycogen synthase kinase-3. *Int J Alzheimers Dis.* 2011;2011:861072.

Mourvaki E, Gizzi S, Rossi R, Rufini S. Passion flower fruit - a "new" source of lycopene? *J Med Food.* 2005;8:104–106.

Moutinho M, Landreth GE. Therapeutic potential of nuclear receptor agonists in Alzheimer's disease. *J Lipid Res.* 2017;58:1937–1949.

Muchow M, Maincent P, Muller RH. Lipid nanoparticles with a solid matrix (SLN, NLC, LDC) for oral drug delivery. *Drug Dev Ind Pharm.* 2008;34:1394–1405.

Niewiadomska-Cimicka A, Krzyzosiak A, Ye T, Podlesny-Drabiniok A, Dembele D, Dolle P, Krezel W. Genome-wide analysis of RARβ transcriptional targets in mouse striatum links retinoic acid signaling with Huntington's disease and other neurodegenerative disorders. *Mol Neurobiol.* 2017;54:3859–3878.

Nishikawa S, Hosokawa M, Miyashita K. Fucoxanthin promotes translocation and induction of glucose transporter 4 in skeletal muscles of diabetic/obese KK-Ay mice. *Phytomedicine*. 2012;19:389–394.

Nolan MJ, Mulcahy R, Power R, Moran R, Howard AN. Nutritional intervention to prevent Alzheimer's disease: potential benefits of xanthophyll carotenoids and omega-3 fatty acids combined. *J Alzheimer's Dis*. 2018;64:367–378.

Obulesu M, Muralidhara Rao D, Bramhachari PV. Carotenoids and Alzheimer's disease: an insight into therapeutic role of retinoids in animal models. *Neurochem Int*. 2011;59:535–541.

Odeberg JM, Lignell A, Pettersson A, Hoglund P. Oral bioavailability of the antioxidant astaxanthin in humans is enhanced by incorporation of lipid based formulations. *Eur J Pharm Sci*. 2003;19:299–304.

Okada T, Nakai M, Maeda H, Hosokawa M, Sashima T, Miyashita K. Suppressive effect of neoxanthin on the differentiation of 3T3-L1 adipose cells. *J. Oleo Sci*. 2008;57:345–351.

Ozawa M, Ninomiya T, Ohara T, Doi Y, Uchida K, Shirota T, Yonemoto K, Kitazono T, Kiyohara Y. Dietary patterns and risk of dementia in an elderly Japanese population: the Hisayama study. *Am J Clin Nutr*. 2013;97:1076–1082.

Peng J, Yuan JP, Wu CF, Wang JH. Fucoxanthin, a marine carotenoid present in brown seaweeds and diatoms: metabolism and bioactivities relevant to human health. *Mar Drugs*. 2011;9:1806–1828.

Power R, Coen RF, Beatty S, Mulcahy R, Moran R, Stack J, Howard AN, Nolan JM. Supplemental retinal carotenoids enhance memory in healthy individuals with low levels of macular pigment in a randomized, double-blind, placebo-controlled clinical trial. *J Alzheimers Dis*. 2018;61:947–961.

Prakash A, Kumar A. Implicating the role of lycopene in restoration of mitochondrial enzymes and BDNF levels in β-amyloid induced Alzheimer's disease. *Eur J Pharmacol*. 2014;741:104–111.

Price AR, Xu G, Siemienski ZB, Smithson LA, Borchelt DR, Golde TE, Felsenstein KM. Comment on "ApoE-directed therapeutics rapidly clear beta-amyloid and reverse deficits in AD mouse models". *Science*. 2013;340:924-d.

Psaltopoulou T, Sergentanis TN, Panagiotakos DB, Sergentanis IN, Kosti R, Scarmeas N. Mediterranean diet, stroke, cognitive impairment, and depression: a metaanalysis. *Ann Neurol*. 2013;74:580–591.

Qu M, Li L, Chen C, Li M, Pei L, Chu F, Yang J, Yu Z, Wang D, Zhou Z. Protective effects of lycopene against amyloid β-induced neurotoxicity in cultured rat cortical neurons. *Neurosci Lett*. 2011;505:286–290.

Rahman SO, Panda BP, Parvez S, Kaundal M, Hussain S, Akhtar M. Neuroprotective role of astaxanthin in hippocampal insulin resistance induced by Aβ peptides in animal model of Alzheimer's disease. *Biomed Pharmacother*. 2019;110:47–58.

Rodriguez-Ruiz V, Salatti-Dorado JA, Barzegari A, Nicolas-Boluda A, Houaoui A, Caballo C. Caballero-Casero N, Sicilia D, Bastias Venegas J, Pauthe E, Omidi Y, Letourneur D, Rubio S, Gueguen V, Pavon-Djavid G. Astaxanthin-loaded nanostructured lipid carriers for preservation of antioxidant activity. *Molecules*. 2018;23(10):2601.

Sachindra NM, Sato E, Maeda H, Hosokawa M, Niwano Y, Kohno M, Miyashita K. Radical scavenging and singlet oxygen quenching activity of marine carotenoid fucoxanthin and its metabolites. *J Agric Food Chem*. 2007;55:8516–8522.

Sandell LL, Sanderson BW, Moiseyev G, Johnson T, Mushegian A, Young K, Rey JP, Ma JX, Staehling-Hampton K, Trainor PA. RDH10 is essential for synthesis of embryonic retinoic acid and is required for limb, craniofacial, and organ development. *Genes Dev*. 2007;21:1113–1124.

Sandhir R, Mehrotra A, Kamboj SS. Lycopene prevents 3-nitropropionic acid induced mitochondrial oxidative stress and dysfunction in the nervous system. *Neurochem Int*. 2010;57:579–587.

Scarmeas N, Stern Y, Mayeux R, Manly JJ, Schupf N, Luchsinger JA. Mediterranean diet and mild cognitive impairment. *Arch Neurol*. 2009;66:216–225.

Scarmeas N, Stern Y, Tang MX, Mayeux R, Luchsinger JA. Mediterranean diet and risk for Alzheimer's disease. *Ann Neurol*. 2006;59:912–921.

Shipley MM, Mangold CA, Szpara ML. Differentiation of the SHSY5Y human neuroblastoma cell line. *J Vis Exp*. 2016;108:709–712.

Singh B, Parsaik AK, Mielke MM, Erwin PJ, Knopman DS, Petersen RC, Roberts RO. Association of Mediterranean diet with mild cognitive impairment and Alzheimer's disease: a systematic review and meta-analysis. *J Alzheimers Dis*. 2014;39:271–282.

Sofi F, Macchi C, Abbate R, Gensini GF, Casini A. Mediterranean diet and health status: an updated meta-analysis and a proposal for a literature-based adherence score. *Public Health Nutr*. 2014;17:2769–2782.

Solfrizzi V, Custodero C, Lozupone M, Imbimbo BP, Valiani V, Agosti P. Relationships of dietary patterns, foods, and micro- and macronutrients with Alzheimer's disease and late-life cognitive disorders: a systematic review. *J Alzheimers Dis*. 2017;59:815–849.

Stewart JS, Lignell A, Pettersson A, Elfving E, Soni M. Safety assessment of astaxanthin-rich microalgae biomass: acute and subchronic toxicity studies in rats. *Food Chem Toxicol.* 2008;46:3030–3036.

Takaichi S. Carotenoids in algae: distributions, biosyntheses and functions. *Mar Drugs.* 2011;9:1101–1118.

Tamjidi F, Shahedi M, Varshosaz J, Nasirpour A. Design and characterization of astaxanthin-loaded nano-structured lipid carriers. *Innov Food Sci Emerg Technol.* 2014;26:366–374.

Tamjidi F, Shahedi M, Varshosaz J, Nasirpour A. Stability of astaxanthin-loaded nanostructured lipid carriers in beverage systems. *J Sci Food Agric.* 2018;98:511–518.

Tesseur I, Lo AC, Roberfroid A, Dietvorst S, Van Broeck B, Borgers B, Gijsen H, Moechars D, Mercken M, Kemp J, D'Hooge R, De Strooper B. Comment on "ApoE-directed therapeutics rapidly clear beta-amyloid and reverse deficits in AD mouse models". *Science.* 2013;340:924-e.

Van den Berg H, Faulks R, Granado HF, Hirschberg J, Olmedilla-Alonso B, Sandmann G, Southon S, Stahl W. The potential for the improvement of carotenoid levels in foods and the likely systemic effects. *J Sci Food Agric.* 2000;80:880–912.

van Het Hof KH, West CE, Weststrate JA, Hautvast JG. Dietary factors that affect the bioavailability of carotenoids. *J Nutr.* 2000;130:503–506.

Veeraraghavalu K, Zhang C, Miller S, Hefendehl JK, Rajapaksha TW, Ulrich J, Jucker M, Holtzman DM, Tanzi RE, Vassar R, Sisodia SS. Comment on "ApoE-directed therapeutics rapidly clear beta-amyloid and reverse deficits in AD mouse models". *Science.* 2013;340:924-f.

Wang C, Cai X, Hu W, Li Z, Kong F, Chen X, Wang D. Investigation of the neuroprotective effects of crocin via antioxidant activities in HT22 cells and in mice with Alzheimer's disease. *Int J Mol Med.* 2019;43:956–966.

Wang HQ, Sun XB, Xu YX, Zhao H, Zhu QY, Zhu CQ. Astaxanthin upregulates heme oxygenase-1 expression through ERK1/2 pathway and its protective effect against beta-amyloid-induced cytotoxicity in SH-SY5Y cells. *Brain Res.* 2010;1360:159–167.

Wang J, Li L, Wang Z, Cui Y, Tan X, Yuan T, Liu Q, Liu Z, Liu X. Supplementation of lycopene attenuates lipopolysaccharide-induced amyloidogenesis and cognitive impairments via mediating neuroinflammation and oxidative stress. *J Nutr Biochem.* 2018;56:16–25.

Wu H, Niu H, Shao A, Wu C, Dixon BJ, Zhang J, Yang S, Wang Y. Astaxanthin as a potential neuroprotective agent for neurological diseases. *Mar Drugs.* 2015;13:5750–5766.

Xiang S, Liu F, Lin J, Chen H, Huang C, Chen L, Zhou Y, Ye L, Zhang K, Jin J. Fucoxanthin inhibits β-amyloid assembly and attenuates β-amyloid oligomer induced cognitive impairments. *J Agric Food Chem.* 2017;65:4092–4102.

Yu L, Wang W, Pang W, Xiao Z, Jiang Y, Hong Y. Dietary lycopene supplementation improves cognitive performances in Tau transgenic mice expressing P301L mutation via inhibiting oxidative stress and Tau hyperphosphorylation. *J Alzheimers Dis.* 2017;57:475–482.

Yuan C, Guo X, Zhou Q, Du F, Jiang W, Zhou X, et al. OAB-14, a bexarotene derivative, improves Alzheimer's disease-related pathologies and cognitive impairments by increasing β-amyloid clearance in APP/PS1 mice. *Biochim Biophys Acta Mol Basis Dis.* 2019;1865:161–180.

Yuan ZZ, Suo Y, Hao X, Wang S, Li G, Wang H. Triterpenic acids from Potentilla Parvifolia Fisch and their protective effects against okadaic acid induced neurotoxicity in differentiated SH-SY5Y cells. *Biol Pharm Bull.* 2018, DOI:10.1248/bpb.b17-01010

Zamroziewicz MK, Paul EJ, Zwilling CE, Johnson EJ, Kuchan MJ, Cohen NJ, Barbey AK. Parahippocampal cortex mediates the relationship between lutein and crystallized intelligence in healthy, older adults. *Front Aging Neurosci.* 2016;8:297.

Zhang XS, Zhang X, Wu Q, Li W, Wang CX, Xie GB, Zhou XM, Shi JX, Zhou ML. Astaxanthin offers neuroprotection and reduces neuroinflammation in experimental subarachnoid hemorrhage. *J Surg Res.* 2014;192:206–213.

Zhao X, Zhang S, An C, Zhang H, Sun Y, Li Y, Pu X. Neuroprotective effect of fucoxanthin on β-amyloid-induced cell death. *J Chin Pharmaceut Sci.* 2015;24:467–474.

Zheng A, Savolainen ER, Koistinen P. All-trans retinoic acid induces apoptosis in acute myeloblastic leukaemia cells. *Apoptosis.* 1997;2:319–329.

Zhu J, Zhuang P, Luan L, Sun Q, Cao F. Preparation and characterization of novel nanocarriers containing krill oil for food application. *J Funct Foods.* 2015;19:902–912.

Index

D

E

F

G

O

P

Q

R

S